T0309111

Current and Future Developments in
Ophthalmology

Current and Future Developments in Ophthalmology

Edited by Ryan Loren

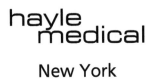

New York

Hayle Medical,
750 Third Avenue, 9ᵗʰ Floor,
New York, NY 10017, USA

Visit us on the World Wide Web at:
www.haylemedical.com

© Hayle Medical, 2023

This book contains information obtained from authentic and highly regarded sources. Copyright for all individual chapters remain with the respective authors as indicated. All chapters are published with permission under the Creative Commons Attribution License or equivalent. A wide variety of references are listed. Permission and sources are indicated; for detailed attributions, please refer to the permissions page and list of contributors. Reasonable efforts have been made to publish reliable data and information, but the authors, editors and publisher cannot assume any responsibility for the validity of all materials or the consequences of their use.

ISBN: 978-1-64647-512-4

Trademark Notice: Registered trademark of products or corporate names are used only for explanation and identification without intent to infringe.

Cataloging-in-Publication Data

Current and future developments in ophthalmology / edited by Ryan Loren
   p. cm.
Includes bibliographical references and index.
ISBN 978-1-64647-512-4
1. Ophthalmology. 2. Eye--Diseases. 3. Ophthalmologists--Guidebooks. I. Loren, Ryan.
RE48 .C55 2023
617.7--dc23

Table of Contents

Preface

The purpose of the book is to provide a glimpse into the dynamics and to present opinions and studies of some of the scientists engaged in the development of new ideas in the field from very different standpoints. This book will prove useful to students and researchers owing to its high content quality.

Ophthalmology is a medical specialty focused on diagnosing and treating eye disorders. This field is focused on treating various eye diseases including cataract, eye tumors, dry eye syndrome, orbital fracture, proptosis, ptosis, retinal detachment, and refractive errors. The examination methods that are utilized for eye examination include visual acuity assessment, slit lamp examination, ocular tonometry, gonioscopy, and dilated fundus examination. The other specialized tests that allow diagnosis of eye related diseases include ultrasonography, corneal topography, visual field testing, electrooculography, and electroretinography. Ocular surgery is a treatment method in ophthalmology, which involves surgery of the eye or associated organs. Ophthalmology has various subspecialties, which aim to treat different diseases of the eye. These subspecialties include ocular oncology, glaucoma, refractive surgery, ophthalmic pathology, neuro-ophthalmology, pediatric ophthalmology, cryotherapy, and vitreo-retinal surgery. The topics included in this book on ophthalmology are of utmost significance and bound to provide incredible insights to the readers. It will prove to be immensely beneficial to students and researchers in this field. The readers would gain knowledge that would broaden their perspective in this area of medicine.

At the end, I would like to appreciate all the efforts made by the authors in completing their chapters professionally. I express my deepest gratitude to all of them for contributing to this book by sharing their valuable works. A special thanks to my family and friends for their constant support in this journey.

Editor

Dry Eye Disease Among Mongolian and Han Older Adults in Grasslands of Northern China: Prevalence, Associated Factors and Vision-Related Quality of Life

Jianhua Wu[1†], Xiaomei Wu[2†], Han Zhang[1†], Xiaoguang Zhang[1], Jie Zhang[3,4], Yanqiu Liu[5], Jun Liu[6], Lu Lu[7], Song Zhang[8], Guisen Zhang[1*] and Lei Liu[9,10,11*]

[1] Inner Mongolia Chaoju Eye Hospital, Inner Mongolia Chaoju Institute of Eye Disease Control, Hohhot, China, [2] Department of Clinical Epidemiology and Center of Evidence-Based Medicine, The First Hospital of China Medical University, Shenyang, China, [3] School of Public Health, Weifang Medical University, Weifang, China, [4] Tobacco Control, Chinese Center for Disease Control and Prevention, Beijing, China, [5] Department of Ophthalmology, Anshan Central Hospital, Anshan, China, [6] Department of Ophthalmology, Changzhi People's Hospital, Changzhi, China, [7] Department of Ophthalmology, The Fourth Affiliated Hospital of China Medical University, Shenyang, China, [8] The First Hospital of China Medical University, Shenyang, China, [9] Department of Ophthalmology, Guangdong Eye Institute, Guangdong Provincial People's Hospital, Guangdong Academy of Medical Sciences, Guangzhou, China, [10] School of Medicine, South China University of Technology, Guangzhou, China, [11] Department of Ophthalmology, The First Affiliated Hospital of China Medical University, Shenyang, China

*Correspondence:
Guisen Zhang
zhangguisen76@sohu.com
Lei Liu
liuleijiao@163.com

[†] These authors have contributed equally to this work

Purpose: Dry eye disease (DED) is projected to have increasing public health burden in China with the aging population. No published studies on the epidemiology of DED have been found in grasslands. We estimated DED prevalence among older adults living in grasslands of northern China and investigated its associated factors and impact on vision-related quality of life (VR-QoL).

Methods: A multistage cluster random sampling technique was used to select Mongolian and Han participants aged over 40 from November 2020 to May 2021 in this area. An assessment of DED was performed with Ocular Surface Disease Index (OSDI) questionnaire, Schirmer's I test (ST), and Tear film break up time (TBUT). All the participants completed the Chinese version of National Eye Institute Visual Function Questionnaire (NEI-VFQ-25) assessing VR-QoL.

Results: Of the 1,400 enumerated residents, 1,287 were examined. The overall age and gender standardized prevalence of DED was 34.5%, of which, 32.6% of Mongolian and 35.4% of Han had DED. In a multivariate model, statistically significant associations were found with advancing age [odds ratio (OR) 1.03, 95% confidence interval (CI) 1.02–1.04], female gender (OR 1.32, 95% CI 1.04–1.68), smoking (OR 0.7, 95% CI 0.5–0.98), anti-fatigue eye-drop use (OR 0.56, 95% CI 0.41–0.77), milk product intake (OR 0.55, 95% CI 0.39–0.77), number of household members (OR 0.8, 95% CI 0.72–0.88). DED was associated with lower scores on VR-QoL ($\beta = -0.14$, $P < 0.01$). Similar results were observed when analyses were stratified by ethnicity.

Conclusions: The novelty-associated factors for DED in the grasslands area were anti-fatigue eye drop use, milk product intake, and number of household members. DED and its components were associated with VR-QoL. Further prospective studies are needed to confirm these findings.

Keywords: dry eye disease, prevalence, associated factors, vision-related quality of life, epidemiology—analytic (risk factors)

INTRODUCTION

Dry eye disease (DED) is an age-related degenerative condition. It is one of the leading reasons for patients seeking eye care, with prevalence estimates ranging from ~5–50% in population-based studies, depending on population studied and diagnostic criteria (1). According to geographic (i.e., high latitude), climatic (i.e., humidity levels), and environmental variations (i.e., ultraviolet radiation) associated with DED, it is more common in Asian populations (2–5). In China, a previous meta-analysis has shown that the pooled prevalence of dry eye syndrome (DES) is 17%, and that subjects living in the Northern and Western China have significantly higher prevalence rates than those living in other areas (6).

The area of grasslands is about 3.84 million square kilometers. The grasslands in northern of China are mainly located in the Inner Mongolia Autonomous Region, and have high latitude, low humidity, increased ultraviolet (UV) light, and windy conditions. Most of the residents living in these grasslands area are herders (Mongolian and Han). Because of their unique living and eating habits (more milk and meat), which lead to differences in diseases, it is very important to understand the eye health of residents in grasslands area.

In 2006, Guo et al. conducted an epidemiology investigation of DED among Chinese Mongolian in Henan county, Qinghai province of China, which showed that the crude prevalence of symptomatic dry eye measured with a six-item validated questionnaire was 50.1%, and that its independent factors included increased age, presence of age-related cataract, and pterygium (7). In addition, to the best of our knowledge, limited data are available on the prevalence and related factors of DED in grasslands area.

Recently, many reports have suggested that DED can affect vision-related quality of life (VR-QoL) (1, 8), but there were only a few population-based studies on the association between DED and VR-QoL worldwide (9–13). Furthermore, the impact of DED on VR-QoL in grasslands populations is relatively unknown.

The aims of this investigation in the grasslands area, which is predominately composed of Chinese Mongolian and Han older adults aged over 40 years, were to determine the prevalence of DED, identify independent associated factors, and quantify their impact on VR-QoL.

METHODS
Study Introduction

This grasslands multiethnic eye disease epidemiological study is a cross-sectional, population-based one in eastern, middle, and western parts of the Inner Mongolia Autonomous Region and Ningxia province, China. This investigation is divided into three parts. The first stage was conducted in the middle grasslands area, and focused on Mongolian and Han ethnicities. The second stage will be conducted in eastern the grasslands area, and will focus on Ewenki, Oroqen, and Daur ethnicities. The third stage will be conducted in the western grasslands area, and will focus on Hui ethnicity. This study is the first stage.

Study Area

Multistage cluster sampling was performed to select two areas (Xilingol and Ulanqab) from the grasslands area located in the northern and middle parts of the Inner Mongolia Autonomous Region, China (Supplementary Figure 1). The three areas (Ujimqin Banner, Sonid Banner, and Siziwang Banner) were chosen by primary cluster sampling, and then relevant county seats were randomly selected by secondary cluster sampling. The county seats were divided into two levels (urban and rural) according to economic conditions. The study area runs from 111° 68 to 117° 58 E in longitude and 41°37 to 44°60N in latitude. The mean annual temperature ranges from 1 to 6°C in 2019. The region is far away from the ocean and resides in a low-humidity wide area. The mean annual precipitation range is between 170 and 350 mm, with 60 −90% falling during the growing season from April to August.

Study Population

According to the data obtained from the 2010 nationwide population census, there are ~0.46 million with two predominant ethnic groups, Mongolian and Han, in the study region. An estimated prevalence of DED of 31.4% was made reference to our sample (2). The formula: $n = Z^2 p(1-p)/q^2$ was used to calculate sample size, whereas $Z = 1.96$, $p = 0.314$, $q = 0.1\ p$. The estimated minimum sample size was 839. We added an additional 15% to the minimum sample size factoring in possible non-compliance rate and targeted 1,258 subjects. The study sample was stratified to include proportions of Mongolian and Han ethnic groups in two grasslands. All the participants gave informed consent. This study was approved by the ethics committee of Inner Mongolia Chaoju Eye Hospital and adhered to the tenets of the Declaration of Helsinki. This study was registered in Chinese Clinical Trial Registry with No. ChiCTR2000040141.

This study was conducted from November 2020 to May 2021. Only Mongolian and Han subjects aged 40 and above were interviewed for the study. Patients who underwent refractive surgery at latest 3 months and those with an active ocular surface disease were excluded.

The Questionnaire

In order to acquire participants-reported questionnaires, Chinese version of the Ocular Surface Disease Index (OSDI) and

National Eye Institute Visual Functioning Questionnaire-25 (NEI-VFQ-25) questionnaire were interviewed by well-trained investigators. Previous studies have revealed that these two Chinese version questionnaires were easily administered, socio-culturally acceptable, and understandable (14, 15). The OSDI questionnaire consists of 12 questions, and each question is graded from 0 (indicating no problem) to 5 (indicating a significant problem). OSDI scores were calculated with the formula (sum of scores) × 25/(12 questions). The NEI-VFQ-25 questionnaire includes 12 subcategories: (i) general health; (ii) general vision; (iii) ocular pain; (iv) near vision; (v) distance vision; (vi) social functioning; (vii) mental health; (viii) role difficulties; (ix) dependency; (x) driving; (xi) color vision; and (xii) peripheral vision. The NEI-VFQ-25 questionnaire was scored by the researcher according to the scoring manual. Its score ranges from 0 to 100, and designates worst state to normal visual function, respectively. Furthermore, socio-demographic characteristics (such as cultural level, family income, and employment), lifestyle, screen exposure, and dietary supplements, as well as medical history were acquired from each participant. Milk product intake was categorized as occasional (<1 time/day) or regular (more than one time/day). Anti-fatigue eye drop was defined as topical medications improving patient comfort, such as eye lubricants and artificial tear drops.

Examination

Tear Film Break Up Time

One drop of topical anesthesia, 0.4% oxybuprocaine hydrochloride ophthalmic solution (Benoxil; Oxybuprocaine, Santen, Japan), was instilled. After 1 min, the subjects were instructed to look up to apply a fluorescein sodium ophthalmic strip into the inferior fornix. Each subject should blink three times, then keep their eyes open as long as possible. The time between the last blink and the first dry spot around the central cornea was recorded under cobalt blue light. The average of three measurements was recorded as the final TBUT.

Schirmer's I Test

Schirmer's I test is a basic tear secretion test without anesthesia and performed with tear strip (30 mm; Jingming Tianjin, China).

The tear strip was placed in the mid-lateral portion of the lower fornix, and the subjects were instructed to close their eyes for 5 min. After that, the length of the wetting strip was recorded as the level of tear secretion.

Definitions

DED in this study was defined as OSDI scores of 13 and above plus one of the items as shown below: (i) Schirmer's I test reading value less than 10 mm (ii) TBUT value less than 10 s.

Statistical Analysis

All data were entered into an Excel form. The SPSS 23.0 (IBM Corp., Armonk, NY, United States) statistical software was applied to analyze the data. For qualitative indicators, we used frequency and percentage for statistical description, and Wilcoxon rank sum test was performed for analysis. The normal distribution continuous data were expressed by the mean ± standard deviation (mean ± SD), and then Students' t-test was performed to determine if there were significant differences between groups. According to the sixth national census of 2010, the prevalence of DED was standardized by age and gender composition data of 40 years and above (http://www.stats.gov.cn/tjsj/pcsj/rkpc/6rp/indexch.htm). After adjusting for age, gender, and other variables, a multivariate logistic regression model was used to estimate the odds ratio (OR) and 95% confidence interval (CI) of DED factors. A Pearson's linear correlation analysis was performed to analyze the relationship between NEI-VFQ-25 scores and OSDI, TBUT as well as Schirmer's I test variables. Multiple linear regression was used, and the VR-QoL subscales were used as dependent variables. DED clinical indicators were used as independent variables and inputted into the multiple linear regression model to detect their impacts on VR-QoL. The test standard is $\alpha = 0.05$ (bilateral), and a P-value of <0.05 was considered statistically significant.

RESULTS

Totally, there were 1,400 participants eligible for this survey. Forty-four subjects declined to participate. Fifty-six subjects were excluded from the study, of which 5 underwent refractive surgery

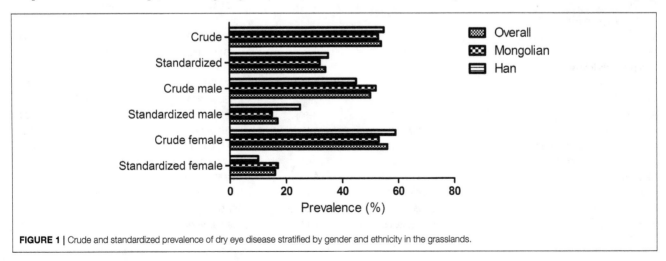

FIGURE 1 | Crude and standardized prevalence of dry eye disease stratified by gender and ethnicity in the grasslands.

TABLE 1 | Characteristics of the participants.

	N/Mean ± sd	Range	DED	No DED	P
Total	1,287	–	697 (54.2%)	590 (45.8%)	
Ethnic					
Mongolian	816	–	437 (53.6%)	379 (46.4%)	0.57
Han	471	–	60 (55.2%)	211 (44.8%)	
Residence					
Rural	404	–	223 (55.2%)	181 (44.8%)	0.61
Urban	883	–	474 (53.7%)	409 (46.3%)	
Gender					
Male	433	–	211 (50.1%)	216 (49.9%)	**0.03**
Female	854	–	481 (56.3%)	373 (43.7%)	
Occupation					
Worker	22	–	10 (45.5%)	12 (54.5%)	0.86
Farmer	490	–	268 (54.7%)	222 (45.3%)	
Staff	60	–	32 (53.3%)	28 (46.7%)	
Other	715	–	386 (54.1%)	329 (45.9%)	
Smoke					
Current	198	–	111 (56.1%)	87 (43.9%)	0.28
Never	1,053	–	563 (53.5%)	490 (46.5%)	
Former	37	–	23 (62.2%)	14 (37.8%)	
Drink					
Current	116	–	57 (49.2%)	59 (50.8%)	0.55
Never	1,135	–	617 (54.4%)	518 (45.6%)	
Former	36	–	20 (55.6%)	16 (44.4%)	
Level of education					
Primary school	689	–	397 (57.6%)	292 (42.4%)	0.11
Junior high school	318	–	162 (50.9%)	156 (49.1%)	
Senior high school	158	–	80 (50.6%)	78 (49.4%)	
College	120	–	57 (47.5%)	63 (52.5%)	
Unclear	2	–	1 (50%)	1 (50%)	
Diabetes					
With	137	–	72 (52.6%)	65 (47.4%)	0.70
Without	1,088	–	587 (54%)	501 (46%)	
Unclear	62	–	35 (56.5%)	27 (43.5%)	
Hypertension					
With	474	–	276 (58.2%)	198 (41.8%)	0.08
Without	768	–	397 (51.7%)	371 (48.3%)	
Unclear	45	–	24 (53.4%)	21 (46.6%)	
Anti-fatigue eye-drop use					
Yes	204	–	132 (64.7%)	72 (35.3%)	**<0.01**
No	1,083	–	564 (52.1%)	519 (47.9%)	
Milk products intake					
Regular	1,028	–	576 (56.1%)	452 (43.9%)	**0.01**
Occasional	259	–	122 (47.2%)	137 (52.8%)	
Age (years)	61.24 ± 9.54	(22–93)	62.71 ± 9.07	59.51 ± 9.80	**<0.01**
Screen exposure per day (h)	2.65 ± 1.81	(0–12)	2.61 ± 1.84	2.69 ± 1.77	0.39
Number of household members (n)	2.58 ± 1.21	(1–11)	2.4 ± 1.19	2.79 ± 1.19	**<0.01**
Annual household incomes (per 10,000 Yuan)	4.07 ± 4.83	(0–60)	3.77 ± 3.91	4.42 ± 5.71	**0.02**
Height (cm)	160.42 ± 8.43	(103–188)	159.57 ± 8.41	161.44 ± 8.35	**<0.01**
Weight (kg)	70.64 ± 14.37	(41–170)	70.22 ± 14.75	71.13 ± 13.90	0.26
BMI	27.35 ± 5.42	(14.88–66.92)	27.56 ± 5.33	27.24 ± 5.17	0.27
Height (cm)	98.25 ± 28.58	(39–171)	99.1 ± 36.78	97.24 ± 13.44	0.25

(Continued)

TABLE 1 | Continued

	N/Mean ± sd	Range	DED	No DED	P
Waist (cm)	86.69 ± 12.63	(15–140)	86.94 ± 12.34	86.4 ± 12.97	0.44
SBP (mmHg)	139.75 ± 24.72	(85–200)	140.2 ± 28.96	139.22 ± 18.52	0.48
DBP (mmHg)	82.22 ± 14.19	(50–144)	81.91 ± 14.06	82.58 ± 14.35	0.40
Hart rate (per minute)	81.38 ± 13.69	(42–122)	81.27 ± 14.01	81.51 ± 13.31	0.76
Schirmer's I test (mm)	8.55 ± 7.34	(0–30)	6.23 ± 5.75	11.28 ± 8.05	**<0.01**
TBUT (s)	5.98 ± 3.99	(0–15)	3.86 ± 2.50	8.48 ± 3.97	**<0.01**
OSDI score	21.82 ± 13.00	(0–100)	26.82 ± 10.99	15.91 ± 12.71	**<0.01**

DED, dry eye disease; BMI, body mass index; SBP, systolic blood pressure; DBP, diastolic blood pressure; TBUT, Tear film break up time; OSDI, ocular surface disease index; SD, standard deviation. Bold values mean statistically significant.

within at latest 3 months, and 51 had an active ocular surface disease. Thirteen subjects were eliminated because of missing data. Finally, there were 1,287 people (age 61.24 ± 9.54 years, 66.4% women) who actually participated in the ophthalmology and medical examinations, and the response rate was 91.93%. There were 816 Mongolian (age 60.46 ± 9.29 years, 64.1% women) and 471 Han (aging 62.59 ± 9.82 years, 70.3% women) participants. Among all the participants, the number of current smokers, never-smokers, and ex-smokers was 198, 1,053, and 37, respectively.

Prevalence

A total of 696 participants fulfilled the diagnostic criteria for DED, with a crude prevalence rate of 54.2%, and the crude prevalence of DED in Mongolian and Han ethnicities was 53.6 and 55.1%, respectively. Based on the 2010 sixth National Census of China, the overall age and gender standardized prevalence rate of DED was 34.5% in the grasslands, and the age- and gender-standardized prevalence of DED in Mongolian and Han ethnicities was 32.6 and 35.4%, respectively. The prevalence of DED is shown in **Figure 1**.

Factors Associated With the Presence of DED

According to the univariate analysis (**Table 1**), participants with DED were more likely to be older, of female gender, shorter in height, and with anti-fatigue eye-drop use, occasional milk intake, less number of household members, less annual household incomes, and lower Schirmer's I test and TBUT but higher OSDI scores (all $P < 0.05$). Unadjusted univariate differences in DED among the Han and Mongolian participants by demographic, lifestyle and other factors are presented in **Supplementary Tables 1, 2**. The multivariate logistic regression demonstrated that advancing age, female gender, no smoke, anti-fatigue eye-drop use, milk product intake, number of household members, and Schirmer's I test, TBUT, and OSDI scores were independently associated with DED (all $P < 0.05$, **Table 2**). Similar factors were found in the ethnic-specific analysis (**Supplementary Tables 3, 4**). However, female gender and milk product intake were not associated with DED among the Chinese Mongolians.

Vision-Related Quality of Life

The correlation between DED characteristics and VR-QoL in all the participants is shown in **Table 3**. Schirmer's I test was significantly correlated with the three NEI-VFQ-25 subscales: general health ($r = -0.06$), general vision ($r = 0.06$), and dependency ($r = 0.06$). TBUT was correlated with the NEIVFQ-25 overall scores ($r = 0.06$), as well as with three subscales: general health ($r = 0.06$), general vision ($r = 0.07$), and driving ($r = 0.1$) in all the participants. Furthermore, OSDI score was correlated with the NEI-VFQ-25 overall score ($r = -0.47$) and all its 12 subscales. Schirmer's I test and TBUT were not correlated with quality of life in the Han participants, while OSDI score was significantly correlated with the NEI-VFQ-25 scores (see **Supplementary Table 5**). Among the Mongolians, Schirmer's I test and TBUT were correlated with general health ($r = -0.08$) and general vision ($r = 0.08$), respectively. Moreover, the OSDI score of the Mongolians was significantly correlated with the all NEI-VFQ-25 scores, except general health (see **Supplementary Table 6**).

The results of multiple linear regression for the overall NEI-VFQ-25 score and subscales are presented in **Table 4**. DED was a predictor for the overall scores ($\beta = -0.14$, $P < 0.01$), and general health ($\beta = -0.06$, $P = 0.03$), general vision ($\beta = -0.18$, $P < 0.01$), ocular pain ($\beta = -0.02$, $P = 0.49$), near activities ($\beta = -0.07$, $P = 0.01$), distance activities ($\beta = -0.09$, $P < 0.01$), and social functioning ($\beta = -0.07$, $P = 0.02$). OSDI score was associated with the overall NEI-VFQ-25 score and all the subscales. Schirmer's I test and TBUT were not associated with NEI-VFQ-25 scores. NEI-VFQ-25 and its subscales are used as dependent variables, and demographic and clinical characteristics are used as predictors to be added to the stepwise multiple linear regression model to screen risk factors. Stratification by ethnicity showed similar results (see **Supplementary Tables 7, 8**).

DISCUSSION

Documented epidemic data on DED among residents in the grasslands area are limited, and, this study sought to determine the prevalence, risk factors of DED, and its role in VR-QoL between the two main ethnicities (Mongolian and Han) in the northern grasslands area in China. The overall age- and

TABLE 2 | Logistic regression analysis of risk factors associated with definite DED.

	Crude			Adjusted*			Adjusted**		
	OR	95% CI	P	OR	95% CI	P	OR	95% CI	P
Age (years)	1.04	1.02–1.05	**<0.01**	1.04	1.03–1.05	**<0.01**	1.03	1.02–1.04	**<0.01**
Gender (female)	1.29	1.02–1.62	**0.03**	1.29	1.02–1.64	**0.03**	1.32	1.04–1.68	**0.02**
Ethnic (Mongolian)	0.94	0.75–1.18	0.57	1.03	0.82–1.30	0.79	1.06	0.83–1.34	0.66
Residence (rural)	1.31	0.74–1.19	0.20	0.99	0.78–1.26	0.92	0.92	0.69–1.21	0.53
Occupation									
Worker	Ref			Ref			Ref		
Farmer	1.45	0.61–3.42	0.40	1.31	0.55–3.11	0.55	1.12	0.46–2.71	0.80
Staff	1.37	0.51–3.66	0.53	1.32	0.49–3.57	0.58	1.18	0.44–3.22	0.74
Other	1.41	0.60–3.31	0.43	1.33	0.56–3.15	0.52	1.11	0.46–2.66	0.82
Smoke									
Current	Ref			Ref			Ref		
Never	0.90	0.66–1.22	0.50	0.70	0.50–0.98	0.04	0.70	0.50–0.98	**0.04**
Former	1.57	0.72–3.41	0.26	1.33	0.60–2.95	0.48	1.36	0.61–3.00	0.45
Drink									
Current	Ref			Ref			Ref		
Never	1.23	0.84–1.81	0.29	0.92	0.60–1.40	0.68	0.92	0.60–1.41	0.70
Former	1.31	0.61–2.83	0.49	1.28	0.58–2.82	0.55	1.25	0.56–2.77	0.58
Screen exposure per day (h)	0.97	0.92–1.03	0.39	1.04	0.98–1.12	0.20	1.04	0.97–1.11	0.27
Anti-fatigue eye-drop use (no)	0.58	0.42–0.80	**<0.01**	1.04	1.03–1.05	**<0.01**	0.56	0.41–0.77	**<0.01**
Milk products intake (regular)	0.69	0.53–0.91	**0.01**	0.64	0.48–0.85	**<0.01**	0.55	0.39–0.77	**<0.01**
Level of education									
Primary school	Ref			Ref			Ref		
Junior high school	0.76	0.59–1.00	0.05	0.87	0.66–1.14	0.31	0.91	0.68–1.20	0.49
Senior high school	0.75	0.53–1.07	0.11	0.92	0.65–1.32	0.66	0.93	0.64–1.33	0.68
College	0.67	0.41–0.98	0.04	0.90	0.60–1.36	0.63	0.91	0.61–1.38	0.66
Unclear	0.74	0.05–11.81	0.83	0.81	0.05–13.27	0.88	0.69	0.04–11.28	0.80
Number of household members (n)	0.76	0.69–0.83	**<0.01**	0.80	0.72–0.88	**<0.01**	0.80	0.72–0.88	**<0.01**
Annual household incomes (per ten thousand yuan)	0.97	0.95–1.00	0.02	0.99	0.97–1.02	0.51	1.00	0.98–1.03	0.99
Diabetes									
Yes	Ref			Ref			Ref		
No	1.06	0.74–1.51	0.76	1.14	0.79–1.64	0.48	1.15	0.80–1.67	0.46
Unclear	1.31	0.69–2.49	0.40	1.42	0.74–2.74	0.29	1.36	0.70–2.64	0.36
Hypertension									
Yes	Ref			Ref			Ref		
No	0.77	0.61–0.97	0.03	0.90	0.71–1.14	0.38	0.93	0.73–1.18	0.54
Unclear	0.83	0.44–1.54	0.55	0.86	0.46–1.63	0.65	0.85	0.45–1.63	0.63
Height (cm)	0.97	0.96–0.99	< 0.01	0.99	0.97–1.00	0.13	0.99	0.97–1.01	0.19
Weight (kg)	1.00	0.99–1.00	0.26	1.00	0.99–1.01	0.83	1.00	0.99–1.01	0.98
BMI	1.01	0.99–1.03	0.21	1.01	0.99–1.03	0.50	1.01	0.99–1.03	0.43
Height (cm)	1.00	1.00–1.01	0.31	1.00	1.00–1.01	0.35	1.00	1.00–1.01	0.37
Waist (cm)	1.00	1.00–1.01	0.44	1.00	0.99–1.01	0.63	1.00	0.99–1.01	0.66
SBP (mmHg)	1.00	1.00–1.01	0.49	1.00	0.99–1.00	0.57	1.00	0.99–1.00	0.61
DBP (mmHg)	1.00	0.99–1.00	0.40	1.00	0.99–1.01	0.41	1.00	0.99–1.00	0.38
Hart rate (per minute)	1.00	0.99–1.01	0.76	1.00	0.99–1.01	0.43	1.00	0.99–1.01	0.38
Schirmer's I test (mm)	0.90	0.88–0.92	**<0.01**	0.90	0.88–0.92	**<0.01**	0.90	0.88–0.92	**<0.01**
TBUT (s)	0.70	0.67–0.72	**<0.01**	0.70	0.67–0.73	**<0.01**	0.69	0.67–0.72	**<0.01**
OSDI score	1.10	1.09–1.12	**<0.01**	1.10	1.08–1.11	**<0.01**	1.10	1.08–1.11	**<0.01**

DED, dry eye disease; BMI, body mass index; SBP, systolic blood pressure; DBP, diastolic blood pressure; TBUT, Tear film break up time; OSDI, ocular surface disease index; OR, odds ratio; CI, confidence interval.
Adjusted with age, gender, and ethnicity.
**Adjusted with age, gender, ethnicity, and number of household members.*
Bold values mean statistically significant.

TABLE 3 | Correlation between DED subscale and NEI-VFQ-25 subscale.

	Overall	General health	General vision	Ocular pain	Near activities	Distance activities	Social functioning	Mental health	Role difficulties	Dependency	Driving	Color vision	Peripheral vision
Schirmer's I test (mm)	−0.01	−0.06*	0.06*	−0.03	0.01	0.03	0.02	−0.02	0.02	0.06*	−0.02	0.01	−0.00
TBUT (s)	0.06*	0.06*	0.07*	−0.03	0.02	0.04	0.03	−0.01	0.05	0.01	0.10*	0.01	0.03
OSDI score	−0.47**	−0.15**	−0.40**	0.10**	−0.09**	−0.26**	−0.24**	−0.09**	−0.22**	−0.48**	−0.55**	−0.12**	−0.21**

DED, Dry eye disease; TBUT, Tear film break up time; OSDI, ocular surface disease index; NEI-VFQ-25, National Eye Institute Visual Functioning Questionnaire-25.
*P < 0.05; **P < 0.01.

gender-standardized prevalence of DED was 34.5%, and, the standardized prevalence in the Mongolian and Han were 32.6 and 35.4%, respectively. In addition, DED was associated with several factors, such as being female and older, smoking, anti-fatigue eye-drop use, regular milk product intake, number of household members, and Schirmer's I test, TBUT, and OSDI scores. Notably, there was a significant correlation between DED components (OSDI, Schirmer's I test, and TBUT) and NEI-VFQ-25 scores. After the multivariate regression analysis, DED and OSDI have significant impacts on VR-QoL among population living in the grasslands.

The prevalence of DED in this study was 54.2%, which is over the range of previous population-based findings (5–50%) (7, 16–20). The participants were relatively older, at 61.24 ± 9.54 years old and with predominance of women (66.4%). However, the age- and gender-standardized prevalence was still higher than that in previous meta-analysis (2). This discrepancy may be due to the special geographical (high latitude) and environmental factors (dust, sand, and drought) as well as the lifestyle of people living in the grasslands area of Northern China. In addition, different techniques used to diagnose DED may also have an impact on this discrepancy. There may be discordance between dry eye signs and symptoms, with the signs being more prevalent and variable than the symptoms (1). Furthermore, there was no significant difference in the prevalence of DED between Mongolian and Han participants in our study.

So far, advancing age, female gender, and smoking are the most common factors associated with DED (21), which were consistent with our findings. However, another population-based investigation in Dubai showed that daily screen time (> 6 h) was positively associated with dry eyes (22, 23), while no association between daily screen exposure time and DED was found in this study. This discrepancy might be due to the different lifestyle of the study participants. Our participants spent most of their time outdoors and, therefore, had low exposure to screen, which might explain the absence of an association between daily screen time and dry eyes in the current study.

It is interesting to note that anti-fatigue eye-drop use was associated with DED. Eye fatigue is a manifestation of DED (24), and many patients were confirmed to use anti-fatigue eye-drops to relieve the syndrome. Furthermore, regular milk product intake might reduce the risk for presence of DED. Recently, a randomized, double-blind, placebo-controlled, parallel group comparative study revealed that H_2-producing milk appeared to retard the decline in tear stability and may prevent short fTBUT-type DED by decreasing oxidative stress in the lacrimal functional unit (25). In addition, it would be a good idea to identify the effects of milk product intake on DED prevention or treatment in future studies. When stratified by ethnicity, the association was still significant in the Han participants rather than the Mongolians. Similar findings were obtained in association between number of household members and presence of DED. However, there is limited direct population-based evidence on this relationship, and the causal direction of the relationship is unclear. Future prospective studies should recruit a larger sample that is more representative of the population of China.

TABLE 4 | Multiple linear regression on dry eye disease and vision-related quality of life based on NEI-VFQ-25 in all the participants.

| | DED | | | | OSDI score | | | | Schirmer's I test (mm) | | | | TBUT (s) | | | |
| | | | 95%CI | | | | 95%CI | | | | 95%CI | | | | 95%CI | |
	β*	P	Low	Up	β*	P	Low	Up	β*	P	Low	Up	β*	P	Low	Up
Overall	-0.14	**<0.01**	-0.19	-0.09	-0.50	**<0.01**	-0.54	-0.45	0.01	0.69	-0.04	0.06	0.02	0.37	-0.03	0.08
General health	-0.06	**0.03**	-0.11	-0.01	-0.11	**<0.01**	-0.16	-0.06	-0.05	0.06	-0.10	0.01	0.03	0.32	-0.03	0.08
General vision	-0.18	**<0.01**	-0.24	-0.13	-0.39	**<0.01**	-0.44	-0.34	0.04	0.13	-0.01	0.09	0.05	0.06	<0.01	0.10
Ocular pain	-0.02	0.49	-0.08	0.04	0.16	**<0.01**	0.11	0.22	0.01	0.88	-0.06	0.05	0.01	0.67	-0.04	0.07
Near activities	-0.07	**0.01**	-0.12	-0.02	-0.24	**<0.01**	-0.29	-0.18	0.01	0.61	-0.04	0.07	0.01	0.95	-0.06	0.05
Distance activities	-0.09	**<0.01**	-0.14	-0.03	-0.29	**<0.01**	-0.34	-0.24	0.02	0.38	-0.03	0.08	0.02	0.56	-0.04	0.07
Social functioning	-0.07	**0.02**	-0.12	-0.01	-0.32	**<0.01**	-0.37	-0.26	-0.01	0.80	-0.06	0.05	0.02	0.56	-0.04	0.07
Mental health	0.05	0.11	-0.01	0.10	-0.14	**<0.01**	-0.19	-0.08	-0.02	0.44	-0.08	0.03	-0.04	0.20	-0.09	0.02
Role difficulties	-0.05	0.06	-0.11	<0.01	-0.24	**<0.01**	-0.29	-0.18	0.02	0.49	-0.04	0.07	0.02	0.60	-0.04	0.07
Dependency	-0.13	**<0.01**	-0.18	-0.07	-0.45	**<0.01**	-0.50	-0.40	0.05	0.08	-0.01	0.10	0.01	0.81	-0.05	0.06
Driving	-0.10	**0.02**	-0.18	-0.02	-0.21	**<0.01**	-0.28	-0.15	-0.02	0.63	-0.10	0.06	0.01	0.98	-0.08	0.08
Color vision	-0.01	0.70	-0.07	0.05	-0.21	**<0.01**	-0.27	-0.15	0.02	0.52	-0.04	0.07	0.01	0.80	-0.05	0.06
Peripheral vision	-0.04	0.19	-0.09	0.02	-0.26	**<0.01**	-0.31	-0.20	-0.03	0.29	-0.09	0.03	0.01	0.94	-0.05	0.06

TBUT, Tear film break up time; OSDI, ocular surface disease index; CI, confidence interval; DED, dry eye disease; NEI-VFQ-25, 25-item National Eye Institute Visual Functioning Questionnaire.
*Adjusted with age, gender, annual household incomes, and diabetes.
Bold values mean statistically significant.

In this study, Schirmer's I test, TBUT, and OSDI scores were correlated with NEI-VFQ-25 scales. After controlling for factors, DED inversely associated with multiple subscales in NEI-VFQ-25 in Han and Mongolian adults. So far, only two large-sample size population-based study investigated the relationship between dry eye and quality of life. In a previous study involving 78,165 participants (19–94 years, 59.2% women) in Netherlands from 2006 to 2013, Morthen et al. found that dry eye is associated with low quality of life measured with SF-36 questionnaire. (11). In another study including 3,275 subjects in the United States from 2014, Paulsen et al. found that dry eye is also associated with low quality of life measured by both SF-36 and vision specific NEI-VFQ-25 questionnaires (13). Both these two previous studies were focused on dry eye symptoms (DES), which defined by a validated dry eye questionnaire, and a question "at least moderately bothersome symptoms present at minimum sometimes and/or treated with eye drops," respectively. In China, a population-based cross-sectional study enrolled 229 subjects from Shanghai city focusing on vision-specific quality of life by NEI-VFQ-25 found that only two subscales, ocular pain and mental health, were related to DED (10). Another cross-sectional comparative study that enrolled 77 outpatients and 77 general participants with DED found that NEI-VFQ-25 composite score had a negative correlation with the OSDI score of all participants. The impairment of VR-QoL has a significant correlation with the severity of DES (26). However, in this study, associations were found between DED and all of the 12 NEI-VFQ subscales, although the effect was greatest on general vision. The effect of DED on all ethnicities in this investigation suggests that the impact of DED on the perception by an individual of their health is substantial and of importance as a public health problem.

This study has some strengths. Although the majority of correlations between DED and its factors were low power, such as age and female gender, to the best of our knowledge, this was the first large population-based study investigating epidemiology on DED among individuals from two ethnicities living in grasslands, which further enabled us to analyze the impacts of DED on VR-QOL. Therefore, our study added to the current knowledge of public health concern on preventive strategies for DED. Nevertheless, our study also has several limitations. First, this study had a cross-sectional design, and as such the causality of any findings between DED and factors as well as VR-QoL cannot be made. Second, in this study, we did not look at the epidemiology characteristics of DED severity. Hence, the diagnosis of DED was done based on both the presence of dry eye symptoms (OSDI) and clinical assessment (TBUT or Schirmer's I test), but did not include ocular surface staining, tear osmolarity, or meibomian dysfunction assessment because of the limited material conditions. In addition, TBUT was performed with topical anesthesia instead of balanced salt solution in this study. Third, causes of visual disturbances in the eligible participants with DED would have allowed this study to investigate if and to what extent reductions in VR-QoL were mediated by reductions in vision quality. Fourth, we did not collect information on menopausal states of the women, which may be associated with DED. Further studies are needed to identify this association among residents living in grasslands. Finally, when correcting for numerous comorbidities, we did not adjust for ocular disorders, such as diabetic retinopathy, age-related macular degeneration, retinal detachment, cataract, and glaucoma, because of the limited validity and reliability of self-report data, which might have overcorrected and, thus, underestimated the true effect of DED on VR-QoL.

In conclusion, both crude and adjusted prevalence of DED was relatively high in this study on Mongolian and Han populations living in the northern grasslands of China. Few studies have investigated DED in this area. Many similar risk factors previously found to be associated with DED were also found in this study and some novelties, such as anti-fatigue eye drop use, milk product intake, and number of household members, warrant further investigation. DED also proved to have a significant impact on VR-QoL, independent of other confounding factors. These findings on elder adults make DED prevention an important public health problem. Further longitudinal, multi-ethnical studies on DED in grasslands are necessary to improve broad representation, establish the causal relationship between factor exposure and onset of disease, and measure the impact of long-term disease on VR-QoL.

AUTHOR CONTRIBUTIONS

All authors listed have made a substantial, direct, and intellectual contribution to the work and approved it for publication.

REFERENCES

1. Stapleton F, Alves M, Bunya VY, Jalbert I, Lekhanont K, Malet F, et al. TFOS DEWS II epidemiology report. *Ocul Surf.* (2017) 15:334–65. doi: 10.1016/j.jtos.2017.05.003

2. Song P, Xia W, Wang M, Chang X, Wang J, Jin S, et al. Variations of dry eye disease prevalence by age, sex and geographic characteristics in China: a systematic review and meta-analysis. *J Glob Health.* (2018) 8:020503. doi: 10.7189/jogh.08.020503

3. Berg EJ, Ying GS, Maguire MG, Sheffield PE, Szczotka-Flynn LB, Asbell PA, et al. Climatic and environmental correlates of dry eye disease severity: a report from the dry eye assessment and management (DREAM) Study. *Transl Vis Sci Technol.* (2020) 9:25. doi: 10.1167/tvst.9.5.25

4. Golden MI, Meyer JJ, Patel BC. *Dry Eye Syndrome.* Treasure Island, FL: StatPearls (2021).

5. Choy CK, Cho P, Benzie IF. Antioxidant content and ultraviolet absorption characteristics of human tears. *Optom Vis Sci.* (2011) 88:507–11. doi: 10.1097/OPX.0b013e31820e9fe2

6. Liu NN, Liu L, Li J, Sun YZ. Prevalence of and risk factors for dry eye symptom in mainland china: a systematic review and meta-analysis. *J Ophthalmol.* (2014) 2014:748654. doi: 10.1155/2014/748654

7. Guo B, Lu P, Chen X, Zhang W, Chen R. Prevalence of dry eye disease in Mongolians at high altitude in China: the Henan eye study. *Ophthalmic Epidemiol.* (2010) 17:234–41. doi: 10.3109/09286586.2010.498659

8. Okumura Y, Inomata T, Iwata N, Sung J, Fujimoto K, Fujio K, et al. A Review of dry eye questionnaires: measuring patient-reported

outcomes and health-related quality of life. *Diagnostics.* (2020) 10:559. doi: 10.3390/diagnostics10080559

9. Na KS, Han K, Park YG, Na C, Joo CK. Depression, stress, quality of life, and dry eye disease in korean women: a population-based study. *Cornea.* (2015) 34:733–8. doi: 10.1097/ICO.0000000000000464

10. Le Q, Zhou X, Ge L, Wu L, Hong J, Xu J. Impact of dry eye syndrome on vision-related quality of life in a non-clinic-based general population. *BMC Ophthalmol.* (2012) 12:22. doi: 10.1186/1471-2415-12-22

11. Morthen MK, Magno MS, Utheim TP, Snieder H, Hammond CJ, Vehof J. The physical and mental burden of dry eye disease: a large population-based study investigating the relationship with health-related quality of life and its determinants. *Ocul Surf.* (2021) 21:107–17. doi: 10.1016/j.jtos.2021.05.006

12. Hossain P, Siffel C, Joseph C, Meunier J, Markowitz JT, Dana R. Patient-reported burden of dry eye disease in the UK: a cross-sectional web-based survey. *BMJ Open.* (2021) 11:e039209. doi: 10.1136/bmjopen-2020-039209

13. Paulsen AJ, Cruickshanks KJ, Fischer ME, Huang GH, Klein BE, Klein R, et al. Dry eye in the beaver dam offspring study: prevalence, risk factors, and health-related quality of life. *Am J Ophthalmol.* (2014) 157:799–806. doi: 10.1016/j.ajo.2013.12.023

14. McAlinden C, Gao R, Wang Q, Zhu S, Yang J, Yu A, et al. Rasch analysis of three dry eye questionnaires and correlates with objective clinical tests. *Ocul Surf.* (2017) 15:202–10. doi: 10.1016/j.jtos.2017.01.005

15. Chan CW, Wong D, Lam CL, McGhee S, Lai WW. Development of a Chinese version of the National Eye Institute Visual Function Questionnaire (CHI-VFQ-25) as a tool to study patients with eye diseases in Hong Kong. *Br J Ophthalmol.* (2009) 93:1431–6. doi: 10.1136/bjo.2009.158428

16. Moss SE, Klein R, Klein BE. Prevalence of and risk factors for dry eye syndrome. *Arch Ophthalmol.* (2000) 118:1264–8. doi: 10.1001/archopht.118.9.1264

17. Chia EM, Mitchell P, Rochtchina E, Lee AJ, Maroun R, Wang JJ, et al. Prevalence and associations of dry eye syndrome in an older population: the Blue Mountains Eye Study. *Clin Exp Ophthalmol.* (2003) 31:229–32. doi: 10.1046/j.1442-9071.2003.00634.x

18. Uchino M, Nishiwaki Y, Michikawa T, Shirakawa K, Kuwahara E, Yamada M, et al. Prevalence and risk factors of dry eye disease in Japan: Koumi study. *Ophthalmology.* (2011) 118:2361–7. doi: 10.1016/j.ophtha.2011.05.029

19. Lekhanont K, Rojanaporn D, Chuck RS, Vongthongsri A. Prevalence of dry eye in Bangkok, Thailand. *Cornea.* (2006) 25:1162–7. doi: 10.1097/01.ico.0000244875.92879.1a

20. Viso E, Rodriguez-Ares MT, Gude F. Prevalence of and associated factors for dry eye in a Spanish adult population (the Salnes Eye Study). *Ophthalmic Epidemiol.* (2009) 16:15–21. doi: 10.1080/09286580802228509

21. Tandon R, Vashist P, Gupta N, Gupta V, Sahay P, Deka D, et al. Association of dry eye disease and sun exposure in geographically diverse adult (>/=40 years) populations of India: the SEED (sun exposure, environment and dry eye disease) study - second report of the ICMR-EYE SEE study group. *Ocul Surf.* (2020) 18:718–30. doi: 10.1016/j.jtos.2020.07.016

22. Alkabbani S, Jeyaseelan L, Rao AP, Thakur SP, Warhekar PT. The prevalence, severity, and risk factors for dry eye disease in Dubai - a cross sectional study. *BMC Ophthalmol.* (2021) 21:219. doi: 10.1186/s12886-021-01978-4

23. Zhu Y, Yu WL, Xu M, Han L, Cao W, Zhang H, et al. [Analysis of risk factors for dry eye syndrome in visual display terminal workers]. *Zhonghua Lao Dong Wei Sheng Zhi Ye Bing Za Zhi.* (2013) 31:597–9.

24. Uchino M, Yokoi N, Uchino Y, Dogru M, Kawashima M, Komuro A, et al. Prevalence of dry eye disease and its risk factors in visual display terminal users: the Osaka study. *Am J Ophthalmol.* (2013) 156:759–66. doi: 10.1016/j.ajo.2013.05.040

25. Kawashima M, Tsuno S, Matsumoto M, Tsubota K. Hydrogen-producing milk to prevent reduction in tear stability in persons using visual display terminals. *Ocul Surf.* (2019) 17:714–21. doi: 10.1016/j.jtos.2019.07.008

26. Le Q, Ge L, Li M, Wu L, Xu J, Hong J, et al. Comparison on the vision-related quality of life between outpatients and general population with dry eye syndrome. *Acta Ophthalmol.* (2014) 92:e124–32. doi: 10.1111/aos.12204

2

Corneal Biomechanics Differences Between Chinese and Caucasian Healthy Subjects

Riccardo Vinciguerra[1]*, Robert Herber[2], Yan Wang[3,4], Fengju Zhang[5], Xingtao Zhou[6], Ji Bai[7], Keming Yu[8], Shihao Chen[9], Xuejun Fang[10], Frederik Raiskup[2] and Paolo Vinciguerra[11,12]

[1] Humanitas San Pio X Hospital, Milan, Italy, [2] Department of Ophthalmology, University Hospital Carl Gustav Carus, Dresden, Germany, [3] Tianjin Eye Hospital, Tianjin Key Laboratory of Ophthalmology and Visual Science, Nankai University Affiliated Eye Hospital, Tianjin, China, [4] Clinical College of Ophthalmology, Tianjin Medical University, Tianjin, China, [5] Beijing Tongren Eye Center, Beijing Tongren Hospital, Beijing Ophthalmology and Visual Sciences Key Lab, Capital Medical University, Beijing, China, [6] EYE & ENT Hospital of Fudan University, Shanghai, China, [7] BAI JI Ophthalmology, Chongqing, China, [8] Zhongshan Ophthalmic Center, Sun Yat-Sen University, Guangzhou, China, [9] Eye Hospital, Wenzhou Medical University, Zhejiang, China, [10] Shenyang Aier Eye Hospital, Shenyang, China, [11] Department of Biomedical Sciences, Humanitas University, Milan, Italy, [12] IRCCS Humanitas Research Hospital, Rozzano, Italy

*Correspondence:
Riccardo Vinciguerra
vinciguerra.riccardo@gmail.com

Purpose: The aim of this study was to evaluate the difference between Caucasian and Chinese healthy subjects with regards to Corvis ST dynamic corneal response parameters (DCRs).

Methods: Two thousand eight hundred and eighty-nine healthy Caucasian and Chinese subjects were included in this multicenter retrospective study. Subsequently, Chinese eyes were matched to Caucasians by age, intraocular pressure (IOP), and Corneal Thickness (CCT) using a case-control matching algorithm. The DCRs assessed were Deformation Amplitude (DA) Applanation 1 velocity (A1v), integrated radius (1/R), deformation amplitude ratio (DAratio), stiffness parameter at applanation 1 (SPA1), ARTh (Ambrósio's Relational Thickness to the horizontal profile), and the novel Stress Strain Index (SSI).

Results: After age-, CCT-, and IOP- matching, 503 Chinese were assigned to 452 Caucasians participants. Statistical analysis showed a statistical significant difference between Chinese and Caucasian Healthy subjects in the values of SPA1 ($p = 0.008$), Arth ($p = 0.008$), and SSI ($p < 0.001$). Conversely, DA, A1v, DAratio, and 1/R were not significantly different between the two ethnical groups ($p > 0.05$).

Conclusion: We found significant differences in the values of the DCRs provided by the Corvis ST between Chinese and Caucasian healthy subjects.

Keywords: biomechanics, cornea, keratoconus, CBI, IOP (intraocular pressure)

INTRODUCTION

Ethnical differences in ocular metrics are well-known since many years and include central corneal thickness (1), corneal curvature (2), anterior chamber depth (3), and axial length (4).

In the last years, corneal biomechanics showed to play an important role for the diagnosis and management of keratoconus (5–9) post refractive surgery ectasia (10), cross-linking effect (11), measurement of intraocular pressure (12, 13), and glaucoma (14, 15).

Two instruments are commercially available to measure corneal biomechanics, the Ocular Response Analyzer (ORA, Reichert Inc., Depew, NY) (16) which measures corneal deformation during a bi-directional applanation method induced by an air jet, and produces appraisals of corneal hysteresis and corneal resistance factor, together with a set of 36 waveform-derived parameters (17–19). The Corvis ST (OCULUS Optikgeräte GmbH; Wetzlar, Germany) evaluates the reaction of the cornea to an air puff *via* an ultra-high speed (UHS) Scheimpflug camera, and uses the acquired image sequence to generate estimates of IOP and deformation response parameters (DCRs) (20).

The native software of the Corvis ST includes normative values for each DCRs which were derived from a mixed south American and Caucasian population (21). Very few population studies have been published with regards to DCRs values in other ethnical populations (22–24) and none of them evaluated the difference between two different ethnical groups.

The aim of this study was to assess the difference between Caucasian and Chinese healthy subjects with regards to Corvis ST DCRs.

METHODS

Two thousand eight hundred and eighty-nine healthy Caucasian and Chinese patients were included in this multicenter retrospective study. Caucasian subjects were recruited from Vincieye Clinic in Milan, Italy and from the Department of Ophthalmology, University Hospital Carl Gustav Carus, Technical University, Dresden, Germany. Conversely, Chinese participants were included from Beijing Tongren Eye Center, Beijing Tongren Hospital, Capital Medical University, Beijing; Shenyang Aier Eye Hospital, Shenyang, Zhongshan Ophthalmic Center, Sun Yat-Sen University, Guangzhou; EYE&ENT Hospital of Fudan University, Shanghai; Eye Hospital, Wenzhou Medical University, Zhejiang; BAI JI Ophthalmology, Chongqing, and Tianjin Eye Hospital,Tianjin.

Each Institutional review board (IRB) either ruled that approval was not required for this record review study or specifically approved the study. The research was conducted according to the ethical standards set in the 1964 Declaration of Helsinki, revised in 2000. All patients signed an informed consent before using their data in the study. All subjects underwent to a complete ophthalmic examination, including the Corvis ST and Pentacam exams. The inclusion criteria of this study were the existence in the database of a Corvis ST and Pentacam exam, a Belin Ambrosio Enhanced Ectasia Index total deviation (BAD-D) <1.6 and a signed informed consent. Exclusion criteria were any earlier ocular surgery or disease, any concurrent or previous glaucoma or hypotonic therapies. All exams with the Corvis ST were acquired by the same experienced technicians and captured by automatic release to ensure the absence of user dependency. Only Corvis ST exams with quality score "OK" were included in the analysis. Only 1 eye per subject was randomly included in the database to exclude the bias of the relationship between bilateral eyes that could influence the analysis result.

The parameters that were included in the analysis were the following: Deformation Amplitude Deformation Amplitude (DA, the largest displacement of corneal apex in the anterior-posterior direction at the moment of highest concavity) Applanation 1 velocity (A1v the velocity of corneal apex at first applanation), integrated radius (1/R the amount of the corneal concave state over the time between applanation 1 and applanation 2), deformation amplitude ratio (DAratio, the ratio between the central deformation and the average of peripheral deformation determined at 2.00 mm), stiffness parameter at applanation 1 [SPA1 is defined as the resultant pressure at inward applanation divided by the corneal displacement (25)], ARTh (Ambrósio's Relational Thickness to the horizontal profile), which is based on the thickness profile in the temporal-nasal direction (26) and the novel Stress Strain Index [SSI, which measures biomechanical behavior of the cornea without influence of corneal thickness and intraocular pressure (27)]. Additonally, the bIOP intraocular pressure estimate was included as a corrected value that is less influenced by age, corneal thickness and other DCR parameters (28).

Statistical Analysis

The statistical analysis was performed with SPSS version 27 (IBM Corp. in Armonk, NY, USA). In this study Chinese eyes were matched by age, bIOP, and Central Corneal Thickness (CCT) using a case-control matching algorithm provided by SPSS (29).

Descriptive statistics were calculated for the DCRs described previously, additionally, differences between data were evaluated with analysis of variance (ANOVA). The chosen level of significance was $p < 0.05$.

RESULTS

After age-, CCT- and bIOP- matching, 503 Chinese were assigned to 452 Caucasians participants. Mean age-, CCT- and bIOP of Chinese were 30.2 ± 6.8 years, 542.7 ± 29.7 μm, and 15.8 ± 2.1 mmHg, respectively, whereas, Caucasians showed 31.1 ± 6.8 years, 547.9 ± 31.8 μm, and 15.6 ± 2.1 mmHg of mean values.

Table 1 shows mean baseline characteristics of the two groups.

Statistical analysis showed a statistical significant difference between Chinese and Caucasian Healthy subjects in the values of SPA1 (**Figure 1**, $p = 0.008$), Arth (**Figure 2**, $p = 0.008$) and SSI (**Figure 3**, $p < 0.001$). Conversely, DA ($p = 0.674$), A1v ($p = 0.373$), DAratio ($p = 0.656$), and 1/R (p

TABLE 1 | Baseline and demographic data of the study population.

Parameter	Caucasians	Chinese
Age	31.1 ± 0.3	30.2 ± 0.3
CCT	547.9 ± 31.8	542.7 ± 29.7
bIOP	15.5 ± 2.2	15.7 ± 2.1
Eye (%Right)	45.1%	49.9%

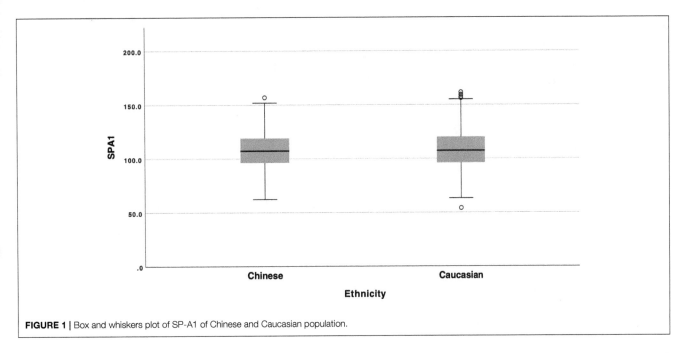

FIGURE 1 | Box and whiskers plot of SP-A1 of Chinese and Caucasian population.

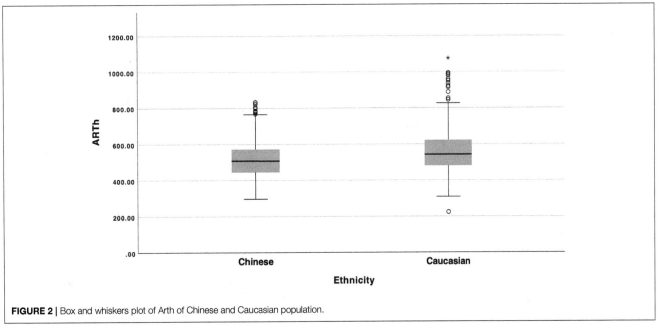

FIGURE 2 | Box and whiskers plot of Arth of Chinese and Caucasian population.

= 0.184) were not significantly different between the two ethnical groups. **Table 2** provides more details of the results of the ANOVA.

DISCUSSION

The evaluation of Ethnical variances in ocular metrics is not only important for the pure scientific knowledge but, more importantly, because a difference between two ethnicities could play a role in disease diagnosis.

The main finding of this study was the evidence that there is a significant difference in the values of the DCRs of the Corvis ST between Chinese and Caucasian population, more in details SPA1 and SSI which are pure biomechanical parameters and Arth which measures the thickness profile in the temporal-nasal direction.

It should be noted that these results are not due to the possible variance in age, IOP or corneal thickness between the two groups as they were specifically matched for these confounding factors. We decided not to match the patients for sex and refractive error to avoid decreasing too much the number of patients and we

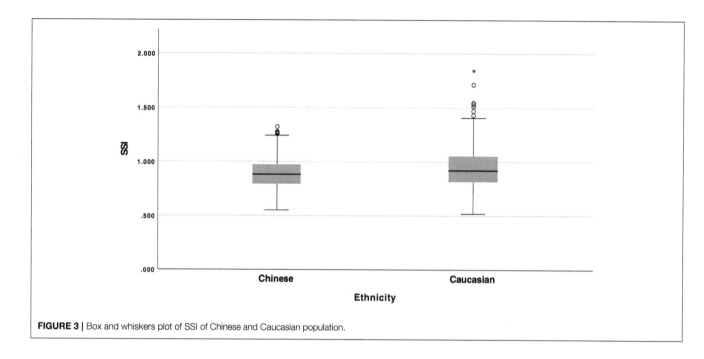

FIGURE 3 | Box and whiskers plot of SSI of Chinese and Caucasian population.

TABLE 2 | Number of cases, mean, standard deviation and p values of Corvis DCRs between Chinese and Caucasian population.

Parameters		N	Mean	Standard deviation	p-value
DA	Chinese	503	1.08485	0.102870	0.674
	Caucasian	452	1.07484	0.100243	
SPA1	Chinese	503	107.844	16.0351	**0.008**
	Caucasian	452	108.456	18.9433	
DARatio	Chinese	503	4.5317	0.45785	0.656
	Caucasian	452	4.3025	0.46629	
ARTh	Chinese	503	518.7264	100.13527	**0.008**
	Caucasian	452	563.2689	120.32852	
1/R	Chinese	503	8.5521	1.05437	0.184
	Caucasian	452	8.2790	1.17436	
A1v	Chinese	503	0.1517	0.01951	0.793
	Caucasian	452	0.1468	0.01883	
SSI	Chinese	503	0.88984	0.137459	**<0.0001**
	Caucasian	452	0.94163	0.186990	

Bold means significant values.

concentrated on age, IOP and CCT which are the most significant confounding factor for corneal biomechanics measurement (26).

It is the first time, to the authors' knowledge, that a large multicenter study was able to show a significant difference in corneal biomechanics (either Corvis ST or ORA) between two ethnical populations.

The importance of these results could be extremely high particularly in the sensitivity and the specificity of the Corvis Biomechanical Index (CBI) which includes all the three indices which were found to be different and was created basing on Caucasian and South American populations (8). We expect that this difference could play a significant role when screening a Chinese patient for refractive surgery that could lead potentially to false positives.

It is worth mentioning though only few studies on Chinese keratoconus patients assessed the sensitivity and specificity values of the CBI when compared to the original publication and they showed similar results (30, 31).

Further work of this group will focus on assessing the sensitivity and the specificity of CBI in Chinese keratoconus and to evaluate whether there is a need to improve the algorithm for this specific ethnic group.

In conclusion, we found significant differences in the values of the DCRs provided by the Corvis ST between Chinese and Caucasian healthy subjects. The presence of a case-control matching confirms this finding and excludes the influence of age, IOP, and CCT as confounding factors.

AUTHOR CONTRIBUTIONS

All authors listed have made a substantial, direct, and intellectual contribution to the work and approved it for publication.

REFERENCES

1. Aghaian E, Choe JE, Lin S, Stamper RL. Central corneal thickness of Caucasians, Chinese, Hispanics, Filipinos, African Americans, and Japanese in a glaucoma clinic. *Ophthalmology.* (2004) 111:2211–9. doi: 10.1016/j.ophtha.2004. 06.013

2. Scheiman M, Gwiazda J, Zhang Q, Deng L, Fern K, Manny RE, et al. Longitudinal changes in corneal curvature and its relationship

to axial length in the Correction of Myopia Evaluation Trial (COMET) cohort. *J Optom.* (2016) 9:13–21. doi: 10.1016/j.optom.2015.10.003

3. Wang D, Qi M, He M, Wu L, Lin S. Ethnic difference of the anterior chamber area and volume and its association with angle width. *Invest Ophthalmol Vis Sci.* (2012) 53:3139–44. doi: 10.1167/iovs.12-9776

4. Wang D, Amoozgar B, Porco T, Wang Z, Lin SC. Ethnic differences in lens parameters measured by ocular biometry in a cataract surgery population. *PLoS One.* (2017) 12:e0179836. doi: 10.1371/journal.pone.0179836

5. Ambrósio R, Correia FF, Lopes B, Salomão MQ, Luz A, Dawson DG, et al. Corneal biomechanics in ectatic diseases: refractive surgery implications. *Open Ophthalmol J.* (2017) 11:176–93. doi: 10.2174/1874364101711010176

6. Ambrosio R Jr, Lopes B, Faria-Correia F, Vinciguerra R, Vinciguerra P, Elsheikh A, et al. Ectasia detection by the assessment of corneal biomechanics. *Cornea.* (2016) 35:e18–20. doi: 10.1097/ICO.0000000000000875

7. Ambrosio R Jr, Lopes BT, Faria-Correia F, Salomao MQ, Buhren J, Roberts CJ, et al. Integration of scheimpflug-based corneal tomography and biomechanical assessments for enhancing ectasia detection. *J Refract Surg.* (2017) 33:434–43. doi: 10.3928/1081597X-20170426-02

8. Vinciguerra R, Ambrósio R, Elsheikh A, Roberts CJ, Lopes B, Morenghi E, et al. Detection of keratoconus with a new biomechanical index. *J Refract Surg.* (2016) 32:803–10. doi: 10.3928/1081597X-20160629-01

9. Vinciguerra R, Ambrósio R, Roberts CJ, Azzolini C, Vinciguerra P. Biomechanical characterization of subclinical keratoconus without topographic or tomographic abnormalities. *J Refract Surg.* (2017) 33:399–407. doi: 10.3928/1081597X-20170213-01

10. Vinciguerra R, Ambrosio R Jr, Elsheikh A, Hafezi F, Yong Kang DS, Kermani O, et al. Detection of post-laser vision correction ectasia with a new combined biomechanical index. *J Cataract Refract Surg.* (2021) 47:1314–8. doi: 10.1097/j.jcrs.000000000000629

11. Vinciguerra R, Romano V, Arbabi EM, Brunner M, Willoughby CE, Batterbury M, et al. *In vivo* early corneal biomechanical changes after corneal cross-linking in patients with progressive keratoconus. *J Refract Surg.* (2017) 33:840–6. doi: 10.3928/1081597X-20170922-02

12. Chen KJ, Eliasy A, Vinciguerra R, Abass A, Lopes BT, Vinciguerra P, et al. Development and validation of a new intraocular pressure estimate for patients with soft corneas. *J Cataract Refract Surg.* (2019) 45:1316–23. doi: 10.1016/j.jcrs.2019.04.004

13. Eliasy A, Chen KJ, Vinciguerra R, Maklad O, Vinciguerra P, Ambrósio R, et al. *Ex-vivo* experimental validation of biomechanically-corrected intraocular pressure measurements on human eyes using the CorVis ST. *Exp Eye Res.* (2018) 175:98–102. doi: 10.1016/j.exer.2018.06.013

14. Qassim A, Mullany S, Abedi F, Marshall H, Hassall MM, Kolovos A, et al. Corneal stiffness parameters are predictive of structural and functional progression in glaucoma suspect eyes. *Ophthalmology.* (2021) 128:993–1004. doi: 10.1016/j.ophtha.2020.11.021

15. Vinciguerra R, Rehman S, Vallabh NA, Batterbury M, Czanner G, Choudhary A, et al. Corneal biomechanics and biomechanically corrected intraocular pressure in primary open-angle glaucoma, ocular hypertension and controls. *Br J Ophthalmol.* (2020) 104:121–6. doi: 10.1136/bjophthalmol-2018-313493

16. Luce DA. Determining *in vivo* biomechanical properties of the cornea with an ocular response analyzer. *J Cataract Refract Surg.* (2005) 31:156–62. doi: 10.1016/j.jcrs.2004.10.044

17. Roberts CJ. Concepts and misconceptions in corneal biomechanics. *J Cataract Refract Surg.* (2014) 40:862–9. doi: 10.1016/j.jcrs.2014.04.019

18. Mikielewicz M, Kotliar K, Barraquer RI, Michael R. Air-pulse corneal applanation signal curve parameters for the characterisation of keratoconus. *Br J Ophthalmol.* (2011) 95:793–8. doi: 10.1136/bjo.2010.188300

19. Hallahan KM, Sinha Roy A, Ambrosio R Jr, Salomao M, Dupps WJ Jr. Discriminant value of custom ocular response analyzer waveform derivatives in keratoconus. *Ophthalmology.* (2014) 121:459–68. doi: 10.1016/j.ophtha.2013.09.013

20. Ambrósio R Jr, Ramos I, Luz A, Faria FC, Steinmueller A, Krug M, et al. Dynamic ultra high speed Scheimpflug imaging for assessing corneal biomechanical properties. *Rev Bras Oftalmol.* (2013) 72:99–102. doi: 10.1590/S0034-72802013000200005

21. Vinciguerra R, Elsheikh A, Roberts CJ, Ambrósio R, Kang DSY, Lopes BT, et al. Influence of pachymetry and intraocular pressure on dynamic corneal response parameters in healthy patients. *J Refract Surg.* (2016) 32:550–61. doi: 10.3928/1081597X-20160524-01

22. Wang W, He M, He H, Zhang C, Jin H, Zhong X. Corneal biomechanical metrics of healthy Chinese adults using Corvis ST. *Cont Lens Anterior Eye.* (2017) 40:97–103. doi: 10.1016/j.clae.2016.12.003

23. Kenia VP, Kenia RV, Pirdankar OH. Age-related variation in corneal biomechanical parameters in healthy Indians. *Indian J Ophthalmol.* (2020) 68:2921–9. doi: 10.4103/ijo.IJO_2127_19

24. Salouti R, Bagheri M, Shamsi A, Zamani M. Corneal parameters in healthy subjects assessed by corvis ST. *J Ophthalmic Vis Res.* (2020) 15:24–31. doi: 10.18502/jovr.v15i1.5936

25. Roberts CJ, Mahmoud AM, Bons JP, Hossain A, Elsheikh A, Vinciguerra R, Vinciguerra P, Ambrosio R Jr. Introduction of two novel stiffness parameters and interpretation of air puff-induced biomechanical deformation parameters with a dynamic scheimpflug analyzer. *J Refract Surg.* (2017) 33:266–73. doi: 10.3928/1081597X-20161221-03

26. Vinciguerra R, Elsheikh A, Roberts CJ, Ambrosio R Jr, Kang DS, Lopes BT, et al. Influence of pachymetry and intraocular pressure on dynamic corneal response parameters in healthy patients. *J Refract Surg.* (2016) 32:550–61.

27. Eliasy A, Chen KJ, Vinciguerra R, Lopes BT, Abass A, Vinciguerra P, et al. Determination of corneal biomechanical behavior *in-vivo* for healthy eyes using CorVis ST tonometry: stress-strain index. *Front Bioeng Biotechnol.* (2019) 7:105. doi: 10.3389/fbioe.2019.00105

28. Joda AA, Shervin MM, Kook D, Elsheikh A. Development and validation of a correction equation for Corvis tonometry. *Comput Methods Biomech Biomed Eng.* (2016) 19:943–53. doi: 10.1080/10255842.2015.1077515

29. Niven DJ, Berthiaume LR, Fick GH, Laupland KB. Matched case-control studies: a review of reported statistical methodology. *Clin Epidemiol.* (2012) 4:99–110. doi: 10.2147/CLEP.S30816

30. Ren S, Xu L, Fan Q, Gu Y, Yang K. Accuracy of new Corvis ST parameters for detecting subclinical and clinical keratoconus eyes in a Chinese population. *Sci Rep.* (2021) 11:4962. doi: 10.1038/s41598-021-84370-y

31. Yang K, Xu L, Fan Q, Zhao D, Ren S. Repeatability and comparison of new Corvis ST parameters in normal and keratoconus eyes. *Sci Rep.* (2019) 9:15379. doi: 10.1038/s41598-019-51502-4

3

In vivo Confocal Microscopic Evaluation of Corneal Dendritic Cell Density and Subbasal Nerve Parameters in Dry Eye Patients

Jing Xu[†], Peng Chen[†], Chaoqun Yu, Yaning Liu, Shaohua Hu and Guohu Di*

School of Basic Medicine, Qingdao University, Qingdao, China

*Correspondence:
Guohu Di
guohu_di@163.com

*[†]These authors have contributed
equally to this work*

Purpose: To conduct a systematic review and meta-analysis of the available research on evaluating changes in corneal dendritic cell density (CDCD) and the main subbasal nerve parameters (SNPs) on the ocular surface and assessing the diagnostic performance of *in vivo* confocal microscopy in patients with dry eye disease.

Methods: A computerized systematic review of literature published in PUBMED, EMBASE, Web of Science, Scopus, and the Cochrane Central Register of Controlled Trials until May 8, 2020 was performed. All statistical analyses were conducted in *RevMan V.5.3* software. The weighted mean differences (WMDs) and standardized mean differences (SMDs) with 95% confidence intervals (CI) between dry eye patients and healthy subjects were presented as results.

Results: A total of 11 studies with 755 participants were recruited, and 931 eyes were included in this meta-analysis. However, not all studies reported both CDCD and SNPs. CDCD in the central cornea was higher (WMD = 51.06, 95% CI = 39.42–62.71), while corneal nerve fiber density (CNFD) and corneal nerve fiber length (CNFL) were lower (WMD = −7.96, 95% CI = −12.12 to −3.81; SMD = −2.30, 95%CI = −3.26 to −1.35) in dry eye patients in comparison with the corresponding values in healthy controls (all $p < 0.00001$).

Conclusion: Taken together, while CNFD and CNFL were lower in dry eye patients, central CDCD showed a significant increase in these patients in comparison with the corresponding values in healthy controls.

Keywords: dry eye, dendritic cell density, subbasal nerve parameters, *in vivo* confocal microscopy, meta-analaysis

INTRODUCTION

Dry eye disease (DED) is the most common ocular surface disorder, with hundreds of millions of people affected throughout the world. The latest and authoritative definition of DED was proposed by the Tear Film and Ocular Surface Society Dry Eye Workshop II (TFOS DEWS II) in 2017. The TFOS DEWS II defined DED as a multifactorial disease that is characterized by the loss of homeostasis of the tear film with ocular discomfort symptoms that involves various etiological factors, such as tear film instability, hyperosmolarity, ocular surface inflammation, and neurosensory abnormalities (1). Due to population growth and aging, the prevalence of DED is increasing worldwide, and it currently ranges widely from 5 to 50%, depending on the populations assessed (2). DED seemingly occurs more frequently in Asia than in Western countries (2–4), and it has been reported to occur more frequently in the older population and among women (5–7). Corneal nerve alteration and inflammation both play key roles in DED development (8). However, the mechanisms underlying the discomfort and pain caused by inflammation and the nerve damage in the ocular surface in DED remain unclear.

In vivo confocal microscopy (IVCM) is a well-designed and non-invasive approach that allows for observation of the ocular surface structure *in vivo* (9). IVCM can be categorized into tandem-scanning confocal microscopy, slit-scanning confocal microscopy, and the newly developed laser-scanning confocal microscopy (10). Using IVCM in clinical assessments, changes in neuromorphic and ocular surface inflammation can be detected and imaged quantitatively (11). The Heidelberg Retinal Tomograph with the Rostock Cornea Module (HRT/RCM) (Heidelberg Engineering, Dossenheim, Germany) is the only commercially available laser-scanning confocal microscope, and is used widely in the diagnosis of DED due to the higher-quality images and the ability to perform serial scanning (10). The differences among previous studies were attributed to the use of various types of IVCM systems. Therefore, in this meta-analysis, we selected studies that used HRT/RCM to evaluate corneal parameters. In comparison with other devices and tests, HRT/RCM allows assessment of the corneal pathology at the cellular level (12). Although changes in the corneal parameters in DED patients have been demonstrated in many studies, conflicting results still exist, especially those pertaining to the density of the subbasal nerve plexus (13). Therefore, this meta-analysis aimed to assess the corneal parameters, mainly the subbasal nerve parameters (SNPs) and corneal dendritic cell density (CDCD), and evaluate the performance of IVCM in diagnosing DED by collecting data from different studies.

METHODS

Search Strategy

Databases, including Pubmed, Scopus, EMBASE, Web of Science, and Cochrane Central Register of Controlled Trials, were searched up to May 8, 2020. We developed a search strategy based on Pubmed and made the necessary modifications for each database. The following strategy was used in Pubmed: (dry eye OR dry eye syndrome OR dry eye disease OR xerophthalmia OR xeroma OR keratoconjunctivitis sicca OR Sjögren's Syndrome) AND (*in vivo* confocal microscopy OR confocal microscopy OR IVCM).

Inclusion and Exclusion Criteria

Inclusion criteria were as follows: (1) at least 10 adults with a definite diagnosis of DED in the test group; (2) a healthy population as the control group; (3) reporting central CDCD and/or at least one corneal nerve parameter (corneal nerve fiber density [CNFD], corneal nerve fiber length [CNFL], corneal nerve branch density [CNBD], or tortuosity coefficient [TC]); (4) using HRT/RCM; and (5) published in English. Studies that met any of the following criteria were excluded: (1) inappropriate types of articles, such as review articles, case reports, editorials, conference papers and abstracts, short surveys, or letters; (2) studies including cases of DED and other ocular disorders simultaneously; (3) studies assessing only animals; (4) studies by the same author (studies with more data, or, in cases involving equal data, the most recently published studies were selected); (5) studies with incomplete raw data; or (6) studies reporting interventions on subjects during trials, such as contact lens wearing, surgery, or anti-inflammatory treatments.

Data Extraction

Before the process of screening, all publications searched were exported to *Endnote* X7. Then, duplicate publications were collated and removed. Two independent reviewers (J.X &Cq.Y) screened eligible titles/abstracts before reading the full article text. Disagreements were resolved via discussion and, if necessary, by consulting a third reviewer (Gh. D). Studies that complied with the inclusion/exclusion criteria were read, and the following information was extracted from the eligible articles: study details (such as the first author's name, year of publication, CDCD, SNPs, and type of IVCM) and patient information (such as mean age, patients' sex, and type of DED). The screening process is summarized in **Figure 1**, and **a-j** in the flow diagram describe the screening protocol.

Assessments of Bias Risks

For this study, we assessed these cross-sectional studies using an 11-item checklist recommended by the Agency for Healthcare Research and Quality (14). Article quality was scored as follows: low quality = 0-3, moderate quality = 4-7, and high quality = 8-11. For case-control studies, the Newcastle-Ottawa Scale was used to rate article quality. This scale assesses studies on three parameters, selection, comparability, and exposure, with a maximum score of nine stars. The studies are rated as follows: low quality = 0-5 stars, medium quality = 6-7 stars, and high quality = 8-9 stars (15).

Investigation of Heterogeneity

Due to the substantial heterogeneity among the studies, subgroup analysis was conducted to investigate heterogeneity as follows: country of research, type of DED, and IVCM images acquisition and analysis (*post-hoc* analyses that were not pre-planned). Based on the references included, more details were shown in **Tables 1–3**.

Statistical Analysis

Review Manager V5.3 (RevMan V.5.3) was used for the meta-analysis. We collected the data for continuous variables; the mean, standard deviation, and sample size were extracted from each study. Weighted mean differences (WMDs) with 95% CI values for continuous variable outcomes were calculated for

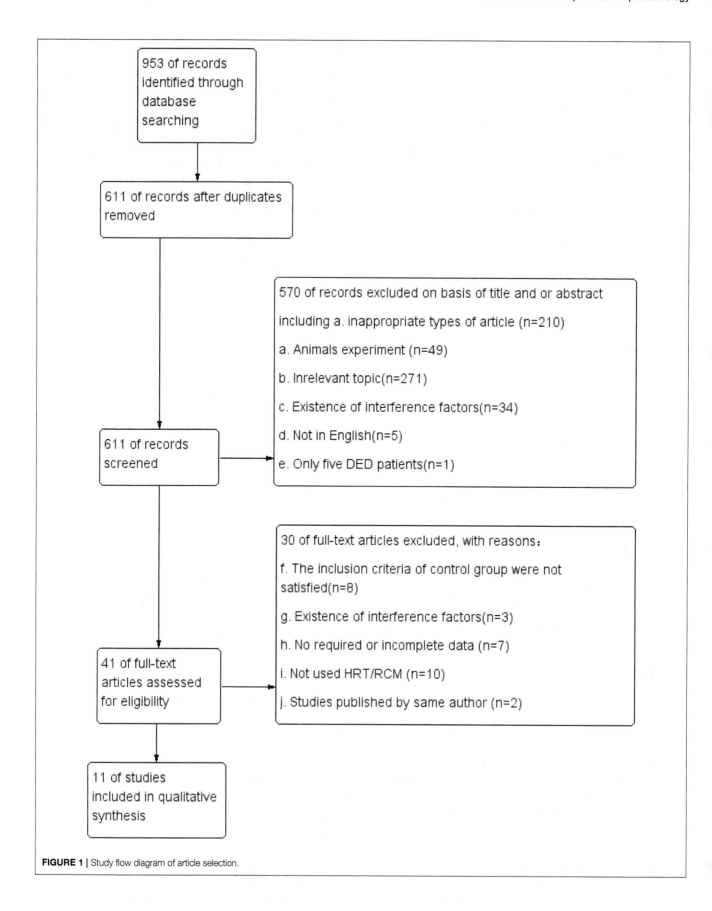

FIGURE 1 | Study flow diagram of article selection.

TABLE 1 | CDCD in the central cornea by various subgroup meta-analyses.

Subgroup	Group by	No of studies	Eyes	Heterogeneity I^2(%)	WMD of CDCD(cells/mm²) (95% CI)	p-value for heterogeneity
Country of study	Western countries	4	305	62%	51.53 [30.79,72.27]	$P = 0.05$
	Asian countries	3	276	95%	51.41 [34.92, 67.89]	$P < 0.00001$
Type of DED	ADDE	5	314	80%	51.00 [34.82, 67.17]	$P = 0.0005$
	EDE	2	207	0%	43.81 [42.95, 44.67]	$P = 0.67$
Illumination intensity	manual	4	277	38%	49.99 [39.27, 60.71]	$P = 0.18$
	automated	1	147	N	43.80 [42.94, 44.66]	N
Number of analyzed images	5	3	244	0%	43.80 [42.94, 44.66]	$P = 0.85$
	3	4	337	83%	56.10 [35.68, 76.53]	$P = 0.0006$
Selecting of analyzed images	randomly	2	107	0%	50.92 [30.01, 71.84]	$P = 0.83$
	subjective judgement	5	474	91%	44.12 [43.27, 44.97]	$P < 0.00001$
Type of counting software	software provided with microscope	4	364	93%	44.10 [43.25, 44.95]	$P < 0.00001$
	Image J	3	217	59%	50.14 [38.32, 61.96]	$P = 0.09$
Location	corneal subbasal plexus	5	424	0.98	3.17 [0.99, 5.36]	$P < 0.00001$
	corneal epithelium	2	157	97%	2.06 [−0.90, 5.02]	$P < 0.00001$

TABLE 2 | CNFD in the central subbasal nerve plexus by various subgroup meta-analyses.

Subgroup	Group by	No of studies	Eyes	Heterogeneity I^2(%)	WMD of CNFD(cells/mm²) (95% CI)	p-value for heterogeneity
Country of study	Western countries	4	312	89%	−9.19 [−14.77, −3.62]	$P < 0.00001$
	Asian countries	2	204	97%	−6.04 [−15.40, 3.33]	$P < 0.00001$
Type of DED	ADDE	4	307	83%	−11.60 [−16.63, −6.58]	$P = 0.0006$
	EDE	2	177	88%	−4.91 [−12.67, 2.84]	$P = 0.004$
Number of analyzed images	5	4	320	93%	−5.02 [−8.69, −1.36]	$P < 0.00001$
	3	1	60	N	−13.10 [−17.60, −8.60]	N
Selecting of analyzed images	randomly	2	194	81%	−2.38 [−4.69, −0.07]	$P = 0.02$
	subjective judgement	4	322	80%	−11.08 [−15.71, −6.46]	$P = 0.002$
Analysis of images	manual or semi-automated	4	300	91%	−10.79 [−16.65, −4.93]	$P < 0.00001$
	automated	2	216	72%	−2.66 [−5.96, 0.63]	$P = 0.06$

CDCD and CNFD. However, for CNFL, one set of data (16) was about 1,000 times larger than the others. Measurement methods and units of measurement were checked, and no substantial differences were found. We adopted standardized mean differences (SMDs) because of the greatly different data for CNFL. In some studies, the CNFD was defined as total length of corneal nerve fiber (mm/mm²), whereas in other studies, it was defined as the number of corneal nerve fibers (n/mm²). In order to facilitate comparison, the total corneal nerve length (mm/mm²) was considered as CNFL. Meanwhile, the sum of corneal nerves within a frame, in units of n/mm², was considered as CNFD. Heterogeneity of the results of the different studies was tested using the I^2 value. If $I^2 > 50\%$ and $p < 0.05$, significant

heterogeneity was indicated statistically. A fixed-effect model was used if $I^2 < 50\%$. Conversely, a random-effects model was applied for significant heterogeneity. Because of the limited number of included studies, bias analysis was not performed.

RESULTS

Characteristics of the Eligible Studies

After the screening process, a total of 10 cross-sectional studies (17–25) and one case-control study (26) were included. The 11 studies assessed a total of 755 participants, and 931 eyes met our criteria and were included. The corneal parameters reported by

TABLE 3 | CNFL in the central subbasal nerve plexus by various subgroup meta-analyses.

Subgroup	Group by	No of studies	Eyes	Heterogeneity I^2(%)	WMD of CNFL (mm/mm²) (95% CI)	p-value for heterogeneity
Country of study	Western countries	4	403	38%	−0.93 [−1.26, −0.61]	$P = 0.18$
	Asian countries	4	315	98%	−6.13 [−10.44, −1.81]	$P < 0.00001$
Type of DED	ADDE	4	321	97%	−1.36 [−3.93, 1.21]	$P < 0.00001$
	EDE	1	147	N	−1.50 [−1.89, −1.10]	N
Number of analyzed images	5	5	411	97%	−3.55 [−5.28, −1.83]	$P < 0.00001$
	3	2	198	0%	−1.12 [−1.48, −0.75]	$p = 0.57$
Analysis of images	manual or semi-automated	6	529	96%	−3.05 [−4.47, −1.64]	$P < 0.00001$
	automated	2	216	90%	−1.00 [−1.99, −0.02]	$p = 0.002$

TABLE 4 | Characteristics of included trials.

Study	Country	N	Eyes	Age (year)	Sex (M/F)	Group	Quality	CDCD(n/mm²)	CNFD (n/mm²)	CNBD(n/mm²)	CNFL (mm/mm²)	TC(rank)
Cardigos et al. (24)	Portugal	54	54	57.8 ± 11.9	54f	pSS	high	✓			✓	
		62	62	60.7 ± 11.0	62f	NSDE						
		20	20	50.9 ± 6.5	20f	Control						
Choi et al. (20)	Korea	44	54	49.3 ± 12.5	19/25	NSDE	moderate				✓	✓
		17	34	52.9 ± 22.3	6/11	Control						
Giannaccare et al. (25)	Italy	39	39	64.3 ± 14.5	14/25	DED	moderate	✓	✓		✓	
		30	30	66.1 ± 10.2	12/18	Control						
Kheirkhah et al. (18)	America	45	90	53.7 ± 9.8	17/28	DED	moderate	✓			✓	
		15	30	50.7 ± 9.8	7/8	Control						
Kobashi et al. (22)	Japan	25	25	61.8 ± 14.9	3/22	NSDE	moderate	✓			✓	
		25	25	61.3 ± 13.6	3/22	Control						
Labbe et al. (16)	China	43	43	46.23 ± 9.74	14/29	NSDE			✓	✓	✓	✓
		14	14	45.40 ± 9.20	6/8	Control						
Lin et al. (17)	China	14	14	43.8 ± 14.7	1/13	SSDE	moderate	✓				
		32	32	47.3 ± 14.9	9/23	NSDE						
		33	33	41.8 ± 16.8	16/17	Control						
Nicolle et al. (23)	France	32	32	50.6 ± 3.4	9/23	DED	moderate	✓	✓			
		15	15	50.7 ± 7.2	6/9	Control						
Shetty et al. (19)	India	52	104	44.5 ± 40	23/29	EDE	moderate	✓	✓	✓	✓	
		43	43	41.0 ± 41.48	14/29	Control						
Tepelus et al. (21)	America	22	44	57.5 ± 8.6	1/21	SSDE	moderate	✓			✓	✓
		12	24	58.9 ± 22.4	1/11	NSDE						
		7	10	59.3 ± 12.7	1/6	Control						
Villani et al. (26)	Italy	15	15	52.1 ± 15.4	4/11	SSDE	medium	✓	✓			✓
		15	15	56.3 ± 9.8	5/10	NSDE						
		15	15	55.3 ± 7.3	5/10	MGD						
		15	15	45.2 ± 15.9	5/10	Control						

the included studies are shown in **Table 4**. In the eligible studies, DED patients and healthy controls were matched for age.

Corneal Dendritic Cell Density

Seven studies (17–19, 21–23, 26) with a total of 581 eyes (DED,410; Controls,171) were included in this meta-analysis. As reported by previous studies (18, 19), corneal dendritic cells were identified as bright single dendritic structures with cell bodies.

The CDCD in DED patients was significantly higher than that in the controls (WMD = 51.06, 95% CI 39.42–62.71, $p < 0.00001$, $I^2 = 87\%$). Further details were provided in **Figure 2**.

Corneal Nerve Fiber Parameters

Six studies (16, 19, 23–26) with 516 eyes (DED, 379; Controls, 137) involved examinations of CNFD using HRT/RCM. The difference in CNFD between DED patients and controls showed

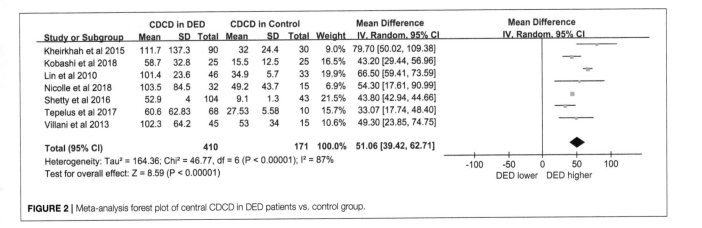

FIGURE 2 | Meta-analysis forest plot of central CDCD in DED patients vs. control group.

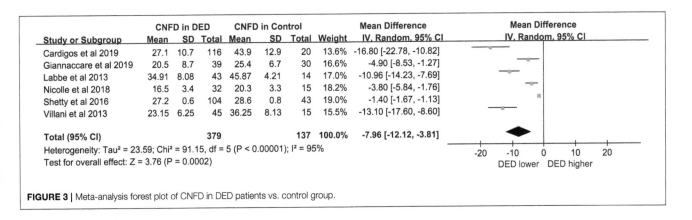

FIGURE 3 | Meta-analysis forest plot of CNFD in DED patients vs. control group.

statistical significance. The DED group showed lower CNFD than controls (WMD = −7.96, 95% CI −12.12 to −3.81, p < 0.00001, I^2 = 95%). For additional details, see **Figure 3**.

Eight studies (16, 19, 23–25) with a total of 745 eyes (DED, 539; Controls, 206) were included in the meta-analysis for CNFL. The CNFL in DED was marginally lower than that in healthy controls (SMD = −2.30, 95% CI −3.26 to −1.35, p< 0.00001, I^2 = 95%). The detailed results can be found in **Figure 4**.

Subgroup Analysis

Due to the high heterogeneity among studies, we performed the following subgroup analyses:

(1) Type of DED: Patients were divided into those with aqueous-deficient dry eye (ADDE) and evaporative dry eye (EDE).
(2) Country: Patients were divided into those from Western and Asian countries.
(3) IVCM images acquisition and analysis: Based on various conditions and different parameters, we did several subgroup analyses.

In assessments based on the type of DED, the high heterogeneity in subgroups for CNFD and CNFL persisted. In subgroup analyses stratified by country, Western countries showed lower heterogeneity than Asian countries for CDCD (I^2 = 62%, p = 0.05 vs. I^2 = 95%, p < 0.00001), CNFD (I^2 = 91%, p <

0.00001 vs. I^2 = 97%, p < 0.00001) and CNFL (I^2 = 38%, p = 0.18 vs. I^2 = 98%, p < 0.00001). However, the overall model showed no significant difference between subgroups in CDCD (p = 0.99) and CNFD (p = 0.57) without heterogeneity (I^2 = 0%). Conversely, there was a subgroup difference in CNFL (I^2 = 81.9%, p = 0.02). The details were shown in **Tables 1–3**.

For the results of IVCM images' acquisition and analysis, manual illumination intensity might be one of source of heterogeneity (I^2=38%, p = 0.18). For analyzing CNFD of images, fully automated analysis might have lower heterogeneity (I^2 = 72%, p = 0.06). Of note, due to the small amount of literature, most of the heterogeneity was not reduced. Thus, the results with low heterogeneity seemed unreliable.

Quality Assessment

The results of the quality assessment were shown in **Table 4**. Among the studies included, most of the studies were moderate quality, although some unsure risk of bias still exists. In this regard, we performed subgroup analysis. Further details were shown in **Tables 1–3**.

DISCUSSION

DED is a typical multifactorial disease with a complex pathophysiology (8). Due to the peculiarity of the cornea, IVCM

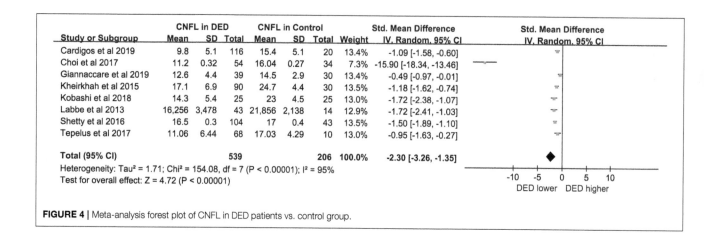

FIGURE 4 | Meta-analysis forest plot of CNFL in DED patients vs. control group.

allows operators to observe corneal nerves and the immune condition in DED and other ocular conditions directly via a non-invasive, quantitative approach. In recent years, growing concern about inflammation and nerve damage has made it important to identify new biomarkers in DED.

Corneal Dendritic Cell Density

The overall results showed significantly increased CDCD in the central corneal region of DED patients (WMD = 51.06, $P < 0.00001$). However, there was substantial heterogeneity ($I^2 > 50\%$). Therefore, we adopted a random effect model, with subgroup analyses performed to explain heterogeneity. For subgroup analyses, the findings indicated no significant difference ($p = 0.99$) without heterogeneity ($I^2 = 0\%$) between subgroups in different countries. Further details were shown in **Figure 2** and **Table 1**. The nationality of patients cannot be considered a source of heterogeneity. Moreover, another study (26) enrolled DED patients, including those with primary Sjögren's syndrome (pSS), non-Sjögren's syndrome dry eye (NSDE), and meibomian gland diseases (MGDs). Thus, the data for the same control groups were used because MGD belongs to EDE, while pSS and NSDE belong to ADDE. However, as previously reported (18), CDCD in ADDE was significantly higher than that in EDE ($p = 0.001$). In some studies (21, 27), a significant increase was observed in CDCD in Sjögren's syndrome dry eye (SSDE) compared to NSDE. Dendritic cells (DCs) play a key role in pSS (28). Other possible factors may contribute to the strong heterogeneity, such as the definition of DCs, diagnostic criteria of DED, and sex ratio of the subjects. However, due to differences in classifications, we could not evaluate these factors.

In the pathogenesis of dry eye, DCs play an important role in inducing the activation of T cells (29), thus triggering an inflammatory cascade reaction. All the CDCD data included in this study pertained to the central cornea. In one study (17), the data for the center and periphery of the cornea were reported simultaneously. To maintain consistency, we selected the data from the central area of the cornea. The density of corneal epithelial DCs in the periphery and the limbus are reported to be higher than those in the central cornea (30, 31). Animal

experiments also confirmed this statement (32). Epithelial DCs are mainly located near the subbasal nerve plexus (11).

Corneal Nerve Parameters

In short, CNFD and CNFL were lower in DED patients compared with healthy controls (WMD = -7.96, $p < 0.00001$; SMD = -2.30, $p < 0.00001$). And the forest plots of CNFL and CNFD both showed statistically great heterogeneity between studies (**Figures 3, 4**). However, in the subgroup analysis of different types of DED, the source of this heterogeneity remained elusive (**Tables 2, 3**). In subgroup analyses, we hypothesized that the pathogenesis of DED patients in Asian countries may be more complicated than that in Western countries. Moreover, in the present study, the exclusion criteria did not include contact lens wearing. Thus, we could not rule out the possibility of DED caused by contact lens wearing. A previous study revealed that wearing contact lenses led to activation and increase in CDCD, as well as a decrease in the subbasal nerve density, indicating that contact lens wear has an impact on the outcome of DED (33).

Only four studies (16, 20, 21, 26) reported corneal nerve TC, and three of those (16, 19, 25) reported CNBD. Therefore, we did not generate the forest plot. Most of the nerve endings that innervate the cornea are located in the SNPs (34). There is no universally agreed definition for corneal nerve parameters, which is one of reasons why changes in corneal nerve parameters varied between different studies. However, there are conflicting results for the difference in CNFD between DED and controls. Some articles (16, 35) have reported a reduction of CNFD in DED, while others reported no difference in SND (36, 37) or a significant increase in corneal nerve density in DED (37, 38). In addition, some studies defined the total length of the nerve fibers per square millimeter as nerve density (18, 20), while others (25, 39, 40) considered the total number of nerves per square millimeter as CNFD. This may be another reason for the conflicting findings. Moreover, variations in nerve density might affect the periods and severity of DED.

IVCM Images Acquisition and Analysis

For IVCM images acquisition and analysis, although the confocal microscope used in included studies was HRTS, the operating and examination procedure of most studies was subjective. We performed a general quality assessment for the included studies, which indicated IVCM examination might be a major source of risks of bias. The operator selection, image capture, and image analysis were different in different studies. Moreover, the software used to quantify the corneal parameters was not the same. It was reported that CNFL analyzed by manual analysis software (CCMetrics) was higher than using semiautomated or automated software (NeuronJ and ACCMetrics). ACCMetrics was more time-efficient and could provide objective results, since it could distinguish nerve fibers with adjacent pixels by fully automated algorithm (41, 42). Of note, one study (43) has developed a quality evaluation form for the examination of corneal nerve parameters, which is meaningful for future studies. However, the images should be selected randomly to minimize subjective bias. Also, a set of standardized operating procedures should be developed with a unified scanning depth range, a fixed position, and other identical image settings. It might be valuable for future research.

Limitations and Future Directions

The present study has some limitations that should be considered. There was considerable heterogeneity in the included studies, such as methods for measuring parameters, examined location for the cornea, and ethnic variation. It is probably one factor of the risk of bias in assessment of corneal parameters between dry eye patients and healthy subjects. And for some corneal parameters (e.g., branch density, fiber area), we could not conduct a meta-analysis because of incomplete reporting of data. This meta-analysis might be meaningful in assessing corneal pathology in DED and future relevant research. The quantification of CDCD and corneal nerve parameters by IVCM might be valuable for

early diagnosis of dry eye, predicting the severity of dry eye, and contributing to clinical evaluation of anti-inflammatory drug efficacy.

CONCLUSION

In summary, the CDCD and SNPs in DED could be examined by IVCM. However, there is still a lack of gold standard criteria for the definitions of parameters and a complete, objective assessment system. In general, CNFD and CNFL were reduced while CDCD showed a significant increase in DED patients. Moreover, IVCM could provide objective markers for diagnosing DED but was not suitable for indicating the subtype of DED.

AUTHOR CONTRIBUTIONS

JX and PC designed the program, searched and reviewed the studies, and were in charge of the manuscript. CY and YL assessed the studies, extracted the data, and wrote the part of the manuscript. SH extracted the data and wrote the part of the manuscript. GD directed the project, contributed to the discussion, reviewed, and edited the manuscript. GD had full access to all the data in the study and had final responsibility for the decision to submit for publication. All authors contributed to the article and approved the submitted version.

ACKNOWLEDGMENTS

We would like to thank Editage (www.editage.com) for English language editing.

REFERENCES

1. Craig J, Nichols K, Akpek E, Caffery B, Dua H, Joo C, et al. TFOS DEWS II definition and classification report. *Ocular Surf.* (2017) 15:276–83. doi: 10.1016/j.jtos.2017.05.008
2. Stapleton F, Alves M, Bunya V, Jalbert I, Lekhanont K, Malet F, et al. TFOS DEWS II epidemiology report. *Ocular Surf.* (2017) 15:334–65. doi: 10.1016/j.jtos.2017.05.003
3. Hyon J, Yang H, Han S. Association between dry eye disease and psychological stress among paramedical workers in Korea. *Sci Rep.* (2019) 9:3783. doi: 10.1038/s41598-019-40539-0
4. Siffel C, Hennies N, Joseph C, Lascano V, Horvat P, Scheider M, et al. Burden of dry eye disease in Germany: a retrospective observational study using German claims data. *Acta Ophthalmol (Copenh).* (2020) 98:e504–12. doi: 10.1111/aos.14300
5. Jie Y, Xu L, Wu Y, Jonas J. Prevalence of dry eye among adult Chinese in the Beijing Eye Study. *Eye.* (2009) 23:688–93. doi: 10.1038/sj.eye.6703101
6. Han SB, Hyon JY, Woo SJ, Lee JJ, Kim TH, Kim KW. Prevalence of dry eye disease in an elderly korean population. *Arch Ophthalmol.* (2011) 129:633–8. doi: 10.1001/archophthalmol.2011.78

7. Mai ELC, Lin C-C, Lian I, Liao R, Chen M, Chang C. Population-based study on the epidemiology of dry eye disease and its association with presbyopia and other risk factors. *Int Ophthalmol.* (2019) 39:2731–9. doi: 10.1007/s10792-019-01117-5
8. Bron AJ, de Paiva CS, Chauhan SK, Bonini S, Gabison EE, Jain S, et al. TFOS DEWS II pathophysiology report. *Ocular Surf.* (2017) 15:438–510. doi: 10.1016/j.jtos.2017.05.011
9. Zhivov A, Stachs O, Kraak R, Stave J, Guthoff RF. *In vivo* confocal microscopy of the ocular surface. *Ocular Surf.* (2006) 4:81–93. doi: 10.1016/S1542-0124(12)70030-7
10. Cruzat A, Qazi Y, Hamrah P. *In vivo* confocal microscopy of corneal nerves in health and disease. *Ocular Surf.* (2017) 15:15–47. doi: 10.1016/j.jtos.2016.09.004
11. Cruzat A, Witkin D, Baniasadi N, Zheng L, Ciolino J, Jurkunas U, et al. Inflammation and the nervous system: the connection in the cornea in patients with infectious keratitis. *Invest Ophthalmol Vis Sci.* (2011) 52:5136–43. doi: 10.1167/iovs.10-7048
12. Lee OL, Tepelus TC, Huang J, Irvine AG, Irvine C, Chiu GB, et al. Evaluation of the corneal epithelium in non-Sjogren's and Sjogren's dry eyes: an *in vivo*

confocal microscopy study using HRT III RCM. *BMC Ophthalmol.* (2018) 18:309. doi: 10.1186/s12886-018-0971-3

13. Belmonte C, Nichols JJ, Cox SM, Brock JA, Begley CG, Bereiter DA, et al. TFOS DEWS II pain and sensation report. *Ocular Surf.* (2017) 15:404–37. doi: 10.1016/j.jtos.2017.05.002

14. Rostom A, Dubé C, Cranney A, Saloojee N, Sy R, Garritty C, et al. *Celiac Disease.* Rockville (MD): Agency for Healthcare Research and Quality (US) (2004). (Evidence Reports/Technology Assessments, No. 104.) Appendix D. Quality Assessment Forms. Available online at: https://www.ncbi.nlm.nih.gov/books/NBK35156/

15. Stang A. Critical evaluation of the Newcastle-Ottawa scale for the assessment of the quality of nonrandomized studies in meta-analyses. *Eur J Epidemiol.* (2010) 25:603–5. doi: 10.1007/s10654-010-9491-z

16. Labbe A, Liang QF, Wang ZQ, Zhang Y, Xu L, Baudouin C, et al. Corneal nerve structure and function in patients with non-Sjogren dry eye: clinical correlations. *Invest Ophthalmol Vis Sci.* (2013) 54:5144–50. doi: 10.1167/iovs.13-12370

17. Lin H, Li W, Dong N, Chen WS, Liu J, Chen LL, et al. Changes in corneal epithelial layer inflammatory cells in aqueous tear-deficient dry eye. *Invest Ophthalmol Vis Sci.* (2010) 51:122–8. doi: 10.1167/iovs.09-3629

18. Kheirkhah A, Saboo US, Abud TB, Dohlman TH, Arnoldner MA, Hamrah P, et al. Reduced corneal endothelial cell density in patients with dry eye disease. *Am J Ophthalmol.* (2015) 159:1022–6.e1022. doi: 10.1016/j.ajo.2015.03.011

19. Shetty R, Sethu S, Deshmukh R, Deshpande K, Ghosh A, Agrawal A, et al. Corneal dendritic cell density is associated with subbasal nerve plexus features, ocular surface disease index, and serum vitamin D in evaporative dry eye disease. *Biomed Res Int.* (2016) 2016:4369750. doi: 10.1155/2016/4369750

20. Choi EY, Kang HG, Lee CH, Yeo A, Noh HM, Gu N, et al. Langerhans cells prevent subbasal nerve damage and upregulate neurotrophic factors in dry eye disease. *PLoS ONE.* (2017) 12:e0176153. doi: 10.1371/journal.pone.0176153

21. Tepelus TC, Chiu GB, Huang JY, Huang P, Sadda SR, Irvine J, et al. Correlation between corneal innervation and inflammation evaluated with confocal microscopy and symptomatology in patients with dry eye syndromes: a preliminary study. *Graefes Arch Clin Exp Ophthalmol.* (2017) 255:1771–8. doi: 10.1007/s00417-017-3680-3

22. Kobashi H, Kamiya K, Sambe T, Nakagawa R. Factors influencing subjective symptoms in dry eye disease. *Int J Ophthalmol.* (2018) 11:1926–31. doi: 10.18240/ijo.2018.12.08

23. Nicolle P, Liang H, Reboussin E, Rabut G, Warcoin E, Brignole-Baudouin F, et al. Proinflammatory markers, chemokines, and enkephalin in patients suffering from dry eye disease. *Int J Mol Sci.* (2018) 19:14. doi: 10.3390/ijms19041221

24. Cardigos J, Barcelos F, Carvalho H, Hipólito D, Crisóstomo S, Vaz-Patto J, et al. Tear meniscus and corneal sub-basal nerve plexus assessment in primary Sjögren syndrome and Sicca syndrome patients. *Cornea.* (2019) 38:221–8. doi: 10.1097/ICO.0000000000001800

25. Giannaccare G, Pellegrini M, Sebastiani S, Moscardelli F, Versura P, Campos EC. *In vivo* confocal microscopy morphometric analysis of corneal subbasal nerve plexus in dry eye disease using newly developed fully automated system. *Graefes Arch Clin Exp Ophthalmol.* (2019) 257:583–9. doi: 10.1007/s00417-018-04225-7

26. Villani E, Magnani F, Viola F, Santaniello A, Scorza R, Nucci P, et al. *In vivo* confocal evaluation of the ocular surface morpho-functional unit in dry eye. *Optom Vis Sci.* (2013) 90:576–86. doi: 10.1097/OPX.0b013e318294c184

27. Machetta F, Fea AM, Actis AG, de Sanctis U, Dalmasso P, Grignolo FM. *In vivo* confocal microscopic evaluation of corneal langerhans cells in dry eye patients. *Open Ophthalmol J.* (2014) 8:51–9. doi: 10.2174/1874364101408010051

28. Hillen M, Ververs F, Kruize A, Van Roon J. Dendritic cells, T-cells and epithelial cells: a crucial interplay in immunopathology of primary Sjögren's syndrome. *Expert Rev Clin Immunol.* (2014) 10:521–31. doi: 10.1586/1744666X.2014.878650

29. Maruoka S, Inaba M, Ogata N. Activation of dendritic cells in dry eye mouse model. *Invest Ophthalmol Vis Sci.* (2018) 59:3269–77. doi: 10.1167/iovs.17-22550

30. Alzahrani Y, Colorado L, Pritchard N, Efron N. Longitudinal changes in Langerhans cell density of the cornea and conjunctiva in contact lens-induced dry eye. *Clin Exp Optom.* (2017) 100:33–40. doi: 10.1111/cxo.12399

31. Mobeen R, Stapleton F, Chao C, Madigan M, Briggs N, Golebiowski B. Corneal epithelial dendritic cell density in the healthy human cornea: a meta-analysis of in-vivo confocal microscopy data. *Ocular Surf.* (2019) 17:753–62. doi: 10.1016/j.jtos.2019.07.001

32. Hamrah P, Huq S, Liu Y, Zhang Q, Dana M. Corneal immunity is mediated by heterogeneous population of antigen-presenting cells. *J Leukoc Biol.* (2003) 74:172–8. doi: 10.1189/jlb.1102544

33. Liu Q, Xu Z, Xu Y, Zhang J, Li Y, Xia J, et al. Changes in corneal dendritic cell and sub-basal nerve in long-term contact lens wearers with dry eye. *Eye Contact Lens.* (2020) 40:238–44. doi: 10.1097/ICL.00000000000 00691

34. Vaishnav YJ, Rucker SA, Saharia K, McNamara NA. Rapid, automated mosaicking of the human corneal subbasal nerve plexus. *Biomed Tech.* (2017) 62:609–13. doi: 10.1515/bmt-2016-0148

35. Erdélyi B, Kraak R, Zhivov A, Guthoff R, Németh J. *In vivo* confocal laser scanning microscopy of the cornea in dry eye. *Graefes Arch Clin Exp Ophthalmol.* (2007) 245:39–44. doi: 10.1007/s00417-006-0375-6

36. Tuominen ISJ, Konttinen YT, Vesaluoma MH, Moilanen JAO, Helinto M, Tervo TMT. Corneal innervation and morphology in primary Sjogren's syndrome. *Invest Ophthalmol Vis Sci.* (2003) 44:2545–9. doi: 10.1167/iovs.02-1260

37. Hosal BM, Ornek N, Zilelioglu G, Elhan AH. Morphology of corneal nerves and corneal sensation in dry eye: a preliminary study. *Eye.* (2005) 19:1276–9. doi: 10.1038/sj.eye.6701760

38. Zhang M, Chen J, Luo L, Xiao Q, Sun M, Liu Z. Altered corneal nerves in aqueous tear deficiency viewed by *in vivo* confocal microscopy. *Cornea.* (2005) 24:818–24. doi: 10.1097/01.ico.0000154402.01710.95

39. Malik RA, Kallinikos P, Abbott CA, van Schie CHM, Morgan P, Efron N, et al. Corneal confocal microscopy: a non-invasive surrogate of nerve fibre damage and repair in diabetic patients. *Diabetologia.* (2003) 46:683–8. doi: 10.1007/s00125-003-1086-8

40. Khamar P, Nair AP, Shetty R, Vaidya T, Subramani M, Ponnalagu M, et al. Dysregulated Tear fluid nociception-associated factors, corneal dendritic cell density, and vitamin D levels in evaporative dry eye. *Invest Ophthalmol Vis Sci.* (2019) 60:2532–42. doi: 10.1167/iovs.19-26914

41. Dehghani C, Pritchard N, Edwards K, Russell AW, Malik RA, Efron N. Fully automated, semiautomated, and manual morphometric analysis of corneal subbasal nerve plexus in individuals with and without diabetes. *Cornea.* (2014) 33:696–702. doi: 10.1097/ICO.00000000000 00152

42. Schaldemose EL, Fontain FI, Karlsson P, Nyengaard JR. Improved sampling and analysis of images in corneal confocal microscopy. *J Microsc.* (2017) 268:3–12. doi: 10.1111/jmi.12581

43. De Silva M, Zhang A, Karahalios A, Chinnery H, Downie L. Laser scanning *in vivo* confocal microscopy (IVCM) for evaluating human corneal sub-basal nerve plexus parameters: protocol for a systematic review. *BMJ Open.* (2017) 7:e018646. doi: 10.1136/bmjopen-2017-018646

4

"Endothelium-Out" and "Endothelium-In" Descemet Membrane Endothelial Keratoplasty (DMEK) Graft Insertion Techniques

Hon Shing Ong[1,2,3]*, Hla M. Htoon[2,3], Marcus Ang[1,2,3] and Jodhbir S. Mehta[1,2,3,4]*

[1] Department of Corneal & External Eye Diseases, Singapore National Eye Centre, Singapore, Singapore, [2] Singapore Eye Research Institute, Singapore, Singapore, [3] Duke-NUS Medical School, Singapore, Singapore, [4] School of Materials Science and Engineering, Nanyang Technological University, Singapore, Singapore

*Correspondence:
Jodhbir S. Mehta
jodmehta@gmail.com
Hon Shing Ong
honshing@gmail.com

Background: We evaluated the visual outcomes and complications of "endothelium-out" and "endothelium-in" Descemet membrane endothelial keratoplasty (DMEK) graft insertion techniques.

Materials and Methods: Electronic searches were conducted in CENTRAL, Cochrane databases, PubMed, EMBASE, ClinicalTrials.gov. Study designs included clinical trials, comparative observational studies, and large case series ($\geq$25 eyes). PRISMA guidelines were used for abstracting data and synthesis. Random-effects models were employed for meta-analyses.

Results: 21,323 eyes (95 studies) were included. Eighty-six studies reported on "endothelium-out" techniques; eight studies reported on "endothelium-in" techniques. One study compared "endothelium-out" to "endothelium-in" techniques. Eighteen "endothelium-out" studies reported that 42.5–85% of eyes achieved best-corrected visual acuity (BCVA) $\geq$20/25 at 6 months; pooled proportion of eyes achieving BCVA $\geq$20/25 at 6 months was 58.7% (95% CI 49.4–67.7%,15 studies). Three "endothelium-in" studies reported that 44.7–87.5% of eyes achieved BCVA of $\geq$20/25 at 6 months; pooled proportion of eyes achieving BCVA $\geq$20/25 at 6 months was 62.4% (95% CI 33.9–86.9%). Pooled mean endothelial cell loss was lower in the *"endothelium-in"* studies (28.1 $\pm$ 1.3%, 7 studies) compared to *"endothelium-out"* studies (36.3 $\pm$ 6.9%,10 studies) at 6 months (p = 0.018). Graft re-bubbling rates were higher in the "endothelium-out" studies (26.2%, 95% CI 21.9–30.9%, 74 studies) compared to "endothelium-in" studies (16.5%, 95% CI 8.5–26.4%, 6 studies), although statistical significance was not reached (p = 0.440). Primary graft failure rates were comparable between the two groups (p = 0.552). Quality of evidence was considered low and significant heterogeneity existed amongst the studies.

Conclusion: Reported rates of endothelial cell loss were lower in "endothelium-in" DMEK studies at 6 months compared to "endothelium-out" studies. Outcomes of "endothelium-in" techniques were otherwise comparable to those reported in "endothelium-out" studies. Given the technical challenges encountered in "endothelium-out" procedures, surgeons may consider "endothelium-in" techniques designed for easier intra-operative DMEK graft unfolding. "Endothelium-in" studies evaluating outcomes at longer time points are required before conclusive comparisons between the two techniques can be drawn.

Keywords: endothelial keratoplasty, Descemet's membrane endothelial keratoplasty, DMEK, bullous keratopathy, cornea, corneal transplants, outcomes, surgical techniques

INTRODUCTION

Background

Loss of vision from diseases of the corneal endothelium is the predominant indication for corneal transplantations (1, 2). Over the past 20 years, selective replacement of damaged corneal endothelium using lamellar keratoplasty procedures has significantly changed the management of endothelial diseases (3–5). The first posterior lamellar keratoplasty procedure was described in the late 1990s (6). In this report, the surgeon only partially replaced the recipient's diseased corneal endothelium, avoiding full-thickness or penetrating keratoplasty (PK). Ensuing developments to the procedure have resulted in more advanced techniques of endothelial keratoplasty (EK), which are associated with better visual outcomes, lower graft rejection risks, and improved graft survival rates (5, 7–9). Unlike PK, these EK techniques avoid full-thickness corneal trephination and intra-operative "open sky" situations associated the risks of severe blinding complications such as suprachoroidal hemorrhage. Endothelial keratoplasties also maintain corneal biomechanics and the overall strength of the globe, important in protecting the eye from external trauma. Data from national corneal graft registries have reported that EK procedures have now overtaken full-thickness PK as the leading procedure for treating corneal endothelial diseases in several countries (1, 2, 10).

Currently, there are two predominant techniques of EK performed worldwide: Descemet's stripping automated endothelial keratoplasty (DSAEK) and Descemet membrane endothelial keratoplasty (DMEK) (3, 4, 11). In DSAEK, the transplanted corneal grafts are comprised of donor endothelium, Descemet's membrane (DM), and some posterior stroma. Advancement of the DSAEK technique, such as the development of devices for graft insertion and techniques to cut thinner grafts, has greatly simplified DSAEK (12–15). With more predictable visual outcomes and faster visual recovery compared to PK (8, 16, 17), many corneal surgeons are now performing DSAEK as the primary technique to treat end-stage corneal endothelial diseases (18, 19).

Descemet membrane endothelial keratoplasty is the more recent advancement in EK surgery (20). In DMEK, only the DM and the corneal endothelium are harvested from donor corneal tissues and transplanted, rendering them anatomically more accurate. As corneal stroma is not transplanted, changes in corneal profiles are avoided. Faster visual recovery and improved visual outcomes compared to DSAEK can thus be achieved (21–25). Lower rates of graft rejection have also been reported in DMEK compared to DSAEK (26).

Rationale for This Review

Current methods of DMEK graft transfer into the anterior chamber involve inserting the graft through a small clear corneal wound. Different surgical instruments have been described for the insertion of DMEK grafts. Examples of such instruments include glass injectors (27, 28) and intraocular lens cartridges (29, 30). All these instruments are designed to shield the DMEK graft scroll from the surgical wound. Nevertheless, the majority of techniques reported in published literature involves the loading and insertion of the DMEK graft with the endothelium on the outer surface ("endothelium-out"). Thus, the grafts are potentially at risk of endothelial cell loss due to endothelial contact with the walls of the injection devices. Furthermore, "endothelium-out" DMEK techniques all involve the injection of the entire scrolled graft into the anterior chamber. The unscrolling of the free floating graft, following its insertion, can be difficult and unpredictable (31, 32). Such challenges have hindered corneal surgeons from adopting DMEK as a primary treatment for corneal endothelial failure (2, 3). In a recent eye banking report, DSAEK still accounted for over 55% of EK procedures performed in the United States (2).

"Endothelium-in" DMEK graft insertion techniques have been described more recently (33–37) (**Figure 1**). In these techniques, the harvested DM is folded and prevented from adopting its natural scroll with its endothelium on the outside. By maintaining the orientation of the DMEK graft during graft insertion, these "endothelium-in" techniques aim to provide more control in graft unscrolling following insertion into the eye. Nevertheless, the differences in surgical outcomes of either technique for DMEK graft insertion, "endothelium-in" or "endothelium-out," remains unclear.

Objectives of This Review

This review aims to evaluate the published literature reporting the visual outcomes and complications of both "endothelium-out" and "endothelium-in" graft insertion techniques for DMEK.

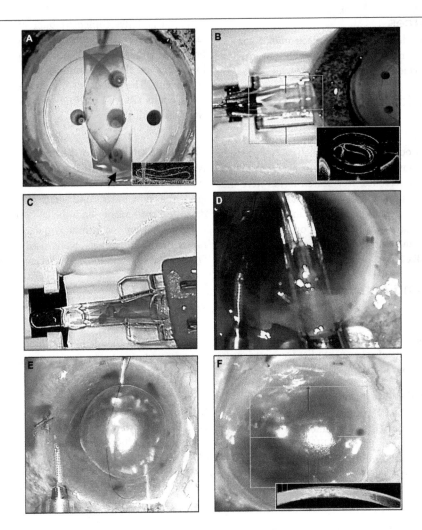

FIGURE 1 | An "endothelium-in" surgical technique of Descemet membrane endothelial keratoplasty (DMEK) using the using the DMEK EndoGlide (Network Medical Products, United Kingdom). **(A)** DMEK graft is folded into a tri-fold with its endothelium in its inner surface; note the asymmetrical orientation marker (arrow); (inset) intraoperative optical coherence tomography (OCT) image of the tri-folded graft – note that the leaves of the tri-fold do not touch. **(B)** Graft is pulled and loaded into the EndoGlide; (inset) OCT image showing the tri-folded graft within the DMEK EndoGlide – note that the leaves of the tri-fold do not touch. **(C)** Customized clip fixed to the back of the EndoGlide; this creates a "closed system" after graft insertion maintaining anterior chamber stability. **(D)** Graft is drawn into the anterior chamber with micro-forceps with its endothelium facing down. **(E)** Unfolding of the graft with its orientation maintained whilst air is injected for tamponade. **(F)** Full air-gas tamponade of graft; (inset) intraoperative OCT showing a fully attached DMEK graft.

MATERIALS AND METHODS

This review was submitted to PROSPERO International prospective register of systematic reviews (reference ID: 160657)[1]. A study protocol for this systematic review is available in **Supplementary Appendix 1.**

Criteria for Considering Studies for This Review
Types of Intervention
We included publications in which the visual outcomes and complications of DMEK performed for the treatment of endothelial dysfunction were reported.

Types of Studies
Study designs included controlled clinical trials, prospective or retrospective comparative observational studies, and large case series (≥25 eyes). Small case series (<25 eyes), letters, reviews, published abstracts, and laboratory-based studies were excluded.

Types of Participants (Study Population)
Studies reporting only surgical outcomes of DMEK performed for graft failure (including repeat DMEK surgery) or specific high-risk disease groups (e.g., glaucoma, cytomegalovirus endotheliitis, herpes simplex) were also excluded. To avoid duplicate reporting of similar study populations, where the same group of investigators published several studies, earlier smaller studies were excluded if more recent larger studies reporting the same outcome measures were available.

---
[1]https://www.crd.york.ac.uk/PROSPERO

Information Sources

Information sources included all applicable electronic databases, all relevant articles in the reference list of any relevant articles, and all relevant articles which cite any relevant articles.

Search Methods for Identification of Studies

Electronic literature searches were conducted in the following databases: CENTRAL, Cochrane Library databases[2], PubMed, EMBASE, ClinicalTrials.gov.[3] No date or language restrictions were set in our electronic searches. Key search terms were the MeSH headings Descemet's membrane endothelial keratoplasty, Descemet membrane endothelial keratoplasty, and DMEK. The last electronic database search was performed on 30 June 2021. The search strategies for the relevant databases can be found in **Supplementary Appendix 2**.

Data Collection and Analysis

Selection of Studies

Citations and abstracts obtained from electronic searches were examined. Replicated studies and evidently irrelevant studies were removed. Full text prints of relevant studies were retrieved; they were assessed against our inclusion criteria for this review.

Data Extraction and Management

Only data from eyes that had received DMEK surgeries were included. Where studies reported on the outcomes of eyes that had undergone surgeries other than DMEK, these eyes were excluded from the review. The following details of each study were extracted for this review: study participants' characteristics, study design, DMEK graft insertion techniques, and surgical outcome measures.

Assessment of Risks of Bias in Included Studies

The study design of each article was assessed and rated according to its level of evidence. A rating scale adapted from the Oxford Centre for Evidence-Based Medicine was used (38) (**Table 1**).

Studies meeting the inclusion criteria were also assessed for risk of bias using Chapter 8 of the *Cochrane Handbook for Systematic Reviews of Intervention* (39). The following domains for potential risk of bias were considered: (a) *selection bias* – random sequence generation, (b) *selection bias* – allocation concealment, (c) *performance/detection bias* – masking of outcome examiners and participants (to determine whether knowledge of the allocated intervention was adequately prevented during the study), (d) *attrition bias* incomplete outcome data, and (e) *reporting bias* – selective outcome reporting. Each study was graded as "low risk" of bias, "high risk" of bias, or "unclear risk." Any differences between the authors were resolved by discussion.

Outcome Measures

Data on the following surgical outcome measures were obtained: visual outcomes, endothelial cell loss, and complications including graft detachment/re-bubbling, graft rejection, and graft failure. For direct comparison of visual outcomes, measures of visual acuities in Snellen were converted to the respective logarithm of the minimum angle of resolution (LogMAR) equivalents. The proportion of eyes that achieved a best-corrected visual acuity (BCVA) of 20/25 or better at a specific time points were also evaluated.

Measures of Treatment Effect

All outcome measures (proportion of eyes achieving ≥20/25 BCVA, re-bubbling rates for graft detachments, graft rejection rates, and graft failure rates) were discrete data, except mean endothelial cell loss where outcome measures were continuous data. Outcomes for eyes rather than individuals were used as the unit of analysis. Studies where both eyes received the same treatment were included.

Managing Missing Data

All relevant data were extracted from the published studies. These included the details of studies and their quantitative results, without having to request these data from the original investigators.

Data Synthesis

Data analyses were performed according to Chapter 9 of the Cochrane Handbook for Systematic Reviews of Interventions (39). As published studies were performed in different institutions at various times, it is likely that variations exist amongst the patient populations included in this review. We therefore employed a random-effects model for our meta-analyses as the true effect size might differ between studies. Where we could not perform a meta-analysis, narrative syntheses describing the directions, magnitude, and consistencies of effects across the studies has been presented. MedCalc software was used for providing the meta-analyses results (MedCalc®

TABLE 1 | Level of evidence used to rate the design of each study (adapted from the Oxford Centre for Evidence-Based Medicine March) (38).

Level of evidence	Study design
1	Well-designed and conducted RCT
2	Cohort studies and low quality RCT (e.g., <80% follow-up)
3	Case-control studies
4	Case-series and poor quality[†] cohort studies or case-control studies

RCT, randomized controlled trials.
[†]Poor quality cohort study indicate one that failed to clearly define comparison groups and/or failed to measure exposures and outcomes in the same (preferably blinded), objective way in both exposed and non-exposed individuals and/or failed to identify or appropriately control known confounders and/or failed to carry out a sufficiently long and complete follow-up of patients; poor quality case-control study indicate one that failed to clearly define comparison groups and/or failed to measure exposures and outcomes in the same (preferably blinded), objective way in both cases and controls and/or failed to identify or appropriately control known confounders.

[2] www.thecochranelibrary.com
[3] www.clinicaltrials.gov

Statistical Software version 20.014; MedCalc Software Ltd., Ostend, Belgium; 2021).[4]

Assessment of Heterogeneity

We identified dissimilarities between published studies which are expected to introduce heterogeneities. As some degree of heterogeneity would always exist due to the diversities in methodologies of studies, where appropriate, we employed the Chi^2 test and I^2 statistic to quantify heterogeneities across reports. Significant heterogeneity was defined as an I^2 statistic of $\geq$50% and a Chi^2 test p-value of <0.1. If all the effects of an outcome measure were in a similar direction, then we considered data-pooling to be acceptable even in the existence of heterogeneities.

RESULTS

Results of Search

Electronic searches generated a total of 1,603 citations. Publications not relevant to the review were removed. After removal of duplicated publications, abstracts of 579 records were screened and a further 463 records were removed. Full text copies of 116 articles were obtained and reviewed. We included 95 studies in this review; 21 studies that failed to meet the inclusion criteria were excluded. The PRISMA flow diagram is illustrated in **Figure 2**.

Characteristics of Included Studies

Studies included in this review are summarized in **Supplementary Table 1**. A total of 21,323 eyes in 95 studies that had undergone DMEK were included. Eighty-six studies (19,945 eyes) reported on "endothelium-out" insertion techniques; eight studies (624 eyes) reported on "endothelium-in" insertion techniques, respectively. Only one study (36) compared "endothelium-out" to "endothelium-in" DMEK graft insertion techniques; this study was a large comparative series of 754 eyes (36).

Levels of Evidence and the Risks of Bias in Included Studies

Using the Oxford Centre for Evidence-Based Medicine rating (38) of the "endothelium-out" studies included, 4/86 (4.7%) were rated level I, 17/86 (19.8%) were rated level II, 22/86 (25.6%) were rated level III, and 43/86 (50.0%) were rated level IV evidence. Of the eight "endothelium-in" studies included, 5/8 (62.5%) were rated level III evidence and 3/8 (37.5%) were rated level IV evidence. The study that included both "endothelium-out" and "endothelium-in" techniques was rated level III evidence.

Figure 3 summarizes the judgments of each risk of bias domain of all studies included. Five of 95 included studies (5.3%) were assessed as "low risk" and 90/95 (94.7%) as "high risk" of random sequence generation (selection bias). Four of 95 studies (4.2%) were assessed as "low risk" and 91/95 (95.8%) as "high risk" of allocation concealment (selection bias). Two of 95 studies

(2.1%) and two studies (2.1%) were assessed as "low risk" of performance bias and detection bias, respectively. Fifty-six of 95 studies (58.9%), 28/95 (29.5%), and 11/76 (11.6%) were assessed as "low risk," "high risk," and "unclear risk" of attrition bias, respectively. When assessing selective reporting (reporting bias), it was noted that all included studies reported results on some of the pre-specified outcome measures for this review. No study reported results for every outcome measure. All included studies did not state whether the published methods used in the analysis of outcomes were pre-specified in a protocol. Thus, 55/95 (57.9%) and 40/95 (42.1%) of studies were assessed as "high risk" or "unclear risk" for selective reporting, respectively. The authors' judgments of each risk of bias item for each included study is found in **Supplementary Appendix 3**.

Visual Outcomes and Complications Reported in Studies

The visual outcomes and complications reported in studies included are summarized in **Supplementary Table 1**.

Follow-Up

The reported mean length of follow-up of all studies ranged from 0 to 60 months (mean 12.8 ± 12.2 months).

Visual Outcomes

"Endothelium-out" studies: Thirty-four of the 87 studies (39.1%) reported the mean BCVA at 6 months after DMEK surgery; BCVA ranged from 0.0 to 0.49 LogMAR.

Fifteen studies (17.2%) reported that 42.5–85% of eyes achieved a BCVA of 20/25 or better at 6 months. The random pooled proportion of eyes achieving BCVA of 20/25 or better at 6 months was 58.7% (95% CI 49.4–67.7%) (15 studies).

"Endothelium-in" studies: Two of the nine studies (22.2%) reported the mean BCVA at 6 months after DMEK surgery; BCVA ranged from 0.09 to 0.10 LogMAR. Three studies (33.3%) reported that 44.7–87.5% of eyes achieved a BCVA of 20/25 or better at 6 months. The random pooled proportion of eyes achieving BCVA of 20/25 or better at 6 months was 62.4% (95% CI 33.9–86.9%) (3 studies).

Endothelial Cell Loss

"Endothelium-out" studies: 67/87 (77.0%) studies reported data on percentage endothelial cell loss following DMEK surgery at various time points. The mean endothelial cell loss ranged from 19 to 53%. One study (40), reported a rate of 5.6–6.4% endothelial cell loss per year. The random pooled mean endothelial cell loss was 36.3 ± 6.4% at 6 months (27 studies) and 38.7 ± 7.2% at 12 months (12 studies).

"Endothelium-in" studies: Percentage endothelial cells loss data following DMEK surgery were reported in eight out of the nine studies (88.9%) at various time points. The reported mean endothelial cell loss range from 26.6 to 56.0%. The random pooled mean endothelial cell loss was 28.1 ± 1.3% at 6 months (7 studies) and 29.6 ± 1.2% at 12 months (1 studies).

Comparing outcomes of *"endothelium-out"* to *"endothelium-in"* techniques, pooled mean endothelial cell loss was lower in the *"endothelium-in"* group, compared to *"endothelium-out"* group

---

[4]https://www.medcalc.org

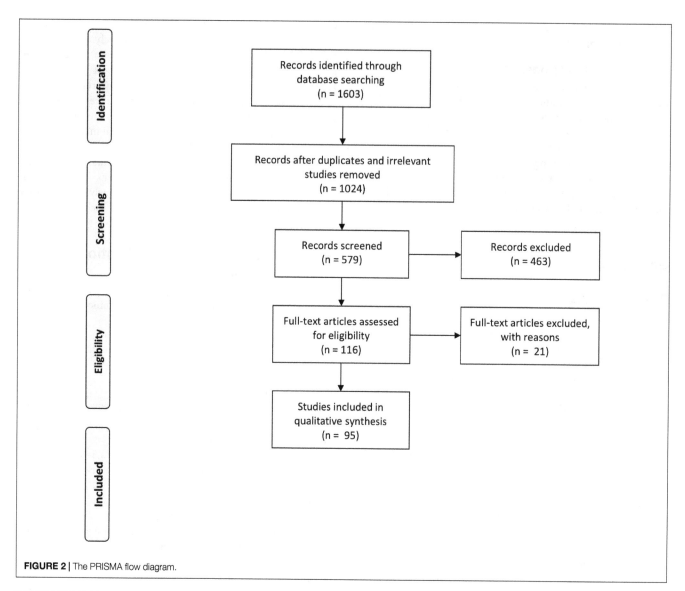

FIGURE 2 | The PRISMA flow diagram.

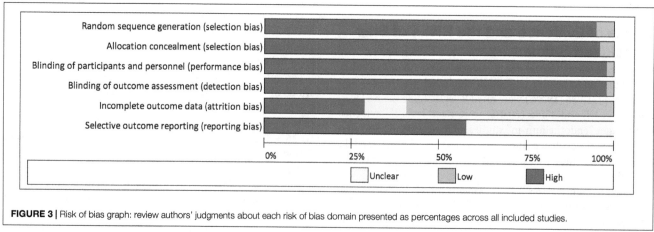

FIGURE 3 | Risk of bias graph: review authors' judgments about each risk of bias domain presented as percentages across all included studies.

at 6 months ($p = 0.018$). However, this was not statistically computable at 12 months as there was only 1 study for the "endothelium in" group.

Rates of Complications

"Endothelium-out" studies: Re-bubbling rates to treat DMEK graft detachments were reported in 77/87 (88.5%) studies and ranged

from 0 to 82%. Fifty-eight (66.7%) studies reported primary graft failure rates which ranged from 0 to 21.0%. Thirty-five (40.2%) studies reported secondary graft failure rates which ranged from 0 to 7.0% at 15.3 ± 13.9 months. Fifty (57.5%) studies reported graft rejection rates; rates ranged from 0 to 7.0%.

"Endothelium-in" studies: Re-bubbling rates to treat DMEK graft detachments were reported in all nine studies and ranged from 4.7 to 45.7%. Six of the nine studies (66.7%) reported primary graft failure rates which ranged from 0 to 3.0%. Three of the nine studies (33.3%) reported on secondary graft failures rates which ranged from 0 to 6.5%.

The random pooled graft re-bubbling rates for *"endothelium-out"* and *"endothelium-in"* techniques were 26.2% (95% CI 21.9–30.9%) (74 studies) and 16.5% (95% CI 8.5–26.4%) (6 studies), respectively. Comparing outcomes of *"endothelium-out"* to *"endothelium-in"* techniques, graft re-bubbling rates were not statistically significant in the "endothelium-out" group ($p = 0.440$). The random pooled primary graft failure rates for *"endothelium-out"* and *"endothelium-in"* techniques were 2.9% (95% CI 2.03–4.02%) (58 studies) and 1.5% (95% CI 0.6–2.7%) (5 studies), respectively. Comparing outcomes of *"endothelium-out"* to *"endothelium-in"* techniques, there was no significant difference in primary graft failure rates between the two groups ($p = 0.552$).

DISCUSSION

Although DMEK offers the advantages of faster visual rehabilitation, better visual and refractive outcomes (21–25), and lower risks of graft rejection compared to DSAEK (26), many transplant surgeons have been slow to adopt DMEK as procedure of choice for the management of endothelial diseases (2, 3). Indeed, DSAEK still accounts for approximately 57% of EK surgeries performed in the United States (2). This has been ascribed to: the technical difficulties in DMEK donor preparation and surgical technique, with the reported higher risks of early complications, namely graft detachment and iatrogenic graft failure due to inadvertent up-side-down graft (25, 26, 31, 41–45) (**Figure 4**). The insertion and un-scrolling of the DMEK graft, once inside the anterior chamber, are indeed the most demanding steps in DMEK. The challenges occur as the DM, once detached from the cornea stromal surface, has an intrinsic propensity to adopt a scrolled configuration with the endothelial surface on its outside (46, 47). This is particularly the case for DMEK grafts harvested from young donors (46). Unlike conventional DSAEK, an alternative surgical skill set is needed by the corneal surgeon (42). The surgeon should understand the different described techniques to unscroll the DMEK graft once in the eye (48–50). Such techniques include methodological approaches to unfolding a double scrolled graft by tapping the cornea in a shallow anterior chamber, and the use of air bubbles to assist in tight or single scrolls (49, 50). In situations, for example tight scrolls or deep anterior chambers, the unscrolling of the graft can be technically demanding (46). Consequently, many corneal surgeons still reserve DMEK for more straightforward cases of endothelial diseases and DSAEK for more challenging cases (e.g., advanced

bullous keratopathy, aphakia, large iris defects, vitrectomized eyes, previous glaucoma filtration surgery) (51–54).

In current clinical practice, the vast majority of DMEK surgeries performed are "endothelium-out" techniques. This was reflected in this systematic review. Of the 21,323 included eyes that underwent DMEK, 19,945 (93.5%) received their grafts through various "endothelium-out" insertion techniques. In these techniques, the DMEK graft is loaded into an injector and inserted into the anterior chamber as a scroll, with the endothelium on its outer surface. Injectors used included modified intraocular lens cartridges, implantable contact lens cartridges, intravenous tubing, or glass injectors (**Supplementary Table 1**). Direct contact of the endothelium of the DMEK graft to the walls of the injectors can potentially cause endothelial cell damage and loss. Studies have indicated that plastic graft injectors are associated with higher rates of post-operative graft detachments, compared to glass devices (55, 56). Such observations have been explained by more damage to the corneal endothelium with plastic materials, and intra-operative alterations in the morphologies of the grafts during insertion and un-scrolling, which may be caused by electro-static forces produced by plastic (55). Nonetheless, not all reports have found similar effects (57).

Moreover, in "endothelium-out" techniques, there is often no control of the scrolled graft during insertion. Despite the use of intraoperative imaging (58), orientation markers such as S-stamps (59) or other asymmetrical indicators (60), determining the orientation of the graft in the anterior chamber can sometimes be difficult. Especially in cases of prolonged surgery, DMEK grafts in the eye can lose their pre-stained trypan blue stains, making visualization of graft orientation even more difficult. This is especially so in patients with dark irides (**Figure 5**).

The unfolding of a scrolled DMEK graft and its central positioning on the recipient's posterior stromal surface can also be problematic and time-consuming. To unfold the DMEK scroll after insertion into the anterior chamber, numerous approaches such as using air bubbles or jets of balanced salt solution in the presence of a shallow anterior chamber and the stroking of the corneal surface have been described (48). To overcome these difficulties of intracameral DMEK graft unfolding, different groups have investigated various alternative techniques. An example of such alternative techniques is the transplantation of DMEK tissue of various shapes (61). Authors have showed that certain DMEK graft shapes, such as the Maltese cross graft design, may be less prone to tight scrolling.

The concept of "endothelium-in" DMEK insertion techniques have been recently introduced (33–37, 44, 45). The grafts are folded, usually in a trifold, with the endothelium on the inside. These "endothelium-in" techniques prevent the DMEK grafts from adopting their natural scrolls with the endothelium on the outside. These "endothelium-in" techniques are believed to have the benefits of minimizing endothelial cell damage from the mechanical stress of the endothelial cells on the walls of the injectors. Moreover, in "endothelium-in" techniques, the grafts are pulled into the eyes with the endothelium facing downward. Once in the eye, the graft begins to unfold to acquire

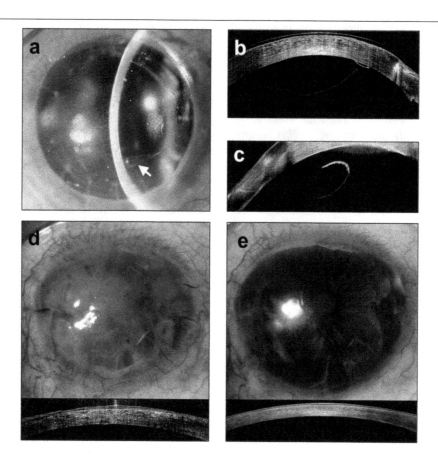

FIGURE 4 | Complications of Descemet membrane endothelial keratoplasty (DMEK). **(a)** Slit lamp image of graft detachment (arrow) at post-operative day 7 and corresponding anterior segment optical coherence tomography (ASOCT) (Optovue, Oculus, CA, United States). Images **(b,c)** showing detached graft. **(d)** Iatrogenic graft failure likely a result of inadvertent graft eversion showing a hazy and thick cornea. **(e)** Repeated DMEK surgery with correct graft orientation showing rapid clearance of cornea and reduction in corneal thickness.

its physiological "endothelium-out" configuration, effectively "aiding" the surgeon in graft unfolding. Pre-clinical laboratory studies have also reported significantly shorter graft unfolding times for "endothelium-in" compared to "endothelium-out" techniques (62). These factors in "endothelium-in" techniques reduce the technical difficulties of intracameral graft orientation and unscrolling, making DMEK procedures more controlled and predictable. Some of these "endothelium-in" techniques also use devices created to mimic DSAEK techniques, which many corneal surgeons are accustomed to (33, 44, 45). Various laboratory studies have reported no significant differences in endothelial cell loss when DMEK grafts were loaded "endothelium-in" and pulled-through or loaded "endothelium-out" and injected-through different graft insertion devices (62–64). In this review, the surgical outcomes of both "endothelium-out" and "endothelium-in" techniques were evaluated.

Summary of Evidence

This review included a total of 95 studies (**Supplementary Table 1**). Eighty-six studies using "endothelium-out" insertion techniques, eight studies using "endothelium-in" insertion techniques, and one study comparing "endothelium-out" to "endothelium-in" techniques. The majority of studies, 73/95

(76.8%), were rated as level III or level IV evidence. Only 4/95 (4.2%) studies were rated as level I evidence.

Evaluating the outcomes of "endothelium-out" techniques, the mean BCVA at 6 months after DMEK surgery ranged from 0.0 to 0.49 LogMAR (34 studies); 42.5–85% of eyes (15 studies) achieved a best-corrected visual acuity (BCVA) of 20/25 or better at 6 months. The mean endothelial cell loss ranged from 19 to 53%. The random pooled mean endothelial cell loss was 36.3 ± 6.4% at 6 months (27 studies) and 38.7 ± 7.2% at 12 months (12 studies). Rates of re-bubbling for graft detachments, primary graft failure rates, secondary graft failure rates, and graft rejection rates ranged from 0 to 82%, 0 to 21.0%, 0 to 7.0%, and 0 to 7.0%, respectively. The random pooled graft re-bubbling rates for "endothelium-out" techniques were 26.2% (95% CI 21.9–30.9%) (74 studies). The random pooled primary graft failure rates for "endothelium-out" techniques was 2.9% (95% CI 2.03–4.02%) (58 studies).

Of the eight "endothelium-in" studies reporting visual acuity data, the mean BCVA at 6 months after DMEK surgery ranged from 0.09 to 0.10 LogMAR (2 studies); 44.7–87.5% of eyes (3 studies) achieved a best-corrected visual acuity (BCVA) of 20/25 or better at 6 months. The mean endothelial cell loss ranged from 26.6 to 56.0% (7 studies). The random pooled mean endothelial cell loss was 28.1 ± 1.3% at 6 months (7 studies) and 29.6 ± 1.2%

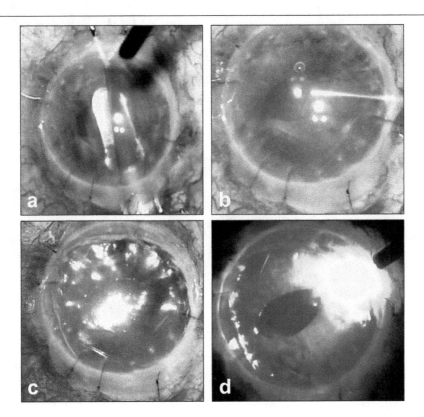

FIGURE 5 | Complex Descemet membrane endothelial keratoplasty (DMEK) surgery performed in an eye with previously failed penetrating keratoplasty graft and iridocorneal endothelial (ICE) syndrome. **(a)** DMEK graft pre-stained with Membrane Blue Dual (D.O.R.C., Netherlands) and inserted into the eye. **(b)** Prolonged surgery has resulted in the loss of the blue stain making visualization of graft orientation and attachment difficult; **(c)** this is made more difficult given the patient's dark iris **(d)** full air-gas tamponade of graft and the use of an external light pipe to assist the surgeon in graft orientation and attachment.

at 12 months (1 study). Graft detachment re-bubbling rates and primary graft failure rates ranged from 4.7 to 45.7% (nine studies) and 0 to 3.0% (six studies), respectively. Only one study reported on secondary graft failure rates in which there were none. None of the studies reporting on "endothelium-in" techniques reported the graft rejection rates. The random pooled graft re-bubbling rates for *"endothelium-in"* techniques was 16.5% (95% CI 8.5–26.4%) (6 studies). The random pooled primary graft failure rates for *"endothelium-in"* techniques was 1.5% (95% CI 0.6–2.7%) (six studies).

Comparing outcomes of *"endothelium-out"* to *"endothelium-in"* techniques, pooled mean endothelial cell loss was lower in the *"endothelium-in"* studies compared to *"endothelium-out"* studies at 6 months ($p = 0.018$); this was not statistically computable at 12 months as there was only 1 study for *"endothelium in"* group. Although re-bubbling rates for graft detachments were higher in the "endothelium-out" studies compared to "endothelium-in" studies, statistical significance was not achieved ($p = 0.440$). There was no significant difference in primary graft failure rates between the two groups ($p = 0.552$).

Limitations of This Review

This review has several limitations. The quality of available evidence was considered low (grade III and IV) with a significant number of studies judged as having high risks of bias (**Figure 3** and **Supplementary Appendix 3**). Significant heterogeneity

existed in the studies, such as study designs, study population, surgical techniques, surgeon experience, outcome measures, and duration of follow-up. Studies published after the date of the pre-defined search strategy have also not been included. Furthermore, there was a smaller number of studies that reported on outcomes using "endothelium-in" DMEK surgeries that met the inclusion criteria for this review. This makes it difficult to provide any definitive conclusions through a comparative meta-analysis, especially in longer post-operative time points. Thus, the evidence to compare "endothelium-out" to "endothelium-in" techniques cannot be considered complete with this review.

CONCLUSION

The rates of endothelial cell loss were reported to be significantly lower in "endothelium-in" DMEK surgeries at 6 months following surgery compared to "endothelium-out" surgeries. Despite the above-mentioned limitations, visual outcomes and rates of complications of "endothelium-in" techniques from the small number of studies were noted to be comparable to those reported in "endothelium-out" studies. Given the intra-operative challenges following graft insertion encountered using "endothelium-out" techniques, surgeons may consider "endothelium-in" techniques designed for easier intra-operative DMEK graft unfolding after graft insertion. However, further well-conducted, adequately powered, randomized controlled trials and studies with longer duration of follow-up are needed before conclusive comparisons between the two techniques can be made.

AUTHOR CONTRIBUTIONS

HO and JM: conceptualization and supervision. HO and HH: data curation. HO, HH, MA, and JM: formal analysis, investigation, methodology, writing draft, and review and editing. All authors approved the manuscript.

REFERENCES

1. Australian Corneal Graft Registry. *The Australian Graft Registry 2018 Report.* Adelaide, SA: Flinders University South Australian Health and Medical Research Institute (2018).

2. EBAA. *Eye Banking Statistical Report 2019.* Washington, DC: Eye Bank Association of America (2020).

3. Park CY, Lee JK, Gore PK, Lim CY, Chuck RS. Keratoplasty in the United States: a 10-year review from 2005 through 2014. *Ophthalmology.* (2015) 122:2432–42. doi: 10.1016/j.ophtha.2015.08.017

4. Tan DT, Dart JK, Holland EJ, Kinoshita S. Corneal transplantation. *Lancet.* (2012) 379:1749–61.

5. Ong HS, Ang M, Mehta JS. Evolution of therapies for the corneal endothelium: past, present and future approaches. *Br J Ophthalmol.* (2020) 105:454–67. doi: 10.1136/bjophthalmol-2020-316149

6. Melles GR, Eggink FA, Lander F, Pels E, Rietveld FJ, Beekhuis WH, et al. A surgical technique for posterior lamellar keratoplasty. *Cornea.* (1998) 17:618–26.

7. Koenig SB, Covert DJ, Dupps WJ Jr, Meisler DM. Visual acuity, refractive error, and endothelial cell density six months after Descemet stripping and automated endothelial keratoplasty (DSAEK). *Cornea.* (2007) 26:670–4. doi: 10.1097/ICO.0b013e3180544902

8. Aung TT, Yam JK, Lin S, Salleh SM, Givskov M, Liu S, et al. Biofilms of pathogenic nontuberculous mycobacteria targeted by new therapeutic approaches. *Antimicrob Agents Chemother.* (2016) 60:24–35. doi: 10.1128/AAC.01509-15

9. Woo JH, Ang M, Htoon HM, Tan DT. Descemet membrane endothelial keratoplasty versus Descemet stripping automated endothelial keratoplasty and penetrating keratoplasty. *Am J Ophthalmol.* (2019) 207:288–303. doi: 10.1016/j.ajo.2019.06.012

10. Guell JL, El Husseiny MA, Manero F, Gris O, Elies D. Historical review and update of surgical treatment for corneal endothelial diseases. *Ophthalmol Ther.* (2014) 3:1–15. doi: 10.1007/s40123-014-0022-y

11. Price FW Jr, Feng MT, Price MO. Evolution of endothelial keratoplasty: where are we headed? *Cornea.* (2015) 34:S41–7. doi: 10.1097/ICO.0000000000000505

12. Ang M, Saroj L, Htoon HM, Kiew S, Mehta JS, Tan D. Comparison of a donor insertion device to sheets glide in Descemet stripping endothelial keratoplasty: 3-year outcomes. *Am J Ophthalmol.* (2014) 157:1163–1169.e3. doi: 10.1016/j.ajo.2014.02.049

13. Ang M, Htoon HM, Cajucom-Uy HY, Tan D, Mehta JS. Donor and surgical risk factors for primary graft failure following Descemet's stripping automated endothelial keratoplasty in Asian eyes. *Clin Ophthalmol.* (2011) 5:1503–8. doi: 10.2147/OPTH.S25973

14. Ang M, Mehta JS, Anshu A, Wong HK, Htoon HM, Tan D. Endothelial cell counts after Descemet's stripping automated endothelial keratoplasty versus penetrating keratoplasty in Asian eyes. *Clin Ophthalmol.* (2012) 6:537–44. doi: 10.2147/OPTH.S26343

15. Ang M, Mehta JS, Lim F, Bose S, Htoon HM, Tan D. Endothelial cell loss and graft survival after Descemet's stripping automated endothelial keratoplasty and penetrating keratoplasty. *Ophthalmology.* (2012) 119:2239–44. doi: 10.1016/j.ophtha.2012.06.012

16. Ang M, Lim F, Htoon HM, Tan D, Mehta JS. Visual acuity and contrast sensitivity following Descemet stripping automated endothelial keratoplasty. *Br J Ophthalmol.* (2016) 100:307–11. doi: 10.1136/bjophthalmol-2015-306975

17. Fuest M, Ang M, Htoon HM, Tan D, Mehta JS. Long-term visual outcomes comparing Descemet stripping automated endothelial keratoplasty and penetrating keratoplasty. *Am J Ophthalmol.* (2017) 182:62–71. doi: 10.1016/j.ajo.2017.07.014

18. Bose S, Ang M, Mehta JS, Tan DT, Finkelstein E. Cost-effectiveness of Descemet's stripping endothelial keratoplasty versus penetrating keratoplasty. *Ophthalmology.* (2013) 120:464–70. doi: 10.1016/j.ophtha.2012.08.024

19. Tan D, Htoon HM, Ang M. Descemet's stripping automated endothelial keratoplasty with anterior chamber intraocular lenses. *Br J Ophthalmol.* (2014) 98:1462.

20. Melles GR, Ong TS, Ververs B, van der Wees J. Descemet membrane endothelial keratoplasty (DMEK). *Cornea.* (2006) 25:987–90.

21. Singh A, Zarei-Ghanavati M, Avadhanam V, Liu C. Systematic review and meta-analysis of clinical outcomes of Descemet membrane endothelial keratoplasty versus Descemet stripping endothelial keratoplasty/Descemet stripping automated endothelial keratoplasty. *Cornea.* (2017) 36:1437–43. doi: 10.1097/ICO.0000000000001320

22. Droutsas K, Lazaridis A, Papaconstantinou D, Brouzas D, Moschos MM, Schulze S, et al. Visual outcomes after Descemet membrane endothelial keratoplasty versus Descemet stripping automated endothelial keratoplasty-comparison of specific matched Pairs. *Cornea.* (2016) 35:765–71. doi: 10.1097/ICO.0000000000000822

23. Tourtas T, Laaser K, Bachmann BO, Cursiefen C, Kruse FE. Descemet membrane endothelial keratoplasty versus descemet stripping automated endothelial keratoplasty. *Am J Ophthalmol.* (2012) 153:1082–90.e2.

24. Guerra FP, Anshu A, Price MO, Price FW. Endothelial keratoplasty: fellow eyes comparison of Descemet stripping automated endothelial keratoplasty and Descemet membrane endothelial keratoplasty. *Cornea.* (2011) 30:1382–6. doi: 10.1097/ICO.0b013e31821ddd25

25. Stuart AJ, Romano V, Virgili G, Shortt AJ. Descemet's membrane endothelial keratoplasty (DMEK) versus Descemet's stripping automated endothelial keratoplasty (DSAEK) for corneal endothelial failure. *Cochrane Database Syst Rev.* (2018) 6:CD012097. doi: 10.1002/14651858.CD012097.pub2

26. Marques RE, Guerra PS, Sousa DC, Goncalves AI, Quintas AM, Rodrigues W. DMEK versus DSAEK for Fuchs' endothelial dystrophy: a meta-analysis. *Eur J Ophthalmol.* (2018) 29:15–22. doi: 10.1177/1120672118757431

27. Dapena I, Moutsouris K, Droutsas K, Ham L, van Dijk K, Melles GR. Standardized "no-touch" technique for Descemet membrane endothelial keratoplasty. *Arch Ophthalmol.* (2011) 129:88–94.

28. Arnalich-Montiel F, Munoz-Negrete FJ, De Miguel MP. Double port injector device to reduce endothelial damage in DMEK. *Eye (Lond).* (2014) 28:748–51. doi: 10.1038/eye.2014.67

29. Kruse FE, Laaser K, Cursiefen C, Heindl LM, Schlotzer-Schrehardt U, Riss S, et al. A stepwise approach to donor preparation and insertion increases safety and outcome of Descemet membrane endothelial keratoplasty. *Cornea.* (2011) 30:580–7. doi: 10.1097/ico.0b013e3182000e2e

30. Kim EC, Bonfadini G, Todd L, Zhu A, Jun AS. Simple, inexpensive, and effective injector for descemet membrane endothelial keratoplasty. *Cornea.* (2014) 33:649–52. doi: 10.1097/ICO.0000000000000121

31. Maier AK, Gundlach E, Schroeter J, Klamann MK, Gonnermann J, Riechardt AI, et al. Influence of the difficulty of graft unfolding and attachment on the outcome in Descemet membrane endothelial keratoplasty. *Graefes Arch Clin Exp Ophthalmol.* (2015) 253:895–900. doi: 10.1007/s00417-015-2939-9

32. Ang M, Ting DSJ, Kumar A, May KO, Htoon HM, Mehta JS. Descemet membrane endothelial keratoplasty in Asian eyes: intraoperative and

postoperative complications. *Cornea*. (2020) 39:940–5. doi: 10.1097/ICO. 0000000000002302

33. Ang M, Mehta JS, Newman SD, Han SB, Chai J, Tan D. Descemet membrane endothelial keratoplasty: preliminary results of a donor insertion pull-through technique using a donor mat device. *Am J Ophthalmol*. (2016) 171:27–34. doi: 10.1016/j.ajo.2016.08.023

34. Busin M, Leon P, D'Angelo S, Ruzza A, Ferrari S, Ponzin D, et al. Clinical outcomes of preloaded Descemet membrane endothelial keratoplasty grafts with endothelium tri-folded inwards. *Am J Ophthalmol*. (2018) 193:106–13. doi: 10.1016/j.ajo.2018.06.013

35. Leon P, Parekh M, Nahum Y, Mimouni M, Giannaccare G, Sapigni L, et al. Factors associated with early graft detachment in primary Descemet membrane endothelial keratoplasty. *Am J Ophthalmol*. (2018) 187:117–24.

36. Price MO, Lisek M, Kelley M, Feng MT, Price FW Jr. Endothelium-in versus endothelium-out insertion with Descemet membrane endothelial keratoplasty. *Cornea*. (2018) 37:1098–101. doi: 10.1097/ ICO.0000000000001650

37. Ong HS, Mehta JS. Descemet's membrane endothelial keratoplasty (DMEK)—why Surgeons should consider adopting endothelium-in techniques. *US Ophthalmic Rev*. (2019) 12:65–8.

38. CEBM. *Oxford Centre for Evidence-Based Medicine – Levels of Evidence*. Oxford: CEBM (2009).

39. Higgins JPT, Altman DG, Sterne JAC. Chapter 8: assessing risk of bias in included studies. In: Higgins JPT, Green S editors. *Cochrane Handbook for Systematic Reviews of Interventions Version 5.1.0*. (London: The Cochrane Collaboration) (2011).

40. Price MO, Scanameo A, Feng MT, Price FW Jr. Descemet's membrane endothelial keratoplasty: risk of immunologic rejection episodes after discontinuing topical corticosteroids. *Ophthalmology*. (2016) 12:1232–6. doi: 10.1016/j.ophtha.2016.02.001

41. Hamzaoglu EC, Straiko MD, Mayko ZM, Sales CS, Terry MA. The first 100 eyes of standardized Descemet stripping automated endothelial keratoplasty versus standardized Descemet membrane endothelial keratoplasty. *Ophthalmology*. (2015) 122:2193–9. doi: 10.1016/j.ophtha.2015.07.003

42. Phillips PM, Phillips LJ, Muthappan V, Maloney CM, Carver CN. Experienced DSAEK Surgeon's transition to DMEK: outcomes comparing the last 100 DSAEK surgeries with the first 100 DMEK surgeries exclusively using previously published techniques. *Cornea*. (2017) 36:275–9. doi: 10. 1097/ICO.0000000000001069

43. Rose-Nussbaumer J, Alloju S, Chamberlain W. Clinical outcomes of Descemet membrane endothelial keratoplasty during the Surgeon learning curve versus Descemet stripping endothelial keratoplasty performed at the same time. *J Clin Exp Ophthalmol*. (2016) 7:599. doi: 10.4172/2155-9570. 1000599

44. Romano V, Kazaili A, Pagano L, Gadhvi KA, Titley M, Steger B, et al. Eye bank versus Surgeon prepared DMEK tissues: influence on adhesion and re-bubbling rate. *Br J Ophthalmol*. (2022) 106:177–83. doi: 10.1136/ bjophthalmol-2020-317608

45. Parekh M, Pedrotti E, Viola P, Leon P, Neri E, Bosio L, et al. Factors affecting the success rate of pre-loaded DMEK with endothelium-inwards technique: a multi-centre clinical study. *Am J Ophthalmol*. (2022). doi: 10.1016/j.ajo.2022. 03.009 [Epub ahead of print].

46. Heinzelmann S, Bohringer D, Haverkamp C, Lapp T, Eberwein P, Reinhard T, et al. Influence of postoperative intraocular pressure on graft detachment after Descemet membrane endothelial keratoplasty. *Cornea*. (2018) 37:1347–50.

47. Tan TE, Devarajan K, Seah XY, Lin SJ, Peh GSL, Cajucom-Uy HY, et al. Lamellar dissection technique for Descemet membrane endothelial keratoplasty graft preparation. *Cornea*. (2019) 39:23–9. doi: 10.1097/ICO. 0000000000002090

48. Ang M, Wilkins MR, Mehta JS, Tan D. Descemet membrane endothelial keratoplasty. *Br J Ophthalmol*. (2016) 100:15–21.

49. Liarakos VS, Dapena I, Ham L, van Dijk K, Melles GR. Intraocular graft unfolding techniques in Descemet membrane endothelial keratoplasty. *JAMA Ophthalmol*. (2013) 131:29–35. doi: 10.1001/2013.jamaophthalmol.4

50. Yoeruek E, Bayyoud T, Hofmann J, Bartz-Schmidt KU. Novel maneuver facilitating Descemet membrane unfolding in the anterior chamber. *Cornea*. (2013) 32:370–3. doi: 10.1097/ICO.0b013e318254fa06

51. Ang M, Ho H, Wong C, Htoon HM, Mehta JS, Tan D. Endothelial keratoplasty after failed penetrating keratoplasty: an alternative to repeat penetrating keratoplasty. *Am J Ophthalmol*. (2014) 158:1221–1227.e1. doi: 10.1016/j.ajo.2014.08.024

52. Ang M, Li L, Chua D, Wong C, Htoon HM, Mehta JS, et al. Descemet's stripping automated endothelial keratoplasty with anterior chamber intraocular lenses: complications and 3-year outcomes. *Br J Ophthalmol*. (2014) 98:1028–32.

53. Ang M, Sng CCA. Descemet membrane endothelial keratoplasty and glaucoma. *Curr Opin Ophthalmol*. (2018) 29:178–84. doi: 10.1097/ICU. 0000000000000454

54. Ang M, Sng CC. Descemet membrane endothelial keratoplasty developing spontaneous 'malignant glaucoma' secondary to gas misdirection. *Clin Exp Ophthalmol*. (2018) 46:811–3. doi: 10.1111/ceo.13150

55. Monnereau C, Quilendrino R, Dapena I, Liarakos VS, Alfonso JF, Arnalich-Montiel F, et al. Multicenter study of descemet membrane endothelial keratoplasty: first case series of 18 Surgeons. *JAMA Ophthalmol*. (2014) 132:1192–8. doi: 10.1001/jamaophthalmol.2014.1710

56. Dirisamer M, van Dijk K, Dapena I, Ham L, Oganes O, Frank LE, et al. Prevention and management of graft detachment in descemet membrane endothelial keratoplasty. *Arch Ophthalmol*. (2012) 130:280–91. doi: 10.1001/ archophthalmol.2011.343

57. Oellerich S, Baydoun L, Peraza-Nieves J, Ilyas A, Frank L, Binder PS, et al. Multicenter study of 6-month clinical outcomes after Descemet membrane endothelial keratoplasty. *Cornea*. (2017) 36:1467–76. doi: 10.1097/ICO. 0000000000001374

58. Ang M, Dubis AM, Wilkins MR. Descemet membrane endothelial keratoplasty: intraoperative and postoperative imaging spectral-domain optical coherence tomography. *Case Rep Ophthalmol Med*. (2015) 2015:506251. doi: 10.1155/2015/506251

59. Veldman PB, Dye PK, Holiman JD, Mayko ZM, Sales CS, Straiko MD, et al. The S-stamp in Descemet membrane endothelial keratoplasty safely eliminates upside-down graft implantation. *Ophthalmology*. (2016) 123:161–4. doi: 10.1016/j.ophtha.2015.08.044

60. Bhogal M, Maurino V, Allan BD. Use of a single peripheral triangular mark to ensure correct graft orientation in Descemet membrane endothelial keratoplasty. *J Cataract Refract Surg*. (2015) 41:2022–4. doi: 10.1016/j.jcrs. 2015.08.005

61. Modabber M, Talajic JC, Mabon M, Mercier M, Jabbour S, Choremis J. The role of novel DMEK graft shapes in facilitating intraoperative unscrolling. *Graefes Arch Clin Exp Ophthalmol*. (2018) 256:2385–90. doi: 10.1007/s00417-018-4145-z

62. Parekh M, Ruzza A, Ferrari S, Ahmad S, Kaye S, Ponzin D, et al. Endothelium-in versus endothelium-out for Descemet membrane endothelial keratoplasty graft preparation and implantation. *Acta Ophthalmol*. (2017) 95:194–8. doi: 10.1111/aos.13162

63. Barnes K, Chiang E, Chen C, Lohmeier J, Christy J, Chaurasia A, et al. Comparison of tri-folded and scroll-based graft viability in preloaded Descemet membrane endothelial keratoplasty. *Cornea*. (2019) 38:392–6. doi: 10.1097/ICO.0000000000001831

64. Romano V, Ruzza A, Kaye S, Parekh M. Pull-through technique for delivery of a larger diameter DMEK graft using endothelium-in method. *Can J Ophthalmol*. (2017) 52:e155–6. doi: 10.1016/j.jcjo.2017.03.006

65. Price MO, Price FW Jr, Kruse FE, Bachmann BO, Tourtas T. Randomized comparison of topical prednisolone acetate 1% versus fluorometholone 0.1% in the first year after Descemet membrane endothelial keratoplasty. *Cornea*. (2014) 33:880–6. doi: 10.1097/ICO.0000000000000206

66. Price MO, Feng MT, Scanameo A, Price FW Jr. Loteprednol etabonate 0.5% Gel Vs. prednisolone acetate 1% solution after Descemet membrane endothelial keratoplasty: prospective randomized trial. *Cornea*. (2015) 34:853–8. doi: 10.1097/ICO.0000000000000475

67. Chamberlain W, Lin CC, Austin A, Schubach N, Clover J, McLeod SD, et al. Descemet endothelial thickness comparison trial: a randomized trial comparing ultrathin Descemet stripping automated endothelial keratoplasty with Descemet membrane endothelial keratoplasty. *Ophthalmology*. (2019) 126:19–26.

68. Dunker SL, Dickman MM, Wisse RPL, Nobacht S, Wijdh RHJ, Bartels MC, et al. Descemet membrane endothelial keratoplasty versus ultrathin

Descemet stripping automated endothelial keratoplasty: a multicenter randomized controlled clinical trial. *Ophthalmology.* (2020) 127:1152–9. doi: 10.1016/j.ophtha.2020.02.029

69. Santander-Garcia D, Peraza-Nieves J, Muller TM, Gerber-Hollbach N, Baydoun L, Liarakos VS, et al. Influence of intraoperative air tamponade time on graft adherence in Descemet membrane endothelial keratoplasty. *Cornea.* (2019) 38:166–72. doi: 10.1097/ICO.0000000000 001795

70. Price MO, Giebel AW, Fairchild KM, Price FW Jr. Descemet's membrane endothelial keratoplasty: prospective multicenter study of visual and refractive outcomes and endothelial survival. *Ophthalmology.* (2009) 116:2361–8. doi: 10.1016/j.ophtha.2009.07.010

71. Rudolph M, Laaser K, Bachmann BO, Cursiefen C, Epstein D, Kruse FE. Corneal higher-order aberrations after Descemet's membrane endothelial keratoplasty. *Ophthalmology.* (2012) 119:528–35. doi: 10.1016/j.ophtha.2011.08.034

72. Feng MT, Burkhart ZN, Price FW Jr, Price MO. Effect of donor preparation-to-use times on Descemet membrane endothelial keratoplasty outcomes. *Cornea.* (2013) 32:1080–2. doi: 10.1097/ICO.0b013e318292a7e5

73. Chaurasia S, Price FW Jr, Gunderson L, Price MO. Descemet's membrane endothelial keratoplasty: clinical results of single versus triple procedures (combined with cataract surgery). *Ophthalmology.* (2014) 121:454–8. doi: 10.1016/j.ophtha.2013.09.032

74. Cabrerizo J, Livny E, Musa FU, Leeuwenburgh P, van Dijk K, Melles GR. Changes in color vision and contrast sensitivity after descemet membrane endothelial keratoplasty for fuchs endothelial dystrophy. *Cornea.* (2014) 33:1010–5. doi: 10.1097/ICO.0000000000000216

75. Guell JL, Morral M, Gris O, Elies D, Manero F. Comparison of sulfur hexafluoride 20% versus air tamponade in Descemet membrane endothelial keratoplasty. *Ophthalmology.* (2015) 122:1757–64. doi: 10.1016/j.ophtha.2015.05.013

76. Heinzelmann S, Maier P, Bohringer D, Huther S, Eberwein P, Reinhard T. Cystoid macular oedema following Descemet membrane endothelial keratoplasty. *Br J Ophthalmol.* (2015) 99:98–102. doi: 10.1136/bjophthalmol-2014-305124

77. Heinzelmann S, Bohringer D, Eberwein P, Reinhard T, Maier P. Outcomes of Descemet membrane endothelial keratoplasty, Descemet stripping automated endothelial keratoplasty and penetrating keratoplasty from a single centre study. *Graefes Arch Clin Exp Ophthalmol.* (2016) 254:515–22. doi: 10.1007/s00417-015-3248-z

78. Schaub F, Enders P, Snijders K, Schrittenlocher S, Siebelmann S, Heindl LM, et al. One-year outcome after Descemet membrane endothelial keratoplasty (DMEK) comparing sulfur hexafluoride (SF6) 20% versus 100% air for anterior chamber tamponade. *Br J Ophthalmol.* (2017) 101:902–8. doi: 10.1136/bjophthalmol-2016-309653

79. Aravena C, Yu F, Deng SX. Outcomes of Descemet membrane endothelial keratoplasty in patients with previous glaucoma surgery. *Cornea.* (2017) 36:284–9. doi: 10.1097/ICO.0000000000001095

80. Tourtas T, Schlomberg J, Wessel JM, Bachmann BO, Schlotzer-Schrehardt U, Kruse FE. Graft adhesion in descemet membrane endothelial keratoplasty dependent on size of removal of host's descemet membrane. *JAMA Ophthalmol.* (2014) 132:155–61. doi: 10.1001/jamaophthalmol.2013.6222

81. Gundlach E, Maier AK, Tsangaridou MA, Riechardt AI, Brockmann T, Bertelmann E, et al. DMEK in phakic eyes: targeted therapy or highway to cataract surgery? *Graefes Arch Clin Exp Ophthalmol.* (2015) 253:909–14. doi: 10.1007/s00417-015-2956-8

82. Rock T, Bramkamp M, Bartz-Schmidt KU, Rock D, Yoruk E. Causes that influence the detachment rate after Descemet membrane endothelial keratoplasty. *Graefes Arch Clin Exp Ophthalmol.* (2015) 253:2217–22.

83. Hoerster R, Stanzel TP, Bachmann BO, Siebelmann S, Felsch M, Cursiefen C. Intensified topical steroids as prophylaxis for macular Edema after posterior lamellar keratoplasty combined with cataract surgery. *Am J Ophthalmol.* (2016) 163:174–179.e2. doi: 10.1016/j.ajo.2015.12.008

84. Schaub F, Pohl L, Enders P, Adler W, Bachmann BO, Cursiefen C, et al. Impact of corneal donor lens status on two-year course and outcome of Descemet membrane endothelial keratoplasty (DMEK). *Graefes Arch Clin Exp Ophthalmol.* (2017) 255:2407–14. doi: 10.1007/s00417-017-3827-2

85. Regnier M, Auxenfans C, Maucort-Boulch D, Marty AS, Damour O, Burillon C, et al. Eye bank prepared versus Surgeon cut endothelial graft tissue for Descemet membrane endothelial keratoplasty: an observational study. *Medicine (Baltimore).* (2017) 96:e6885. doi: 10.1097/MD.0000000000006885

86. Botsford B, Vedana G, Cope L, Yiu SC, Jun AS. Comparison of 20% sulfur hexafluoride with air for intraocular tamponade in Descemet membrane endothelial keratoplasty (DMEK). *Arq Bras Oftalmol.* (2016) 79:299–302. doi: 10.5935/0004-2749.20160086

87. Rickmann A, Opitz N, Szurman P, Boden KT, Jung S, Wahl S, et al. Clinical comparison of two methods of graft preparation in Descemet membrane endothelial keratoplasty. *Curr Eye Res.* (2018) 43:12–7. doi: 10.1080/02713683.2017.1368086

88. Schrittenlocher S, Bachmann B, Cursiefen C. Impact of donor tissue diameter on postoperative central endothelial cell density in Descemet membrane endothelial keratoplasty. *Acta Ophthalmol.* (2018) 97:e618–22. doi: 10.1111/aos.13943

89. Brockmann T, Brockmann C, Maier AB, Schroeter J, Bertelmann E, Torun N. Primary Descemet's membrane endothelial keratoplasty for fuchs endothelial dystrophy versus bullous keratopathy: histopathology and clinical results. *Curr Eye Res.* (2018) 43:1221–7. doi: 10.1080/02713683.2018.1490773

90. Kocluk Y, Kasim B, Sukgen EA, Burcu A. Descemet membrane endothelial keratoplasty (DMEK): intraoperative and postoperative complications and clinical results. *Arq Bras Oftalmol.* (2018) 81:212–8. doi: 10.5935/0004-2749.20180043

91. Rickmann A, Szurman P, Jung S, Boden KT, Wahl S, Haus A, et al. Impact of 10% SF6 gas compared to 100% air tamponade in descemet's membrane endothelial keratoplasty. *Curr Eye Res.* (2018) 43:482–6. doi: 10.1080/02713683.2018.1431286

92. von Marchtaler PV, Weller JM, Kruse FE, Tourtas T. Air versus sulfur hexafluoride gas tamponade in Descemet membrane endothelial keratoplasty: a fellow eye comparison. *Cornea.* (2018) 37:15–9. doi: 10.1097/ICO.0000000000001413

93. Rickmann A, Wahl S, Hofmann N, Haus A, Michaelis R, Petrich T, et al. Precut DMEK using dextran-containing storage medium is equivalent to conventional DMEK: a prospective pilot study. *Cornea.* (2019) 38:24–9. doi: 10.1097/ICO.0000000000001778

94. Shahnazaryan D, Hajjar Sese A, Hollick EJ. Endothelial cell loss after Descemet's membrane endothelial keratoplasty for Fuchs' endothelial dystrophy: DMEK compared to triple DMEK. *Am J Ophthalmol.* (2020) 218:1–6. doi: 10.1016/j.ajo.2020.05.003

95. Koechel D, Hofmann N, Unterlauft JD, Wiedemann P, Girbardt C. Descemet membrane endothelial keratoplasty (DMEK): clinical results of precut versus Surgeon-cut grafts. *Graefes Arch Clin Exp Ophthalmol.* (2021) 259:113–9. doi: 10.1007/s00417-020-04901-7

96. Potts LB, Bauer AJ, Xu DN, Chen SY, Alqudah AA, Sanchez PJ, et al. The last 200 Surgeon-loaded descemet membrane endothelial keratoplasty tissue versus the first 200 preloaded descemet membrane endothelial keratoplasty tissue. *Cornea.* (2020) 39:1261–6. doi: 10.1097/ICO.0000000000002400

97. Bohm MS, Wylegala A, Leon P, Ong Tone S, Ciolino JB, Jurkunas UV. One-year clinical outcomes of preloaded descemet membrane endothelial keratoplasty versus non-preloaded descemet membrane endothelial keratoplasty. *Cornea.* (2021) 40:311–9. doi: 10.1097/ICO.0000000000002430

98. Zwingelberg SB, Buscher F, Schrittenlocher S, Rokohl AC, Loreck N, Wawer-Matos P, et al. Long-term outcome of descemet membrane endothelial keratoplasty in eyes with fuchs endothelial corneal dystrophy versus pseudophakic bullous keratopathy. *Cornea.* (2021) 41:304–9. doi: 10.1097/ICO.0000000000002737

99. Jansen C, Zetterberg M. Descemet membrane endothelial keratoplasty versus Descemet stripping automated keratoplasty – outcome of one single Surgeon's more than 200 initial consecutive cases. *Clin Ophthalmol.* (2021) 15:909–21. doi: 10.2147/OPTH.S289730

100. Fajardo-Sanchez J, de Benito-Llopis L. Clinical outcomes of descemet membrane endothelial keratoplasty in pseudophakic eyes compared with triple-DMEK at 1-year follow-up. *Cornea.* (2021) 40:420–4. doi: 10.1097/ICO.0000000000002636

101. Guerra FP, Anshu A, Price MO, Giebel AW, Price FW. Descemet's membrane endothelial keratoplasty: prospective study of 1-year visual outcomes, graft

survival, and endothelial cell loss. *Ophthalmology*. (2011) 118:2368–73. doi: 10.1016/j.ophtha.2011.06.002

102. Laaser K, Bachmann BO, Horn FK, Cursiefen C, Kruse FE. Descemet membrane endothelial keratoplasty combined with phacoemulsification and intraocular lens implantation: advanced triple procedure. *Am J Ophthalmol*. (2012) 154:47–55e2. doi: 10.1016/j.ajo.2012.01.020

103. Parker J, Dirisamer M, Naveiras M, Tse WH, van Dijk K, Frank LE, et al. Outcomes of Descemet membrane endothelial keratoplasty in phakic eyes. *J Cataract Refract Surg*. (2012) 38:871–7.

104. Anshu A, Price MO, Price FW Jr. Risk of corneal transplant rejection significantly reduced with Descemet's membrane endothelial keratoplasty. *Ophthalmology*. (2012) 119:536–40. doi: 10.1016/j.ophtha.2011.09.019

105. Gorovoy MS. DMEK complications. *Cornea*. (2014) 33:101–4.

106. Burkhart ZN, Feng MT, Price FW Jr, Price MO. One-year outcomes in eyes remaining phakic after Descemet membrane endothelial keratoplasty. *J Cataract Refract Surg*. (2014) 40:430–4. doi: 10.1016/j.jcrs.2013.08.047

107. Maier AK, Wolf T, Gundlach E, Klamann MK, Gonnermann J, Bertelmann E, et al. Intraocular pressure elevation and post-DMEK glaucoma following Descemet membrane endothelial keratoplasty. *Graefes Arch Clin Exp Ophthalmol*. (2014) 252:1947–54. doi: 10.1007/s00417-014-2757-5

108. Feng MT, Price MO, Miller JM, Price FW Jr. Air reinjection and endothelial cell density in Descemet membrane endothelial keratoplasty: five-year follow-up. *J Cataract Refract Surg*. (2014) 40:1116–21. doi: 10.1016/j.jcrs. 2014.04.023

109. Deng SX, Sanchez PJ, Chen L. Clinical outcomes of descemet membrane endothelial keratoplasty using eye bank-prepared tissues. *Am J Ophthalmol*. (2015) 159:590–6. doi: 10.1016/j.ajo.2014.12.007

110. Rodriguez-Calvo-de-Mora M, Quilendrino R, Ham L, Liarakos VS, van Dijk K, Baydoun L, et al. Clinical outcome of 500 consecutive cases undergoing Descemet's membrane endothelial keratoplasty. *Ophthalmology*. (2015) 122:464–70. doi: 10.1016/j.ophtha.2014.09.004

111. Bhandari V, Reddy JK, Relekar K, Prabhu V. Descemet's stripping automated endothelial keratoplasty versus descemet's membrane endothelial keratoplasty in the fellow eye for fuchs endothelial dystrophy: a retrospective study. *Biomed Res Int*. (2015) 2015:750567. doi: 10.1155/2015/75 0567

112. Schoenberg ED, Price FW Jr, Miller J, McKee Y, Price MO. Refractive outcomes of descemet membrane endothelial keratoplasty triple procedures (combined with cataract surgery). *J Cataract Refract Surg*. (2015) 41:1182–9. doi: 10.1016/j.jcrs.2014.09.042

113. Gorovoy IR, Gorovoy MS. Descemet membrane endothelial keratoplasty postoperative year 1 endothelial cell counts. *Am J Ophthalmol*. (2015) 159:597–600e2. doi: 10.1016/j.ajo.2014.12.008

114. Ham L, Dapena I, Liarakos VS, Baydoun L, van Dijk K, Ilyas A, et al. Midterm results of descemet membrane endothelial keratoplasty: 4 to 7 years clinical outcome. *Am J Ophthalmol*. (2016) 171:113–21. doi: 10.1016/j.ajo.2016.08. 038

115. Siggel R, Adler W, Stanzel TP, Cursiefen C, Heindl LM. Bilateral descemet membrane endothelial keratoplasty: analysis of clinical outcome in first and fellow eye. *Cornea*. (2016) 35:772–7. doi: 10.1097/ICO.0000000000000811

116. van Dijk K, Rodriguez-Calvo-de-Mora M, van Esch H, Frank L, Dapena I, Baydoun L, et al. Two-year refractive outcomes after descemet membrane endothelial keratoplasty. *Cornea*. (2016) 35:1548–55. doi: 10.1097/ICO. 0000000000001022

117. Schlogl A, Tourtas T, Kruse FE, Weller JM. Long-term clinical outcome after descemet membrane endothelial keratoplasty. *Am J Ophthalmol*. (2016) 169:218–26.

118. Bhandari V, Reddy JK, Chougale P. Descemet's membrane endothelial keratoplasty in south Asian population. *J Ophthalmic Vis Res*. (2016) 11:368–71. doi: 10.4103/2008-322X.194072

119. Debellemaniere G, Guilbert E, Courtin R, Panthier C, Sabatier P, Gatinel D, et al. Impact of surgical learning curve in descemet membrane endothelial keratoplasty on visual acuity gain. *Cornea*. (2017) 36:1–6. doi: 10.1097/ICO. 0000000000001066

120. Peraza-Nieves J, Baydoun L, Dapena I, Ilyas A, Frank LE, Luceri S, et al. Two-year clinical outcome of 500 consecutive cases undergoing descemet membrane endothelial keratoplasty. *Cornea*. (2017) 36:655–60. doi: 10.1097/ ICO.0000000000001176

121. Showail M, Obthani MA, Sorkin N, Einan-Lifshitz A, Boutin T, Borovik A, et al. Outcomes of the first 250 eyes of descemet membrane endothelial keratoplasty: canadian centre experience. *Can J Ophthalmol*. (2018) 53:510–7. doi: 10.1016/j.jcjo.2017.11.017

122. Basak SK, Basak S, Pradhan VR. Outcomes of descemet membrane endothelial keratoplasty (DMEK) using Surgeon's prepared donor DM-roll in consecutive 100 Indian eyes. *Open Ophthalmol J*. (2018) 12:134–42. doi: 10.2174/1874364101812010134

123. Kurji KH, Cheung AY, Eslani M, Rolfes EJ, Chachare DY, Auteri NJ, et al. Comparison of visual acuity outcomes between nanothin descemet stripping automated endothelial keratoplasty and descemet membrane endothelial keratoplasty. *Cornea*. (2018) 37:1226–31. doi: 10.1097/ICO. 0000000000001697

124. Fajgenbaum MAP, Kopsachilis N, Hollick EJ. Descemet's membrane endothelial keratoplasty: surgical outcomes and endothelial cell count modelling from a UK centre. *Eye (Lond)*. (2018) 32:1629–35. doi: 10.1038/ s41433-018-0152-x

125. Newman LR, DeMill DL, Zeidenweber DA, Mayko ZM, Bauer AJ, Tran KD, et al. Preloaded descemet membrane endothelial keratoplasty donor tissue: surgical technique and early clinical results. *Cornea*. (2018) 37:981–6.

126. Price DA, Kelley M, Price FW Jr, Price MO. Five-year graft survival of descemet membrane endothelial keratoplasty (EK) versus descemet stripping EK and the effect of donor sex matching. *Ophthalmology*. (2018) 125:1508–14. doi: 10.1016/j.ophtha.2018.03.050

127. Schrittenlocher S, Schaub F, Hos D, Siebelmann S, Cursiefen C, Bachmann B. Evolution of consecutive descemet membrane endothelial keratoplasty outcomes throughout a 5-year period performed by two experienced Surgeons. *Am J Ophthalmol*. (2018) 190:171–8. doi: 10.1016/j.ajo.2018.03.036

128. Droutsas K, Lazaridis A, Giallouros E, Kymionis G, Chatzistefanou K, Sekundo W. Scheimpflug densitometry after dmek versus dsaek-two-year outcomes. *Cornea*. (2018) 37:455–61. doi: 10.1097/ICO.0000000000001483

129. Godin MR, Boehlke CS, Kim T, Gupta PK. Influence of lens status on outcomes of descemet membrane endothelial keratoplasty. *Cornea*. (2019) 38:409–12.

130. Rickmann A, Wahl S, Katsen-Globa A, Szurman P. Safety analysis and results of a borosilicate glass cartridge for no-touch graft loading and injection in descemet membrane endothelial keratoplasty. *Int Ophthalmol*. (2019) 39:2295–301. doi: 10.1007/s10792-018-01067-4

131. Sarnicola C, Sabatino F, Sarnicola E, Perri P, Cheung AY, Sarnicola V. Cannula-assisted technique to unfold grafts in descemet membrane endothelial keratoplasty. *Cornea*. (2019) 38:275–9. doi: 10.1097/ICO. 0000000000001827

132. Brockmann T, Pilger D, Brockmann C, Maier AB, Bertelmann E, Torun N. Predictive factors for clinical outcomes after primary descemet's membrane endothelial keratoplasty for fuchs' endothelial dystrophy. *Curr Eye Res*. (2019) 44:147–53. doi: 10.1080/02713683.2018.1538459

133. Schaub F, Gerber F, Adler W, Enders P, Schrittenlocher S, Heindl LM, et al. Corneal densitometry as a predictive diagnostic tool for visual acuity results after descemet membrane endothelial keratoplasty. *Am J Ophthalmol*. (2019) 198:124–9. doi: 10.1016/j.ajo.2018.10.002

134. Livny E, Bahar I, Levy I, Mimouni M, Nahum Y. "PI-less DMEK": results of DESCEMET'S membrane endothelial keratoplasty (DMEK) without a peripheral iridotomy. *Eye (Lond)*. (2019) 33:653–8.

135. Basak SK, Basak S, Gajendragadkar N, Ghatak M. Overall clinical outcomes of descemet membrane endothelial keratoplasty in 600 consecutive eyes: a large retrospective case series. *Indian J Ophthalmol*. (2020) 68:1044–53. doi: 10.4103/ijo.IJO_1563_19

136. Siddharthan KS, Shet V, Agrawal A, Reddy JK. Two-year clinical outcome after descemet membrane endothelial keratoplasty using a standardized protocol. *Indian J Ophthalmol*. (2020) 68:2408–14.

137. Lekhanont K, Pisitpayat P, Cheewaruangroj N, Jongkhajornpong P, Nonpassopon M, Anothaisintawee T. Outcomes of descemet membrane endothelial keratoplasty in Bangkok, Thailand. *Clin Ophthalmol*. (2021) 15:2239–51. doi: 10.2147/OPTH.S310873

138. Marchand M, El-Khoury J, Harissi-Dagher M, Robert MC. Outcomes of first cases of DMEK at a canadian university hospital centre. *Can J Ophthalmol*. (2021) 57:214–5. doi: 10.1016/j.jcjo.2021.05.010

139. Studeny P, Hlozankova K, Krizova D, Netukova M, Veith M, Mojzis P, et al. Long-term results of a combined procedure of cataract surgery and descemet membrane endothelial keratoplasty with stromal rim. *Cornea.* (2021) 40:628–34. doi: 10.1097/ICO.00000000000 02574

140. Tan TE, Devarajan K, Seah XY, Lin SJ, Peh GSL, Cajucom-Uy HY, et al. Descemet membrane endothelial keratoplasty with a pull-through insertion device: surgical technique, endothelial cell loss, and early clinical results. *Cornea.* (2020) 39:558–65. doi: 10.1097/ICO.0000000000002268

141. Yu AC, Myerscough J, Spena R, Fusco F, Socea S, Furiosi L, et al. Three-year outcomes of tri-folded endothelium-in descemet membrane endothelial keratoplasty with pull-through technique. *Am J Ophthalmol.* (2020) 219:121–31. doi: 10.1016/j.ajo.2020.07.004

142. Woo JH, Htoon HM, Tan D. Hybrid descemet membrane endothelial keratoplasty (H-DMEK): results of a donor insertion pull-through technique using donor stroma as carrier. *Br J Ophthalmol.* (2020) 104:1358–62. doi: 10.1136/bjophthalmol-2019-314932

143. Ighani M, Dzhaber D, Jain S, De Rojas JO, Eghrari AO. Techniques, outcomes, and complications of preloaded, trifolded descemet membrane endothelial keratoplasty using the DMEK endoglide. *Cornea.* (2021) 40:669–74. doi: 10.1097/ICO.0000000000002648

144. Jabbour S, Jun AS, Shekhawat NS, Woreta FA, Krick TW, Srikumaran D. Descemet membrane endothelial keratoplasty using a pull-through technique with novel infusion forceps. *Cornea.* (2021) 40:387–92. doi: 10.1097/ICO.0000000000002558

5

Use of Amniotic Membrane for Tectonic Repair of Peripheral Ulcerative Keratitis with Corneal Perforation

Maryam Eslami [1*], Blanca Benito-Pascual [2,3], Saadiah Goolam [2,3], Tanya Trinh [2,3,4] and Greg Moloney [1,2,3,4]

[1] Department of Ophthalmology and Visual Sciences, University of British Columbia, Vancouver, BC, Canada, [2] Sydney Eye Hospital, Sydney, NSW, Australia, [3] Save Sight Institute, University of Sydney, Sydney, NSW, Australia, [4] Mosman Eye Centre and Narellan Eye Specialists, Sydney, NSW, Australia

*Correspondence:
Maryam Eslami
maryam.eslami@alumni.ubc.ca

Purpose: To provide a perspective and surgical video demonstration of peripheral corneal ulceration and perforation managed with multilayered amniotic membrane transplantation.

Case Reports: Case 1 describes a 48-year-old female with progressive redness and pain, and an inferonasal corneal thinning and perforation in the left eye from peripheral ulcerative keratitis. She underwent conjunctival recession with amniotic membrane inlay and onlay (Sandwich technique) transplantation. The amniotic membrane integrated well, and her Snellen visual acuity improved from 6/21 preoperatively to 6/9 at 3 months post op. Case 2 describes a 78-year-old male with redness and pain with temporal corneal thinning bilaterally and perforation in the right eye from peripheral ulcerative keratitis. Both eyes underwent similar surgical intervention with smooth integration of the amniotic membrane in the cornea and improvement in the visual acuity. Both patients were also started on systemic immunosuppression in collaboration with the rheumatology team.

Conclusion: We report successful use of multilayered amniotic membrane transplantation for the treatment of corneal ulceration and perforation. The authors believe the simplicity of the surgical technique, easier access to amniotic membrane tissue, and lower induced post-operative astigmatism all provide advantages over alternative treatment modalities.

Keywords: amniotic membrane transplantation, corneal perforation, peripheral ulcerative keratitis, corneal ulceration, tectonic graft repair

INTRODUCTION

Various corneal pathologies can lead to corneal perforation, including infectious keratitis (bacterial, viral, fungal or parasitic), inflammatory keratitis (Mooren's ulcer, rheumatoid arthritis, systemic lupus erythematosus), neurotrophic keratitis, peripheral corneal thinning (pellucid marginal degeneration, Terrien's marginal degeneration), trauma, and chemical injuries (1–3).

The management of corneal perforation varies from non-surgical treatments such as bandage contact lenses or tissue adhesives, to surgical modalities like corneal suturing, conjunctival flaps, amniotic membrane (AM) transplantation and ultimately tectonic corneal patch graft (2, 3). The treatment chosen often depends on the size, location, and etiology of the corneal perforation, as well as the surgeon's experience and availability of donor tissues (amniotic membrane or donor cornea) (3, 4).

AM may be used as a graft (inlay), patch (onlay) or both for the management of corneal ulcers and perforations (5). It is not immunogenic, prevents apoptosis and has antimicrobial, antifibrotic, anti-inflammatory and antiangiogenic properties (3, 6). AM enhances epithelialisation by facilitating migration and differentiation of epithelial cells, reinforcing adhesion of basal epithelial cells, and regulating proliferation of normal corneal, conjunctival, and limbal fibroblasts (3).

In this paper, we present two cases of corneal perforation secondary to peripheral ulcerative keratitis managed with a sandwich technique of AM transplantation demonstrated in the **Supplementary Video**. Informed consent was obtained from both patients for publication of this case report.

CASE 1

A 48-year-old female presented with progressive pain, redness, and foreign body sensation in the left eye (LE) over the past 6 months. She had a history of peripheral ulcerative keratitis in the right eye (RE) requiring systemic immunosuppression and tectonic lamellar keratoplasty to reconstruct the area of the corneal thinning 15 years ago. Her systemic workup (complete cell blood count, electrolytes, urea, creatinine, liver function test, thyroid function test, C reactive protein (CRP), erythrocyte sedimentation rate (ESR), rheumatoid factor, antinuclear antibodies (ANA), antineutrophil cytoplasmic antibodies (ANCA), extractable nuclear antigens, anti-citrullinated protein antibody, syphilis, herpetic and hepatitis serologies) was negative 15 years prior. Her systems review at that point revealed a chronically inflamed elbow; therefore, she was started on oral cyclosporine up to 100 mg oral BID and Felodipine 2.5 mg oral daily for presumed seronegative rheumatoid arthritis. This systemic management was successfully tapered off 4 years ago with no recurrence of symptoms in the eye or the elbow joint.

On examination, she had uncorrected Snellen visual acuity of 6/30 on the right and 6/21 on the left. RE revealed an uninflamed tectonic lamellar keratoplasty. The LE was acutely inflamed inferonasally adjacent to an area of peripheral corneal ulceration without perforation. The anterior chamber was deep and quiet bilaterally at this point. She had trace nuclear sclerosis in both eyes.

She was commenced on oral ascorbic acid, topical moxifloxacin QID andprednisolone acetate 1% QID in the LE, and advised to use an eye shield at night. The rheumatology team was consulted again, and she was started on oral prednisone 60 mg daily as well as oral mycophenolate mofetil 1 g BID. On repeat assessment a week later, she had not yet started systemic treatment and had not been using her eye shield. She was found

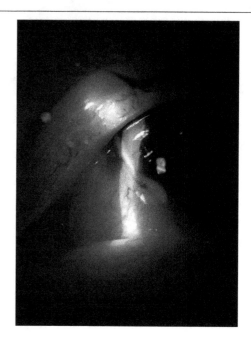

FIGURE 1 | Inferonasal corneal ulceration with adjacent inflammation of the left eye.

to have a perforation within the area of thinning with a flat anterior chamber (**Figure 1**).

A bandage contact lens was put on the LE as a temporizing measure before surgical management. She was continued on topical moxifloxacin and prednisolone acetate in the LE. Two days later, a conjunctival recession, amniotic membrane transplant and a temporary tarsorrhaphy was performed under retrobulbar anesthesia. A single piece of folded, multi-layered, fresh frozen amniotic membrane was packed and sutured into the LE corneal defect and held in place using fibrin glue. An overlying large single layer of amniotic membrane with the epithelial side down was sutured with interrupted sutures of 10.0 nylon with tension over the temporal ocular surface in a bandage fashion (**Supplementary Video**). A medial temporary tarsorrhaphy was carried out using bolsters and 6-0 nylon. Subconjunctival antibiotics of cefazolin and dexamethasone were injected at the end of the procedure. Postoperatively the patient was commenced on moxifloxacin eye drops QID, prednisolone acetate 1% QID and preservative-free lubricants 2-hourly.

The patient had an uneventful post-operative course without further episodes of ulceration, melt or inflammation. The AM patch integrated well into the corneal stroma at the 1-month postoperative visit with Snellen visual acuity of 6/15 and a quiet ocular surface (**Figure 2A**). Her uncorrected Snellen visual acuity improved to 6/9 at 3-months post op (**Figure 2B**).

CASE 2

A 78-year-old male from rural New South Wales presented to the Sydney Eye Hospital emergency department with a RE corneal perforation following a 4-day history of severe right ocular pain.

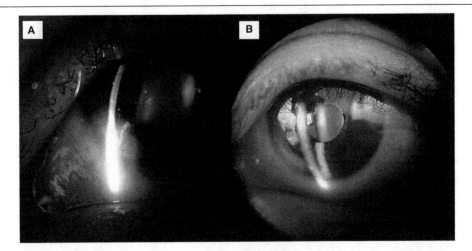

FIGURE 2 | (A) 1-month post-op image showing integration of the amniotic membrane patch in the inferonasal corneal stroma. (B) 3-month post-op image demonstrating smooth integration and an uninflamed left eye.

Past ocular history included LE pseudophakia and bilateral pterygium excision several years ago as well as bilateral dry age-related macular degeneration. He had a medical history of hypertension and ischemic heart disease with no other systemic complaints.

Examination on presentation revealed Snellen visual acuities of 6/38 in the RE and 6/24 in the LE. Intraocular pressure (IOP) was 13 and 11 mmHg in the right and left eye, respectively. Conjunctiva were bilaterally injected without any scleritic foci or evidence of scleromalacia. Corneas bilaterally were found to have temporal peripheral ulcerative keratitis (PUK) (6.5 mm in the RE and 7 mm in the LE), with RE corneal perforation of 2 mm with iris prolapse and LE thinning of ~80–90% within the area of ulceration (**Figures 3A,B**). RE Anterior chamber was almost flat with 3+ cells and a fibrinous reaction. LE anterior chamber was deep with 2+ cells. Other examination findings included pseudoexfoliative cataract in the RE and pseudophakia in the LE.

A cautious corneal scrape and swab of the RE ulcer bed excluded a superimposed microbial keratitis. Blood tests mentioned above, quantiferon gold test and a chest X-Ray were ordered to exclude infective and inflammatory/autoimmune causes of peripheral ulcerative keratitis. Blood tests were positive for a raised ESR (18 mm/h) and ANA (1:320 speckled); the remaining blood tests were unremarkable.

The patient was admitted on an initial treatment regimen of fortified topical antibiotics (gentamicin 0.9% and Cefazolin 5%) hourly in the RE and QID in the LE, topical prednisolone sodium phosphate preservative free 0.5% twice a day in both eyes, oral anti-collagenolytic agents (ascorbic acid 2 grams daily, doxycycline 100 mg twice a day), oral prednisolone 60 mg daily, oral ciprofloxacin 750 mg twice a day and valacyclovir 500 mg three times a day.

Gluing of the corneal perforation as a temporizing measure was not possible due to the significant area of perforation and degree of iris prolapse. For the RE, a conjunctival recession, amniotic membrane transplants and tarsorrhaphy was

performed. A single piece of folded, multi-layered, fresh frozen amniotic membrane was packed and sutured into the RE corneal defect and an overlying large single layer of amniotic membrane with the epithelial side down was sutured with tension over the temporal ocular surface with interrupted sutures of 10.0 nylon. A nasal paracentesis was used to reform the anterior chamber and reposit the iris. A second layer of amniotic membrane was then applied to the entire ocular surface with a purse-string suture.

The LE had conjunctival recession and 3 glue patches applied to the area of melt before a layer of amniotic membrane was glued over the area of thinning incorporating the area of conjunctival recession. Subconjunctival antibiotics of cefazolin and dexamethasone were injected bilaterally at the end of the procedures.

Postoperatively the patient was commenced on preservative-free chloramphenicol 0.5% drops QID, cyclosporine 1% BID and preservative-free lubricants 2-hourly. Topical steroids and fortified antibiotics were ceased. The rheumatology team was consulted as part of the multidisciplinary management of this patient's idiopathic immune-mediated corneal disease. 3 cycles of intravenous methyl prednisolone 500 mg and intravenous cyclophosphamide 650 mg were administered, followed by a tapering dose of the oral prednisone and initiation of long-term immunosuppression with oral mycophenolate 360 mg twice daily.

The patient had an uneventful post-operative course without further episodes of ulceration, melt or inflammation. Snellen visual acuity at the 1-month postoperative visit was 6/90 in RE (with cataract) and 6/9 in LE with normal intraocular pressures and a quiet ocular surface (**Figures 4A,B**).

Topical and systemic immunosuppressants were reduced as the patient continued on a stable postoperative course. At the 4-month post-operative visit the patient had similar visual acuity, and was maintained on topical preservative free lubricants and Mycophenolate 500 mg BD (**Figures 4C,D**).

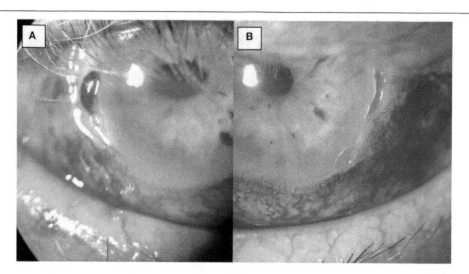

FIGURE 3 | (A) Pre-operative image of the right eye with temporal thinning and perforation, iris prolapse and surrounding inflammation. **(B)** pre-operative image of the left eye with temporal thinning and surrounding inflammation but no corneal perforation.

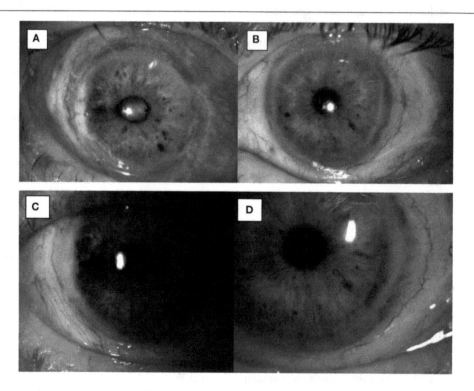

FIGURE 4 | 1-month post-op image showing integration of the amniotic membrane patch in the temporal corneal stroma of the right eye **(A)** and the left eye **(B)**. 3-month post-op image showing uninflamed eyes and a smooth integration of the amniotic membrane patch in the temporal corneal stroma of the right eye **(C)** and the left eye **(D)**.

DISCUSSION

In this article, we present two cases of peripheral ulcerative keratitis (3 eyes) with corneal perforation treated with multi-layered amniotic membrane transplantation using cigar technique demonstrated in the **Supplementary Video**. We found the AM integrated well into the host cornea in all 3 eyes with rapid visual recovery in all eyes but one, in which the reduced vision was attributed to cataract formation.

To replace the corneal tissue defect and fill in the corneal ulceration, the main options are fibrin glue, conjunctival and tenons tissue, donor corneal tissue, and AM (6–8). Fibrin glue,

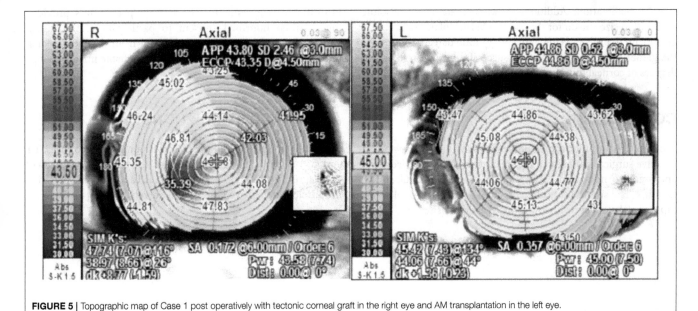

FIGURE 5 | Topographic map of Case 1 post operatively with tectonic corneal graft in the right eye and AM transplantation in the left eye.

TABLE 1 | A comparison of advantages and preferred utilization of AM transplantation and tectonic corneal graft.

	AM transplantation	Tectonic corneal graft
Advantages:	• Rapid recovery • Relative availability and ease of access • Relative simplicity of surgical technique • Less induced astigmatism • Less risk of rejection and ongoing melt	• Transparent tissue • Superior structural integrity with less potential for dislodgement
The technique may be preferred in:	• Peripheral corneal melt • Large areas of thinning with small or medium-sized perforation • Inflamed eye • Rheumatic etiology of corneal melt	• Large-sized perforation • Central disease • Intraocular tissue involvement

although a valuable tool in small perforations, is often ineffective on its own in filling the entire depth of corneal ulceration in large defects and may prolong wound healing and closure of epithelial defect (7). Conjunctival tissue often leads to neovascularization, scarring and conjunctivilization of the epithelium (7). Donor corneal tissue is often in short supply or may not be immediately available for the treatment of corneal perforation (7). It also has an increased risk of rejection and ongoing melt due to the inflamed host cornea and the underlying rheumatic disease (8). Many studies have reported on the successful use of AM in the treatment of corneal perforation (1–4, 6, 7). Some authors believe AM transplantation to be superior to alternatives due to AM's antifibrotic, anti-inflammatory and antiangiogenic properties that not only fills the defect and restores the globe's integrity,

but also prevents further tissue loss (3, 6, 7). This technique does require a tightly "packed" scroll of AM into a "cigar" shape—we find that this contour lends itself well to simultaneously filling in the central "bulk" for the largest portion of the defect alongside tapered "ends" and each pole of the "cigar", allowing for a gradual filling of crescenteric defects at superior and inferior ends. The initial placement of sutures from the host-AM-host requires replacing with tighter tension as the walls of the crevice become more and more closely apposed.

In our cases, we found the rapid visual rehabilitation and low induced astigmatism to be superior to tectonic corneal graft as well. The first case previously required a tectonic lamellar keratoplasty in the right eye for the same indication with an induced astigmatism of 6.5 diopters, while the left eye of the same patient treated with AM transplantation described above had a cylinder of 0.75 diopters at 3 months (**Figure 5**). This is consistent with prior studies with some authors reporting declining astigmatism with time as the AM continues to integrate into the host cornea (1, 3).

Lastly, the simplicity of the surgical technique (**Supplementary Video**) and the relative ease of availability of AM compared to donor cornea makes this an attractive choice for the management of corneal ulcers and perforations. This was also highlighted in a study by Ngan and Chau (9) on Mooren ulcers in Vietnam where systemic immunosuppressive medications are not readily available. Indeed, the management of corneal melting and perforation can be complex, and the treatment modality chosen may vary significantly depending on the clinical picture, other ocular comorbidities, and the size, location, and etiology of corneal thinning (**Table 1**). The authors agree that AM transplantation may not be suitable as the sole treatment of central corneal ulceration, as it leads to corneal opacity once healed and may degrade visual acuity. However, it may be an appropriate temporizing measure to allow for an uninflamed and quiet eye prior to donor corneal graft transplantation, thereby increasing success for visual rehabilitation. Additionally, while there is no absolute perforation size cut-off for the use of AM transplantation, it may be difficult to pack and close large perforation defects and restore the globe's integrity. However, its successful use in large or 360 degrees of corneal thinning has been previously reported (9).

CONCLUSION

Multi-layered amniotic membrane transplantation may be an effective surgical modality in the treatment of corneal ulceration and small to mid-sized perforation from peripheral ulcerative keratitis. The surgical technique is simple and leads to relatively rapid visual recovery with low induced astigmatism.

institutional requirements. The patients/participants provided their written informed consent to participate in this study. Written informed consent was obtained from the individual(s) for the publication of any potentially identifiable images or data included in this article.

AUTHOR CONTRIBUTIONS

ME, BB-P, and SG drafted the manuscript and the two cases. TT and GM were supervisors, performed the surgeries, and edited the manuscript and the surgical video. All authors contributed to the article and approved the submitted version.

REFERENCES

1. Namba H, Narumi M, Nishi K, Goto S, Hayashi S, Yamashita H. "Pleats fold" technique of amniotic membrane transplantation for management of corneal perforations. *Cornea*. (2014) 33:653–7. doi: 10.1097/ICO.0000000000000128

2. Yokogawa H, Kobayashi A, Yamazaki N, Masaki T, Sugiyama K. Surgical therapies for corneal perforations: 10 years of cases in a tertiary referral hospital. *Clin Ophthalmol*. (2014) 8:2165–70. doi: 10.2147/OPTH.S71102

3. Krysik K, Dobrowolski D, Wylegala E, Lyssek-Boron A. Amniotic membrane as a main component in treatments supporting healing and patch grafts in corneal melting and perforations. *J Ophthalmol*. (2020) 2020:4238919–7. doi: 10.1155/2020/4238919

4. Chan E, Shah AN, O'Brart DPS. "Swiss roll" amniotic membrane technique for the management of corneal perforations. *Cornea*. (2011) 30:838–41. doi: 10.1097/ICO.0b013e31820ce80f

5. Meller D, Pauklin M, Thomasen H, Westekemper H, Steuhl KP. Amniotic membrane transplantation in the human eye. *Dtsch Arztebl Int*. (2011) 108:243–48. doi: 10.3238/arztebl.2011.0243

6. Malhotra C, Jain AK. Human amniotic membrane transplantation: different modalities of its use in ophthalmology. *World J Transplant*. (2014) 4:111–21. doi: 10.5500/wjt.v4.i2.111

7. Hanada K, Shimazaki J, Shimmura S, Tsubota K. Multilayered amniotic membrane transplantation for severe ulceration of the cornea and sclera. *Am J Ophthalmol*. (2001) 131:324–31. doi: 10.1016/S0002-9394(00)00825-4

8. Solomon A, Meller D, Prabhasawat P, John T, Espana EM, Steuhl KP, et al. Amniotic membrane grafts for nontraumatic corneal perforations, descemetoceles, and deep ulcers. *Ophthalmology*. (2002) 109:694–703. doi: 10.1016/S0161-6420(01)01032-6

9. Ngan ND, Chau HT. Amniotic membrane transplantation for Mooren's ulcer: amniotic membrane for Mooren's ulcer. *Clin Exp Ophthalmol*. (2011) 39:386–92. doi: 10.1111/j.1442-9071.2010.02479.x

6

Ophthalmology Consultation Plan in the Context of 2019-nCoV

Shuang Song[1], Yidan Chen[1], Ying Han[2], Feng Wang[1]* and Ying Su[1]*

[1] Department of Ophthalmology, The First Affiliated Hospital of Harbin Medical University, Harbin, China, [2] Department of Geriatric, The First Affiliated Hospital of Harbin Medical University, Harbin, China

Keywords: SARS-CoV-2, ophthalmology, consultation, transmission, guidelines

*Correspondence:
Feng Wang
wangfd@126.com
Ying Su
suying0511@126.com

INTRODUCTION

Since December 2019, new coronavirus pneumonia (2019-nCoV) has been spread globally. At first it concentrated outbreak in China, and now reported all over the world, particularly in America and Europe (1, 2). 2019-nCoV is a new virus that everyone can be infected and was labeled as a pandemic by the World Health Organization (WHO) (3). A study in Wuhan reported of 535 patients, 27 patients (5.0%) presented with conjunctival congestion and 4 patients had conjunctival congestion as the initial symptom (4). Besides, a recent paper found that Several infected cases presented firstly with conjunctivitis before the onset of pneumonia, implying that the ocular route might be the potential transmission route of SARS-CoV-2 virus under certain conditions (5). An effective barrier protecting the eye is of paramount importance because the droplets and body fluids have a high probability to get onto the conjunctiva surface (6). Hence safety goggles identified to reduce ocular transmission but ophthalmologists need to close contact with the patients (conjunctival, tear secretions and aerosol secretions) during the fundus examination and other operations, so Ophthalmologists are a high-risk category (7, 8). For large medical centers their daily outpatient clinic and emergency lists have a high patient volume, which also increases the risk of cross-transmission between medical staff and patients (7, 8).

Due to different national conditions and cultures, the measures to respond to the pandemic are also different, so summary the diagnosis and treatment experience of 2019-nCoV and formulating a guideline suitable for the diagnosis and treatment of ophthalmic patients have very important clinical significance for epidemic prevention and control. In this review, we have combined our two experiences in fighting 2019-nCoV and the latest literature to propose rational recommendations for patients with eye diseases during the epidemic, and provide reference opinions for ophthalmology clinics and surgical procedures.

ADVICE FOR OPHTHALMIC PATIENTS

As a regional eye diagnosis and treatment center, our outpatient waiting room is often overcrowded. Risk assessment of patients to achieve patient diversion and avoiding the gathering of patients in large hospitals is an effective means to reduce human-to-human transmission. At this time, the patient needs to know what kind of eye diseases can be treated conservatively at home? Doctors also need to know which eye diseases can be recommended for patients to treat at home when the patient consults? During the epidemic period according to our experience, ophthalmic diseases that can be treated later include (8–11):

- Refractive errors, strabismus and amblyopia. For example, the child's refractive error is usually checked every 6 months. During the epidemic, the check can be post-poned, but if the check is necessary; parents can stagger the holidays because it is the peak period for consultation.
- Patients with eye discomfort such as dry eyes, foreign body sensation, but no eye pain, and vision loss can use artificial tears first.
- Ocular surfacepartial bleeding without other symptoms may be subconjunctival hemorrhage, just observe.
- The long-term gradual decline of visual without pain in the elderly may be age-related cataract, which does not change much in the short term;
- Poor vision, deformed vision, and no significant changes in recent symptoms (such as age-related macular degeneration);
- Glaucoma with good drug control;
- Floaters without obvious changes and without affecting vision.

During home isolation, if eye discomfort such as redness and itching occurs, you can consult an ophthalmologist free of charge on the official website, take medication under the guidance of a physician, and stay away from crowded hospitals based on the principle of maximum benefit. However, it is recommended to go to the doctor in time in the following situations (9, 12, 13):

- Moderate to severe eye trauma: such as chemical burns, thermal burns, eyeball ruptures, etc.
- Redness and pain with obvious loss of vision: This condition may be inflammation of the eye such as keratitis, glaucoma, and iritis.
- Painless sudden drop in vision: such as sudden loss of vision for no apparent reason, fixed black shadow in front of the eyes and gradually enlarged.

OUTPATIENT MANAGEMENT PLAN

Management of Outpatient Hygiene Environment

- Places that can be ventilated, open windows, 3 times a day, no <30 min each time, In a place without ventilation, irradiate with ultraviolet light twice a day, 30~60 min each time (14).
- The floor and wall should be cleaned with chlorine-containing disinfectant first. Use 1,000 mg/L to disinfect 3 times a day, each action is 30 min, and it will be disinfected at any time if it is contaminated; the contaminated area should be disinfected 3 times a day, and the action is 30 min (14-16).
- Seventy-five percentage ethanol wipe disinfection is the first choice for high-frequency contact surfaces, followed by wiping with 1,000 mg/L chlorine disinfectant, which is disinfected 3 times a day. The mobile phones of medical staff should be wiped frequently with 75% ethanol disinfectant, at least once a day (14-16).

Medical Equipment Disinfection

- Use disposable medical equipment, instruments and articles as much as possible, and treat them as infectious medical waste after use (14).

- Reusable medical equipment: Depending on whether the reused medical equipment is corrosion-resistant or not, wipe with 75% ethanol disinfectant or soak with 1,000 mg/L chlorine disinfectant (14).

Patient Management

- Ophthalmology patients register online to reduce queuing, and show a health QR code to prove that they have not been to high-risk areas.
- Everyone must wear a mask, measure the temperature, and disinfect their hands (8).
- Infrared fever detectors and thermometers (guns) are used to monitor the temperature of patients, and patients with fever are transferred to fever clinics (8, 11).
- Keep patients in the waiting area at least 1 m away from each other (11).
- Careful screening of the visiting patients as shown in **Figure 1**.

Patients who require oral or topical drugs after consultation can contact the doctor for consultation by phone or WeChat, tell your doctor about your condition, and guide medication through the network.

Outpatient Staff Management

- Epidemic theory knowledge training, protective equipment use training (8).
- Strictly require hand hygiene.
- Correctly select the protection level according to the exposure risk classification.
- Handling abnormalities of protective equipment quickly (such as damaged protective clothing, damaged gloves, fogging of goggles, loose masks) (14).

Special Attention of Ophthalmologists

Since the ophthalmologists in the outpatient clinic will inevitably come into contact with the patient's body fluids during the diagnosis and treatment (such as fundus examination), we must pay more attention to self-protection than ordinary staff.

- Ophthalmologists need third-level protection [Work clothes, medical protective clothing (disposable), isolation gowns, medical protective masks, work caps, protective visor/goggles, double gloves, hand hygiene] (8, 17, 18).
- Wash hands before and after treating patients.
- One room, one doctor and one patient. Strictly limit the number of people in the outpatient clinic (8).
- It is best for ophthalmologists to wear a face barriers instead of goggles, because the face barriers can well isolate the patient's body fluids or respiratory droplets during close examinations.
- It is best to use a non-contact tonometer or single-use disposable tonometer tip, and it is better to use indirect inspection methods rather than direct contact with the patient. All instruments used must be cleaned with 75% alcohol or chlorine-containing disinfectant in time (17, 18).
- A protective barriers can be added to inspection machines such as slit lamps and clean the contamination on the patient side in time (17, 18).

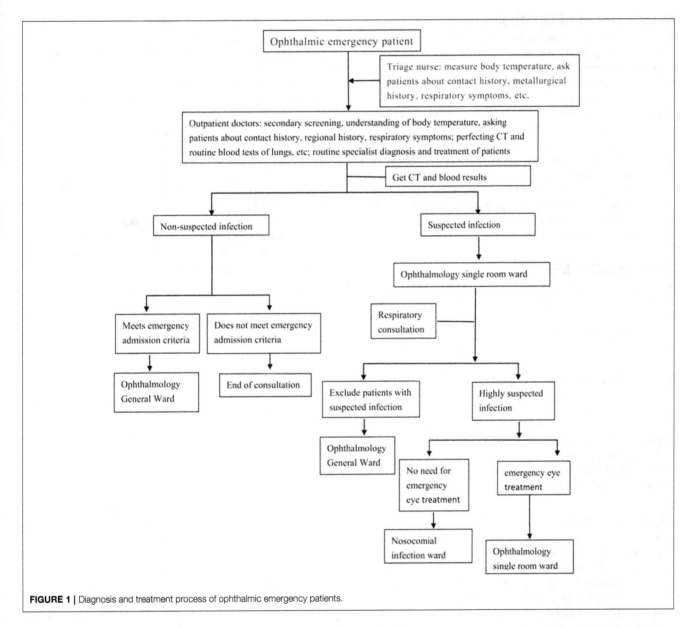

FIGURE 1 | Diagnosis and treatment process of ophthalmic emergency patients.

- Keep the examination limited to that required to make a clinical decision special tests requested (visual field, optical coherence tomography, corneal topography, ultrasound) only when critical to making a clinical decision.

Doctor Wang, a member of the national expert panel on pneumonia, was infected with 2019-nCoV in Wuhan (5). He wore a N95 mask but did not wear anything to protect his eyes. A few days before the onset of pneumonia, he developed redness and other conjunctival infections. Therefore, it is highly suspected that 2019-nCoV is first invaded by the conjunctiva, leading to respiratory infections. In addition, ophthalmologists have many inspections and operations during the diagnosis and treatment, and the distance between the doctor and the patient is very close during the inspection (8). The above reasons lead to a higher risk of infection by the ophthalmologist, and any improper protection is extremely easy to infect. Therefore, strict screening of patients is necessary at the time of their visit, and at the same time try to reduce the relevant examinations as much as possible, and doctors must perform secondary protection for necessary inspections and tertiary protection for high-risk operations. In the face of new coronary pneumonia, any prudent self-protection by ophthalmologists is reasonable.

Surgical Procedure for n-2019-nCoV Patients

In principle, only emergency ophthalmic surgery is performed during the epidemic, limited-period surgery should delay the operation time. During the hospitalization period, minimize the number of escorts and reduce the flow of personnel. All hospitalized patients and escorts need nucleic acid test for pathogenic screening of new coronary pneumonia.

Management of Ophthalmology Ward

- Set up general departments and isolation departments to isolate patients suspected or diagnosed with new coronavirus pneumonia (8, 14).
- Buffer wards are set up in normal departments for suspicious patients.
- If suspected or confirmed patients are found in the ward, relevant emergency plans and work procedures will be activated and transferred to a specific area for treatment (18).
- All hospitalized patients are checked for 2019-nCoV nucleic acid, questionnaire about upper respiratory symptoms, fever, myalgia and anosmia, domicile or traveling in hot areas, and contact history with confirmed or suspected COVID-19 patients within the past 14 days (8, 19).
- Hygienic environment of the normal ward reference 3.1

Pre-operative Management

- Not infected patients are normally prepared for eye surgery.
- For patients who are diagnosed or suspected and must be operated, an independent negative pressure operating room should be arranged. If there is no negative pressure operating room, an independent clean room with relatively independent spatial location should be selected (8, 14, 19).
- If 2 or more suspected or confirmed infections occur at the same time, surgery should be performed for the more critically ill patients (19).
- Disposable medical supplies are preferred. Non-disposable equipment and items must have a clear cleaning and disinfection process.
- Perform detailed inspections of surgical supplies before surgery to reduce the activities of personnel during surgery.

Intraoperative Management

- Most ophthalmic operations are not general anesthesia, patients can continue to wear surgical masks during the operation; if it is general anesthesia, it is recommended to place a disposable filter between the tracheal intubation and the breathing circuit to reduce the pollution of the breathing circuit, the anesthesia machine Strictly disinfect after use (20).
- Ordinary goggles seriously impede microsurgery, replaced it with homemade goggles by sealing the own glasses or flat lenses around the eyes with plastic wrap and remove the plastic wrap from the center of the lens to get protection and clear vision during the ophthalmic microsurgery (21, 22).
- Protective shields can be added to the slit lamp microscope to reduce the risk of close face-to-face contact between doctors and patients (21–23).
- Adjust the examination light from weak to strong, increasing gradually to avoid tears or a reflex sneeze.
- The third level of protection for surgeons in the whole process: hand-brushing clothing, medical protective clothing (disposable), surgical gown (disposable), medical protective masks, work caps, protective visor/goggles, double gloves (23).
- The number of people in the room is limited to the minimum number of patients required for care and surgery.

Post-operative Management

- Medical staff escorting the patient should do a tertiary level of protection, and the patient must wear a mask all the way.
- A special transfer flat car should be used to achieve "one person, one use, one disinfection," and the transfer elevator should also be disinfected on the surface. During the transfer of patients, attention should be paid to the protection of public areas and public appliances. Transfer patients according to the transfer route specified by the hospital and the special transfer route in the negative pressure operating room (14, 19).
- Disposal of surgical supplies, reusable medical supplies are placed separately and transported to disinfection supply center for centralized processing. Disposable items used in patients need to be handed over separately, delivered directly, and processed uniformly. A new coronavirus label is prominently placed on the outside of the pathological specimen bag and delivered by special personnel (14, 19).

Isolation Observation of Medical Staff

All medical staff involved in the operation of suspected or infected patients should be isolated for medical observation after surgery. If the suspected case excludes infection, release the isolation of the surgical staff; if it is an infected person, continue to isolate and observe until 14 day. And pay attention to observe whether the clinical manifestations of the new coronary pneumonia mentioned above, and report to the competent department.

SUMMARY

2019-nCoV is a global biochemical crisis. Ophthalmologists should remind patients to pay attention to eye protection and hand hygiene to prevent the eyes from becoming a gateway to viral infection. Prevent mutual infection between patients and patients, and between patients and doctors, disinfection and isolation of departments and operating rooms, and establish a simple and effective diagnosis and treatment process is necessary. In this review, we clearly told patients with eye diseases which conditions can be post-poned for medical treatment, which conditions require urgent medical attention, and provide our experience on the protective measures in the outpatient and ward. We have experienced two local outbreaks of the epidemic, and the infection rate is zero. It is difficult to determine which method is the most important, but in the face of infectious diseases, every detail is very important. China's success in fighting the epidemic shows that these methods are effective. In the context of the normalization of the global epidemic, we hope that our experience can help ophthalmologists.

AUTHOR CONTRIBUTIONS

FW designed the article. YS drafted important content. SS wrote the manuscript. YC and YH provided important intellectual comment during revising the article. All authors listed have made a substantial, direct and intellectual contribution to the work, and approved it for publication.

REFERENCES

1. Wang Y, Liu Y, Struthers J, Lian M. Spatiotemporal characteristics of the COVID-19 epidemic in the United States. *Clin Infect Dis.* (2021) 72:643–51. doi: 10.1093/cid/ciaa934

2. Andelić N, Baressi Šegota S, Lorencin I, Car Z. Estimation of COVID-19 epidemic curves using genetic programming algorithm. *Health Inform J.* (2021) 27:1460458220976728. doi: 10.1177/1460458220976728

3. *WHO Timeline-COVID-19.* Available online at: https://www.who.int/news-room/detail/27-04-2020-who-timeline-covid-19 (accessed June 20, 2020).

4. Chen L, Deng C, Chen X, Zhang X, Chen B, Yu H, et al. Ocular manifestations and clinical characteristics of 535 cases of COVID-19 in Wuhan, China: a cross-sectional study. *Acta Ophthalmol.* (2020) 98:e951–9. doi: 10.1111/aos.14472

5. Lu CW, Liu XF, Jia ZF. 2019-nCoV transmission through the ocular surface must not be ignored. *Lancet.* (2020) 395:e39. doi: 10.1016/S0140-6736(20)30313-5

6. Qing H, Yang Z, Shi M, Zhang Z. New evidence of SARS-CoV-2 transmission through the ocular surface. *Graefes Arch Clin Exp Ophthalmol.* (2020). doi: 10.1007/s00417-020-04726-4. [Epub ahead of print].

7. Jørstad ØK, Moe MC, Eriksen K, Petrovski G, Bragadóttir R. Coronavirus disease 2019 (COVID-19) outbreak at the department of ophthalmology, Oslo University Hospital, Norway. *Acta Ophthalmol.* (2020) 98:e388–9. doi: 10.1111/aos.14426

8. Romano MR, Montericcio A, Montalbano C, Raimondi R, Allegrini D, Ricciardelli G, et al. Facing COVID-19 in ophthalmology department. *Curr Eye Res.* (2020) 45:653–8. doi: 10.1080/02713683.2020.1752737

9. Bourdon H, Jaillant R, Ballino A, Kaim PE, Debillon L, Bodin S, et al. Teleconsultation in primary ophthalmic emergencies during the COVID-19 lockdown in Paris: experience with 500 patients in March and April 2020. *J Fr Ophtalmol.* (2020) 43:577–85. doi: 10.1016/j.jfo.2020.05.005

10. Muir KW, Gupta C, Gill P, Stein JD. Accuracy of international classification of diseases, ninth revision, clinical modification billing codes for common ophthalmic conditions. *JAMA Ophthalmol.* (2013) 131:119–20. doi: 10.1001/jamaophthalmol.2013.577

11. Wang Q, Wang X, Lin H. The role of triage in the prevention and control of COVID-19. *Infect Control Hosp Epidemiol.* (2020) 41:772–76. doi: 10.1017/ice.2020.185

12. Sobol EK, Carter KL, Ibrahim K, Alfaro C, Patel E, Pasquale LR, et al. A Convergence of ophthalmic and life-threatening emergencies: acute angle closure glaucoma and subarachnoid hemorrhage. *J Glaucoma.* (2019) 28:e151–2. doi: 10.1097/IJG.0000000000001310

13. Shah SM, Khanna CL. Ophthalmic emergencies for the clinician. *Mayo Clin Proc.* (2020) 95:1050–8. doi: 10.1016/j.mayocp.2020.03.018

14. National Health Commission WS/T511-2016 *Nosocomial Infection Prevention and Control Regulations for Airborne Diseases.* Available online at: http://www.nhc.gov.cn/ (accessed January 17, 2017).

15. Scaggs Huang F, Schaffzin JK. Rewriting the playbook: infection prevention practices to mitigate nosocomial severe acute respiratory syndrome coronavirus 2 transmission. *Curr Opin Pediatr.* (2021) 33:136–43. doi: 10.1097/MOP.0000000000000973

16. Wang Y, Wang L, Zhao X, Zhang J, Ma W, Zhao H, et al. A semi-quantitative risk assessment and management strategies on COVID-19 infection to outpatient health care workers in the post-pandemic period. *Risk Manag Healthc Policy.* (2021) 14:815–25. doi: 10.2147/RMHP.S293198

17. Reda AM, Ahmed WM. Standard precaution measurements during ophthalmology practice in the pandemic stage of COVID-19. *Int J Ophthalmol.* (2020) 13:1017–22. doi: 10.18240/ijo.2020.07.01

18. Nagesh S, Chakraborty S. Saving the frontline health workforce amidst the COVID-19 crisis: challenges and recommendations. *J Glob Health.* (2020) 10:010345. doi: 10.7189/jogh.10.010345

19. Tognetto D, Pastore MR, De Giacinto C, Cecchini P, Agolini R, Giglio R, et al. Managing ophthalmic practices in a referral emergency COVID-19 hospital in north-east Italy. *Acta Ophthalmol.* (2020) 98:e1057–8. doi: 10.1111/aos.14488

20. Smith F, Lee K, Binnie-McLeod E, Higgins M, Irvine E, Henderson A, et al. Identifying the World Health Organization's fifth moment for hand hygiene: infection prevention in the operating room. *J Infect Prev.* (2020) 21:28–34. doi: 10.1177/1757177419879996

21. WHO. *Infection Prevention and Control During Health Care When Novel Coronavirus (nCoV) Infection is Suspected Interim Guidance.* Geneva: World Health Organization (2020).

22. Du H, Zhang M, Zhang H, Sun X. Practical experience on emergency ophthalmic surgery during the prevalence of COVID-19. *Graefes Arch Clin Exp Ophthalmol.* (2020) 258:1831–33. doi: 10.1007/s00417-020-04692-x

23. Hydén D, Arlinger S. On light-induced sneezing. *Eye (Lond).* (2009) 23:2112–4. doi: 10.1038/eye.2009.165

7

Effects of Combined Cataract Surgery on Outcomes of Descemet's Membrane Endothelial Keratoplasty

*Kai Yuan Tey [1,2], Sarah Yingli Tan [2], Darren S. J. Ting [3,4], Jodhbir S. Mehta [1,5,6] and Marcus Ang [1,5,6]**

[1] Singapore Eye Research Institute, Singapore, Singapore, [2] Tasmanian Medical School, University of Tasmania, Hobart, TAS, Australia, [3] Academic Ophthalmology, Division of Clinical Neuroscience, University of Nottingham, Nottingham, United Kingdom, [4] Department of Ophthalmology, Queen's Medical Centre, Nottingham, United Kingdom, [5] Singapore National Eye Center, Singapore, Singapore, [6] Duke-National University Singapore Graduate Medical School, Singapore, Singapore

Correspondence:
Marcus Ang
marcus.ang@snec.com.sg

Objective: A systematic review and meta-analysis of literature-to-date regarding the effects of combined cataract surgery on outcomes of DMEK.

Methods: Multiple electronic databases were searched, including Cochrane Library databases, PubMed, Web of Science, and ClinicalTrials.gov. The final search was updated on 10th February 2022. We included randomized controlled trials (RCTs), non-randomized studies and large case series (≥25 eyes) of DMEK (pseudophakic/phakic) and "triple DMEK". A total of 36 studies were included in this study. Meta-analyses were done with risk differences (RD) computed for dichotomous data and the mean difference (MD) for continuous data via random-effects model. Primary outcome measure: postoperative re-bubbling rate; secondary outcome measures: complete/partial graft detachment rate, best-corrected visual acuity (BCVA), endothelial cell loss (ECL), primary graft failure, and cystoid macular edema (CMO).

Results: A total of 11,401 eyes were included in this review. Based on non-randomized studies, triple DMEK demonstrated a better BCVA at 1-month postoperative than DMEK alone (MD 0.10 logMAR; 95% CI: 0.07–0.13; $p < 0.001$), though not statistically significant at 3–6 months postoperative (MD 0.07 logMAR; 95% CI: −0.01 to 0.15; $p = 0.08$). There was no significant difference in rebubbling, ECL, graft failures, and CMO postoperatively between the two groups ($p = 0.07$, $p = 0.40$, 0.06, and 0.54 respectively).

Conclusion: Our review suggests that DMEK has a similar post-operative complication risk compared to "triple DMEK" (low-quality evidence), with comparable visual outcome and graft survival rate at 6 months postoperative. High-quality RCTs specifically studying the outcomes of combined vs. staged DMEK are still warranted.

Systematic Review Registration: https://www.crd.york.ac.uk/prospero/display_record.php?ID=CRD42020173760, identifier: CRD42020173760.

Keywords: DMEK, cataract surgery, systematic review & meta-analysis, staged surgery, combined surgery, Descemet's membrane endothelial keratoplasty

INTRODUCTION

Cataract surgery is the most commonly performed elective surgery in the world, with >10 millions of cases being carried out each year (1). In addition, age-related corneal endothelial diseases (e.g., Fuchs endothelial corneal dystrophy; FECD) are common causes of visual impairment, and represent a leading indication for corneal transplantation (2–4). Therefore, with the aging global population, it is becoming increasingly common for patients to require treatment for co-existing age-related ocular diseases such as cataract and FECD.

FECD can lead to endothelial cell loss (ECL) with resultant corneal edema, ocular discomfort, and visual impairment (5). Once corneal decompensation sets in, corneal transplant serves as the mainstay of treatment for restoring the vision (6). In recent years, selective endothelial keratoplasty (EK) has been the treatment choice for managing corneal endothelial diseases (3, 4, 7). In EKs, the donor corneal tissue is inserted, and positioned against the posterior surface of the host cornea (8–10). In particular, Descemet's membrane endothelial keratoplasty (DMEK) involves the use of a manually prepared partial-thickness donor cornea containing only endothelium and Descemet membrane (11–13). DMEK has been shown to have superior postoperative visual acuity and lower graft rejection rate (14–17). Despite the established benefits, the adoption of DMEK is gaining popularity albeit slowly, owing to its steep surgical learning curve (16, 18–20).

The approach in managing a concomitant cataract with FECD can be done in various ways. One of the commonest approaches is to perform a combined DMEK and cataract surgery (i.e., "triple DMEK"). When compared to a staged DMEK procedure (i.e., cataract surgery followed by DMEK, or DMEK followed by cataract surgery), "triple DMEK" offers advantages such as improved cost-effectiveness, better intraoperative corneal clarity (due to simultaneous removal of the diseased and thickened endothelium and elimination of the risk of post-cataract surgery-induced corneal edema) and comparable clinical outcomes (8, 21). It was however also found that "triple DMEK" may be associated with a higher rate of postoperative complications such as graft detachment requiring postoperative re-bubbling (22–24). Overall, there is no consensus on whether to stage or combine DMEK with cataract surgery in patients who present with visually significant cataracts and FECD.

Thus, we performed a systematic review to appraise and compare the published evidence on the surgical outcomes of DMEK and "triple DMEK" procedures, which could help inform the future clinical practice on managing patients with co-existing corneal endothelial diseases and cataract. As graft detachment requiring postoperative re-bubbling is one of the most complications of DMEK, we have studied this as the main outcome measure of our systematic review.

MATERIALS AND METHODS

Eligibility Criteria for Considering Studies for This Review

We included publications in which the surgical outcomes of DMEK performed for the treatment of corneal endothelial dysfunction were reported. Studies that reported on the outcomes of eyes that had undergone surgeries other than DMEK or "triple DMEK" were excluded from the review. Studies that solely reported on the clinical outcomes of DMEK performed for previous graft failures (including repeat DMEK surgery) or specific high-risk disease groups (e.g., glaucoma, previous glaucoma filtration surgeries, cytomegalovirus retinitis, herpes simplex virus) were excluded. There were no restrictions on age, gender, or ethnic group. To avoid any duplication of the reporting of similar study populations, where the same group of investigators published several studies, earlier smaller studies were excluded if more recent larger studies reporting the same outcome measures were available. We included all randomized controlled trials (RCTs), non-randomized studies, and large prospective and retrospective case series ($n \geq 25$ eyes). Small case series (<25 eyes), letter, reviews, published abstracts, and laboratory-based studies were excluded from this review. The main outcome measure was the postoperative re-bubbling rate (at 0–6 months). Secondary outcome measures included graft detachment (including partial and complete detachment at 0–6 months), BCVA (at 1–6 months; in logarithm of the minimum angle of resolution, logMAR), graft failure (at 1–6 months), ECL (at 1–6 months), and cystoid macular edema (CME; at 1–6 months). Analysis of the literature and writing of the manuscript were performed in accordance with the Preferred Reporting Items for Systematic Reviews and Meta-Analyses (PRISMA) guidelines (http://www.prisma-statement.org/).

Search Methods for Identifying Studies

We conducted a literature search in multiple electronic databases, including Cochrane Library databases, PubMed, Web of Science, and ClinicalTrials.gov (www.clinicaltrials.gov). We did not set any restrictions on the date, language, or publication status in our electronic search. The search strategies for the relevant databases can be found in **Supplementary Appendix 1**. We also performed manual searches by reviewing the reference lists of relevant reports and reviews. The final search was updated on 10th February 2022. The protocol was registered at the Prospective Register for Systematic Reviews (PROSPERO; registration number: CRD42020173760). Distiller Systematic

Review (DSR) was used to manage the records identified and eligibility status.

Study Selection

The reviewers (K.Y.T and M.A) independently screened the titles and abstracts. Full reports of all titles that met the inclusion criteria or where there was uncertainty were obtained. Reviewers (K.Y.T and S.Y.T) then screened the full-text reports and additional information from the original investigators were sought after where necessary to resolve questions about the eligibility. We resolved any disagreement through discussion and any unresolved discussion was adjudicated by M.A. Reasons for excluding studies were recorded.

Data Collection and Risk of Bias Assessment

The following details of each study were extracted for this review: study participants' characteristics, location of study, study design, DMEK sub-groups, funding support (if any), and surgical outcome measures. Data on the following surgical outcome measures were included: re-bubbling rate, best-corrected visual acuity (BCVA), postoperative ECL, and complications including graft detachment. If only absolute numbers of the EC count were described, ECL was calculated by the method described by Hwang et al. (25). For descriptive and analytic purposes, visual outcome reported in Snellen visual acuity (VA) was converted to the respective logMAR (26). All outcome measures were ordinal data, except for mean BCVA and mean ECL (continuous data). The preferred unit of analysis was outcomes for eyes rather than individuals as some individuals had unilateral treatment or different treatments in each eye. For results that were reported in median, range and/or interquartile range, the mean and standard deviation were calculated using the method described by Luo et al. (27) and Wan et al. (28). Missing data were dealt per protocol, which is available in **Supplementary Appendix 2**.

Risk of bias was assessed by two authors (K.Y.T and S.Y.T) independently and any disagreement was adjudicated by M.A. Included randomized controlled trials (RCT) were assessed for risk of bias using Chapter 8 of the Cochrane Handbook for Systematic Reviews of Intervention (29). For non-randomized studies, we utilized the tool—Risk of Bias in non-randomized Studies—of Intervention (ROBINS-I) to evaluate the risk of bias in estimates (30). The study design of each article was also assessed and rated according to its level of evidence using a rating scale adapted from the Oxford Centre for Evidence-based Medicine (31). Funnel plots were analyzed to evaluate publication bias and small-study effects.

RCTs were judged for the selection bias, performance bias, detection bias, attrition bias, reporting bias and other sources of bias. Non-randomized studies were judged for confounding bias, selection bias, bias in classification of interventions, bias in deviation from intended interventions, bias due to missing data, bias in measurement of outcome and bias in selection of the reported results. Non-comparative case series was not assessed for risk of bias in view of the inherent high risk of bias.

Quality of evidence of each study was assessed by one author (K.Y.T) using the Grading of Recommendations Assessment, Development and Evaluation (GRADE) tool (32). Each study was graded as either high, moderate, low or very low based on the study design, study limitations, consistency of results, directness of evidence, precision, treatment effect and reporting bias.

Data Synthesis and Analysis

A meta-analysis was performed if there were sufficient similarities in the reporting of outcome measures in different studies. The meta-analyses for comparison between both "triple DMEK" and DMEK alone were performed using Review Manager (Version 5.3) by Cochrane. Meta-analyses were done by computing the risk differences for dichotomous data and the mean difference for continuous data using a random-effects model. For single-arm studies (i.e., "triple DMEK" or DMEK alone), the overall effect was studied using Open Meta-Analyst [OpenMetaAnalyst for Windows 8 (64-bit) (built 04/06/2015) by Brown University]. Random-effects model was used in view of the anticipated heterogeneity in study design, patient cohort and surgical aspects (including surgeon's experience and surgical technique). Where zeros caused problems with the computation of effects or standard errors, 0.5 was added to all cells for that study. Statistical heterogeneity (I^2) was defined as mild (0–40%), moderate (30–60%), substantial (50–90%), and considerable (75–100%) (33).

RESULTS

Literature Search and Study Characteristics

The electronic searches yielded a total of 873 records, and 42 additional records were identified through manual hand searching of bibliography (see **Figure 1** for the PRISMA flow diagram). After deduplication, 815 abstracts were screened and a further 683 records were removed. Full-text copies of 132 articles were obtained and reviewed. After excluding 96 ineligible studies, 36 studies ($n = 11,401$ eyes) were included in this systematic review. These included 17 non-randomized studies comparing DMEK alone to "triple DMEK" ($n = 8,304$ eyes) with a mean follow-up duration of 12.8 ± 15.9 months (ranged, 6–60 months) (21, 22, 34–48), 14 studies on DMEK ($n = 2,609$ eyes) with a mean follow-up duration of 20.0 ± 21.9 months (ranged, 3–42 months) (49–62), and five studies on "triple DMEK" ($n = 495$ eyes) with a mean follow-up duration of 8.0 ± 3.4 months (ranged, 6–12 months) (63–67). Studies included were conducted at The Netherland (12 studies), Germany (nine studies), United States of America (seven studies), Canada (two studies), Egypt (one study), France (one study), Italy (one study), Nepal (one study), Spain (one study), United Kingdom (one study), and a multicenter study (23 countries). The surgical outcomes reported in studies included are summarized in **Supplementary Appendix 3**. Subgroup analysis comparing "triple DMEK" with phakic DMEK or pseudophakic DMEK alone was not possible due to due to limited numbers and heterogeneous study design (21, 34–36, 44).

Level of Evidence, Quality of Evidence and the Risks of Bias of Included Studies

The level of evidence assessed could be found in **Supplementary Appendix 3**. Of all the 17 studies that compared

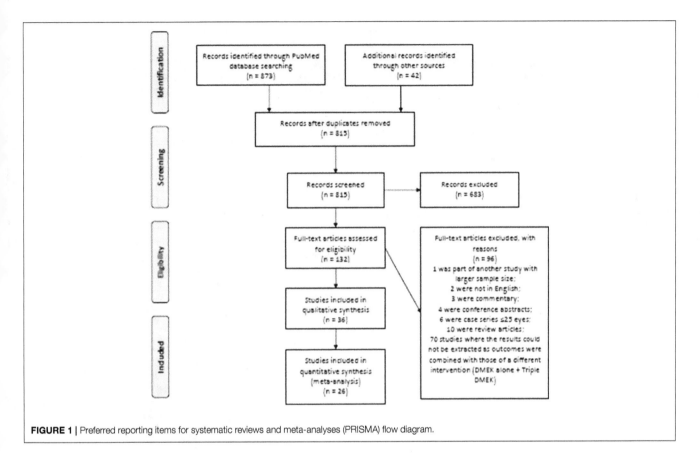

FIGURE 1 | Preferred reporting items for systematic reviews and meta-analyses (PRISMA) flow diagram.

DMEK alone and "triple DMEK", eight (47.1%) were rated as level II evidence, three (17.6%) were rated as level III evidence, and six (35.3%) were rated as level IV evidence. Of all the 14 DMEK alone studies, two (14.3%) were rated as level II evidence and 12 (85.7%) were rated as level IV evidence. Of all the five "triple DMEK" studies, all (100%) were rated as level IV evidence.

Similarly, the quality of evidence assessed could be found in **Supplementary Appendix 3**. Of all the 17 studies that compared DMEK alone and "triple DMEK", nine (52.9%) were graded as moderate quality of evidence and eight (47.1%) were graded as low quality. Of all the DMEK alone studies, 14 (100%) were graded as low quality evidence, and of all the five "triple DMEK" studies, all (100%) were graded as low quality.

Based on all 17 non-randomized studies, the risk of bias assessment considered one (5.9%) study as low risk, 13 (76.5%) studies as moderate risk, and three (17.6%) studies as high risk. **Figure 2** summarizes the judgments of each risk of bias domain presented as overall percentages across all included studies and **Figure 3** summarizes the authors' judgments of each risk of bias item for each included comparative study.

Surgical Outcomes

Summary of the outcomes of meta-analysis of various surgical outcomes could be found in **Table 1** (for non-randomized studies) and **Table 2** (for non-comparative studies).

Postoperative Re-bubbling Rate

Eight comparative studies ($n = 2,799$ eyes), which included 1,408 DMEK eyes and 1,391 "triple DMEK" eyes, reported the postoperative re-bubbling rate (21, 22, 34, 35, 39, 43, 45, 48). Re-bubbling was reported in 316 (22.4%) DMEK eyes and 381 (27.4%) "triple DMEK" eyes. The meta-analysis demonstrated that there was no statistical difference between DMEK alone and "triple DMEK" in terms of postoperative re-bubbling rate (RD -0.06; 95% CI: -0.13 to 0.00; $I^2 = 73\%$; $p = 0.07$; **Figure 4A**). Based on the findings of non-comparative studies, the overall re-bubbling rate following DMEK was estimated at 3.9% (95% CI: 1.9–5.8; $n = 950$ eyes from five studies; **Figure 4B**) (52, 55, 58, 59, 62). No relevant data was available from "triple DMEK" studies.

Graft Detachment

There was insufficient data regarding graft detachment among the comparative studies for meta-analysis. One study, which included 131 DMEK and 101 "triple DMEK" eyes, reported 12.9 and 10.1% of partial and complete graft detachment following DMEK, respectively, whilst there were 10.7 and 11.9% eyes with partial and complete graft detachment following "triple DMEK", respectively, with no statistical difference observed between both groups ($p = 0.78$) (43).

Amongst the non-comparative DMEK studies, four studies ($n = 1,085$ eyes) and five studies ($n = 1,152$ eyes) that reported the rate of complete and partial graft detachments postoperatively respectively (52, 58, 59, 61, 62). The overall rate of complete and

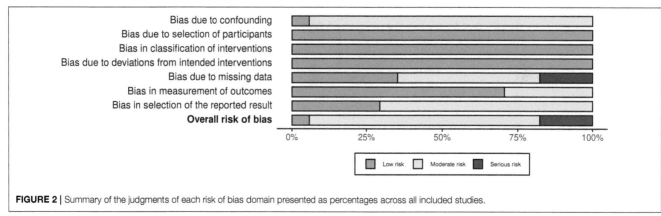

FIGURE 2 | Summary of the judgments of each risk of bias domain presented as percentages across all included studies.

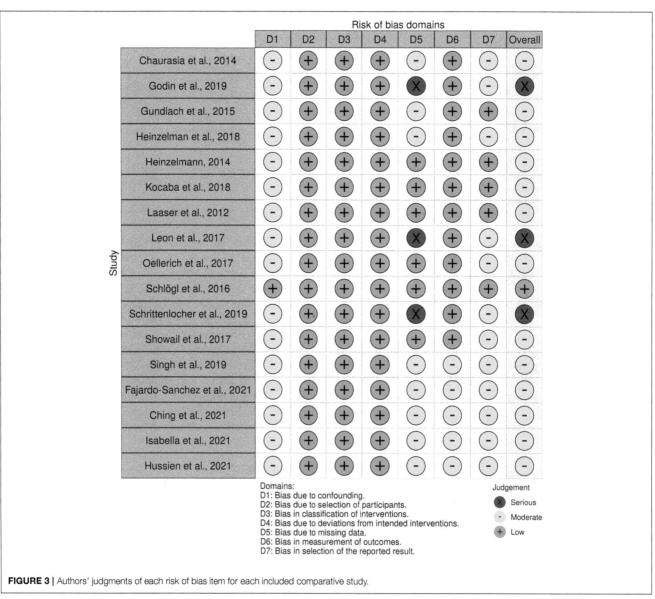

FIGURE 3 | Authors' judgments of each risk of bias item for each included comparative study.

partial graft detachment was 8.3% (95% CI: 4.2–12.4) and 8.3% (95% CI: 5.1–11.5), respectively (**Figures 4C,D**). There was no data on graft detachment amongst the non-comparative "triple DMEK" studies.

TABLE 1 | Summary of meta-analysis result of each surgical outcomes in the non-randomized studies (non-randomized studies).

Surgical outcomes	Number of studies, n	Number of eyes included, n (DMEK only vs. "triple DMEK")	Effect Measure, MD/RD (95% CI)	I^2, %	p-value	Level of evidences
Postoperative re-bubbling rate	8	2,799 (1,408 vs. 1,391)	RD −0.06 (−0.13 to 0.00)	76	0.07	6 Level 2 2 Level 3 2 Level 4
Best corrected visual acuity, LogMAR at 1-month	2	435 (243 vs. 192)	MD 0.10 (0.07–0.13)	0	<0.001	1 Level 2 1 Level 4
Best corrected visual acuity, LogMAR at 3–6 month	5	769 (393 vs. 376)	MD 0.07 (−0.01 to 0.15)	88	0.08	2 Level 2 1 Level 1 2 Level 2
Endothelial cell loss at 3- month	2	154 (60 vs. 94)	MD −3.24 (−9.30 to 2.81)	78	0.29	1 Level 2 1 Level 4
Endothelial cell loss at 6-month	2	297 (142 vs. 155)	MD 2.93 (−3.94 to 9.79)	49	0.40	1 Level 2 1 Level 4
Primary graft failure	7	1,414 (807 vs. 607)	MD 0.01 (−0.02 to 0.05)	34	0.44	4 Level 2 1 Level 3 2 Level 4
Cystoid macular edema	5	1,013 (573 vs. 440)	RD 0.00 (−0.02 to 0.01)	0	0.70	3 Level 2 1 Level 3 1 Level 4
Posterior capsular rupture	2	235 (117 vs. 118)	RD −0.04 (−0.08 to 0.01)	0	0.15	1 Level 2 1 Level 3

DMEK, Descemet's membrane endothelial keratoplasty; MD, mean difference; RD, risk difference.

TABLE 2 | Summary of meta-analysis result of each surgical outcomes in the non-comparative studies.

Surgical outcomes	Number of studies, n	DMEK Alone or "triple" DMEK	Number of eyes included n	Overall effect (95% CI)	I^2, %
Postoperative re-bubbling rate	6	DMEK Alone	950	3.9% (1.9–5.8)	43
Complete graft detachment	4	DMEK Alone	1,085	8.3% (4.2–12.4)	84
Partial graft detachment	5	DMEK Alone	1,152	8.3 (5.1–11.5)	73
Best corrected visual acuity, LogMAR at 3-month	3	DMEK Alone	107	0.15 (0.10–0.20)	54
Best corrected visual acuity, LogMAR at 6- month	4	DMEK Alone	838	0.15 (0.09–0.22)	97
Best corrected visual acuity, LogMAR at 1-month	3	"Triple" DMEK	123	0.20 (0.12–0.29)	95
Best corrected visual acuity, LogMAR at 3-month	4	"Triple" DMEK	275	0.15 (0.11–0.19)	87
Endothelial cell loss at 6- month	2	DMEK Alone	549	33.1 (24.89–41.25)	92
Cataract development postoperative	7	DMEK Alone	465	13.5% (5.4–21.7)	91

DMEK, Descemet's membrane endothelial keratoplasty.

Best Corrected Visual Acuity

Five comparative studies (n = 822 eyes) reported BCVA at 1–6 months postoperatively (21, 35, 42–44). "Triple DMEK" was shown to have a better BCVA compared to DMEK at 1 month postoperative (MD 0.10 logMAR; 95% CI: 0.07–0.13; I^2 = 0%; p < 0.001; **Figure 5A**). Whilst the MD of BCVA between "triple DMEK" and DMEK at 3–6 months was insignificant, we however found that the result was highly heterogenous (MD 0.07 logMAR; 95% CI: −0.01 to 0.15; I^2 = 88%; p = 0.08; **Figure 5B**).

A total of seven DMEK studies (n = 692 eyes) (49, 54, 56, 60, 62, 68), and three "triple DMEK" studies (n = 275 eyes) reported BCVA at 1–6 months postoperative (64, 65, 67). The mean BCVA following DMEK was 0.50 logMAR (reported by one study), 0.14 (95% CI: 0.10–0.20) logMAR, and 0.07 (95% CI: 0.09–0.22) logMAR at 1-, 3-, and 6-month postoperative,

respectively (**Figures 5C,D**), whereas the mean BCVA following "triple DMEK" was 0.19 (95% CI: 0.12–0.29) logMAR, 0.15 (95% CI: 0.11–0.19) logMAR, and 0.19 logMAR (reported by one study) at 1, 3, and 6 months postoperative, respectively (**Figures 5E,F**).

Endothelial Cell Loss

Three non-randomized studies (n = 394 eyes), which included 191 DMEK eyes and 203 "triple DMEK" eyes, reported the ECL at 3–6 months postoperative (35, 42, 43). Based on non-randomized studies, the rate of ECL was similar between DMEK and "triple DMEK" at 3 months postoperative (MD −3.24%; 95% CI: −9.30 to 2.81; I^2 = 78%; p = 0.29) and at 6 months postoperative (MD 2.93%; 95% CI: −3.94 to 9.79; I^2 = 49%; p = 0.40; **Figures 6A,B**).

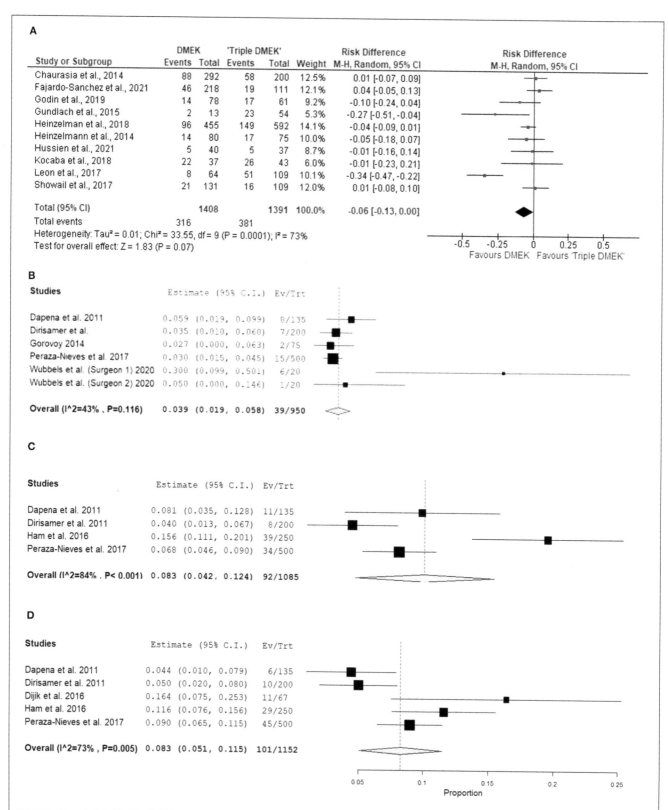

FIGURE 4 | Forest plot of (A,B) re-bubbling rates and (C,D) graft detachments (complete and partial) in comparative Descemet's membrane endothelial keratoplasty (DMEK) vs. "Triple DMEK" studies (comparative meta-analysis), and non-comparative DMEK alone studies (single-arm meta-analysis).

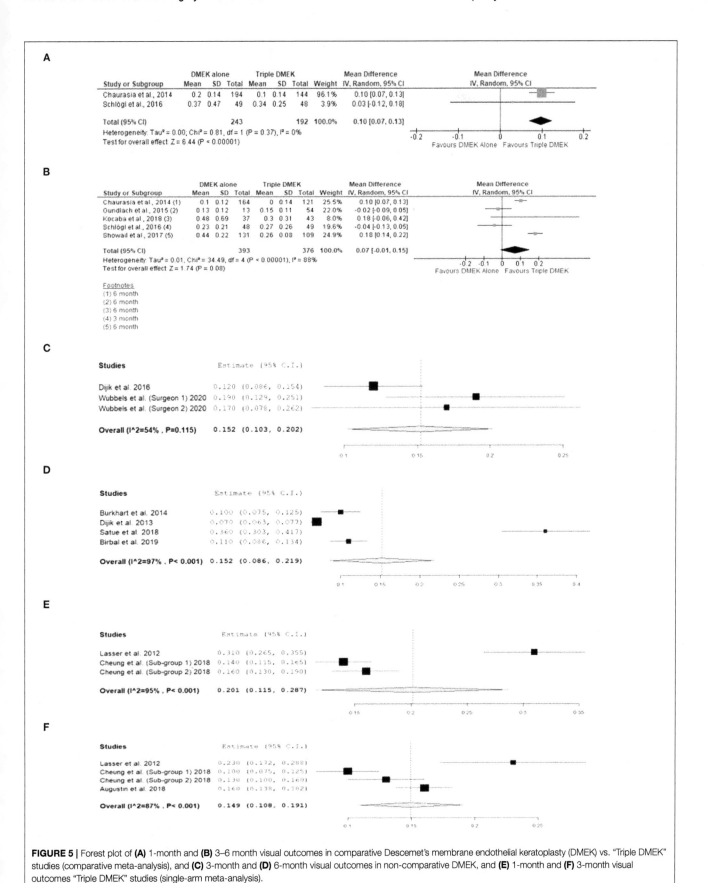

FIGURE 5 | Forest plot of **(A)** 1-month and **(B)** 3–6 month visual outcomes in comparative Descemet's membrane endothelial keratoplasty (DMEK) vs. "Triple DMEK" studies (comparative meta-analysis), and **(C)** 3-month and **(D)** 6-month visual outcomes in non-comparative DMEK, and **(E)** 1-month and **(F)** 3-month visual outcomes "Triple DMEK" studies (single-arm meta-analysis).

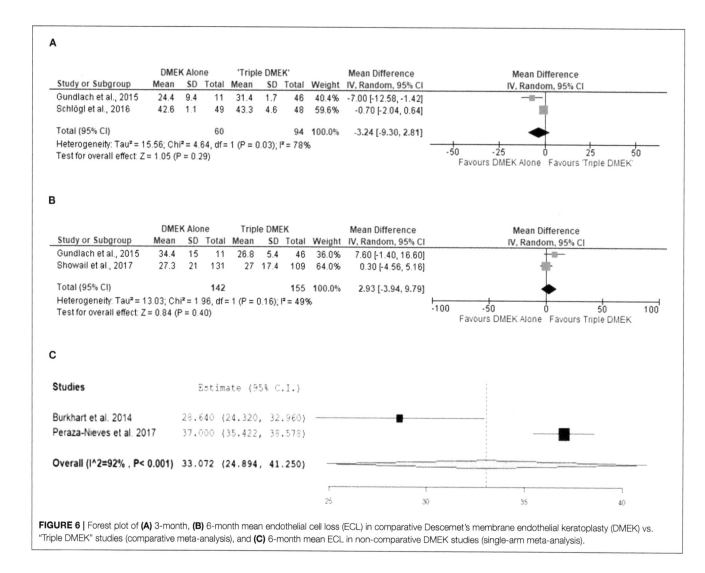

FIGURE 6 | Forest plot of **(A)** 3-month, **(B)** 6-month mean endothelial cell loss (ECL) in comparative Descemet's membrane endothelial keratoplasty (DMEK) vs. "Triple DMEK" studies (comparative meta-analysis), and **(C)** 6-month mean ECL in non-comparative DMEK studies (single-arm meta-analysis).

A total of three DMEK studies ($n = 572$ eyes) reported the postoperative ECL at 1–6 months postoperative (49, 51, 58). The mean ECL following DMEK was 37% (reported by one study) and 33.1% (95% CI: 24.9–41.3) at 1 and 6 months postoperative, respectively (**Figure 6C**). Data regarding mean ECL was not available in the non-comparative "triple DMEK" studies.

Primary Graft Failure

Seven non-randomized studies ($n = 1,414$ eyes) reported the primary graft failure rate, which was similar between DMEK and "triple DMEK" (RD 0.01; 95% CI: −0.02 to 0.05; $I^2 = 34\%$; $p = 0.44$; **Figure 7A**) (21, 34, 35, 43–45, 48). There was no data available regarding primary graft failures among non-comparative DMEK and "triple DMEK" studies.

Cystoid Macular Edema

Five non-randomized studies reported the development of CME postoperatively (21, 36, 44, 46, 48). The risk of CME was similar between DMEK and "triple DMEK" (RD = −0.00; 95% CI: −0.02 to 0.01; $I^2 = 0\%$; $p = 0.70$; **Figure 7B**). Data regarding CME

was not available in the non-comparative DMEK and "triple DMEK" studies.

Other Complications

Amongst the non-randomized studies, two studies reported the development of posterior capsular rupture (PCR) intraoperatively (36, 44). The risk of PCR was similar between DMEK and "triple DMEK" (RD = −0.03; 95% CI = −0.08 to −0.01; $I^2 = 0\%$; $p = 0.15$; **Figure 7C**). One study with 11 phakic DMEK eyes and 46 "triple DMEK" eyes reported elevated intraocular pressures in 18.2 and 8.7% of the eyes, respectively (35). In addition, 18.2% of the phakic DMEK eyes developed cataracts by 6 months' postoperative (35). Hyphaema were reported in 31% of the DMEK eyes and 49.8% of the "triple DMEK" eyes, with triple DMEK eyes having a 1.5 times (95% CI = 1.2–1.9) higher risk of developing hyphema (38).

For non-comparative DMEK studies, seven studies ($n = 465$) phakic eyes reported 68 eyes developed cataracts postoperatively (47, 50–52, 58, 59, 68). The overall risk of cataract development

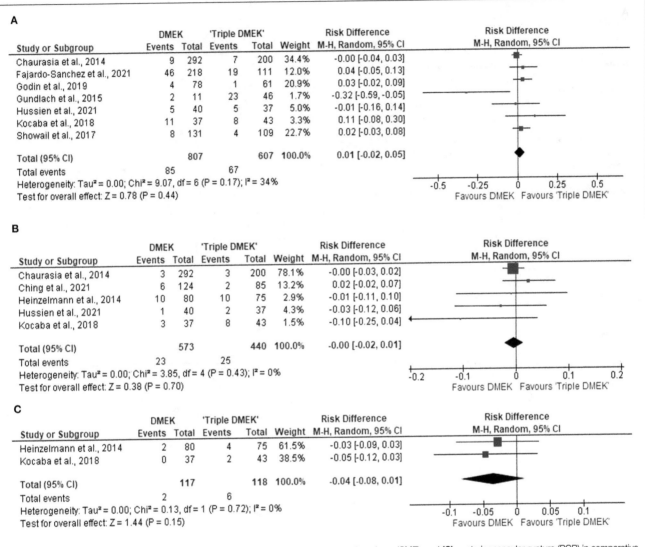

FIGURE 7 | Forest plot of other complications—**(A)** primary graft failures, **(B)** cystoid macular edema (CME), and **(C)** posterior capsular rupture (PCR) in comparative Descemet's membrane endothelial keratoplasty (DMEK) vs. "Triple DMEK" studies (comparative meta-analysis).

was 13.5% (95% CI = 5.4–21.7; **Figure 8A**). Specifically, four studies ($n = 170$ eyes) reported 20 eyes developed cataracts post-operatively within the first year, with an overall risk of 10.0% (95% CI = 0.01–0.20; **Figure 8B**) (49, 50, 52, 59), two studies ($n = 186$) reported 27 at 2 years follow-up with an overall risk of 20.5% in developing cataracts postoperatively (95% CI = −0.174 to 0.584; **Figure 8C**) (47, 58), and one study ($n = 124$) reported 21 at 5-year follow-up (68).

DISCUSSION

In this systematic review, we aimed to compare the surgical outcomes and safety between DMEK alone and "triple DMEK", with 36 studies and 11,401 eyes being included in this review. "Triple DMEK" demonstrated a better BCVA at 1-month postoperative (0.10 logMAR better) than DMEK, albeit non-significant at 3–6 months (0.07 logMAR better, $p = 0.08$). There

was no significant difference in the rate of ECL and other postoperative complications such as re-bubbling rate, primary graft failure, CME, and PCR.

Our meta-analysis suggested that DMEK has a comparable rate of postoperative re-bubbling to "triple DMEK" (RD = −0.06; 95% CI: −0.13 to 0.00; $p = 0.07$). Whilst the difference in re-bubbling rate was statistically insignificant, it is important to highlight that there was a substantial heterogeneity ($I^2 = 73\%$) among the included studies. The heterogeneity is likely ascribed to multiple confounding factors such as patient factors (e.g., age, lens status, depth of anterior chamber, and compliance to postoperative management like posturing), indication, surgeon's experience, surgical technique, choice of tamponade agent, and criteria for re-bubbling, amongst others. For instance, Dapena et al. (52) demonstrated that the graft detachment rate of DMEK reduced from 20% in the first 45 cases to 4.4% in the 91–135 cases. In addition, the use of 20% SF_6 for intraocular tamponade

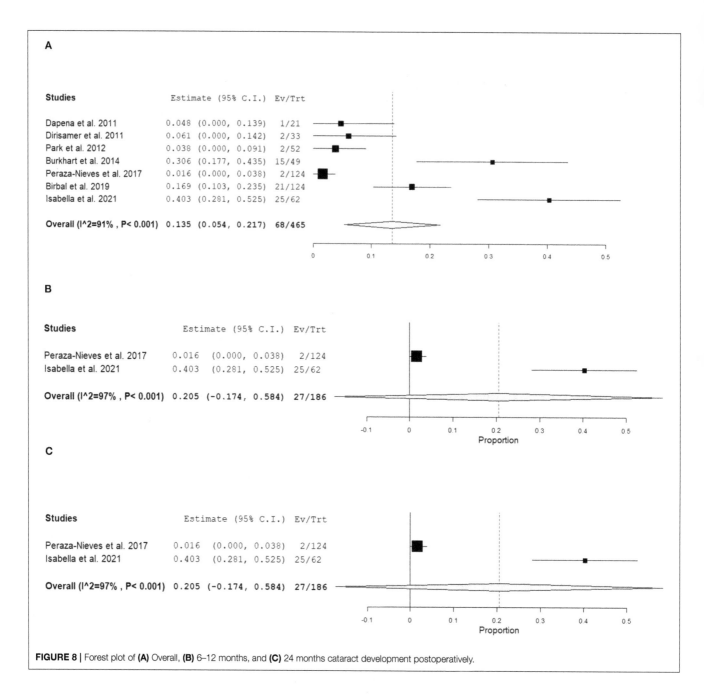

FIGURE 8 | Forest plot of **(A)** Overall, **(B)** 6–12 months, and **(C)** 24 months cataract development postoperatively.

in DMEK has been reported to reduce the rate of partial graft detachment significantly when compared with air (69).

As direct comparative studies were lacking, we performed a meta-analysis of non-comparative DMEK studies to examine the difference in reported graft detachment comparing combined cataract surgery with DMEK and standalone DMEK. We found that in DMEK alone, the overall total and partial graft detachment rates were both 8.2%. Showail et al. reported no significant difference in graft detachment between both approaches ($p = 0.78$) (43) and similar observations were made by other studies (34, 39, 41). Contrary to that, Leon et al. (22) and Gundlach et al. (35) have identified triple DMEK as an independent risk factor for early graft detachment. These studies, however, do

demonstrate significant heterogeneity with various confounders, e.g., age, surgeons' techniques, indications for DMEK and pre-operative lens status (phakic vs. pseudophakic) which may have led to varying outcomes of the studies. Our meta-analyses are also affected by several outliers which may reflect the learning curve of DMEK—e.g. surgeon 1 from Wubbels et al. (62) demonstrated a much higher rate of re-bubbling compared to other studies as the aim of the study was to establish the learning curve from the first 40 consecutive cases of DMEK performed.

In terms of visual outcome, our meta-analysis of existing literature suggests that "triple DMEK" offered better visual outcomes at 1 month postoperative, though non-statistically significant at 3–6 months postoperative. It is, however, important to note that the visual outcome at 1 month postoperative was based on only two studies, with significant weightage (96%) placed on one study (21). Chaurasia et al. (21) observed that "triple DMEK" resulted in a better BCVA (0.10 logMAR better) than DMEK at 1–6 months postoperative; however their finding was confounded by the higher rate of ocular co-morbidities and non-FECD cases in the latter group. Whilst there was limited long-term BCVA data available, a study by Schlogl et al. (42) evaluated the long-term outcomes of 250 eyes and found no significant difference between both approaches up to 5 years postoperatively. On the other hand, the ECL was shown to be comparable (0.8% difference) between the two approaches at 6 months postoperative, and the similarity was maintained at 5 years postoperative according to one study (42).

It is important to note that of the 17 studies that compared both approaches, four studies did not specify the preoperative lens status of DMEK eyes (39, 41–43), two studies reported a mix of pseudophakic and phakic DMEK surgeries but did not analyze them separately (37, 40). Similarly, Godin et al. (34) have reported a mix of pseudophakic and phakic DMEK surgeries and the group analyzed them independently. Four studies compared "triple DMEK" directly with pseudophakic DMEK surgeries (21, 36, 38, 44), whilst one study compared "triple DMEK" with phakic DMEK (35). These studies concluded that the surgical outcomes are comparable regardless of preoperative lens status and approaches, except for Crew et al. (38) who reported intraoperative hyphema was more common in "triple DMEK" compared to pseudophakic DMEK. Between approaches, both shared similar complication rates in terms of primary graft failure, CME and PCR.

One sequala to phakic DMEK is accelerated cataract progression, which may be secondary to surgical manipulation, air injection and postoperative topical steroid use (35). It was observed that cataract progression occurred in 72% of the phakic eyes post-DMEK and patients above the age of 50 have a higher risk of cataract progression when compared to younger patients (83 vs. 40%) (49). This differs from our meta-analysis where we observed a considerably lower (but highly variable) risk of cataract development in phakic eyes post-DMEK (mean 9.3%, ranged 0.4–72%) (49, 50, 52, 58, 59, 68). This could be attributed to several factors such as patient cohort and follow-up duration. The mean age of included studies reported cataract progression ranged from 50 to 68 years old, and the youngest patient included was 20 years old, whereas the oldest was 96 years old. Furthermore, follow-up duration was highly heterogeneous amongst studies as well, ranging from 6 to 60 months. These factors combined could lead to variable detection rates of cataract post-DMEK. Whilst doing a staged "DMEK followed by cataract surgery" offers several advantages such as more accurate biometry and potential ability to use a wider variety of intraocular lenses, anecdotally, staged "DMEK then cataract surgery" is less commonly performed due to the potential of damaging the in-situ DMEK (70, 71).

We have also attempted to further compare phakic DMEK (i.e., DMEK in phakic eyes) vs. "triple DMEK", and pseudophakic DMEK (i.e., DMEK in pseudophakic eyes) vs. "triple DMEK". However, this was not possible due to the lack of data and the heterogeneity in study design. Whilst we did not quantitatively evaluate the accommodation and refractive outcomes of either approach, Gundlach et al. (35) have suggested that phakic DMEK (i.e., DMEK in phakic eyes) may be beneficial in younger patients as accommodation power can be preserved. In addition, a hyperopic shift may occur following triple DMEK (65, 66), and this can be potentially avoided if cataract surgery is performed after DMEK. Given the low incidence of cataract development post-DMEK, the decision to conduct a targeted DMEK surgery or triple/sequential DMEK should consider the patient's age, preferences, refractive need, and social circumstances.

This review has several limitations. There was no RCT available in the literature that directly compared the outcome of DMEK alone and triple DMEK. In addition, the level and quality of the available evidence were mostly level 3 or 4, and low respectively, with a significant number of studies judged as having moderate to high risks of bias (**Figures 2, 3**). Furthermore, significant heterogeneity existed in the studies, such as study design, study population, surgical techniques, outcome measures, methods of reporting, and duration of follow-up; and we could not study other factors or important complications such as glaucoma (72), which was not routinely reported. Risk of bias is high as the indication for DMEK included not only FECD but also other causes of corneal endothelial dysfunction such as PBK, complex eyes and re-grafts (73), which have been shown to have a prognostic impact on the surgical outcome (21). There were also inadequate longitudinal studies that compared DMEK alone and triple DMEK, hence making it difficult to provide a meaningful comparison regarding the long-term clinical outcomes of both approaches. With the reasons cited above, whilst meta-analysis could be done with the limited literature available at this juncture, it is hard to make a conclusive assessment on these two approaches.

Overall, our review showed that "triple DMEK" and DMEK alone surgeries are largely comparable in surgical outcomes, sharing similar ECL and complication rates, except for re possible graft detachment rates (lower in DMEK only eyes), which are important clinical points that should be discussed with patients prior to surgery. Looking at the existing evidences, sequential DMEK surgery (cataract surgery followed by DMEK) in patients with endothelial disease who are above the age of 50 years old or have concurrent cataracts could potentially avoid graft detachment. Targeted DMEK alone may be considered in younger patients with no evidence of cataract formation. The decision should, however, be guided by other factors such as patient's preference, social circumstances, surgeon's experience, and availability of operating theaters. Finally, there exists gap in current literature and further adequately powered, randomized controlled trials specifically looking at the long-term outcomes of combined and staged DMEK (with cataract surgery) are warranted for a definitive comparison of the two approaches.

AUTHOR CONTRIBUTIONS

JM and MA conceptualized and supervised the study. KT, ST, and MA conducted the literature review and curated the data. KT, ST, DT, and MA conducted the formal analysis of the data. All authors wrote, reviewed, edited and approved the manuscript.

REFERENCES

1. Allen Foster. Vision 2020: the cataract challenge. *Comm Eye Health.* (2000) 13:17–9.
2. Price MO, Mehta JS, Jurkunas UV, Price FW Jr. Corneal endothelial dysfunction: Evolving understanding and treatment options. *Prog Retin Eye Res.* (2020) 100904. doi: 10.1016/j.preteyeres.2020.100904
3. Park CY, Lee JK, Gore PK, Lim CY, Chuck RS. Keratoplasty in the United States: A 10-Year Review from 2005 through 2014. *Ophthalmology.* (2015) 122:2432–42. doi: 10.1016/j.ophtha.2015.08.017
4. Ting DS, Sau CY, Srinivasan S, Ramaesh K, Mantry S, Roberts F. Changing trends in keratoplasty in the West of Scotland: a 10-year review. *Br J Ophthalmol.* (2012) 96:405–8. doi: 10.1136/bjophthalmol-2011-300244
5. Nanda GG, Alone DP. REVIEW: Current understanding of the pathogenesis of Fuchs' endothelial corneal dystrophy. *Mol Vis.* (2019) 25:295–310.
6. Vedana G, Villarreal G Jr, Jun AS. Fuchs endothelial corneal dystrophy: current perspectives. *Clin Ophthalmol.* (2016) 10:321–30. doi: 10.2147/OPTH.S83467
7. Tan D, Ang M, Arundhati A, Khor WB. Development of Selective Lamellar Keratoplasty within an Asian Corneal Transplant Program: The Singapore Corneal Transplant Study (An American Ophthalmological Society Thesis). *Trans Am Ophthalmol Soc.* (2015) 113:T10.
8. Price FW Jr, Price MO. Combined Cataract/DSEK/DMEK: Changing Expectations. *Asia Pac J Ophthalmol.* (2017) 6:388–92. doi: 10.22608/APO.2017127
9. Bose S, Ang M, Mehta JS, Tan DT, Finkelstein E. Cost-effectiveness of Descemet's stripping endothelial keratoplasty versus penetrating keratoplasty. *Ophthalmology.* (2013) 120:464–70. doi: 10.1016/j.ophtha.2012.08.024
10. Ang M, Soh Y, Htoon HM, Mehta JS, Tan D. Five-year graft survival comparing Descemet stripping automated endothelial keratoplasty and penetrating keratoplasty. *Ophthalmology.* (2016) 123:1646–52. doi: 10.1016/j.ophtha.2016.04.049
11. Melles GRJ, Lander F, Rietveld FJR. Transplantation of DESCEMET's membrane carrying viable endothelium through a small scleral incision. *Cornea.* (2002) 21:415–8. doi: 10.1097/00003226-200205000-00016
12. Melles GRJ, Ong TS, Ververs B, van der Wees J. Descemet membrane endothelial keratoplasty (DMEK). *Cornea.* (2006) 25:987–90. doi: 10.1097/01.ico.0000248385.16896.34
13. Ang M, Mehta JS, Newman SD, Han SB, Chai J, Tan D. Descemet membrane endothelial keratoplasty: preliminary results of a donor insertion pull-through technique using a donor mat device. *Am J Ophthalmol.* (2016) 171:27–34. doi: 10.1016/j.ajo.2016.08.023
14. Marques RE, Guerra PS, Sousa DC, Gonçalves AI, Quintas AM, Rodrigues W. DMEK versus DSAEK for Fuchs' endothelial dystrophy: a meta-analysis. *Eur J Ophthalmol.* (2019) 29:15–22. doi: 10.1177/1120672118757431
15. Deng SX, Lee WB, Hammersmith KM, Kuo AN, Li JY, Shen JF, et al. Descemet membrane endothelial keratoplasty: safety and outcomes: a report by the American Academy of Ophthalmology. *Ophthalmology.* (2018) 125:295–310. doi: 10.1016/j.ophtha.2017.08.015
16. Stuart AJ, Romano V, Virgili G, Shortt AJ. Descemet's membrane endothelial keratoplasty (DMEK) versus Descemet's stripping automated endothelial keratoplasty (DSAEK) for corneal endothelial failure. *Cochr Database Syst Rev.* (2018) 6. doi: 10.1002/14651858.CD012097.pub2
17. Woo JH, Ang M, Htoon HM, Tan D. Descemet membrane endothelial keratoplasty versus Descemet stripping automated endothelial keratoplasty and penetrating keratoplasty. *Am J Ophthalmol.* (2019) 207:288–303. doi: 10.1016/j.ajo.2019.06.012

18. Ang M, Wilkins MR, Mehta JS, Tan D. Descemet membrane endothelial keratoplasty. *Br J Ophthalmol.* (2016) 100:15–21. doi: 10.1136/bjophthalmol-2015-306837
19. Tan TE, Devarajan K, Seah XY, Lin SJ, Peh GSL, Cajucom-Uy HY, et al. Lamellar dissection technique for Descemet membrane endothelial keratoplasty graft preparation. *Cornea.* (2020) 39:23–9. doi: 10.1097/ICO.0000000000002090
20. Tan TE, Devarajan K, Seah XY, Lin SJ, Peh GSL, Cajucom-Uy HY, et al. Descemet membrane endothelial keratoplasty with a pull-through insertion device: surgical technique, endothelial cell loss, and early clinical results. *Cornea.* (2020) 39:558–65. doi: 10.1097/ICO.0000000000002268
21. Chaurasia S, Price FW, Jr., Gunderson L, Price MO. Descemet's membrane endothelial keratoplasty: clinical results of single versus triple procedures (combined with cataract surgery). *Ophthalmology.* (2014) 121:454–8. doi: 10.1016/j.ophtha.2013.09.032
22. Leon P, Parekh M, Nahum Y, Mimouni M, Giannaccare G, Sapigni L, et al. Factors associated with early graft detachment in primary Descemet membrane endothelial keratoplasty. *Am J Ophthalmol.* (2018) 187:117–24. doi: 10.1016/j.ajo.2017.12.014
23. Deshmukh R, Nair S, Ting DSJ, Agarwal T, Beltz J, Vajpayee RB. Graft detachments in endothelial keratoplasty. *Br J Ophthalmol.* (2021) 106:1–13. doi: 10.1136/bjophthalmol-2020-318092
24. Ang M, Ting DSJ, Kumar A, May KO, Htoon HM, Mehta JS. Descemet membrane endothelial keratoplasty in asian eyes: intraoperative and postoperative complications. *Cornea.* (2020) 39:940–5. doi: 10.1097/ICO.0000000000002302
25. Hwang HB, Lyu B, Yim HB, Lee NY. Endothelial cell loss after phacoemulsification according to different anterior chamber depths. *J Ophthalmol.* (2015) 2015:210716. doi: 10.1155/2015/210716
26. Tiew S, Lim C, Sivagnanasithiyar T. Using an excel spreadsheet to convert Snellen visual acuity to LogMAR visual acuity. *Eye.* (2020) 34:2148–49. doi: 10.1038/s41433-020-0783-6
27. Luo D, Wan X, Liu J, Tong T. Optimally estimating the sample mean from the sample size, median, mid-range, and/or mid-quartile range. *Stat Methods Med Res.* (2018) 27:1785–805. doi: 10.1177/0962280216669183
28. Wan X, Wang W, Liu J, Tong T. Estimating the sample mean and standard deviation from the sample size, median, range and/or interquartile range. *BMC Med Res Methodol.* (2014) 14:135. doi: 10.1186/1471-2288-14-135
29. Higgins JP, Savović J, Page MJ, Elbers RG, Sterne JA. Chapter 8: assessing risk of bias in a randomized trial. In: Higgins JP, Thomas J, Chandler J, Cumpston M, Li T, Page MJ, editors. *Cochrane Handbook for Systematic Reviews of Interventions version 60.* 6th ed. Chichester: Cochrane (2019) 82.
30. Sterne JA, Hernán MA, Reeves BC, Savović J, Berkman ND, Viswanathan M, et al. ROBINS-I: a tool for assessing risk of bias in non-randomised studies of interventions. *BMJ.* (2016) 355:i4919. doi: 10.1136/bmj.i4919
31. CEBM. *Oxford Centre for Evidence-based Medicine – Levels of Evidence.* (2009). Available from: https://www.cebm.net/2009/06/oxford-centre-evidence-based-medicine-levels-evidence-march-2009/ (accessed January 1, 2022).
32. Guyatt GH, Oxman AD, Vist GE, Kunz R, Falck-Ytter Y, Alonso-Coello P, et al. GRADE: an emerging consensus on rating quality of evidence and strength of recommendations. *BMJ.* (2008) 336:924–6. doi: 10.1136/bmj.39489.470347.AD
33. Higgins JPT, Thomas J, Chandler J, Cumpston M, Page MJ. Identifying and Measuring Heterogeneity. In: Deeks JJ, Higgins JPT, Altman DG, on behalf of the Cochrane Statistical Methods Group editors. *Cochrane Handbook for Systematic Reviews of Interventions Cochrane.* Chichester: Cochrane (2020).

34. Godin MR, Boehlke CS, Kim T, Gupta PK. Influence of lens status on outcomes of Descemet membrane endothelial keratoplasty. *Cornea.* (2019) 38:409–12. doi: 10.1097/ICO.0000000000001872

35. Gundlach E, Maier A-KB, Tsangaridou M-A, Riechardt AI, Brockmann T, Bertelmann E, et al. DMEK in phakic eyes: targeted therapy or highway to cataract surgery? *Graefes Arch Clin Exp Ophthalmol.* (2015) 253:909–14. doi: 10.1007/s00417-015-2956-8

36. Heinzelmann S, Maier P, Böhringer D, Hüther S, Eberwein P, Reinhard T. Cystoid macular oedema following Descemet membrane endothelial keratoplasty. *Br J Ophthalmol.* (2015) 99:98–102. doi: 10.1136/bjophthalmol-2014-305124

37. Singh SK, Sitaula S. Visual outcome of Descemet membrane endothelial keratoplasty during the learning curve in initial fifty cases. *J Ophthalmol.* (2019) 2019:5921846. doi: 10.1155/2019/5921846

38. Crews JW, Price MO, Lautert J, Feng MT, Price FW Jr. Intraoperative hyphema in Descemet membrane endothelial keratoplasty alone or combined with phacoemulsification. *J Cataract Refract Surg.* (2018) 44:198–201. doi: 10.1016/j.jcrs.2017.11.015

39. Heinzelmann S, Bohringer D, Haverkamp C, Lapp T, Eberwein P, Reinhard T, et al. Influence of postoperative intraocular pressure on graft detachment after Descemet membrane endothelial keratoplasty. *Cornea.* (2018) 37:1347–50. doi: 10.1097/ICO.0000000000001677

40. Schrittenlocher S, Bachmann B, Tiurbe AM, Tuac O, Velten K, Schmidt D, et al. Impact of preoperative visual acuity on Descemet Membrane Endothelial Keratoplasty (DMEK) outcome. *Graefes Arch Clin Exp Ophthalmol.* (2019) 257:321–9. doi: 10.1007/s00417-018-4193-4

41. Oellerich S, Baydoun L, Peraza-Nieves J, Ilyas A, Frank L, Binder PS, et al. Multicenter study of 6-month clinical outcomes after Descemet membrane endothelial keratoplasty. *Cornea.* (2017) 36:1467–76. doi: 10.1097/ICO.0000000000001374

42. Schlogl A, Tourtas T, Kruse FE, Weller JM. Long-term clinical outcome after Descemet membrane endothelial keratoplasty. *Am J Ophthalmol.* (2016) 169:218–26. doi: 10.1016/j.ajo.2016.07.002

43. Showail M, Obthani MA, Sorkin N, Einan-Lifshitz A, Boutin T, Borovik A, et al. Outcomes of the first 250 eyes of Descemet membrane endothelial keratoplasty: Canadian centre experience. *Can J Ophthalmol.* (2018) 53:510–7. doi: 10.1016/j.jcjo.2017.11.017

44. Kocaba V, Mouchel R, Fleury J, Marty A-S, Janin-Manificat H, Maucort-Boulch D, et al. Incidence of cystoid macular edema after Descemet membrane endothelial keratoplasty. *Cornea.* (2018) 37:277–82. doi: 10.1097/ICO.0000000000001501

45. Fajardo-Sanchez J, de Benito-Llopis L. Clinical outcomes of Descemet membrane endothelial keratoplasty in pseudophakic eyes compared with triple-DMEK at 1-year follow-up. *Cornea.* (2021) 40:420–4. doi: 10.1097/ICO.0000000000002636

46. Ching G, Covello AT, Bae SS, Holland S, McCarthy M, Ritenour R, et al. Incidence and outcomes of cystoid macular edema after Descemet membrane endothelial keratoplasty (DMEK) and DMEK combined with cataract surgery. *Curr Eye Res.* (2021) 46:678–82. doi: 10.1080/02713683.2020.1818260

47. Moshiri I, Karimi-Golkar D, Schrittenlocher S, Cursiefen C, Bachmann B. Outcomes of pseudophakic, phakic, and triple DMEK. *Cornea.* (2021) 40:1253–7. doi: 10.1097/ICO.0000000000002723

48. Hussien A, Elmassry A, Ghaith AA, Goweida MBB. Descemet's membrane endothelial keratoplasty and phacoemulsification: combined versus sequential surgery. *J Curr Ophthalmol.* (2021) 33:277–84. doi: 10.4103/joco.joco_188_20

49. Burkhart ZN, Feng MT, Price FW, Jr., Price MO. One-year outcomes in eyes remaining phakic after Descemet membrane endothelial keratoplasty. *J Cataract Refract Surg.* (2014) 40:430–4. doi: 10.1016/j.jcrs.2013.08.047

50. Parker J, Dirisamer M, Naveiras M, Tse WH, van Dijk K, Frank LE, et al. Outcomes of Descemet membrane endothelial keratoplasty in phakic eyes. *J Cataract Refract Surg.* (2012) 38:871–7. doi: 10.1016/j.jcrs.2011.11.038

51. Birbal RS, Tong CM, Dapena I, Parker JS, Parker JS, Oellerich S, et al. Clinical outcomes of Descemet membrane endothelial keratoplasty in eyes with a glaucoma drainage device. *Am J Ophthalmol.* (2019) 199:150–8. doi: 10.1016/j.ajo.2018.11.014

52. Dapena I, Ham L, Droutsas K, van Dijk K, Moutsouris K, Melles GR. Learning curve in Descemet's membrane endothelial keratoplasty:

53. first series of 135 consecutive cases. *Ophthalmology.* (2011) 118:2147–54. doi: 10.1016/j.ophtha.2011.03.037

53. Ham L, Dapena I, Moutsouris K, Balachandran C, Frank LE, van Dijk K, et al. Refractive change and stability after Descemet membrane endothelial keratoplasty: effect of corneal dehydration-induced hyperopic shift on intraocular lens power calculation. *J Catar Refract Surg.* (2011) 37:1455–64. doi: 10.1016/j.jcrs.2011.02.033

54. Satue M, Idoipe M, Gavin A, Romero-Sanz M, Liarakos VS, Mateo A, et al. Early changes in visual quality and corneal structure after DMEK: does DMEK approach optical quality of a healthy cornea? *J Ophthalmol.* (2018) 2018:2012560. doi: 10.1155/2018/2012560

55. Gorovoy MS. DMEK complications. *Cornea.* (2014) 33:101–4. doi: 10.1097/ICO.0000000000000023

56. van Dijk K, Parker J, Liarakos VS, Ham L, Frank LE, Melles GR. Incidence of irregular astigmatism eligible for contact lens fitting after Descemet membrane endothelial keratoplasty. *J Cataract Refract Surg.* (2013) 39:1036–46. doi: 10.1016/j.jcrs.2013.02.051

57. Baydoun L, Ham L, Borderie V, Dapena I, Hou J, Frank LE, et al. Endothelial survival after Descemet membrane endothelial keratoplasty: effect of surgical indication and graft adherence status. *JAMA Ophthalmol.* (2015) 133:1277–85. doi: 10.1001/jamaophthalmol.2015.3064

58. Peraza-Nieves J, Baydoun L, Dapena I, Ilyas A, Frank LE, Luceri S, et al. Two-year clinical outcome of 500 consecutive cases undergoing Descemet membrane endothelial keratoplasty. *Cornea.* (2017) 36:655–60. doi: 10.1097/ICO.0000000000001176

59. Dirisamer M, Ham L, Dapena I, Moutsouris K, Droutsas K, van Dijk K, et al. Efficacy of Descemet membrane endothelial keratoplasty: clinical outcome of 200 consecutive cases after a learning curve of 25 cases. *Arch Ophthalmol.* (2011) 129:1435–43. doi: 10.1001/archophthalmol.2011.195

60. van Dijk K, Rodriguez-Calvo-de-Mora M, van Esch H, Frank L, Dapena I, Baydoun L, et al. Two-year refractive outcomes after Descemet membrane endothelial keratoplasty. *Cornea.* (2016) 35:1548–55. doi: 10.1097/ICO.0000000000001022

61. Ham L, Dapena I, Liarakos VS, Baydoun L, van Dijk K, Ilyas A, et al. Midterm results of Descemet membrane endothelial keratoplasty: 4 to 7 years clinical outcome. *Am J Ophthalmol.* (2016) 171:113–21. doi: 10.1016/j.ajo.2016.08.038

62. Wubbels RJ, Remeijer L, Engel A, van Rooij J. The learning curve for Descemet membrane endothelial keratoplasty performed by two experienced corneal surgeons: a consecutive series of 40 cases. *Acta Ophthalmol.* (2020) 98:74–9. doi: 10.1111/aos.14152

63. Schoenberg ED, Price FW, Jr., Miller J, McKee Y, Price MO. Refractive outcomes of Descemet membrane endothelial keratoplasty triple procedures (combined with cataract surgery). *J Cataract Refract Surg.* (2015) 41:1182–9. doi: 10.1016/j.jcrs.2014.09.042

64. Laaser K, Bachmann BO, Horn FK, Cursiefen C, Kruse FE. Descemet membrane endothelial keratoplasty combined with phacoemulsification and intraocular lens implantation: advanced triple procedure. *Am J Ophthalmol.* (2012) 154:47–55.e2. doi: 10.1016/j.ajo.2012.01.020

65. Cheung AY, Chachare DY, Eslani M, Schneider J, Nordlund ML. Tomographic changes in eyes with hyperopic shift after triple Descemet membrane endothelial keratoplasty. *J Cataract Refract Surg.* (2018) 44:738–44. doi: 10.1016/j.jcrs.2018.04.040

66. Fritz M, Grewing V, Böhringer D, Lapp T, Maier P, Reinhard T, et al. Avoiding hyperopic surprises after Descemet membrane endothelial keratoplasty in fuchs dystrophy eyes by assessing corneal shape. *Am J Ophthalmol.* (2019) 197:1–6. doi: 10.1016/j.ajo.2018.08.052

67. Augustin VA, Weller JM, Kruse FE, Tourtas T. Can we predict the refractive outcome after triple Descemet membrane endothelial keratoplasty? *Eur J Ophthalmol.* (2019) 29:165–70. doi: 10.1177/1120672118785282

68. Birbal RS, Ni Dhubhghaill S, Bourgonje VJA, Hanko J, Ham L, Jager MJ, et al. Five-year graft survival and clinical outcomes of 500 consecutive cases after Descemet membrane endothelial keratoplasty. *Cornea.* (2020) 39:290–7. doi: 10.1097/ICO.0000000000002120

69. Botsford B, Vedana G, Cope L, Yiu SC, Jun AS. Comparison of 20% sulfur hexafluoride with air for intraocular tamponade in Descemet membrane endothelial keratoplasty (DMEK). *Arq Bras Oftalmol.* (2016) 79:299–302. doi: 10.5935/0004-2749.20160086

70. Bailey TC, Zaidman GW, Mirochnik B, Naadimuthu R. The incidence of cataract extraction following corneal transplantation in young and middle-aged patients. *Invest Ophthalmol Vis Sci.* (2009) 50:2207.

71. Chaurasia S, Ramappa M, Sangwan V. Cataract surgery after Descemet stripping endothelial keratoplasty. *Indian J Ophthalmol.* (2012) 60:572–4. doi: 10.4103/0301-4738.103803

72. Ang M, Sng CCA. Descemet membrane endothelial keratoplasty and glaucoma. *Curr Opin Ophthalmol.* (2018) 29:178–84. doi: 10.1097/ICU.0000000000000454

73. Ang M, Tan D. Anterior segment reconstruction with artificial iris and Descemet membrane endothelial keratoplasty: a staged surgical approach. *Br J Ophthalmol.* (2021). doi: 10.1136/bjophthalmol-2020-317906

8

Cost of Myopia Correction: A Systematic Review

Li Lian Foo [1,2,3], Carla Lanca [2,4,5], Chee Wai Wong [1,2,3], Daniel Ting [1,2,3], Ecosse Lamoureux [2,3], Seang-Mei Saw [2,3,6] and Marcus Ang [1,2,3]*

[1] Singapore National Eye Centre, Singapore, Singapore, [2] Singapore Eye Research Institute, Singapore, Singapore, [3] Duke–NUS Medical School, National University of Singapore, Singapore, Singapore, [4] Escola Superior de Tecnologia da Saúde de Lisboa (ESTeSL), Instituto Politécnico de Lisboa, Lisboa, Portugal, [5] Comprehensive Health Research Center (CHRC), Escola Nacional de Saúde Pública, Universidade Nova de Lisboa, Lisboa, Portugal, [6] NUS Saw Swee Hock School of Public Health, Singapore, Singapore

*Correspondence:
Marcus Ang
marcus.ang@singhealth.com.sg

Myopia is one of the leading causes of visual impairment globally. Despite increasing prevalence and incidence, the associated cost of treatment remains unclear. Health care spending is a major concern in many countries and understanding the cost of myopia correction is the first step eluding to the overall cost of myopia treatment. As cost of treatment will reduce the burden of cost of illness, this will aid in future cost-benefit analysis and the allocation of healthcare resources, including considerations in integrating eye care (refractive correction with spectacles) into universal health coverage (UHC). We performed a systematic review to determine the economic costs of myopia correction. However, there were few studies for direct comparison. Costs related to myopia correction were mainly direct with few indirect costs. Annual prevalence-based direct costs for myopia ranged from $14-26 (USA), $56 (Iran) and $199 (Singapore) per capita, respectively (population: 274.63 million, 75.15 million and 3.79 million, respectively). Annually, the direct costs of contact lens were $198.30-$378.10 while spectacles and refractive surgeries were $342.50 and $19.10, respectively. This review provides an insight to the cost of myopia correction. Myopia costs are high from nation-wide perspectives because of the high prevalence of myopia, with contact lenses being the more expensive option. Without further interventions, the burden of illness of myopia will increase substantially with the projected increase in prevalence worldwide. Future studies will be necessary to generate more homogenous cost data and provide a complete picture of the global economic cost of myopia.

Keywords: myopia, costs, spectacles, contact lenses, refractive surgeries declaration

INTRODUCTION

Myopia is one of the leading causes of visual impairment in the world (1, 2). The prevalence of myopia ranges from 15 to 49% in adult populations, and ranges from 20 to 90% in children, adolescents and young adults (3–7). Studies estimate that myopia will affect 50% (4.7 billion) of the world's population by 2050, with 10% (1 billion) having high myopia ($\leq$-5.00 Dioptres) (8–10) Correction of myopia with spectacles, contact lenses and refractive surgeries therefore play an increasingly important role in society, as uncorrected myopia results in reduction of visual acuity leading to impaired visual functioning (11).

However, there are significant costs associated with optical correction, treatment to retard myopia progression and treatment of myopia related complications, including pathologic myopia, cataract, glaucoma and retinal detachment (12–16). With increasing demand for the limited healthcare resources globally, an understanding of the economic cost associated with the treatment of myopia is important for further cost-benefit analysis and policy making decisions. This will aid and justify in the allocation of invaluable healthcare resources to the treatment of myopia, in order to reduce the economic burden of this illness.

We aim to perform an evidence-based review of the economic costs associated with the correction of myopia.

SOURCES AND METHODS OF LITERATURE SEARCH

We conducted a systematic review of relevant literature articles in accordance with the Preferred Reporting Items for Systematic Reviews and Meta-analysis (PRISMA) guidelines (17). Several electronic databases (PubMed, ScienceDirect, Cochrane Library, and Web of Science databases) were searched to identify English language articles up to 29 February 2020 on costs associated with myopia correction treatment. The search used the keywords "myopia," "short-sightedness" or "near-sightedness" combined with "cost" or "economic burden." Original full-text articles in English were included if costs were quantified in relation to myopia correction, including: myopia correction (spectacles, contact lenses, refractive surgeries). 8,492 titles were retrieved through database searching. Forty five relevant records were reviewed with 12 records excluded (9 duplicates and 3 with no full-text available). Fifteen full-text articles were assessed for eligibility with 2 non-English articles excluded (articles in German). Articles that did not fulfill the inclusion criteria were excluded. Five eligible full-text articles were included in this review (18–22). The review article selection process is illustrated as a flowchart in **Figure 1**. The Asian studies comprised of 2 from Singapore while the non-Asian studies comprised of one from each of the following countries: United States of America (USA), Iran and Spain.

A 20-items Consensus Health Economic Criteria (CHEC)-extended checklist was used to evaluate the overall quality of included studies (23, 24). Scoring was performed by assigning a score of 1 (yes), 0 (no), 2 (not applicable) to each item and the total scores were summed to generate the overall quality score (0–100%). The total quality score for each study was categorized into low, moderate, good and excellent with cut-off value of <50, 51–75, 76–95 and >95, respectively. Only moderate, good and excellent quality studies were included as higher scores denote lower risk of bias. Two independent reviewers conducted the assessment (LLF and CL) and the interrater-agreement was evaluated using κ from STATA/IC 11.1 (25). The interpretation of the κ was based on a scale which indicates poor, slight, fair, moderate, substantial and perfect agreement with κ levels <0.0, 0.0–0.20, 0.21–0.40, 0.41–0.60, 0.61–0.80 and ≥0.81, respectively (26). Of the included studies,

4 were good in quality (76.5–95) and 1 was excellent (100). The interrater-reliability κ was moderate in 1 study (0.44), substantial in 2 studies (0.63, 0.64) and perfect in 2 studies (1, 1).

Examples of costs assessed included optical correction devices/procedures (spectacles, contact lenses, refractive surgeries), visits to professional services (transportation and fees) and time spent and loss of productivity while seeking treatment.

All costs are quoted in US dollars ($). Conversion rate used was Euro to USD = 1:1.12 (22, 27) and Pound sterling to USD = 1:1.31 (28), using average 2019 exchange rates (29).

RESULTS

The costs for myopia correction are shown in **Table 1**.

The average direct costs of myopia correction in Singapore children aged 12–17 years from the SCORM study (Singapore Cohort study of the Risk factors of Myopia) were $147.80 per year per myopia patient, $82.10 per pair of spectacles and $378.10 per year for contact lenses (18).

In Singapore adults aged ≥40 years, the mean direct cost of myopia correction was $709 per year per patient. This estimate translates into an annual economic burden of $755 million in Singapore. Refractive correction, comprising of optometry visits, spectacles and contact lenses, were the most significant, accounting for 65.2% of the total costs (19). The remaining costs comprise of refractive surgeries and complications related to it as well as contact lens use.

In USA, the annual direct country-wide cost of correcting distance vision impairment was estimated to be between $3.9 and $7.2 billion, with $780 million per annum for persons >age 65 years (33). The National Health and Nutrition Examination Survey (NHANES) was an ongoing, nationally representative survey of 14,203 participants aged ≥ 12 years (32, 33). The cost calculations were based on single-vision spectacles, without including other refractive correction options. Hence, this cost would be much higher if contact lenses and refractive surgeries were taken into account. As the annual costs from the earlier Singapore study were based on all forms of corrections, direct comparison is inequitable. In addition, due to the study's methodology for distant vision correction, subjects with pure astigmatism without myopia were also included in the cost calculations.

In two other studies (21, 22), the costs of refractive correction were computed by including other refractive errors (hyperopia and astigmatism). While the costs of each modality for myopia correction alone could not be determined, they provide insights to the general cost for refractive correction in the country.

In a Spanish study, the direct cost of spectacles, contact lenses and LASIK were evaluated (22). It was reported that the total direct (medical and non-medical) cost over 10, 20, and 30 years (5% discount rate) for contact lens was $3019.64; 4723.21; 5779.46, LASIK was $3341.96; 3368.75; 3385.71 and spectacles was $1091.07; 1623.21; 1960.71 (22). This was a

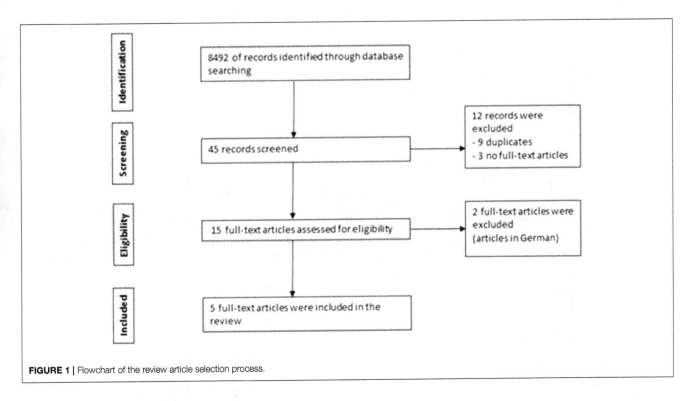

FIGURE 1 | Flowchart of the review article selection process.

small study of 40 subjects from one city in Alicante, with 80% myopes (12.5% hyperopes and 42.5% astigmatic). This study was conducted in 2002 and hence costs might not be representative of the current market, particularly the cost of cleaning and fitting contact lens and transport system with technological advancements.

In a recent Iranian study, 120 subjects aged ≥ 23 years were interviewed in a hospital and the lifetime direct costs of spectacles, contact lenses and refractive surgeries were $9373.50, $5203.10, and $568.10, respectively (21). The annual direct costs of refractive correction per patient and for each of the three modalities were $309, $342.50, $198.30, and $19.10, respectively. Annually, direct cost of myopia correction was estimated to be $4.2 billion in Iran. Indirect costs in this study were estimated using the human capital approach, by ascertaining lost productivity due to the complication, maintenance, repair and travel costs as a measure of patient's and caregiver's lost earnings (34). Annually, the indirect costs were $12112.10, $3045.20, and $113.60, respectively with the main bulk contributed by patient's and caregiver's opportunity cost. However, it was not clear from the study regarding the basis and role of caregiver's costs calculation in optical correction and no justification was offered for the high indirect costs from spectacles, considering it is least prone to complications. In addition, cost calculations for each refractive correction modality were generalized to all forms of refractive errors, it was challenging to estimate the cost generated from myopia only.

Out of the three groups of myopia correction modalities reported in the studies (18, 21, 22), contact lens and spectacles appeared to be generally more costly than refractive surgeries

(**Figure 2**). Annually, the direct costs of contact lens and spectacles were $198.30-$378.10 and $342.50, respectively while refractive surgeries was $19.10 (18, 21).

In Singapore, while the annual direct cost of myopia correction to the individual is the lowest compared to diabetic retinopathy and wet age-related macular degeneration (AMD) (18, 19, 35, 36), the nation's annual direct cost of myopia correction ($755 million) alone far exceeded other ocular diseases including acute primary angle closure glaucoma ($0.26-0.29 million), dry eyes ($1.51-1.52 million) and wet AMD ($96.8-120.7 million) (**Table 2**) (18, 19, 35, 36, 41, 42).

DISCUSSION

In this review, we found 5 studies addressing the cost of myopia correction (18, 19, 21, 22, 33), which are generally direct costs from spectacles, contact lens and refractive surgeries. The per capita annual cost of myopia correction was low in USA, moderate in Iran and high in Singapore. Indirect costs in myopia correction are mainly related to complications, particularly with contact lens use, including cost of treatment, loss of productivity secondary to complications and its associated travel costs (21). We found that the annual direct costs of myopia correction in USA, Iran and Singapore were substantial at $3.9-7.2 billion, $4.2 billion and $755 million, respectively. This translated to $14-26 (USA), $56 (Iran) and $199 (Singapore) per capita, respectively (population: 274.63 million, 75.15 million and 3.79 million, respectively) (19, 21, 43). Most costs related to myopia correction were direct costs, with contact lens appearing to be generally more costly compared to other modalities.

TABLE 1 | Summary table of reviewed articles (treatment of Myopia-Myopia correction: $n = 5$).

No	References	Year	Country	Type of study	Costs	Sample size (n)	Age (Years)	Method of ascertaining cost	Prevalence of Myopia (%)	Direct cost ($)	Indirect cost ($)
									Treatment of Myopia (Myopia correction)		
1	Ruiz-Moreno and Roura (27)	2009	Singapore	Cross-sectional study	Myopia correction	301	12–17	Parent and Self questionnaire	NA	Annual direct cost Mean (Per patient) = $147.8 ± 209.1 (CI, $124.3–172.1) Median (Per patient) = $83.3 Mean cost per pair of spectacles $82.1 ± 40.8 (CI, $77.8–86.5) Mean annual cost of contact lenses $378.1 ± 377.1 (CI, $281.4–474.6).	NA
2	Zheng YF et al. (30)	2013	Singapore	Cross-sectional study	Myopia correction	113	52.6 ± 7.8	Questionnaire	Age 0–4 = 10% 5–9 = 30% 10–14 = 60% 15–24 = 80% 25–39 = 90% 40–49 = 45% 50–59 = 35% 60–80+ =30%	Annual direct cost Mean (Per patient) = $709 Annual direct cost Singapore = $755 million Urban Asia = $328 billion Lifetime per capita cost (disease of 0–80 years) $232–17,020	
3	Vitale S et al. (31)	2006	USA	Cross-sectional	Myopia correction	13211	≥12	NHANES and fees schedule and expenditure data	NA	Annual direct cost All = $3.9–7.2 billion Persons age > 65 = $780 million	NA
4	Morgan et al. (7)	2002	Spain	Cross-sectional	Myopia correction	40 (80% Myopia)	Mean 32	Questionnaire markov model	NA	Total direct cost* (10, 20 and 30 years) LASIK = $ 3341.96; 3368.75; 3385.71 Spectacles = $ 1091.07; 1623.21; 1960.71 Contact lens = $ 3019.64; 4723.21; 5779.46	NA

(Continued)

TABLE 1 | Continued

No	References	Year	Country	Type of study	Costs	Sample size (n)	Age (Years)	Method of ascertaining cost	Prevalence of Myopia (%)	Direct cost ($)	Indirect cost ($)
										Treatment of Myopia (Myopia correction)	
5	Malec et al. (32)	2018	Iran	Cross-sectional	Myopia correction	120 (60.83% Myopia)	≥23	Interview	Age < 14 = 3.6% 15–19 = 16.5% 20–29 = 22.0% >60 = 32.8%	Total annual direct cost* Spectacles = $342.5 ± 8.41 Contact lenses = $198.30 ± 0.12 Refractive surgery = $19.10 ± 1.2 Lifetime direct cost* Spectacles = $9373.5 ± 230.1 Contact lenses = $5203.10 ± 256.3 Refractive surgery = $568.1 ± 64.6 Annual direct cost* Mean (Per patient) = $309 Annual direct cost All ages = $4.2 billion Persons age < 14 = $196 million Persons age 15–19 = $337 million Persons age 20–29 = $3043 million Persons age > 60 = $628.55 million Annual and lifetime total costs* (direct and indirect) Spectacles = $12454.6; 340754.10, Contact lenses = $3243.5; 84965.30 Refractive surgery = $132.7; 3357.20	Total annual indirect cost* Spectacles = $12112.10 Contact lenses = $3045.20 Refractive surgery = $113.60 Lifetime indirect cost* Spectacles = $331380.60 Contact lenses = $79762.20 Refractive surgery = $2789.10

*Include all types of refractive error (myopia, hyperopia and astigmatism).

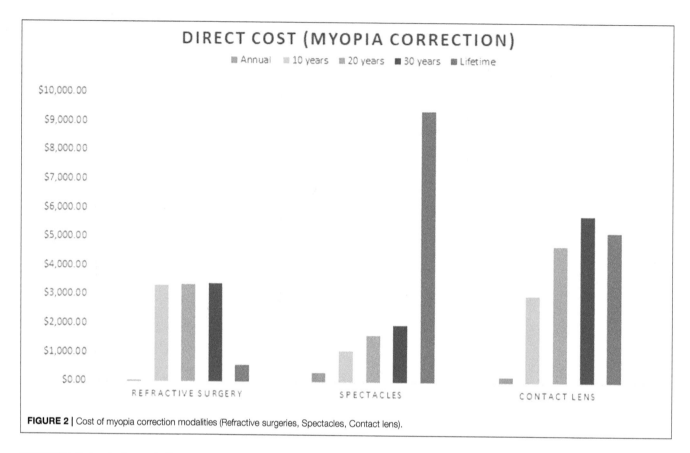

FIGURE 2 | Cost of myopia correction modalities (Refractive surgeries, Spectacles, Contact lens).

TABLE 2 | Cost of ocular diseases in Singapore.

Eye diseases in Singapore	Annual direct cost in Singapore ($)	Mean annual direct cost per patient ($)
Diabetic retinopathy (37)	NA	$863.65–2660.15
Acute primary angle closure glaucoma (38)	$0.26–0.29 million	NA
Dry eyes (39)	$1.51–1.52 million*	NA
Wet AMD (40)	$96.8–120.7 million	$6902.20
Myopia correction (27, 30)	$755 million	$147.80–709

*Singapore National Eye Centre only.

We found few studies to adequately address this topic and limited studies using similar costs definitions for comparison. Firstly, there was a limited representation of studies globally, with 2 from Asia (Singapore) and 3 from Europe (Spain), USA and Middle East (Iran), respectively. Secondly, different methodologies and cost definitions were used for cost calculations and many studies did not assessed indirect costs in detail.

The World Health Organization (WHO) considers spectacles or contact lenses as functioning interventions (44), with spectacles being also considered as an assistive device which is part of the WHO Priority Assistive Products List (45). As health care spending is a major concern in many countries, understanding the cost of myopia correction is the first step eluding to the overall cost of myopia treatment. Moreover, among the worldwide population with moderate or severe vision

impairment, uncorrected refractive error was the highest at 116.3 to 123.7 million (46, 47), with the cost of coverage gap for unaddressed refractive error and cataract estimated to be $14.3 billion globally (45). As cost of treatment will reduce the burden of cost of illness, this will aid in future cost-benefit analysis and the allocation of healthcare resources, including considerations in integrating eye care (refractive correction with spectacles) into universal health coverage (UHC) (45). This is particularly important in Asian developing countries where there is high prevalence of myopia with low accessibility to spectacles.

Although the cost of myopia to an individual may not be very high, the cost of myopia to the nation is one of the highest as the prevalence of myopia is higher than many other diseases. The high prevalence of myopia plays an important role in determining the economic cost of the treatment of myopia in each country. In East and Southeast Asia, the prevalence of myopia was reported to be as high as 80–90% in adolescents of age of 17–18 (7). In contrast, 20–40% was reported in developed western countries (7, 20, 40, 48–50). Hence while the magnitude of direct cost of refractive correction was greater in USA and Iran than in Singapore, the per capita cost was lesser at $14–26 and $56 vs. $199 (19, 31).

Other factors that could account for variation in costs include country-specific costs, different methodologies, study subject's characteristics (including age), timeline, varying costs of living and socioeconomic status. However, due to limited studies available, it would be challenging to explore the influence of these factors. As the governments in most countries are unlikely to be able to monitor spectacle or contact lens sales, future cost data can be obtained by considering cross-sectional rapid assessment protocols, targeting for instance high schools.

In Singapore, although the annual direct cost of myopia correction to the individual is lowest amongst diabetic retinopathy and wet AMD (18, 19, 35, 36), the nation's annual direct cost of myopia correction alone far exceeded other ocular diseases including acute primary angle closure glaucoma, dry eyes and AMD (18, 19, 35, 36, 41, 42). This finding is not surprising and is attributed to the high prevalence of myopia in the country, with myopia expected to remain as the most common ocular condition with 2.393 million cases in 2040 (51).

Out of the three groups of myopia correction modalities, contact lens and spectacles seemed to be generally more costly than refractive surgery (18, 21, 22), with the exception of 1 study which did not justify the inclusion of high patient and caregiver opportunity costs from spectacles use (21). This is excluding the indirect costs of contact lens related complications (e.g., infective keratitis), including cost of treatment, loss of productivity secondary to complications and its associated travel costs. However, this cost is expected to be dynamic in view of technological advancement, economic forces, occupational and recreational requirements, individuals paying premium for factors such as aesthetics and quality as well as free or subsidized refractive correction by the government.

Contact lenses were mainly prescribed for the correction of myopia, with proportion as high as 94% (52). The three key cost components of contact lens wear are the professional fees, the cost of lenses and the cost of lens care solutions (38, 39). Spherical lenses have the lowest overall cost, followed by toric and multifocal lenses (39), with the true cost of lens wear (cost-per-wear) dependent on the frequency of use (38, 39). Generally, daily replacement contact lenses are more cost-effective on a part-time usage, while reusable lenses are more cost-effective on a full-time usage (38). With contact lens gaining popularity among the teenagers and young adults (52), together with the high prevalence of myopia in this age-group (3–7), the nation-wide costs of contact lenses are expected to rise in the near future.

We have reviewed the costs of optical correction of myopia. However, since the cost and burden to the nation is high, treatments to slow myopia progression and measures to prevent myopia and high myopia (including outdoor programs) are important to reduce the prevalence of myopia and subsequent costs of illness, including burden related to its complications.

Atropine eyedrops have shown strong evidence in myopia control while Orthokeratology, myopic defocus multizone contact lenses and spectacles have shown some effect (30, 37, 53–57). However, there is currently no literature reporting the treatment costs generated from Atropine use in children (53, 54). The use of myopia control treatment modalities will inevitably incur costs including equipment, professional services and the management of complications, particularly infective keratitis with contact lens use. Further studies, including cost-effectiveness randomized control trials of treatments for myopia progression will be necessary to evaluate this knowledge deficit.

LIMITATIONS

For myopia correction, differentiating costs of optometry visits and refractive correction devices was difficult due to difference in studie's methodology. Another limitation includes the presence recall and non-response bias from retrospective design studies and the use of questionnaires/interviews. In addition, cost data reported in older studies may not be a reliable reflection of today's costs, due to various economic factors. Details of indirect costs were lacking. There were few studies available in the literature with limited representation globally.

FURTHER STUDIES

Future studies will be necessary to generate a more homogenous cost data and provide a more complete picture of the global economic cost of myopia treatment. These include cost of illness analysis, programmatic costs of spectacles correction in rural areas by non-governmental organizations and cost-effectiveness randomized control trials of treatments for myopia progression.

CONCLUSION

Our systematic review provides insight on the costs of myopia correction. Annual prevalence-based direct costs for myopia correction are substantial, ranging from US$14–26 (USA), $56 (Iran) to $199 (Singapore) per capita. In Singapore, the annual direct cost of myopia correction alone far exceeded the costs of other ocular diseases including acute primary angle closure glaucoma, dry eyes and wet AMD due to high prevalence of disease. Without further interventions, the economic burden of illness of myopia will increase substantially with the projected increase in prevalence worldwide. Hence, myopia control treatment in children and measures to prevent myopia and high myopia will play an increasingly important role to reduce prevalence and costs of illness. Future studies will be necessary to generate a more homogenous cost data and provide a complete picture of the global economic cost of myopia.

AUTHOR CONTRIBUTIONS

LF, CL, and S-MS: conception and design of study. LF, CL, CW, DT, EL, and MA: analysis and/or interpretation of data. LF, CL, S-MS, and MA: drafting the manuscript. CW, DT, EL, S-MS, and MA: revising the manuscript critically for important intellectual content. All authors contributed to the article and approved the submitted version.

REFERENCES

1. Pararajasegaram R. VISION 2020-the right to sight: from strategies to action. *Am J Ophthalmol.* (1999) 128:359–60. doi: 10.1016/S0002-9394(99)00251-2

2. Holden BA, Wilson DA, Jong M, Sankaridurg P, Fricke TR, Smith EL, et al. Myopia: a growing global problem with sight-threatening complications. *Community eye health.* (2015) 28:35.

3. Pan CW, Ramamurthy D, Saw SM. Worldwide prevalence and risk factors for myopia. *Ophthalmic Physiol Opt.* (2012) 32:3–16. doi: 10.1111/j.1475-1313.2011.00884.x

4. Lim DH, Han J, Chung TY, Kang S, Yim HW, Epidemiologic Survey Committee of the Korean Ophthalmologic Society. The high prevalence of myopia in Korean children with influence of parental refractive errors: the 2008-2012 Korean national health and nutrition examination survey. *PLoS ONE.* (2018) 13:e0207690. doi: 10.1371/journal.pone.0207690

5. Belete GT, Anbesse DH, Tsegaye AT, Hussen MS. Prevalence and associated factors of myopia among high school students in Gondar town, northwest Ethiopia, 2016. *Clinical optometry.* (2017) 9:11–8. doi: 10.2147/OPTO.S120485

6. Xie Z, Long Y, Wang J, Li Q, Zhang Q. Prevalence of myopia and associated risk factors among primary students in Chongqing: multilevel modeling. *BMC Ophthalmol.* (2020) 20:146. doi: 10.1186/s12886-020-01410-3

7. Morgan IG, Ohno-Matsui K, Saw SM. Myopia. *Lancet.* (2012) 379:1739–48. doi: 10.1016/S0140-6736(12)60272-4

8. Modjtahedi BS, Ferris FL, Hunter DG, Fong DS. Public health burden and potential interventions for myopia. *Ophthalmology.* (2018) 125:628–30. doi: 10.1016/j.ophtha.2018.01.033

9. Holden BA, Fricke TR, Wilson DA, Jong M, Naidoo KS, Sankaridurg P, et al. Global prevalence of myopia and high myopia and temporal trends from 2000 through 2050. *Ophthalmology.* (2016) 123:1036–42. doi: 10.1016/j.ophtha.2016.01.006

10. Chia A, Lu QS. Tan D. Five-year clinical trial on atropine for the treatment of myopia 2: myopia control with atropine 001% eyedrops. *Ophthalmology.* (2016) 123:391–9. doi: 10.1016/j.ophtha.2015.07.004

11. Naidoo KS, Fricke TR, Frick KD, Jong M, Naduvilath TJ, Resnikoff S, et al. Potential lost productivity resulting from the global burden of myopia: systematic review, meta-analysis, and modeling. *Ophthalmology.* (2019) 126:338–46. doi: 10.1016/j.ophtha.2018.10.029

12. Marcus MW, de Vries MM, Junoy Montolio FG, Jansonius NM. Myopia as a risk factor for open-angle glaucoma: a systematic review and meta-analysis. *Ophthalmology.* (2011) 118:1989–94. doi: 10.1016/j.ophtha.2011.03.012

13. Bechrakis NE, Dimmer A. [Rhegmatogenous retinal detachment: Epidemiology and risk factors]. *Ophthalmologe.* (2018) 115:163–78. doi: 10.1007/s00347-017-0647-z

14. Praveen MR, Vasavada AR, Jani UD, Trivedi RH, Choudhary PK. Prevalence of cataract type in relation to axial length in subjects with high myopia and emmetropia in an Indian population. *Am J Ophthalmol.* (2008) 145:176–81. doi: 10.1016/j.ajo.2007.07.043

15. Saw SM, Gazzard G, Shih-Yen EC, Chua WH. Myopia and associated pathological complications. *Ophthalmic Physiol Opt.* (2005) 25:381–91. doi: 10.1111/j.1475-1313.2005.00298.x

16. Saw SM, Matsumura S, Hoang QV. Prevention and management of myopia and myopic pathology. *Invest Ophthalmol Vis Sci.* (2019) 60:488–99. doi: 10.1167/iovs.18-25221

17. Moher D, Liberati A, Tetzlaff J, Altman DG, Group P. Preferred reporting items for systematic reviews and meta-analyses: the PRISMA statement. *J Clin Epidemiol.* (2009) 62:1006–12. doi: 10.1016/j.jclinepi.2009.06.005

18. Lim MC, Gazzard G, Sim EL, Tong L, Saw SM. Direct costs of myopia in Singapore. *Eye.* (2009) 23:1086–9. doi: 10.1038/eye.2008.225

19. Zheng YF, Pan CW, Chay J, Wong TY, Finkelstein E, Saw SM. The economic cost of myopia in adults aged over 40 years in Singapore. *Invest Ophthalmol Vis Sci.* (2013) 54:7532–7. doi: 10.1167/iovs.13-12795

20. Vitale S, Ellwein L, Cotch MF, Ferris FL, Sperduto R. Prevalence of refractive error in the United States, 1999-2004. *Arch Ophthalmol.* (2008) 126:1111–9. doi: 10.1001/archopht.126.8.1111

21. Mohammadi SF, Alinia C, Tavakkoli M, Lashay A, Chams H. Refractive surgery: the most cost-saving technique in refractive errors correction. *Int J Ophthalmol.* (2018) 11:1013–9.

22. Berdeaux G, Alio JL, Martinez JM, Magaz S, Badia X. Socioeconomic aspects of laser *in situ* keratomileusis, eyeglasses, and contact lenses in mild to moderate myopia. *J Cataract Refract Surg.* (2002) 28:1914–23. doi: 10.1016/S0886-3350(02)01496-7

23. Evers S, Goossens M, de Vet H, van Tulder M, Ament A. Criteria list for assessment of methodological quality of economic evaluations: consensus on health economic criteria. *Int J Technol Assess Health Care.* (2005) 21:240–5. doi: 10.1017/S0266462305050324

24. *Consensus Health Economic Criteria-CHEC list.* Available online: https://hsr. mumc.maastrichtuniversity.nl/consensus-health-economic-criteria-chec-list.

25. Brennan RL, Prediger DJ. Coefficient kappa: some uses, misuses, and alternatives. *Educ Psychol Meas.* (1981) 41:687–99. doi: 10.1177/001316448104100307

26. Landis JR, Koch GG. The measurement of observer agreement for categorical data. *Biometrics.* (1977) 33:159–74. doi: 10.2307/2529310

27. Ruiz-Moreno JM, Roura M. en representacion del grupo del estudio M. Cost of myopic patients with and without myopic choroidal neovascularization. *Arch Soc Esp Oftalmol.* (2016) 91:265–72. doi: 10.1016/j.oftal.2016.01.013

28. Claxton L, Malcolm B, Taylor M, Haig J, Leteneux C. Ranibizumab, verteporfin photodynamic therapy or observation for the treatment of myopic choroidal neovascularization: cost effectiveness in the UK. *Drugs Aging.* (2014) 31:837–48. doi: 10.1007/s40266-014-0216-y

29. *Monetary Authority of Singapore (MAS).* Available online at: https://www.mas.gov.sg/

30. Pineles SL, Kraker RT, VanderVeen DK, Hutchinson AK, Galvin JA, Wilson LB, et al. Atropine for the prevention of myopia progression in children: a report by the American Academy of Ophthalmology. *Ophthalmology.* (2017) 124:1857–66. doi: 10.1016/j.ophtha.2017.05.032

31. *Worldometer Elaboration of data by United Nations, Department of Economic and Social Affairs, Population Division.*

32. Malec D, Davis WW, Cao X. Model-based small area estimates of overweight prevalence using sample selection adjustment. *Stat Med.* (1999) 18:3189–200. doi: 10.1002/(sici)1097-0258(19991215)18:23<3189::aid-sim309>3.0.co;2-c

33. Vitale S, Cotch MF, Sperduto R, Ellwein L. Costs of refractive correction of distance vision impairment in the United States, 1999-2002. *Ophthalmology.* (2006) 113:2163–70. doi: 10.1016/j.ophtha.2006.06.033

34. Kigozi J, Jowett S, Lewis M, Barton P, Coast J. Estimating productivity costs using the friction cost approach in practice: a systematic review. *Eur J Health Econ.* (2016) 17:31–44. doi: 10.1007/s10198-014-0652-y

35. Saxena N, George PP, Hoon HB, Han LT, Onn YS. Burden of wet age-related macular degeneration and its economic implications in Singapore in the year

2030. *Ophthalmic Epidemiol.* (2016) 23:232–7. doi: 10.1080/09286586.2016.11 93617

36. Zhang X, Low S, Kumari N, Wang J, Ang K, Yeo D, et al. Direct medical cost associated with diabetic retinopathy severity in type 2 diabetes in Singapore. *PLoS ONE.* (2017) 12:e0180949. doi: 10.1371/journal.pone.0 180949

37. Joachimsen L, Bohringer D, Gross NJ, Reich M, Stifter J, Reinhard T, et al. A pilot study on the efficacy and safety of 0.01% atropine in German school children with progressive myopia. *Ophthalmol Ther.* (2019) 8:427–33. doi: 10.1007/s40123-019-0194-6

38. Efron SE, Efron N, Morgan PB, Morgan SL, A. theoretical model for comparing UK costs of contact lens replacement modalities. *Cont Lens Anterior Eye.* (2012) 35:28–34. doi: 10.1016/j.clae.2011.07.006

39. Efron N, Efron SE, Morgan PB, Morgan SL, A. 'cost-per-wear' model based on contact lens replacement frequency. *Clin Exp Optom.* (2010) 93:253–60. doi: 10.1111/j.1444-0938.2010.00488.x

40. Vitale S, Sperduto RD, Ferris FL, III. Increased prevalence of myopia in the United States between 1971–1972 and 1999–2004. *Arch Ophthalmol.* (2009) 127:1632–9. doi: 10.1001/archophthalmol.2009.303

41. Waduthantri S, Yong SS, Tan CH, Shen L, Lee MX, Nagarajan S, et al. Cost of dry eye treatment in an Asian clinic setting. *PLoS ONE.* (2012) 7:e37711. doi: 10.1371/journal.pone.0037711

42. Wang JC, Chew PT. What is the direct cost of treatment of acute primary angle closure glaucoma? the Singapore model. *Clin Exp Ophthalmol.* (2004) 32:578–83. doi: 10.1111/j.1442-9071.2004.00906.x

43. Klein RJ SC. Age adjustment using the 2000 projected U.S. population. *Healthy People 2010 Stat Notes.* (2001) 20:1–10. doi: 10.1037/e583772012-001

44. WHO. *Western Pacific Regional Strategy for Health Systems Based on the Values of Primary Health Care.* World Health Organization (2010).

45. World Health Organization. *World Report on Vision Switzerland.* (2019).

46. Flaxman SR, Bourne RRA, Resnikoff S, Ackland P, Braithwaite T, Cicinelli MV, et al. Global causes of blindness and distance vision impairment 1990-2020: a systematic review and meta-analysis. *Lancet Glob Health.* (2017) 5:e1221–34. doi: 10.1016/S2214-109X(17)30393-5

47. Bourne RRA, Flaxman SR, Braithwaite T, Cicinelli MV, Das A, Jonas JB, et al. Magnitude, temporal trends, and projections of the global prevalence of blindness and distance and near vision impairment: a systematic review and meta-analysis. *Lancet Glob Health.* (2017) 5:e888–97. doi: 10.1016/S2214-109X(17)30293-0

48. Cumberland PM, Bao Y, Hysi PG, Foster PJ, Hammond CJ, Rahi JS, et al. Frequency and distribution of refractive error in adult life: methodology and findings of the UK Biobank Study. *PLoS ONE.* (2015) 10:e0139780. doi: 10.1371/journal.pone.0139780

49. Pan CW, Dirani M, Cheng CY, Wong TY, Saw SM. The age-specific prevalence of myopia in Asia: a meta-analysis. *Optom Vis Sci.* (2015) 92:258–66. doi: 10.1097/OPX.0000000000000516

50. Williams KM, Verhoeven VJ, Cumberland P, Bertelsen G, Wolfram C, Buitendijk GH, et al. Prevalence of refractive error in Europe: the European Eye Epidemiology (E(3)) Consortium. *Eur J Epidemiol.* (2015) 30:305–15. doi: 10.1007/s10654-015-0010-0

51. Ansah JP, Koh V, de Korne DF, Bayer S, Pan C, Thiyagarajan J, et al. Projection of eye disease burden in Singapore. *Ann Acad Med Singapore.* (2018) 47:13–28.

52. Yung AM, Cho P, Yap M, A. market survey of contact lens practice in Hong Kong. *Clin Exp Optom.* (2005) 88:165–75. doi: 10.1111/j.1444-0938.2005.tb06690.x

53. Huang J, Wen D, Wang Q, McAlinden C, Flitcroft I, Chen H, et al. efficacy comparison of 16 interventions for myopia control in children: a network meta-analysis. *Ophthalmology.* (2016) 123:697–708. doi: 10.1016/j.ophtha.2015.11.010

54. Weiss RS, Park S. Recent updates on myopia control: preventing progression 1 diopter at a time. *Curr Opin Ophthalmol.* (2019) 30:215–9. doi: 10.1097/ICU.0000000000000571

55. Chia A, Chua WH, Cheung YB, Wong WL, Lingham A, Fong A, et al. Atropine for the treatment of childhood myopia: safety and efficacy of 0.5%, 01%, and 001% doses (Atropine for the Treatment of Myopia 2). *Ophthalmology.* (2012) 119:347–54. doi: 10.1016/j.ophtha.2011.07.031

56. Li FF, Yam JC. Low-concentration atropine eye drops for myopia progression. *Asia Pac J Ophthalmol.* (2019) 8:360–5. doi: 10.1097/APO.0000000000000256

57. Sacchi M, Serafino M, Villani E, Tagliabue E, Luccarelli S, Bonsignore F, et al. Efficacy of atropine 0.01% for the treatment of childhood myopia in European patients. *Acta Ophthalmol.* (2019) 97:e1136–40. doi: 10.1111/aos

9

Benefits of Integrating Telemedicine and Artificial Intelligence into Outreach Eye Care

Mark A. Chia[1,2] and Angus W. Turner[1,3]*

[1] Lions Outback Vision, Lions Eye Institute, Nedlands, WA, Australia, [2] Institute of Ophthalmology, Faculty of Brain Sciences, University College London, London, United Kingdom, [3] Centre for Ophthalmology and Visual Science, University of Western Australia, Nedlands, WA, Australia

Telemedicine has traditionally been applied within remote settings to overcome geographical barriers to healthcare access, providing an alternate means of connecting patients to specialist services. The coronavirus 2019 pandemic has rapidly expanded the use of telemedicine into metropolitan areas and enhanced global telemedicine capabilities. Through our experience of delivering real-time telemedicine over the past decade within a large outreach eye service, we have identified key themes for successful implementation which may be relevant to services facing common challenges. We present our journey toward establishing a comprehensive teleophthalmology model built on the principles of collaborative care, with a focus on delivering practical lessons for service design. Artificial intelligence is an emerging technology that has shown potential to further address resource limitations. We explore the applications of artificial intelligence and the need for targeted research within underserved settings in order to meet growing healthcare demands. Based on our rural telemedicine experience, we make the case that similar models may be adapted to urban settings with the aim of reducing surgical waitlists and improving efficiency.

*Correspondence:
Angus W. Turner
angus.turner@gmail.com

Keywords: telemedicine, ophthalmology (MeSH), rural health services, indigenous health services, quality of health care (MeSH), artificial intelligence

INTRODUCTION

The delivery of equitable eye services for rural and remote communities represents a unique challenge to healthcare providers. Within Western Australia (WA), the integration of teleophthalmology into service delivery has played a pivotal role in addressing these challenges. Lions Outback Vision was established in 2010 at the Lions Eye Institute in Perth and now serves 51 communities with visiting optometry and/or ophthalmology. This article presents an overview of our journey toward the development of an integrated teleophthalmology model over the past decade, with a focus on the key lessons for building an effective telemedicine service. Beyond telemedicine, we consider the role of recent advancements in artificial intelligence (AI) and the pathway toward harnessing this technology for more equitable service provision in under-resourced settings. Finally, we make the case that outreach telemedicine models may be translated into urban areas to address the problem of burgeoning surgical waitlists. The coronavirus 2019 (COVID-19) pandemic has accelerated telemedicine capabilities across the globe and catapulted its applications beyond traditional geographic barriers to healthcare.

TELEMEDICINE INTEGRATION FOR OUTREACH EYE CARE

With an area of 2.65 million square kilometers, the state of WA would feature within the top 10 countries by size worldwide. Ninety percent of the population live within the southwest corner of the state, centered around the capital city where all tertiary services are located. The remaining population is scattered sparsely across outback WA, representing a significant challenge for eye care providers. Remote health services are frequently affected by high staff turnover, impacting on long-term stability. Furthermore, rural areas have a high proportion of Indigenous patients compared to metropolitan areas. Patient rurality and Indigenous status are both associated with a higher burden of vision impairment coupled with reduced access to eye care services (1).

Given the unique demography of WA, teleophthalmology has been a key and growing service element within Lions Outback Vision through both real-time videoconferencing and "store and forward" modalities (**Figure 1**). In 2021, 25% ($n = 1,825$) of all ophthalmology appointments at our service were conducted though telemedicine. During face-to-face outreach specialist visits, 62% ($n = 3,442$) of appointments required specialist procedural management, representing a highly efficient clinical triage through collaboration with optometrists. The ability to waitlist surgical patients via videoconference at the time of primary-care assessment eliminates the waiting time for the initial specialist appointment with attendant logistical and cost implications. Moreover, teleophthalmology can also be delivered safely utilizing the correct expertise and case-selection, with a systematic review finding that diagnostic accuracy for real-time teleophthalmology was comparable to face-to-face consultation (2).

We believe that our experience in delivering real-time videoconference consults over the last decade may provide useful lessons for similar regions around the world. Through our history of service delivery, we have identified several key lessons in our journey. These include: 1) a focus on coordination of services at both regional and local community levels, 2) engagement with government funding agencies to align telemedicine-related financial incentives with the benefits they deliver, and 3) reducing barriers to telemedicine uptake through a range of service modifications, education, and support initiatives.

Coordination of Eye Services

Coordination between ophthalmology and optometry has been identified as an essential part of delivering effective outreach eye care. A cross-sectional case study of rural eye services in Australia demonstrated that higher levels of integration between optometrists and ophthalmologists led to improved surgical case rates, with trends toward increased clinical activity and reduced wait times (3). The primary screening and triage provided by optometrists funneled more patients with a higher concentration of pathology requiring procedural intervention to the limited number of specialist visits. Important elements of coordination were highlighted including: 1) service integration with optometry services to facilitate primary screening and triage, 2) involvement

of local health staff such as Aboriginal Health Workers to support patient attendance, and 3) appointment of a Rural Eye Health Coordinator (REHC) to liaise between primary healthcare, regional hospitals, and visiting eye services.

In 2011, Lions Outback Vision implemented real-time videoconference teleophthalmology services that linked patients to an ophthalmologist and was facilitated by their primary healthcare provider. To build an evidence base, we conducted a series of studies designed to evaluate our service and found that several of the themes highlighted above regarding eye service coordination were also critical for telemedicine. A prospective clinical audit of 100 telemedicine consultations showed that 60% of referrals emanated from optometrists, despite there being no reimbursement for referral at that time, and the remainder of the referrals were generated from general practitioners (4). A survey of 109 patients who took part in telemedicine consultations found a high level of satisfaction, with 94% of patients indicating they were "satisfied" or "very satisfied" (5). Qualitative analysis of the factors contributing to satisfaction revealed that familiarity with staff at the patient-end was important, in part making up for any perceived impersonality due to the absence of face-to-face interaction. This again highlights the essential part that local community staff play in facilitating effective teleophthalmology.

The key role of REHCs has been demonstrated within our diabetic retinopathy screening program, which operates using a store-and-forward model (6). Following a period of declining screening activity in WA's Kimberley region, an REHC was appointed with the aim of providing high-level support for retinal screening and staff training. A retrospective audit comparing the period before and after the REHC's appointment showed an increase in screening coverage from 9 to 30%, with the number of screening sites increasing from 4 to 17 (6). This illustrates the positive impact that regional coordination can have on the effective delivery of teleophthalmology.

Alignment of Funding Incentives

A high degree of engagement with government funding bodies has been critical to the success of our telemedicine program, with the aim of ensuring that reimbursement sustains services and reflects the costs of high-quality service delivery. In 2011, the Commonwealth government introduced Medicare funding for both the referring doctor and specialist, with ~50% loading above equivalent face-to-face visits to reflect the additional resources required for telemedicine consults. Limited reimbursement in the United States is a frequently cited reason for reduced uptake of teleophthalmology (7). In 2019, only 10 of 50 states had payment parity between telemedicine and office visits (7). In response to COVID-19, telemedicine was made more widely available through reimbursement at the same rate as in-person visits regardless of setting. Similarly, in Australia regulations have been temporarily relaxed to include funding for audio-only consultations as well as metropolitan settings.

Despite the introduction of sustainable funding, telemedicine uptake in WA was initially low, falling 74% below government targets in the first year that incentives became available (8). Our group conducted an analysis of structural and economic drivers within WA eye care services with the aim of increasing the impact

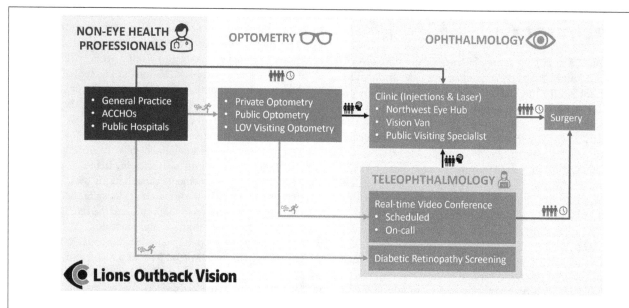

FIGURE 1 | Clinical pathway demonstrating the role of teleophthalmology within Lions Outback Vision. Teleophthalmology enables fast-track access (green) for patients to specialist care compared to traditional referral pathways which are congested (red). By diverting referrals from non-eye care professionals via optometry and diabetic retinal screening, specialist clinics can manage well-triaged pathology (brown). ACCHOs, Aboriginal Community Controlled Health Organizations; LOV, Lions Outback Vision.

of teleophthalmology in Australia (9). Based on clinical audits of 5,456 eye visits, an estimated 15% of urgent transfers and 24% of outreach consultations were assessed as being suitable for telemedicine, leading to an estimated annual cost-saving of $1.1 million. Additionally, to determine the initial capital expenditure required to facilitate basic teleophthalmology, we conducted a survey of ocular diagnostic and teleconference equipment available at optometrists, primary-care practices, and hospitals. Setup costs for primary-care practices were estimated at $20,500, compared to negligible costs for already well-equipped optometry practices.

Based on this finding, along with the reduced need for further eye-specific clinical training for optometrists, we concluded that facilitating optometrist-led teleophthalmology provided the most compelling economic case. A strategy document was created with recommendations for teleophthalmology in Australia and submitted to the Royal Australian and New Zealand College of Ophthalmologists and Optometry Australia. Amongst other strategic initiatives, successful advocacy resulted in the approval of new Medicare codes for optometrist-led rural telemedicine referrals in 2015. In the first year following approval, Lions Outback Vision received 709 teleophthalmology referrals facilitated by optometrists (10).

Addressing Barriers to Telemedicine Uptake

Despite the demonstrated benefits of telemedicine, there are numerous barriers that can limit widespread uptake. In addition to the financial barriers previously outlined, there are also a range of technical and logistical obstacles. Taking a proactive approach to addressing these challenges has been critical to developing

our service model. We found that introducing a multi-faceted intervention increased teleophthalmology uptake at our service (11). Key elements of this intervention included awareness raising, educational resources, logistical support, an updated online booking system, and a funding mechanism to simulate Medicare payments prior to government implementation.

In the United States, restrictions on permitted videoconferencing software emerged as an important barrier to telemedicine uptake in the context of COVID-19 (7). In response, the Centers for Medicare and Medicaid Services removed penalties for technologies that were previously considered non-compliant, such as Facetime, Skype, and Google Hangout. In contrast, these types of technologies have been used for telemedicine in Australia since 2011. Our existing service remains agnostic to videoconference platforms in order to minimize barriers for the referrer. Multiple audits of our service have shown that freely available voice-over-Internet-Protocol services such as Skype and Facetime are commonly chosen by referrers, supporting the idea that familiarity and useability are critical factors (10, 11).

Scheduling three parties (patient, referrer and specialist) for synchronous telemedicine relies on availability and timeliness of participants to ensure minimal disruption to clinical workflow. In 2017, our service introduced on-call teleophthalmology services to complement the existing online booking system. When an optometrist is visiting a community or a patient has traveled a significant distance for an assessment, there is limited opportunity for a scheduled future telemedicine appointment. This alternative provided immediate access to the ophthalmologist, resulting in improved access for rural and Indigenous patients. A clinical audit showed that the proportion of Indigenous patients in the on-call telemedicine cohort was 51.4%, compared to 8.7% in the online-booking telemedicine group (12). We found similar improvements in access for the most remote regions of WA, with 79.0% in the on-call service compared to 26.1% in the online-booking cohort. Of all telemedicine consultations in 2018, 27.8% made use of the on-call service, demonstrating high demand for the more flexible booking arrangement.

BEYOND TELEMEDICINE: THE ROLE OF AI IN RURAL EYE CARE

Rapid progress in AI technology has attracted interest due to its potential to perform complex medical tasks with supra-human performance. Deep learning is a type of AI utilizing multiple processing layers to learn representation of data with multiple levels of abstraction (13). Deep learning is particularly well-suited to image analysis tasks; hence, image-driven specialties like ophthalmology have become the frontrunners for medical AI. Advances in AI hold promise in helping bridge the widening gap between population eye care needs and trained human resources to meet these needs, particularly for underserved rural communities. A well-known limitation of AI is the tendency for algorithms to generalize poorly outside their research milieu (14). AI systems must therefore be trained on data from diverse populations and then rigorously validated within their intended settings.

Autonomous Diabetic Retinopathy Screening

Ophthalmic AI applications exist for numerous conditions, most commonly for diabetic retinopathy (DR), glaucoma, and age-related macular degeneration (AMD) (13). DR represents a growing burden for outreach eye services due to increasing prevalence, requirement for expensive imaging equipment, and the need for regular specialist intervention for optimal outcomes. It is therefore reassuring that much of the most promising progress toward real-world AI implementation has been for autonomous DR screening. Currently, two autonomous DR screening systems have been approved for use by Food and Drug Administration, following pivotal trials showing strong performance in real-world settings (15, 16). Both studies were conducted in the United States within majority white populations.

Our group was recently involved with a real-world validation study of a separate autonomous DR screening system evaluating 236 diabetic patients from Aboriginal Medical Services and endocrinology outpatient clinics (17). In addition to identifying referable DR, the system was also designed to screen for AMD and glaucoma, although performance was only assessed for DR screening. The system achieved a sensitivity and specificity of 96.9 and 87.7%, respectively, in detecting referable DR. Apart from investigating an at-risk ethnic group, other novel aspects of the study included: 1) the use of an offline AI system rather than a cloud-based system, as the latter is a notable barrier in some rural settings, 2) use of several types of retinal camera,

and 3) evaluation of patient and clinician acceptability, which is frequently cited as a major limitation to AI uptake. Of 207 participants who completed a satisfaction questionnaire, 93.7% stated that they were either "satisfied" or "extremely satisfied". Clinicians most frequently noted that the AI system was easy to use, and that the real-time diagnostic report was helpful.

Research Potential at Australia's First Remote Eye Center

Despite the progress of ophthalmic AI applications, further study is required to ensure that AI technology delivers benefit to patients. In 2021, Lions Outback Vision opened the Northwest Eye Hub in the remote Kimberley town of Broome. As Australia's first permanent dedicated eye center located in a remote region, it holds significant potential for furthering AI research in this high-risk but under-studied population. Our decade-long history of working in partnership with local community leaders and health organizations means we are well-positioned to develop further collaborative research partnerships. The hub is equipped with state-of-the-art diagnostic equipment, which, in many cases, surpasses that of tertiary eye clinics. The center is staffed by two full-time ophthalmologists and a range of other health staff including Aboriginal Health Workers and optometrists. Our team is currently engaged in several AI projects focusing on DR screening, detecting macular edema, (18) and analyzing optical coherence tomography angiography linking systemic risk factors.

TRANSLATIONAL TELEMEDICINE: OUTBACK SOLUTIONS TO BIG CITY PROBLEMS

A significant "hidden" waitlist has been recently highlighted in Australia—the waiting time for initial specialist assessment (19). This pre-specialist assessment waiting time is often not publicly available and yet masks a burden of preventable diseases silently resulting in unknown levels of permanent blindness or unnecessarily prolonged visual impairment. An audit of cataract referrals from two metropolitan public hospitals in New South Wales found that two-thirds of patients were yet to have their initial hospital appointment in the year following referral (20).

The COVID-19 pandemic has elevated telemedicine in the consciousness of all health service providers attempting to bridge barriers to healthcare. The imperative for telemedicine in outback Australia over the last decade and the robust supporting evidence-base can be translated rapidly to urban settings. For eye care in Australia, optometrists represent an accessible, publicly funded, and well-equipped resource to help tackle population eye health needs. Collaborative care models involving community-based optometrists and virtual review by an ophthalmologist using "store-and-forward" telemedicine modalities have been demonstrated for glaucoma and diabetes clinics in Australia, leading to cost-savings and reduced wait times (21, 22). Exploring options for upscaling these models has the potential to further improve the capacity of public eye services.

Synchronous videoconferencing may also be utilized to consent patients for surgical management during their first in-person contact point with the specialist, as shown within Lions Outback Vision. An audit of outreach surgery found that patients assessed through telemedicine waited half the length of time compared to those assessed in traditional outpatient clinics (23). Urban centers in the United Kingdom have explored comparable models involving community optometrists and telemedicine consultations to enable "one stop cataract surgery," demonstrating similar benefits (24, 25). Adapting these models to the Australian context will require careful consideration to safeguard informed consent, rigorous surgical risk-assessment, and effective use of theater-time, however the benefits warrant further exploration. Telemedicine provides a seamless path from primary care to surgical management, and enables expert medical input where required, establishing a cornerstone to collaborative care.

CONCLUSION

Within WA, integration of teleophthalmology has been a crucial component in enabling Lions Outback Vision to make progress toward equitable eye care delivery. Much of this headway has relied upon establishing collaborative care models with regional optometrists, maximizing the efficiency of in-person specialist visits. Key lessons from our service have the potential to be applied to areas that share similar geographical and logistical challenges. Looking forward, advances in AI have shown promise toward bridging the gap between expanding eye care demands and limited resources; however, further investigation within under-resourced settings is critical to future progress. Finally, following the acceleration of global telemedicine capabilities triggered by COVID-19, lessons from rural services may be applied to urban centers to curb rapidly growing surgical wait lists. There is a clarion call to harness telemedicine advances in collaborative care to preserve sight in both urban and rural settings.

AUTHOR CONTRIBUTIONS

MC and AT were involved in planning, researching, and drafting the manuscript. The final manuscript was reviewed and approved by both authors.

REFERENCES

1. Foreman J, Xie J, Keel S, van Wijngaarden P, Sandhu SS, Ang GS, et al. The prevalence and causes of vision loss in indigenous and non-indigenous Australians: the national eye health survey. *Ophthalmology.* (2017) 124:1743–52. doi: 10.1016/j.ophtha.2017.06.001
2. Tan IJ, Dobson LP, Bartnik S, Muir J, Turner AW. Real-time teleophthalmology versus face-to-face consultation: a systematic review. *J Telemed Telecare.* (2017) 23:629–38. doi: 10.1177/1357633X16660640
3. Turner AW, Mulholland WJ, Taylor HR. Coordination of outreach eye services in remote Australia. *Clin Experiment Ophthalmol.* (2011) 39:344–9. doi: 10.1111/j.1442-9071.2010.02474.x
4. Johnson KA, Meyer J, Yazar S, Turner AW. Real-time teleophthalmology in rural Western Australia. *Aust J Rural Health.* (2015) 23:142–9. doi: 10.1111/ajr.12150
5. Host BK, Turner AW, Muir J. Real-time teleophthalmology video consultation: an analysis of patient satisfaction in rural Western Australia. *Clin Exp Optom.* (2018) 101:129–34. doi: 10.1111/cxo.12535
6. Moynihan V, Turner A. Coordination of diabetic retinopathy screening in the Kimberley region of Western Australia. *Aust J Rural Health.* (2017) 25:110–5. doi: 10.1111/ajr.12290
7. Kalavar M, Hua H-U, Sridhar J. Teleophthalmology: an essential tool in the era of the novel coronavirus 2019. *Curr Opin Ophthalmol.* (2020) 31:366–73. doi: 10.1097/ICU.0000000000000689
8. Turner A, Razavi DH, Copeland S. *Increasing the Impact of Eye Telehealth in Rural and Remote Western Australia.* (2014). Available online at: https://www.outbackvision.com.au/wp-content/uploads/2020/04/increasing-the-impact-of-telehealth-for-eye-care-in-rural-and-remote-western-australia.pdf (accessed December 01, 2021).
9. Razavi H, Copeland SP, Turner AW. Increasing the impact of teleophthalmology in Australia: Analysis of structural and economic drivers in a state service. *Aust J Rural Health.* (2017) 25:45–52. doi: 10.1111/ajr.12277
10. Bartnik SE, Copeland SP, Aicken AJ, Turner AW. Optometry-facilitated teleophthalmology: an audit of the first year in Western Australia. *Clin Exp Optom.* (2018) 101:700–3. doi: 10.1111/cxo.12658
11. O'Day R, Smith C, Muir J, Turner A. Optometric use of a teleophthalmology service in rural Western Australia: comparison of two prospective audits. *Clin Exp Optom.* (2016) 99:163–7. doi: 10.1111/cxo.12334
12. Nguyen AA, Baker A, Turner AW. On-call telehealth for visiting optometry in regional Western Australia improves patient access to eye care. *Clin Exp Optom.* (2020) 103:393–4. doi: 10.1111/cxo.12979
13. Wang Z, Keane PA, Chiang M, Cheung CY, Wong TY, Ting DSW. Artificial intelligence and deep learning in ophthalmology. *Artif Intell Med.* (2021) 1–34. doi: 10.1007/978-3-030-58080-3_200-1
14. Ting DSW, Pasquale LR, Peng L, Campbell JP, Lee AY, Raman R, et al. Artificial intelligence and deep learning in ophthalmology. *Br J Ophthalmol.* (2019) 103:167–75. doi: 10.1136/bjophthalmol-2018-313173
15. Abràmoff MD, Lavin PT, Birch M, Shah N, Folk JC. Pivotal trial of an autonomous AI-based diagnostic system for detection of diabetic retinopathy in primary care offices. *Npj Digit Med.* (2018) 1:1–8. doi: 10.1038/s41746-018-0040-6
16. Ipp E, Liljenquist D, Bode B, Shah VN, Silverstein S, Regillo CD, et al. Pivotal evaluation of an artificial intelligence system for autonomous detection of referrable and vision-threatening diabetic retinopathy. *JAMA Netw Open.* (2021) 4:e2134254. doi: 10.1001/jamanetworkopen.2021.34254
17. Scheetz J, Koca D, McGuinness M, Holloway E, Tan Z, Zhu Z, et al. Real-world artificial intelligence-based opportunistic screening for diabetic retinopathy in endocrinology and indigenous healthcare settings in Australia. *Sci Rep.* (2021) 11:15808. doi: 10.1038/s41598-021-94178-5
18. Liu X, Ali TK, Singh P, Shah A, McKinney SM, Ruamviboonsuk P, et al. Deep learning to detect optical coherence tomography-derived diabetic macular edema from retinal photographs: a multicenter validation study. *Ophthalmol Retina.* (2022) : doi: 10.1016/j.oret.2021.12.021. [Epub ahead of print].
19. Huang-Lung J, Angell B, Palagyi A, Taylor H, White A, McCluskey P, et al. The true cost of hidden waiting times for cataract surgery in Australia. *Public Health Res Pract.* (2021) doi: 10.17061/phrp31342116. [Epub ahead of print].
20. Do VQ, McCluskey P, Palagyi A, Stapleton FJ, White A, Carnt N, et al. Are cataract surgery referrals to public hospitals in Australia poorly targeted? *Clin Experiment Ophthalmol.* (2018) 46:364–70. doi: 10.1111/ceo.13057

21. Ford BK, Angell B, Liew G, White AJR, Keay LJ. Improving patient access and reducing costs for glaucoma with integrated hospital and community care: a case study from Australia. *Int J Integr Care.* (2019) 19:5. doi: 10.5334/ijic.4642

22. Tahhan N, Ford BK, Angell B, Liew G, Nazarian J, Maberly G, et al. Evaluating the cost and wait-times of a task-sharing model of care for diabetic eye care: a case study from Australia. *BMJ Open.* (2020) 10:e036842. doi: 10.1136/bmjopen-2020-036842

23. McGlacken-Byrne A, Turner AW, Drinkwater J. Review of cataract surgery in rural north Western Australia with the Lions Outback Vision. *Clin Experiment Ophthalmol.* (2019) 47:802–3. doi: 10.1111/ceo.13481

24. Gaskell A, McLaughline A, Young E, McCristal K. Direct optometrist referral of cataract patients into a pilot 'one-stop'cataract surgery facility. *J R Coll Surg Edinb.* (2001) 46:1.

25. Dhillon N, Ghazal D, Harcourt J, Kumarasamy M. A proposed redesign of elective cataract services in Scotland – pilot project. *Eye.* (2021) 1–6. doi: 10.1038/s41433-021-01810-9

Widefield Optical Coherence Tomography in Pediatric Retina: A Case Series of Intraoperative Applications using a Prototype Handheld Device

Thanh-Tin P. Nguyen[1], Shuibin Ni[1,2], Guangru Liang[1,2], Shanjida Khan[1,2], Xiang Wei[1,2], Alison Skalet[1,3,4,5], Susan Ostmo[1], Michael F. Chiang[6], Yali Jia[1,2], David Huang[1,2], Yifan Jian[1,2] and J. Peter Campbell[1]*

[1] Casey Eye Institute, Oregon Health and Science University, Portland, OR, United States, [2] Department of Biomedical Engineering, Oregon Health and Science University, Portland, OR, United States, [3] Knight Cancer Institute, Oregon Health and Science University, Portland, OR, United States, [4] Department of Radiation Medicine, Oregon Health and Science University, Portland, OR, United States, [5] Department of Dermatology, Oregon Health and Science University, Portland, OR, United States, [6] National Eye Institute, National Institutes of Health, Bethesda, MD, United States

Correspondence:
J. Peter Campbell
campbelp@ohsu.edu

Optical coherence tomography (OCT) has changed the standard of care for diagnosis and management of macular diseases in adults. Current commercially available OCT systems, including handheld OCT for pediatric use, have a relatively narrow field of view (FOV), which has limited the potential application of OCT to retinal diseases with primarily peripheral pathology, including many of the most common pediatric retinal conditions. More broadly, diagnosis of all types of retinal detachment (exudative, tractional, and rhegmatogenous) may be improved with OCT-based assessment of retinal breaks, identification of proliferative vitreoretinopathy (PVR) membranes, and the pattern of subretinal fluid. Intraocular tumors both benign and malignant often occur outside of the central macula and may be associated with exudation, subretinal and intraretinal fluid, and vitreoretinal traction. The development of wider field OCT systems thus has the potential to improve the diagnosis and management of myriad diseases in both adult and pediatric retina. In this paper, we present a case series of pediatric patients with complex vitreoretinal pathology undergoing examinations under anesthesia (EUA) using a portable widefield (WF) swept-source (SS)-OCT device.

Keywords: retina, pediatric retina, optical coherence tomography, handheld optical coherence tomography, optical coherence tomography with angiography

INTRODUCTION

Optical coherence tomography (OCT) is an essential diagnostic tool in the management of retinal disease. There are trade-offs in the acquisition of OCT images between speed of acquisition, field of view (FOV), and image resolution and quality. Over the last two decades, despite significant advances in imaging speed and the transition from time-domain to spectral domain (SD)-OCT, the vast majority of OCT applications are for macular diseases in adults. OCT has proven ability to detect subclinical disease, often resulting in new disease classifications and earlier treatment, facilitate objective assessment of macular thickness and pathologic fluid, and improve visualization of the vitreoretinal interface. As a result, it is not possible to provide the standard of care for many adult retinal diseases without OCT.

These same advances in clinical diagnosis and management would likely benefit pediatric retina patients. In retinopathy of prematurity (ROP), the most common pediatric retinal disease, OCT has revealed the normal spectrum of macular development in prematurely born infants (1, 2), identified the presence of intraretinal fluid (3, 4), and demonstrated the ability to objectively assess changes at the vitreoretinal interface (5). However, early work has been limited by the specifications of commercially available devices. Over the past few years, a number of groups have explored the advantages of arm-mounted SD-OCT (6) and prototype swept-source (SS)-OCT in pediatric retinal diseases (7–10). With the versatility of a handheld probe and faster image acquisition times, SS-OCT has improved the ease of imaging in both awake and sedated children.

We have developed a handheld SS-OCT device with two imaging configurations, one with a 55° FOV and higher resolution for OCTA imaging (11), and one with a 105° FOV for OCT structural imaging only (12). Our 55° FOV system generates OCTA volumes concurrently with OCT, and both imaging configurations allow for real time en face visualization to allow the physician to position the probe optimally for image acquisition. The 105° FOV system has potential to provide objective diagnosis in pediatric retinal diseases with predominantly extramacular pathology, like ROP, and contribute to new insight in these disease processes. We recently described our experience using these devices for ROP screening in the neonatal intensive care unit (NICU) in awake infants (13, 14). Here, we present a review of the potential clinical benefits and applications of widefield (WF) and ultra-widefield (UWF) handheld OCT in pediatric retina patients undergoing examinations under anesthesia (EUA) for a variety of conditions.

MATERIALS AND METHODS

This study was approved by the Institutional Review Board (IRB) at Oregon Health and Science University (OHSU) and adheres to all tenets of the Declaration of Helsinki. Consent for imaging was obtained from parents. Pupils were pharmacologically dilated per routine clinical care. Infants were imaged in the operating room (OR) after the induction of general anesthesia and placement of an eyelid speculum with a 400-kHz portable handheld SS-OCT system, shown in **Figure 1**, using a modular lens system providing up to a 105° FOV. A display screen on the probe provides real-time en face visualization of the retina and allows for efficient positioning of the probe (15–17). The probe was operated by the examining ophthalmologist, whilst another operator

controlled the software. Image acquisition time was 1.5 s per volume. Patients were imaged between November of 2020 to October 2021.

Optical coherence tomography volumes were processed and presented in linear scale. Mean-intensity en face projections were calculated with custom software coded in MATLAB (18). B-scans presented in this manuscript were produced via image registration and averaging of adjacent B-scans. Three-dimensional image rendering was performed via the Volume Viewer plugin of Fiji, a distribution of ImageJ after pre-processing using a combination of thresholding and manual image segmentation (19). OCTA images were generated using a novel phase-stabilized complex-decorrelation methodology (20), with automated segmentation performed using a guided bidirectional graph search method (21), both of which were designed specifically for use in swept-source, widefield applications.

RESULTS

During the study period, we obtained images in 20 patients undergoing EUA in the operating room, as seen in **Table 1**. Here, we present a variety of pathologies and examples to illustrate some potential applications in pediatric retina.

Retinal Detachments
Portable widefield OCT facilitates the evaluation of tractional, exudative, rhegmatogenous (and combined mechanism) retinal detachments (RDs) in children. The most common visualization of OCT is the cross-sectional scan (B-scan) that reveals axial anatomy within a single imaging slice. However, SS-OCT can facilitate real-time en-face visualization of the entire imaging range. **Figure 2** reveals en face and selected B-scans from several children with tractional retinal detachment (TRD). TRDs are most commonly related to peripheral epiretinal neovascularization with fibrosis, with the resulting vitreoretinal traction leading to macular dragging (as seen in **Figure 2A**), distortion of the normal retinal architecture, and if there is sufficient anterior-posterior traction, separation of the retina from the retinal pigment epithelium (RPE). OCT is more sensitive for detection of this spectrum of changes, as seen in **Figure 2C** which reveals an early stage 4a detachment in ROP with the selected B-scan demonstrating tractional schisis but no subretinal fluid. It is important to note that the transverse resolution of these B-scans is relatively low, the result of expanding FOV while maintaining efficient imaging time (1.5 s). Resolution can be improved with either longer imaging time, which is challenging in children, or narrower FOV, as previously seen with our 55° FOV prototype (11). **Figure 3** demonstrates a rhegmatogenous retinal detachment (RRD) with a large temporal retinal break in a 5-year-old girl. Exudative retinal detachments (ERDs) may be relatively more common in pediatric retinal diseases such as in ROP after laser treatment or in severe Coats' disease, which means they are often diagnosed clinically rather than with OCT imaging due to

TABLE 1 | Patient ages and diagnoses.

	Diagnosis	Figure	Age
Case 1	Tractional retinal detachment (TRD) secondary to Familial Exudative Vitreoretinopathy (FEVR)	2A	3 years, 6 months
Case 2	TRD secondary to incontinentia pigmenti (IP)	2B, 8A	2B: 1 year, 6 months; 8A: 1 year
Case 3	TRD secondary to retinopathy of prematurity (ROP), Stage 4A	2C	4 months
Case 4	Rhegmatogenous retinal detachment (RRD)	3	5 years, 10 months
Case 5	Tractional and exudative retinal detachment (ERD) secondary to vasoproliferative lesion	4A	15 years
Case 6	Chronic exudative retinopathy	4B	16 years
Case 7	ERD secondary to ROP after laser	4C	5 months
Case 8	Coats disease	5	2 years, 3 months
Case 9	Retinoblastoma with calcified, partially calcified, and atrophic regressed tumors after completion of therapy	6A	3 years
Case 10	Retinoblastoma with partially calcified tumor in patient undergoing chemotherapy	6B	5 months
Case 11	Retinoblastoma with vitreous seeding and multifocal tumors	6C	7 months
Case 12	X-linked retinoschisis (XLRS)	7A	8 years
Case 13	Chorioretinal scarring with retinal traction secondary to non-accidental trauma (NAT)	7B	7 months
Case 14	ROP with regressed Stage 3 ROP with vitreoretinal traction	7C	2 months
Case 15	Persistent fetal vasculature (PFV)	7D	1 year, 7 months
Case 16	IP with peripheral avascular retina and neovascularization	8B	2 years, 7 months
Case 17	Hemangioblastomas in the setting of Von Hippel Lindau syndrome	9	15 years
Case 18	Central cataract in the setting of PFV	10A, 10B	6 months
Case 19	Retained silicone oil in the anterior chamber	10C	14 years
Case 20	TRD secondary to FEVR	11	4 months

Patient ages are at the time of OCT imaging.

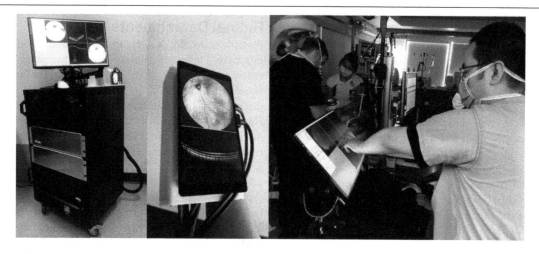

FIGURE 1 | Handheld, SS-OCT device. From left: portable prototype device, imaging probe with real-time *en face* display, and process of obtaining OCT volumes of an infant in the NICU.

the limitations of existing commercially available devices. Yet accurate diagnosis is critical because the management of exudative detachments is often different than if the primary mechanism is tractional or rhegmatogenous. **Figure 4** provides several examples ERDs and combined tractional and exudative RDs in children.

Macular Exudation

While WF-OCT is critical for visualization of the retinal periphery, it can still be used to diagnose and monitor exudation in the macula in many diseases. **Figure 5** demonstrates several examples of the visualization of

subretinal exudative in Coats' disease, including the potential benefit of *en face* visualization with topographic volume rendering. There are many previous publications focusing on the role of OCT in pediatric macular disease (2, 3, 22).

Intraocular Tumors

A number of retinal tumors can present in childhood including retinoblastoma (RB), retinal hemangioblastoma as part of Von-Hippel Lindau (VHL) disease, vasoproliferative tumor, and a variety of benign hamartomas such as choroidal hemangioma and congenital hypertrophy of the retina and RPE. The

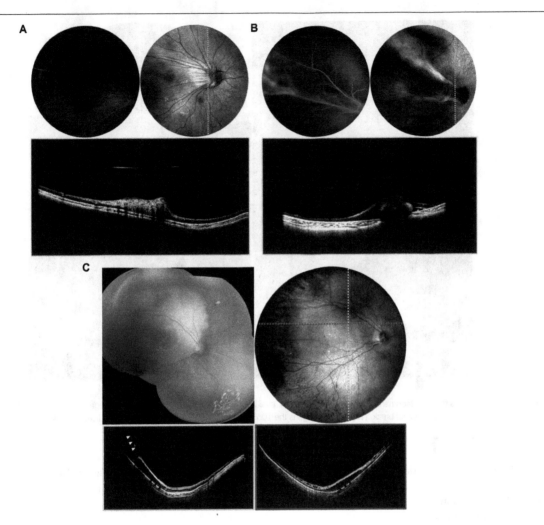

FIGURE 2 | Tractional retinal disease evaluated *via* OCT. **(A)** Tractional retinal fold secondary to FEVR in a 3-year-old patient. **(B)** Tractional fold with peripheral detachment secondary to IP in a 1-year-old patient. For **(A,B)**, top left is the FA, top right is the mean-intensity *en face* projection taken with the 55° FOV configuration, and bottom is the B-scan corresponding to the dotted line. **(C)** Stage 4a ROP in a 4-month-old born at 24 weeks gestation. Top left image is a montage of fundus photographs. Top right is a 105° FOV OCT *en face* with dotted lines indicating the locations of the color-coded B-scans in the bottom row. Vitreoretinal traction is indicated by white arrows, and areas of schisis are indicated by black arrows.

most serious of these is RB, which is both vision- and life-threatening. The current standard of care requires careful documentation of all tumors in the retina, including their size, location and the presence of any associated vitreous seeding, and subretinal fluid. Fundus photos are used to document these findings. Commercially available OCT systems are also widely used in retinoblastoma care, but have significant limitations due to their narrow field of view and narrow depth of focus (23–26). Retinoblastoma tumors are often highly elevated, multifocal and arise in the peripheral retina as well as the posterior pole. There is considerable potential for the use of WF-OCT in retinoblastoma care. **Figure 6** demonstrates several examples of RB documented with our device during routine RB EUAs. The WF-OCT system was successful in capturing three dimensional images of elevated tumors, including those in the far periphery, and provided better images than traditional fundus photography in the setting of

diffuse vitreous seeding (**Figure 6C**). WF-OCT was also able to identify very small subclinical tumors (27), indicating that it may prove useful in surveillance for new tumors in children with known RB or in those being screened due to family history of the disease.

Vitreoretinal Interface Disorders

Changes at the vitreoretinal interface are better diagnosed with OCT than ophthalmoscopy and are common in pediatric proliferative retinopathies, some inherited retinal degenerations, and disorders of ocular development. **Figure 7A** shows an example of X-linked retinoschisis (XLRS), in which retinoschisis may manifest both in the macula and periphery. Many conditions demonstrate an abnormally adherent vitreoretinal interface. An abnormal vitreoretinal interface may be associated with prior trauma, as in **Figure 7B**, and regressed neovascularization in ROP, as in **Figure 7C**. Finally, in persistent fetal vasculature

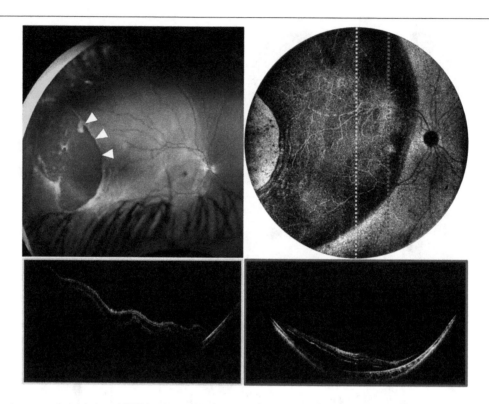

FIGURE 3 | Rhegmatogenous retinal detachment (RRD) in a 5-year-old girl, evaluated using widefield OCT. **(Top left)** Image is an ultra-widefield fundus photograph, with white arrows indicating a large temporal break. **(Top right)** Image is the 105° FOV OCT *en face*, with dotted lines indicating the locations of the color-coded B-scans shown below.

(PFV), there is a cellular connection through the vitreous cavity that connects the retina to the anterior segment, which can be associated with traction at the nerve or in an extramacular location, as seen in **Figure 7D**.

Vascular Disorders

Obtaining high quality OCTA is challenging even in cooperative adults, more so in children, and even more so with wider field of view. Nonetheless, particularly under anesthesia, it is possible to explore the potential role OCTA may play in the diagnosis of pediatric retinal diseases when used in conjunction with structural OCT (**Figure 8A**). **Figure 8B** demonstrates an OCTA taken during an EUA for a child with incontinentia pigmenti (IP), revealing both non-perfusion and neovascularization without the need for fluorescein dye. **Figure 9** demonstrates several VHL tumors visualized with *en face* OCT and OCTA.

Anterior Segment Optical Coherence Tomography

Anterior segment (AS)-OCT has demonstrated a number of potential uses in adults, including evaluation of corneal curvature and pathology, angle structures, and iris and lens abnormalities (28). We have included a few examples of AS-OCT obtained in our practice, but believe that the most significant potential application of this imaging may be in the evaluation and management of pediatric glaucoma in which anterior segment

dysgenesis is typical (29). **Figure 10** reveals *en face* and cross-sectional AS-OCT in several patients with both preoperative and post-operative abnormalities of the anterior segment.

DISCUSSION

In this paper, we reviewed our experience using WF-OCT in the management of patients with a variety of pediatric retinal diseases undergoing EUA. Compared to the highest resolution commercially available adult OCT devices, our prototype uses a faster, swept-source laser, which facilitates efficient imaging of the retina even in awake neonates and children. These results demonstrate the tradeoff between FOV and resolution, which is necessary when trying to keep imaging time to a minimum.

Retinopathy of Prematurity

The diagnosis of ROP relies on subjective assessment of clinical features on ophthalmoscopic exam or fundus photography, despite significant inter-observer variability in diagnosis, practice, and outcomes. Most of the early work using OCT work has focused on macular manifestations of ROP, such as the presence of macular edema, vitreous opacities, and the presence of retinoschisis posterior to the ridge (3, 4, 30). Widefield OCT has demonstrated the potential to provide real-time *en face* visualization, objective assessment of the peripheral stage, longitudinal monitoring of disease progression and regression,

Widefield Optical Coherence Tomography in Pediatric Retina: A Case Series of Intraoperative Applications...

85

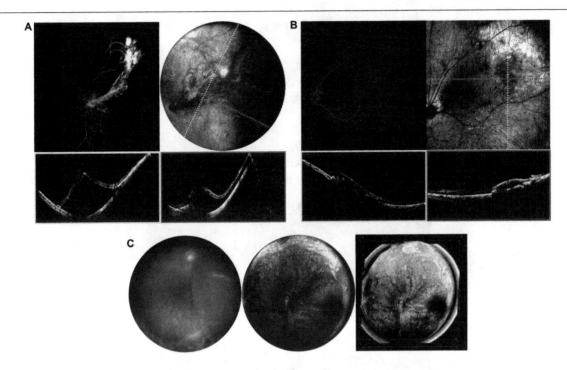

FIGURE 4 | Tractional and exudative retinal detachments. **(A)** ERD in a 15-year-old girl in the setting of a vasoproliferative lesion. **(B)** Chronic exudative retinopathy in a 16-year-old girl. For **(A,B)**, top left image is fluorescein angiography (FA), top right is the mean-intensity *en face* projection [105° FOV for panel **(A)** and 40° FOV for panel **(B)**], with dotted lines indicating the locations of the color-coded B-scans shown below. **(C)** ERD in a 5-month-old patient with ROP. From left: fundus photograph, 105° FOV OCT en face, and three-dimensional rendering of the same OCT volume.

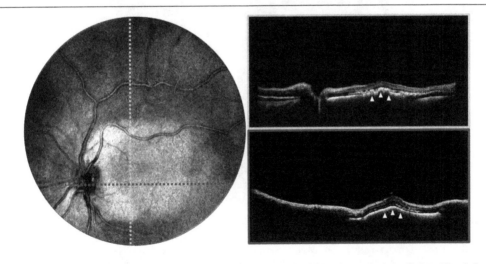

FIGURE 5 | Macular exudation in a 2-year-old with Coats disease. **(Left)** Image shows 55° FOV OCT *en face* projection, with dotted lines indicating the locations of the color-coded B-scans shown on the **(right)**. White arrows point to the area of subretinal exudation.

and detection of early vitreoretinal interface abnormalities (13, 14, 31).

Tractional, Exudative, and Rhegmatogenous Retinal Detachments

Differentiating the cause of retinal detachment is key for proper management of retinal detachments in children, and OCT may be a pivotal tool. RRD repair depends on accurate identification

of breaks, and the identification and management of proliferative vitreoretinopathy (PVR) membranes, which may be above or below the retinal surface. The standard of care is to carefully observe the entire retina with ophthalmoscopy and scleral depression for the presence of breaks. However, clinical diagnosis is not perfect and OCT may be superior for identification of peripheral pathology (32, 33). In this paper, we have presented several examples of tractional, rhegmatogenous, and exudative

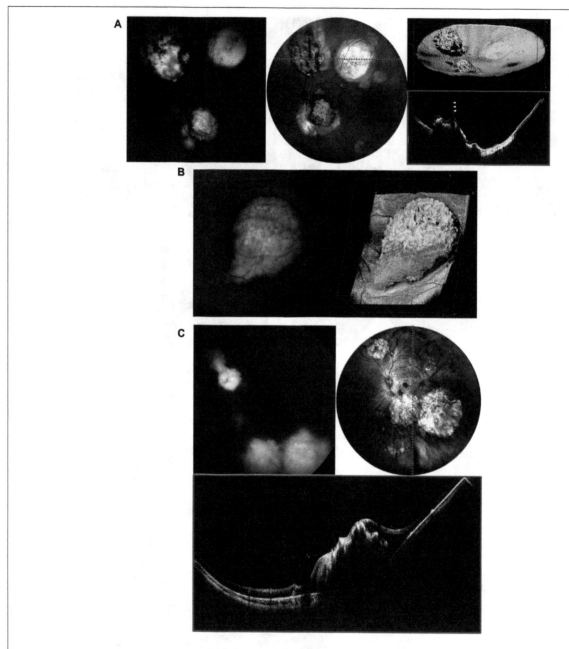

FIGURE 6 | Retinoblastoma evaluated with OCT in three patients with bilateral disease. **(A)** 3-year-old with multifocal RB in the left eye who has completed therapy. Left image is the fundus photograph, middle image is the 105° FOV OCT *en face* projection showing multiple regressed tumors, with dashed purple line corresponding to the location of the B-scan on the bottom right. White arrows point toward a vitreous band, while black arrows point to an area of retinal atrophy. Top right image shows three-dimensional rendering of the same volume shown in the middle panel. **(B)** Large partially calcified retinoblastoma in a 5-month-old patient undergoing systemic chemotherapy. Fundus photograph is shown on the left, and three-dimensional rendering of 40° FOV, high-resolution OCT volume is shown on the right. **(C)** 7-month-old undergoing systemic chemotherapy with active RB including diffuse vitreous seeding and multifocal tumors in the left eye. Top left image shows the fundus photograph, top right shows the 105° FOV OCT *en face* projection, with dashed purple line corresponding to the B-scan below.

detachments and highlighted ways in which WF-OCT may be utilized in the diagnosis and monitoring of these diseases in the future. One example of a potential use of WF-OCT is in monitoring the resolution of subretinal fluid following RD surgery. **Figure 11** reveals pre- and post-operative *en face* OCT and B-scans for a child with familial exudative vitreoretinopathy (FEVR) who presented shortly after birth with bilateral retinal

folds and tractional-exudative RDs. Post-operative scans reveal improved exudation and subretinal fluid.

Intraocular Tumors

In retinoblastoma (RB), the most common primary intraocular malignancy in children, the value of OCT has been demonstrated, however, there are known challenges

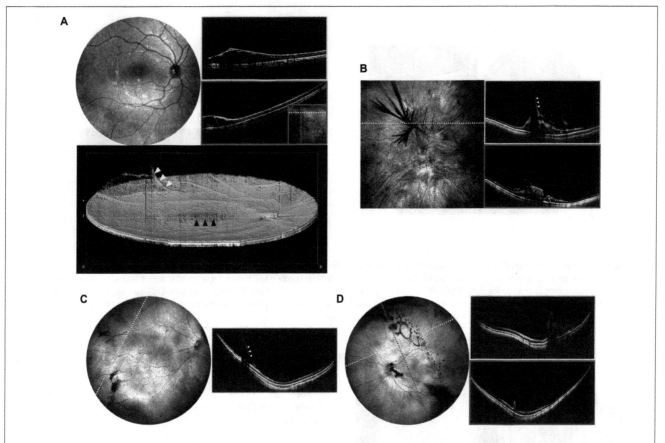

FIGURE 7 | Peripheral retinal and vitreoretinal interface abnormalities. **(A)** OCT evaluation in an 8-year-old patient with XLRS. Top left shows the 55° FOV *en face* projection, with corresponding volume rendering shown below. White arrows denote a blood vessel extending into the area of vitreoschisis (vitreous veils) and black arrows denote the area of foveoschisis. Top right images show high-resolution scans of an area of retinoschisis taken with 40° FOV. The inset in the bottom-right corner of the purple B-scan shows the locations of the cross-sections in dotted lines. **(B)** OCT evaluation of 7-month-old patient with history of non-accidental trauma, displaying disorganization of the retinal architecture, as well as vitreoretinal traction in region of prior breakthrough vitreous hemorrhage. Left image shows a 40° FOV *en face* projection, with dashed yellow and purple lines denoting the location of the corresponding B-scans on the right. White arrows denote vitreoretinal traction. **(C)** Vitreoretinal traction in a 2-month-old at site of regressed stage 3 extraretinal neovascularization in ROP. Left image shows 105° FOV *en face* view with dashed line indicating the location of the cross-sectional B-scan pictured on the right. White arrows denote vitreoretinal traction. **(D)** 1-month-old with ectopic PFV. Top left image shows the 105° FOV *en face* projection with complex oval-shaped vitreoschisis. Dotted lines correspond to B-scan locations demonstrating retinal fold through the macula.

with commercially available OCT systems (23–26). The potential value for WF-OCT to image and document tumor location and size, to monitor treatment response to laser, cryotherapy and chemotherapy, and to evaluate for newly emerging tumors is clear. A system which could combine structural images with OCTA would be of particular interest. House et al. (34) utilized OCTA to evaluate irregular tumor vasculature, with the advantage of depth resolution compared to fluorescein angiography (FA). As tumor vascular density in RB has been found to correlate significantly with a greater risk of metastasis (35), OCTA imaging could be useful in providing prognostic information. Beyond RB, there is considerable potential for WF-OCTA in the management of a wide variety of elevated and/or peripheral tumors involving the choroid and retina. In retinal hemangioblastomas, which may be associated with Von Hippel Lindau (VHL) syndrome, OCTA has been useful to differentiate non-vascular lesions from the vascular tumors, but the limited FOV has been a comparative disadvantage versus FA (36).

Inherited Retinal Dystrophies and Congenital Anomalies

In the realm of inherited retinal dystrophies (IRDs), OCT has been useful in identifying prognostic indicators, such as foveal cavitation (37), and the extent of photoreceptor atrophy. Spectral-domain (SD-OCT) technology has provided adequate axial resolution to evaluate X-linked retinoschisis in greater detail, elucidating the precise layers where retinal separation tends to occur (38). OCTA has also been utilized to evaluate choroidal neovascularization in IRDs, with advances in automated image segmentation capable of accurately delineating vascular plexuses even

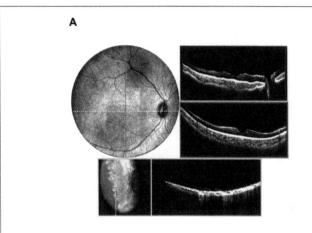

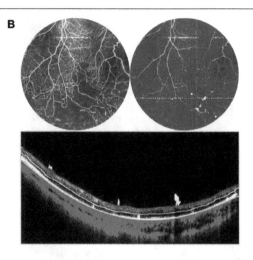

FIGURE 8 | Incontinentia pigmenti (IP). **(A)** OCT volume of a 1-year-old with IP. Top left image is the OCT 55° FOV *en face* projection. Corresponding color-coded B-scans at top right show irregularities in the nerve fiber layer and retinal surface. Bottom image in teal shows the retina after laser treatment, with *en face* view on the left, and corresponding B-scan on the right. **(B)** OCTA evaluation of a 2-year-old patient with IP. Top left image shows the OCTA en face projection with 55° FOV, while top right image shows the same volume with extraretinal neovascularization highlighted in bright yellow. Bottom image is the B-scan corresponding to the dashed yellow line above, showing automated segmentation of capillary plexus layers.

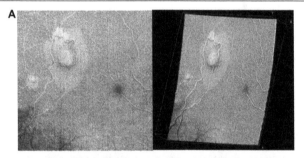

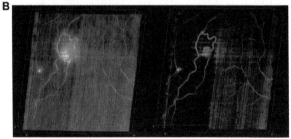

FIGURE 9 | Retinal hemangioblastomas in the setting of Von Hippel Lindau (VHL) syndrome. **(A)** Volume rendering of retinal hemangioblastomas in a 15-year-old. Left image shows an *en face* of a three-dimensional volume rendering of the tumors taken with a 40° FOV, while image on the right shows an angled view of the same volume. **(B)** Three-dimensional visualization of vessels generated from OCTA of the same volume as in panel **(A)**. The image on the left shows a three-dimensional rendering of the OCTA volume, showing flow signal within the tumors. Image on the right shows the same volume with higher contrast between vessels and surrounding tissue.

detect optic nerve head dragging and associated vitreous bands (41, 42). In IP, OCT has illustrated subclinical change to foveal structure, including inner and outer retinal thinning associated with retinal ischemia in IP (43–46).

Limitations of Widefield Optical Coherence Tomography Imaging

As mentioned throughout, there is a tradeoff between FOV, resolution, and acquisition speed, therefore the transverse resolution is lower for a given laser when expanding the FOV for a given amount of imaging time. Practically speaking, that means that individual B-scans may be lower resolution using this approach compared to commercially available systems with narrower FOV, such as the Heidelberg Flex system, although the acquisition time is faster (6). Other limitations to this approach overlap with those found in comparable commercial OCT systems, and include motion artifacts and shadow which often necessitate the capture of multiple redundant volumes per region of interest. Current OCT systems are also limited by the potential axial imaging range, which limits the ability to obtain UWF imaging in larger eyes.

CONCLUSION

In summary, the use of WF-OCT has several potential advantages compared to the clinical exam and fundus photography in the setting of pediatric retinal diseases. As in adults, the axial resolution is superior to what our eyes can see, enabling earlier detection of retinal abnormalities in multiple diseases. *En face* visualization can provide the same benefit as fundus

in the setting of distorted retinal architecture (39). In FEVR, OCTA has shown vascular abnormalities in the deep and superficial vascular complexes (40), and for both FEVR and PFV, handheld OCT has been used to

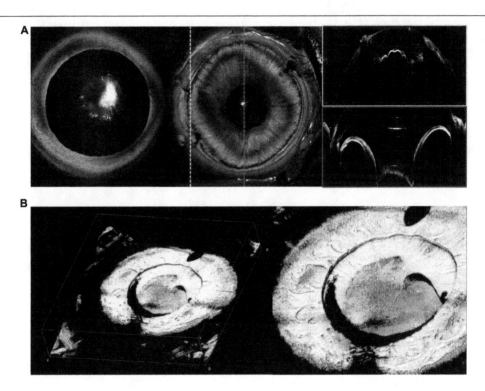

FIGURE 10 | Anterior segment (AS)-OCT. **(A)** AS-OCT in a 6-month-old with PFV. Leftmost *en face* OCT demonstrates good pupillary dilation and central cataract. Middle image shows *en face* of AS-OCT, with corresponding color-coded B-scans on the right. The scan outlined in yellow was taken at the limbus, providing visualization of the ciliary body. The scan outlined in purple shows the iris, with a reflection artifact affecting the cornea. **(B)** Silicone oil in the anterior chamber on AS-OCT in a 14-year-old. Leftmost image shows three-dimensional rendering of the iris and anterior chamber, while rightmost image shows a close up of retained oil above the lens. Both **(A,B)** were captured with a 105° FOV.

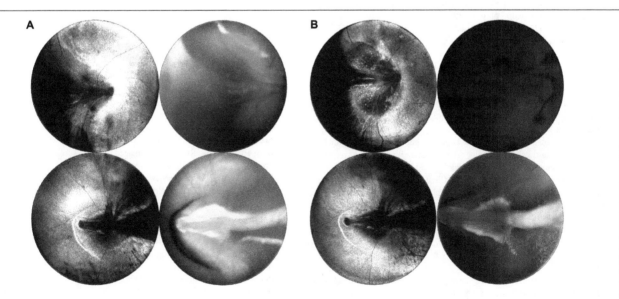

FIGURE 11 | Longitudinal monitoring of a patient with familial exudative vitreoretinopathy (FEVR). **(A)** Pre-surgical repair of bilateral tractional retinal detachments secondary to FEVR in a 4-month-old patient taken with 55° FOV device. **(B)** Post-surgical repair images, with OCT *en face* taken 1 week after surgery, and fundus photographs taken 3 months after surgery. For panels **(A,B)**, left column are OCT en face projections, whilst right column are color fundus photographs.

photography, but with volumetric structural and angiographic information as well. Finally, OCT facilitates objective assessment of retinal structures that can be used to monitor disease stability.

The challenges to widespread adoption of this technology remain the lack of commercially available OCT devices of sufficient speed and FOV to be effective in capturing images outside of the macula. As the costs of lasers come down with time, our hope is that the market will facilitate the routine use of this technology in the care of children with retinal disease.

AUTHOR CONTRIBUTIONS

JC, MC, DH, YaJ, and YiJ designed the study and obtained the funding. SO developed and maintained the patient database and consented all patients. AS contributed to the data and critically reviewed the manuscript. T-TN, GL, SN, SK, and XW identified, processed, and contributed to the images to the final manuscript. All authors reviewed and approved of the final version of the manuscript.

REFERENCES

1. Maldonado RS, O'Connell RV, Sarin N, Freedman SF, Wallace DK, Cotten CM, et al. Dynamics of human foveal development after premature birth. *Ophthalmology.* (2011) 118:2315–25. doi: 10.1016/j.ophtha.2011.05.028

2. Lee H, Proudlock FA, Gottlob I. Pediatric optical coherence tomography in clinical practice—recent progress. *Invest Ophthalmol Vis Sci.* (2016) 57:OCT69–79. doi: 10.1167/iovs.15-18825

3. Vinekar A, Avadhani K, Sivakumar M, Mahendradas P, Kurian M, Braganza S, et al. Understanding clinically undetected macular changes in early retinopathy of prematurity on spectral domain optical coherence tomography. *Invest Ophthalmol Vis Sci.* (2011) 52:5183–8. doi: 10.1167/iovs.10-7155

4. Muni RH, Kohly RP, Charonis AC, Lee TC. Retinoschisis detected with handheld spectral-domain optical coherence tomography in neonates with advanced retinopathy of prematurity. *Arch Ophthalmol.* (2010) 128:57–62. doi: 10.1001/archophthalmol.2009.361

5. Joshi MM, Trese MT, Capone A Jr. Optical coherence tomography findings in stage 4A retinopathy of prematurity: a theory for visual variability. *Ophthalmology.* (2006) 113:657–60. doi: 10.1016/j.ophtha.2006.01.007

6. Hsu ST, Ngo HT, Stinnett SS, Cheung NL, House RJ, Kelly MP, et al. Assessment of macular microvasculature in healthy eyes of infants and children using OCT angiography. *Ophthalmology.* (2019) 126:1703–11. doi: 10.1016/j.ophtha.2019.06.028

7. Viehland C, Chen X, Tran-Viet D, Jackson-Atogi M, Ortiz P, Waterman G, et al. Ergonomic handheld OCT angiography probe optimized for pediatric and supine imaging. *Biomed Opt Express.* (2019) 10:2623–38. doi: 10.1364/BOE.10.002623

8. Jin P, Zou H, Zhu J, Xu X, Jin J, Chang TC, et al. Choroidal and retinal thickness in children with different refractive status measured by swept-source optical coherence tomography. *Am J Ophthalmol.* (2016) 168:164–76.

9. Campbell JP, Nudleman E, Yang J, Tan O, Chan RP, Chiang MF, et al. Handheld optical coherence tomography angiography and ultra–wide-field optical coherence tomography in retinopathy of prematurity. *JAMA Ophthalmol.* (2017) 135:977–81.

10. Chen X, Viehland C, Carrasco-Zevallos OM, Keller B, Vajzovic L, Izatt JA, et al. Microscope-integrated optical coherence tomography angiography in the operating room in young children with retinal vascular disease. *JAMA Ophthalmol.* (2017) 135:483–6. doi: 10.1001/jamaophthalmol.2017.0422

11. Ni S, Wei X, Ng R, Ostmo S, Chiang MF, Huang D, et al. High-speed and widefield handheld swept-source OCT angiography with a VCSEL light source. *Biomed Opt Express.* (2021) 12:3553–70. doi: 10.1364/BOE.425411

12. Ni S, Nguyen T-TP, Ng R, Khan S, Ostmo S, Jia Y, et al. 105° field of view non-contact handheld swept-source optical coherence tomography. *Opt Lett.* (2021) 46:5878–81. doi: 10.1364/OL.443672

13. Nguyen T-TP, Ni S, Khan S, Wei X, Ostmo S, Chiang MF, et al. Advantages of widefield optical coherence tomography in the diagnosis of retinopathy of prematurity. *Front Pediatr.* (2022) 9:797684. doi: 10.3389/fped.2021.797684

14. Scruggs BA, Ni S, Nguyen T-TP, Ostmo S, Chiang MF, Jia Y, et al. Peripheral optical coherence tomography assisted by scleral depression in retinopathy of prematurity. *Ophthalmol Sci.* (2021) 2:100094. doi: 10.1016/j.xops.2021.100094

15. Borkovkina S, Camino A, Janpongsri W, Sarunic MV, Jian Y. Real-time retinal layer segmentation of OCT volumes with GPU accelerated inferencing using a compressed, low-latency neural network. *Biomed Opt Exp.* (2020) 11:3968–84. doi: 10.1364/BOE.395279

16. Jian Y, Wong K, Sarunic MV. Graphics processing unit accelerated optical coherence tomography processing at megahertz axial scan rate and high resolution video rate volumetric rendering. *J Biomed Opt.* (2013) 18:026002. doi: 10.1117/1.JBO.18.2.026002

17. Xu J, Wong K, Jian Y, Sarunic MV. Real-time acquisition and display of flow contrast using speckle variance optical coherence tomography in a graphics processing unit. *J Biomed Opt.* (2014) 19:026001. doi: 10.1117/1.JBO.19.2.026001

18. MathWorks. *MATLAB and Statistics Release.* Natick, MA: The MathWorks Inc (2021).

19. Abràmoff MD, Magalhães PJ, Ram SJ. Image processing with ImageJ. *Biophotonics Int.* (2004) 11:36–42.

20. Wei X, Hormel TT, Jia Y. Phase-stabilized complex-decorrelation angiography. *Biomed Opt Express.* (2021) 12:2419–31. doi: 10.1364/BOE.420503

21. Guo Y, Camino A, Zhang M, Wang J, Huang D, Hwang T, et al. Automated segmentation of retinal layer boundaries and capillary plexuses in wide-field optical coherence tomographic angiography. *Biomed Opt Exp.* (2018) 9:4429–42. doi: 10.1364/BOE.9.004429

22. Ecsedy M, Szamosi A, Karkó C, Zubovics L, Varsányi B, Németh J, et al. A comparison of macular structure imaged by optical coherence tomography in preterm and full-term children. *Invest Ophthalmol Vis Sci.* (2007) 48:5207–11.

23. Cao C, Markovitz M, Ferenczy S, Shields CL. Hand-held spectral-domain optical coherence tomography of small macular retinoblastoma in infants before and after chemotherapy. *J Pediatr Ophthalmol Strabismus.* (2014) 51:230–4. doi: 10.3928/01913913-20140603-01

24. Rootman DB, Gonzalez E, Mallipatna A, VandenHoven C, Hampton L, Dimaras H, et al. Hand-held high-resolution spectral domain optical coherence tomography in retinoblastoma: clinical and morphologic considerations. *Br J Ophthalmol.* (2013) 97:59–65. doi: 10.1136/bjophthalmol-2012-302133

25. Nadiarnykh O, McNeill-Badalova NA, Gaillard MC, Bosscha MI, Fabius AW, Verbraak FD, et al. Optical coherence tomography (OCT) to image active and inactive retinoblastomas as well as retinomas. *Acta Ophthalmol.* (2020) 98:158–65. doi: 10.1111/aos.14214

26. Soliman SE, VandenHoven C, MacKeen LD, Héon E, Gallie BL. Optical coherence tomography–guided decisions in retinoblastoma management. *Ophthalmology.* (2017) 124:859–72. doi: 10.1016/j.ophtha.2017.01.052

27. Skalet AH, Campbell JP, Jian Y. Ultra-widefield Optical Coherence Tomography for Retinoblastoma. *Ophthalmology*. (2022). 129:718.

28. Ang M, Baskaran M, Werkmeister RM, Chua J, Schmidl D, Dos Santos VA, et al. Anterior segment optical coherence tomography. *Prog Retin Eye Res*. (2018) 66:132–56.

29. Pilat AV, Proudlock FA, Shah S, Sheth V, Purohit R, Abbot J, et al. Assessment of the anterior segment of patients with primary congenital glaucoma using handheld optical coherence tomography. *Eye*. (2019) 33:1232–9. doi: 10.1038/s41433-019-0369-3

30. Legocki AT, Zepeda EM, Gillette TB, Grant LE, Shariff A, Touch P, et al. Vitreous findings by handheld spectral-domain oct correlate with retinopathy of prematurity severity. *Ophthalmol Retina*. (2020) 4:1008–15. doi: 10.1016/j.oret.2020.03.027

31. Chen X, Mangalesh S, Dandridge A, Tran-Viet D, Wallace DK, Freedman SF, et al. Spectral-domain OCT findings of retinal vascular–avascular junction in infants with retinopathy of prematurity. *Ophthalmol Retina*. (2018) 2:963–71. doi: 10.1016/j.oret.2018.02.001

32. Ansari WH, Blackorby BL, Shah GK, Blinder KJ, Dang S. OCT Assistance in identifying retinal breaks in symptomatic posterior vitreous detachments. *Ophthalmic Surg Lasers Imaging Retina*. (2020) 51:628–32.

33. Choudhry N, Golding J, Manry MW, Rao RC. Ultra-widefield steering-based spectral-domain optical coherence tomography imaging of the retinal periphery. *Ophthalmology*. (2016) 123:1368–74. doi: 10.1016/j.ophtha.2016.01.045

34. House RJ, Hsu ST, Thomas AS, Finn AP, Toth CA, Materin MA, et al. Vascular findings in a small retinoblastoma tumor using OCT angiography. *Ophthalmol Retina*. (2019) 3:194. doi: 10.1016/j.oret.2018.09.018

35. Rössler J, Dietrich T, Pavlakovic H, Schweigerer L, Havers W, Schüler A, et al. Higher vessel densities in retinoblastoma with local invasive growth and metastasis. *Am J Pathol*. (2004) 164:391–4. doi: 10.1016/S0002-9440(10)63129-X

36. Sagar P, Rajesh R, Shanmugam M, Konana VK, Mishra D. Comparison of optical coherence tomography angiography and fundus fluorescein angiography features of retinal capillary hemangioblastoma. *Indian J Ophthalmol*. (2018) 66:872.

37. Parodi MB, Cicinelli MV, Iacono P, Bolognesi G, Bandello F. Multimodal imaging of foveal cavitation in retinal dystrophies. *Graefes Arch Clin Exp Ophthalmol*. (2017) 255:271–9.

38. Yu J, Ni Y, Keane PA, Jiang C, Wang W, Xu G. Foveomacular schisis in juvenile X-linked retinoschisis: an optical coherence tomography study. *Am J Ophthalmol*. (2010) 149:973–978.e2. doi: 10.1016/j.ajo.2010.01.031

39. Patel RC, Gao SS, Zhang M, Alabduljalil T, Al-Qahtani A, Weleber RG, et al. Optical coherence tomography angiography of choroidal neovascularization in four inherited retinal dystrophies. *Retina*. (2016) 36:2339–47. doi: 10.1097/IAE.0000000000001159

40. Hsu ST, Finn AP, Chen X, Ngo HT, House RJ, Toth CA, et al. Macular microvascular findings in familial exudative vitreoretinopathy on optical coherence tomography angiography. *Ophthalmic Surg Lasers Imaging Retina*. (2019) 50:322–9.

41. Lee J, El-Dairi MA, Tran-Viet D, Mangalesh S, Dandridge A, Jiramongkolchai K, et al. Longitudinal changes in the optic nerve head and retina over time in very young children with familial exudative vitreoretinopathy. *Retina*. (2019) 39:98. doi: 10.1097/IAE.0000000000001930

42. De la Huerta I, Mesi O, Murphy B, Drenser KA, Capone A Jr, Trese MT. Spectral domain optical coherence tomography imaging of the macula and vitreomacular interface in persistent fetal vasculature syndrome with posterior involvement. *Retina*. (2019) 39:581–6. doi: 10.1097/IAE.0000000000001993

43. Mangalesh S, Chen X, Tran-Viet D, Viehland C, Freedman SF, Toth CA. Assessment of the retinal structure in children with incontinentia pigmenti. *Retina*. (2017) 37:1568.

44. McClintic SM, Wilson LB, Campbell JP. Novel macular findings on optical coherence tomography in incontinentia pigmenti. *JAMA Ophthalmol*. (2016) 134:e162751. doi: 10.1001/jamaophthalmol.2016.2751

45. Kim SJ, Yang J, Liu G, Huang D, Campbell JP. Optical coherence tomography angiography and ultra-widefield optical coherence tomography in a child with Incontinentia pigmenti. *Ophthalmic Surg Lasers Imaging Retina*. (2018) 49:273–5. doi: 10.3928/23258160-20180329-11

46. Kunkler AL, Patel NA, Russell JF, Fan KC, Al-Khersan H, Iyer PG, et al. Intraoperative optical coherence tomography angiography in children with Incontinentia pigmenti. *Ophthalmol Retina*. (2022) 6:330–2. doi: 10.1016/j.oret.2022.01.001

11

Publication Trends of Research on Retinoblastoma During 2001–2021

Xiang Gu [1,2†], Minyue Xie [1,2†], Renbing Jia [1,2*] and Shengfang Ge [1,2*]

[1] Department of Ophthalmology, Ninth People's Hospital, Shanghai JiaoTong University School of Medicine, Shanghai, China,
[2] Shanghai Key Laboratory of Orbital Diseases and Ocular Oncology, Shanghai JiaoTong University School of Medicine, Shanghai, China

*Correspondence:
Renbing Jia
renbingjia@sjtu.edu.cn
Shengfang Ge
geshengfang@sjtu.edu.cn

[†] These authors have contributed equally to this work

Background: Retinoblastoma is the most common primary intraocular malignancy of childhood. Despite high survival and eye salvage as the result of various types of therapies, retinoblastoma remains a disease that places a considerable burden on developing countries. Our study attempted to analyse the research trends in retinoblastoma research and compare contributions from different countries, institutions, journals, and authors.

Methods: We extracted all publications concerning retinoblastoma from 2001 to 2021 from the Web of Science database. Microsoft Excel and VOSviewer were employed to collect publication data, analyse publication trends, and visualize relevant results.

Results: A total of 1,675 publications with 30,148 citations were identified. The United States contributed the most publications (643) and citations (16,931 times) with the highest H-index value (67) as of February 4, 2021. China ranked second in the number of publications (259), while ranking fourth in both citations (2,632 times) and the H-index (26) ranked fourth. The *British Journal of Ophthalmology* was the most productive journal concerning retinoblastoma, and Abramson DH had published the most papers in the field. Keywords were categorized into three clusters; tumor-related research, clinical research, and management-related research. The keywords "intravitreal," "intraarterial," and "intravenous" appeared the most frequently, with the average appearing year being 2018.1, 2017.7, and 2017.1, respectively. Management-related research has been recognized as a heavily researched topic in the field.

Conclusion: We conclude that the United States, China, and India made the most exceptional contributions in the field of retinoblastoma research, while China still has a disparity between the quantity and quality of publications. Management-related research, including intravitreal, intraarterial, and intravenous chemotherapy was considered as a potential focus for future research.

Keywords: retinoblastoma, publication trends, bibliometric analysis, chemotherapy, citations

INTRODUCTION

Retinoblastoma, the most common primary intraocular malignancy of childhood, is initiated by mutation of both *RB1* alleles in a single susceptible developing retinal cell, undergoes the limited proliferation of an $RB1^{-/-}$ retinal cell to form a non-malignant retinal tumor and consequently experiences uncontrolled proliferation and malignant transformation based on genetic or epigenetic alterations (1).

The incidence of retinoblastoma is constant without race or gender differences at one case every 15,000 to 20,000 live births worldwide (2). Asia and Africa, which experience large populations and high birth rates, bear the greatest burden of retinoblastoma (3). They also carry the highest mortality of 40 to 70%, compared with 3 to 5% in Europe, Canada, and the USA, which contributes to the delay in diagnosis and the lack of access to canonical treatment (4–6).

The diagnosis of retinoblastoma is often based on special signs and clinical examinations. Leukocoria is the most common clinical feature of retinoblastoma, in which the normal pupillary is replaced by a whitish discoloration as a result of abnormal growth and calcification of the developing intraocular tumor, followed by strabismus, owing to loss of central vision from the growing tumor. Advanced retinoblastoma may manifest with iris color change, enlarged cornea, or non-infective orbital inflammation (7). Commonly, it is sufficient to make the diagnosis employing indirect ophthalmoscopy with the pupil pharmacologically dilated. In addition, ocular ultrasonography can be used to detect calcification and magnetic resonance imaging (MRI) can be used to evaluate invasion of the optic nerve and the existence of trilateral retinoblastoma (8). Owing to the risk of metastasis brought by biopsy, diagnosis of retinoblastoma does not depend on histopathologic examination (9). However, histological examination after enucleation is a way of assessing high-risk features and establish pathological staging to assist the management of retinoblastoma (10).

The management of retinoblastoma underwent dramatic evolution in a short period of time. Enucleation was the major treatment for retinoblastoma until the emergence of external beam radiotherapy (EBRT) in the 1950s. However, radiation considerably enhances the risk of developing a second malignancy in survivors of retinoblastoma, consequently leading to its replacement by chemotherapy in the 1990s (11). Chemotherapy was originally administered intravenously with vincristine, etoposide, and carboplatin as the most common agents, and intravenous chemotherapy (IVC) combined with local treatments achieved over 90% tumor control rates in Group

A-C retinoblastoma eyes (12). Notably, subsequent targeted chemotherapy, such as intraarterial chemotherapy (IAC) and intravitreal chemotherapy (IVitC), was introduced to diminish the systemic side effects related to IVC and to increase the salvage rate of advanced intraocular retinoblastoma eyes (13, 14). The reported eye salvage rate for Group D retinoblastoma increased from 47 to 85% thanks to the unitality of IAC (15). Various therapies guarantee that the retinoblastoma patients to choose the optimal management according to their conditions. Sound knowledge of the individual conditions and careful monitoring for recurrences are pivotal for the management of retinoblastoma patients.

Bibliometrics is an optimal choice to evaluate particular research trends concerning a certain field over time (16). Bibliometrics plays an important role in analyzing the quantity and quality of publications, including books and journal articles, by employing a literature system and literature metrology (17). Furthermore, the analysis contributes to characterizing and predicting the development in a specific field and comparing contributions among countries, institutions, journals, and authors (18). Remarkably, bibliometrics has been increasingly prevalent based on its importance in governing policy-making, clinical guidelines and research trends (19–21). However, there have so far been few bibliometric studies in the field of ophthalmology, and even fewer in the field of ocular tumors (22).

The study manifests a general analysis of the present state of global retinoblastoma research based on Web of Science (WOS) data. Bibliometrics was applied to uncover the trends in retinoblastoma research and explore its potential hotspots.

METHODS

Data Sources and Search Strategies

Based on the fact that the Science Citation Index-Expanded (SCI-E) of WOS was considered the optimal database for bibliometric analysis, a literature search was conducted for the years 2001 to 2021 using the WOS database.

All searches were performed on a single day, February 4, 2021, to avoid biases introduced by daily database renewal. The search strategies were integrated as follows: TI= (retinoblastoma) AND TS= (eye OR ocular OR oculus OR optical OR ophthalmic OR ophthalmology OR intraocular OR optic OR retinal OR retina) AND Language = English. Despite various types of manuscripts, only the original articles and reviews in the core database were included. Detailed procedures of the enrolment and screening were illustrated in **Figure 1**.

Data Collection

The data were extracted carefully from all eligible publications, including titles, keywords, publication dates, countries and regions, institutions, authors, publishing journals, sums of citations, and H-indexes. Subsequently, the data were imported into Microsoft Excel 2010 (Redmond, Washington, USA) and VOSviewer (Leiden University, Leiden, the Netherlands) and analyzed both quantitatively and qualitatively.

Abbreviations:
AAY, Average appearing year; CeRNA, Competing endogenous RNA; CircRNAs, Circular RNAs; CKS1B, Cyclin-dependent kinase regulatory subunit 1B; EBRT, External beam radiotherapy; IAC, Intraarterial chemotherapy; IVC, Intravenous chemotherapy; IVitC, Intravitreal chemotherapy; MRI, Magnetic resonance imaging; RRI, Relative research interest; SCARA5, Scavenger receptor class A member 5; SCI-E, Science Citation Index-Expanded; STAT3, Signal transducer and activator of transcription 3; VEGF, Vascular endothelial growth factor; WOS, Web of Science.

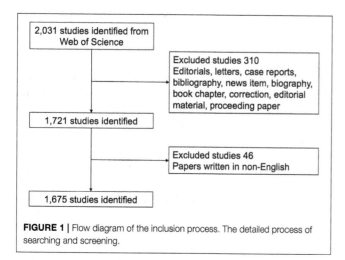

FIGURE 1 | Flow diagram of the inclusion process. The detailed process of searching and screening.

Bibliometric Analysis

Contribution of Countries to Global Publications

WOS was used to describe and examine the characteristics of all included publications. Microsoft Excel 2010 was applied to assess and rank the number of publications among different countries. To determine the global attention to the field, Relative research interest (RRI), which was defined as the number of publications in a specific field divided by all publications across all fields per year, was calculated.

Citations and H-Index

The information related to citations was acquired from the WOS database. The H-index means a scholar, a country or an author published H papers that have been cited in other publications at least H times, considered widely to reflect the scientific research impact of a scholar, a country, or an author (23).

Growth Trends of Publications

To predict the growth trends of publications in the field, Microsoft Excel 2010 was applied to generate the prediction model $f(x) = ax^3 + bx^2 + cx + d$ to calculate cumulative publications, by which we predicted future publication trends. In this formula, x represents time (year) and f (x) denotes the cumulative volume of publications in a certain year (24).

Journals, Institutions, and Authors Publishing Research

The top journals, institutions and authors and their number of publications were retrieved from WOS and Microsoft Excel 2010 was employed to illustrate the results.

Analysis of Keywords

VOSviewer was employed to map and visualize the network of keywords related to retinoblastoma research. Keywords were classified into disparate clusters according to co-occurrence analysis and simultaneously color-coded by time course. Furthermore, the average appearing year (AAY) was defined to estimate the novelty of a keyword (25).

RESULTS

Assessment of Countries Contributing to Global Publications

A total of 1,675 articles from 2001 to 2021 met the search criteria. The United States ranked first in the number of publications (643, 38.4%), followed by China (259, 15.5%) and India (202, 12.1%) (**Figure 2A**). In relation to the number of publications per year, the year with the most publications was 2020 (182, 10.9%). Taking all-field publications into consideration, the global attention to this field based on the RRI value was ~0.005% before 2012, maintaining 0.006% from 2013 to 2019, and rising to 0.008% in 2019 (**Figure 2B**). While before 2011, China published no more than 6 papers in this field per year, the proportion of Chinese publications has increased rapidly over the last decade. Of note, China (66, 36.3%) exceeded the United States (48, 26.4%) in the number of annual publications each year for the first time in 2020.

Citations and H-Index Analysis

Based on the citation report retrieved from the WOS database, all publications related to retinoblastoma have been cited 30,148 times since 2001 (15,469 citations without self-citations), with an average citing frequency of 18 times per paper. The most regularly cited papers were the papers from the United States, accounting for 56.2% of all citations (16,931 citations and 12,612 citations without self-citations) with an H-index of 67. Canada ranked second with a citation frequency of 2,864 (2,571 citations without self-citations) and an H-index of 27, followed by India with 2,829 citations (2,460 citations without self-citations) and an H-index of 27. Despite the second rank of China in the number of publications, the citation frequency ranked the fourth with 2,632 citations (2,230 citations without self-citations), and fourth with an H-index of 26 (**Figure 2A**).

Growth Trends Prediction

Model fitting curves of the growth in retinoblastoma publication demonstrated a significant correlation between time and a cumulative number of publications (**Figure 3**). Furthermore, publication trends for the following 5 years were estimated according to cumulative publication numbers over the past two decades. The volume of global publications increased at a steady and slow curve (**Figure 3A**), which is in accord with several major countries such as the United States and India (**Figures 3B,D**), while China has manifested an obviously faster growth (**Figure 3C**).

Journals Publishing Research on Retinoblastoma

More than one-third of the papers within this field were published in the 20 journals listed in **Figure 4A** (826, 38.7%), the *British Journal of Ophthalmology* published the most with 83 papers (5.0%), followed by *Ophthalmology* with 68 papers (3.9%). In addition, the number of papers published in the journal *Pediatric Blood Cancer* and *Investigative Ophthalmology Visual Science* was 66 (3.5%) and 59 (2.9%) records, ranking the third and the fourth, respectively. Other journals with

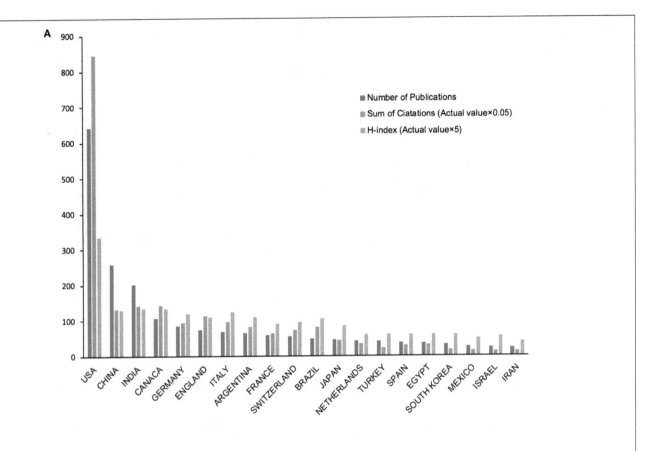

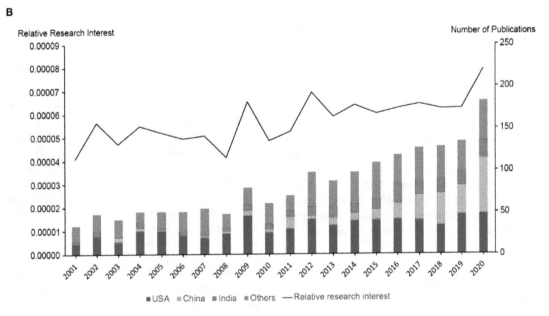

FIGURE 2 | Contributions of different countries/regions to retinoblastoma research. **(A)** The number of publications, sum of citations (×0.05), and H-index (×5) of the top 20 countries or regions; **(B)** The number of publications worldwide and the top 3 countries per year are shown in the histogram. The time course of relative research interest is shown in the line chart.

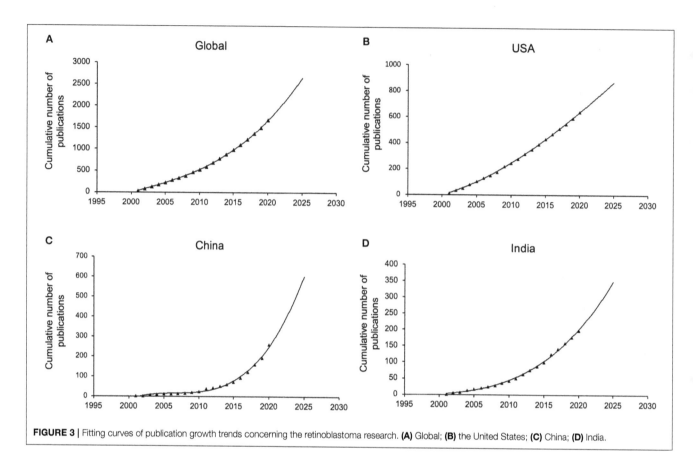

FIGURE 3 | Fitting curves of publication growth trends concerning the retinoblastoma research. **(A)** Global; **(B)** the United States; **(C)** China; **(D)** India.

high impacts, such as *Nature*, published three pieces of high-quality research in the related field, *Cell* published two and *Lancet* published one.

Institutions Publishing Research on Retinoblastoma

Publications from the top 20 institutes accounted for 77.2% of all literature on retinoblastoma research (**Figure 4B**). Memorial Sloan Kettering Cancer Center in the United States had the highest number of publications (117, 7.0%) followed by Jefferson University in the United States (115, 6.9%). Within the top 20 institutions identified in the field, eleven are in the United States, three are Canadian institutions, two are in Argentina, two are in France, and one is in India.

Authors Publishing Research on Retinoblastoma

A total of 598 papers were published by the top 10 authors, accounting for 35.7% of all literature in the field. Abramson DH of Memorial Sloan Kettering Cancer Center had published 114 papers related to retinoblastoma, ranking first in the number of publications (**Table 1**). Shields CL of Jefferson University ranked second with 103 publications; however, she had the highest H-index of 36. Shields JA of Jefferson University published 59 papers, ranking third. Among the top 10 authors, seven are from

the United States, and the remaining three are from Argentina, Canada, and India, respectively.

Analysis of Keywords in Retinoblastoma Publications

Keywords that occurred more than 25 times in the titles and abstracts extracted from 1675 publications were analyzed by using VOSviewer. After merging words with the same meaning words and excluding meaningless words, 81 keywords were identified and classified into tumor-related research, clinical research, and management-related research clusters (**Figure 5A**). Within the tumor-related research cluster, mentioned keywords were as follows: apoptosis (106 times), proliferation (87 times), and progression (72 times). With regard to the clinical research cluster, invasion (100 times), survival (103 times), and diagnosis (92 times) were the primary keywords. As with the management-related research cluster, the most common keywords comprised chemoreduction (316 times), intraarterial chemotherapy (309 times), and radiotherapy (123 times).

In addition, keywords were subsequently colored according to the AAY subsequently by VOSviewer (**Figure 5B**). Keywords that appeared relatively earlier were in blue, and keywords with a more recent appearance were in yellow. Keywords such as intravitreal (cluster 3, AAY of 2018.1), intraarterial (cluster 3, AAY of 2017.7), and intravenous (cluster 3, AAY of 2017.1) have emerged recently, while radiotherapy (cluster 3, AAY of 2010.0) was the major topic during the early stage. In addition, migration

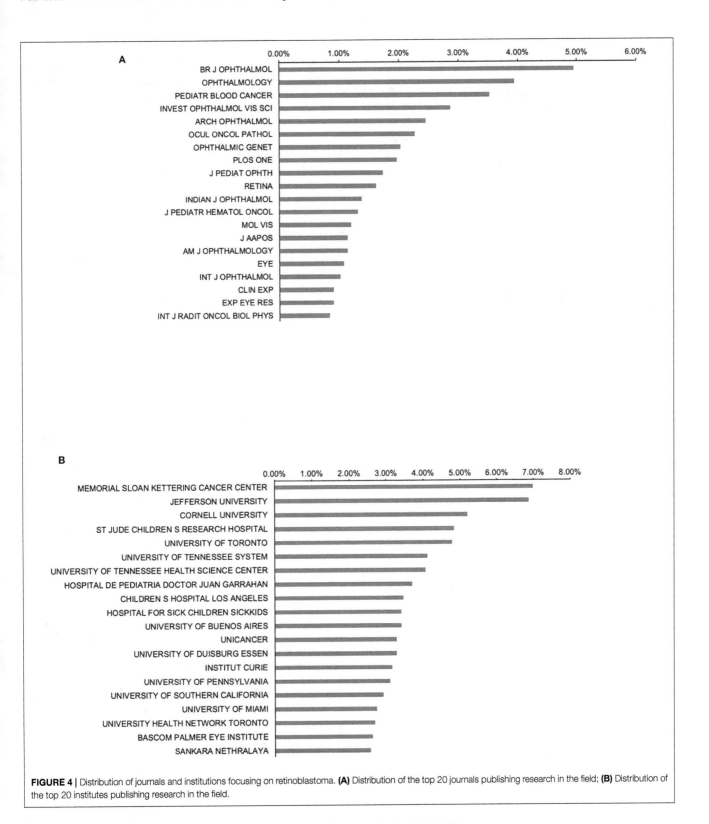

FIGURE 4 | Distribution of journals and institutions focusing on retinoblastoma. **(A)** Distribution of the top 20 journals publishing research in the field; **(B)** Distribution of the top 20 institutes publishing research in the field.

(cluster 1, AAY of 2017.6) and cell-proliferation (cluster 1, AAY of 2017.2) were the two newest words in the tumor-related research cluster. Of note, the most newly appearing words in the management-related research cluster indicate its trend in future investigation.

DISCUSSION

Trends in Retinoblastoma Research

As is documented, the United States ranked first in terms of the total number of citations and H-index values in

TABLE 1 | Top 10 authors with the most publications in retinoblastoma research.

Author	Country	Affiliation	No. of publications	No. of citations
ABRAMSON DH	USA	Memorial Sloan Kettering Cancer Center	114	3,768
SHIELDS CL	USA	Jefferson University	103	3,738
SHIELDS JA	USA	Jefferson University	59	2,949
DUNKEL IJ	USA	Memorial Sloan Kettering Cancer Center	56	2,070
FRANCIS JH	USA	Memorial Sloan Kettering Cancer Center	49	655
GALLIE BL	Canada	University of Toronto	47	1,826
CHANTADA GL	Argentina	Hospital De Pediatria Doctor Juan Garrahan	43	1,354
KRISHNAKUMAR S	India	Sankara Nethralaya	43	589
RODRIGUEZ-GALINDO C	USA	St Jude Children S Research Hospital	42	1,827
WILSON MW	USA	University of Tennessee Health Science Center	42	1,171

the field of retinoblastoma research, and undoubtedly, the United States contributed the most. Although retinoblastoma was first described as a distinct clinical entity by a Scottish surgeon in 1809, American scholars dedicated researching the disease earlier than researchers in the rest of the countries (11). In addition, the two-hit hypothesis was initially proposed by Alfred Knudson, an American physician and cancer geneticist, in 1971 (26), which shifted the concept of the cause of cancer from oncogene activation to tumor-suppressor loss of function, indicating that American scholars took the lead in comprehensively understanding the pathogenesis of retinoblastoma and developing early genetic testing and screening programmes. Moreover, the superior condition of both basic and clinical research in the United States provided adequate funding, advanced equipment, standardized systems and professional researchers. The fact that India ranked second in the sum of citations and H-index values may result from the largest burden of retinoblastoma carried by India, with almost 1,500 new cases every year (27).

Notably, China ranked second in the total number of publications; however, it ranked fourth in the sum of citations and H-index values, suggesting that the quality of research in the field of retinoblastoma still needs to be improved. The contradiction between the quantity and quality may be attributed to the lack of a standardized academic evaluation system, uneven competencies in clinical and scientific research among multiple institutions and the deficiency of high-quality multicenter randomized clinical trials (RCTs).

As illustrated in the time curve, steady growth in the cumulative number of publications concerning global retinoblastoma research was observed over time. In contrast to the United States, which maintained the annual publication quantity within a stable range as the global trend, China sustained a rapid development in the number of publications per year, which may be attributed to improved research conditions, increasingly dense academic networks and growing attention given to the disease over the last decade. Significantly, China accounted for one-third of the global number of publications in 2020, indicating the gradually indispensable position of China in the field.

Within the top 20 institutions in research regarding retinoblastoma, 11 institutions were from the United States, demonstrating its dominant status in the field. The fact that the United States occupies the most productive institutions across the world may partially explain why the United States consistently maintains its high quantity and quality of publications. Although China ranked next to the United States in the total publication quantity, none of the institutions in China was in the top 20, indicating the lack of institutions with professional and research stature with regard to retinoblastoma in China.

Remarkably, journals in the field of ophthalmology such as the *British Journal of Ophthalmology*, *Ophthalmology*, and *Investigative Ophthalmology Visual Science* were the primary journals involved in the publication of research on retinoblastoma. Therefore, it is reasonably concluded that future developments in the field are more likely to be published in these journals.

In relation to authors, Abramson DH of Memorial Sloan Kettering Cancer Center, Shields CL, and Shields JA of Jefferson University had published the most papers on retinoblastoma research. Abramson DH mainly evaluated and developed the management of retinoblastoma (28–30), and similarly, Shields CL focused on the investigation of optimizing the treatment for retinoblastoma patients but paid more attention to the establishment of an international classification to predict chemoreduction success (12). These scholars were considered leaders within the scope of retinoblastoma and their studies will continue to influence future research development and guide the cutting edge research on retinoblastoma.

Focus in Retinoblastoma Research

Published papers that are cited frequently possess tremendous academic impact. The 10 publications with the highest citation frequency in retinoblastoma research are listed in **Table 2**. A paper entitled "Inactivation of the p53 pathway in retinoblastoma" published in *Nature* has been cited 427 times and is the most frequently cited paper in the field. The paper discovered the inactivation of the p53 pathway in retinoblastoma and revealed that the origin of retinoblastoma

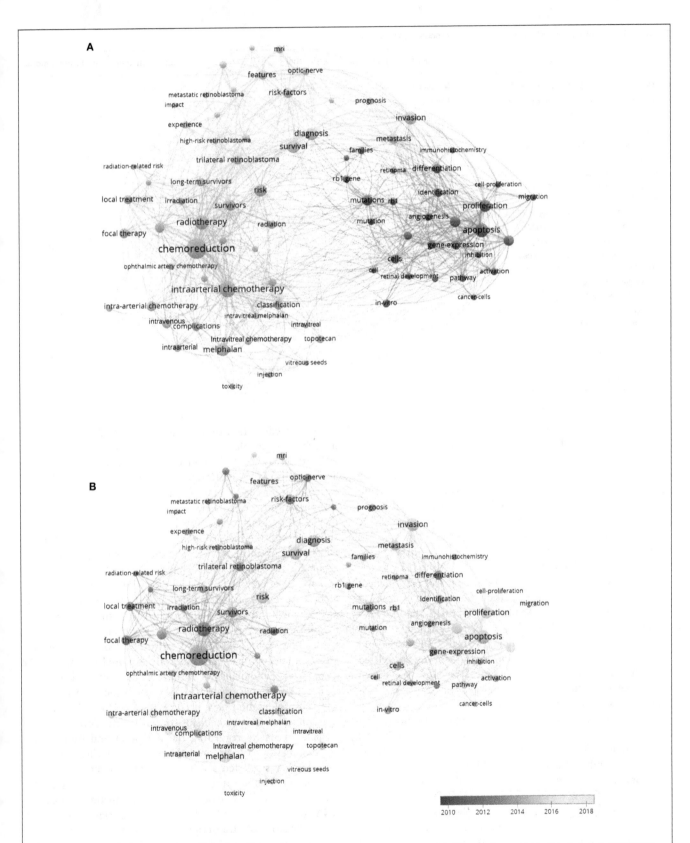

FIGURE 5 | Analysis of keywords in publications of retinoblastoma. **(A)** Mapping of the keywords in the field. All keywords were divided into 3 clusters and colored differently: tumor-related research (left in green), clinical research (right in red), and management-related research (up in purple). The circle with a larger size indicates a higher frequency of the keyword; **(B)** Distribution of keywords on the basis of the average appearance time. Yellow represents a recent appearance, and blue represents an early appearance. The line between two keywords represents their co-occurrence in the same publication, with a thicker line indicating a closer relationship.

TABLE 2 | Top 10 publications with the most citations in retinoblastoma research.

Title	Corresponding authors	Journal	Publication year	Total citations
Inactivation of the p53 pathway in retinoblastoma	Michael A. Dyer	Nature	2006	427
A novel retinoblastoma therapy from genomic and epigenetic analyses	Michael A. Dyer James R. Downing Richard K. Wilson	Nature	2012	289
Retinoblastoma	Gallie, BL	Lancet	2012	288
The international classification of retinoblastoma predicts chemoreduction success	Shields, CL	Ophthalmology	2006	279
A phase I/II study of direct intraarterial (ophthalmic artery) chemotherapy with melphalan for intraocular retinoblastoma - Initial results	Abramson, DH	Ophthalmology	2008	259
Intra-arterial Chemotherapy for the Management of Retinoblastoma Four-Year Experience	Gobin, YP	Archives of Ophthalmology	2011	239
Cell-specific effects of RB or RB/p107 loss on retinal development implicate an intrinsically death-resistant cell-of-origin in retinoblastoma	Bremner, R	Cancer Cell	2004	200
Lifetime risks of common cancers among retinoblastoma survivors	Peto, J	Jnci-Journal of the National Cancer Institute	2004	174
Intravitreal chemotherapy for vitreous disease in retinoblastoma revisited: from prohibition to conditional indications	Munier, FL	British Journal of Ophthalmology	2012	173
Retinoblastoma management: advances in enucleation, intravenous chemoreduction, and intra-arterial chemotherapy	Shields, CL	Current Opinion in Ophthalmology	2010	169

does not originate from intrinsically death-resistant cells, as previously thought (31). This perspective was in contrast to the prevailing theory proposed in *Cancer Cell* that retinoblastoma arises from extendedly proliferative cells with an intrinsically death-resistant capacity, which was cited 200 times as the seventh papers on the list (32). The second most highest cited paper, also published in *Nature* in 2012, supposed that the epigenetic deregulation of key cancer pathways caused by *RB1* loss may lead to the rapid development of retinoblastoma (33). In addition, a review entitled "retinoblastoma" and published in *Lancet* in 2012 presented the lessons learned about the management of retinoblastoma and proposed straightforward approaches to improve the survival chances and quality of life of children with retinoblastoma, which obtained the third most cited ranking (1).

Respecting the latest hotspot, intravitreal, intraarterial and intravenous chemotherapy from the management-related research cluster has emerged the most recently. As shown in **Figures 5A,B**, the cluster of management-related research achieved more attention than the other two clusters, suggesting that the management of retinoblastoma was continuously and extensively explored. With the emergence of IAC and IVitC, the indications for IVC are confined to patients with bilateral disease, confirmed germline mutation, family history or suspected optic nerve or choroidal invasion; IVC is also used as "bridge therapy" for patients weighing <6 kg awaiting IAC (34). Researchers have identified that IAC presented superior globe salvage in contrast to IVC for unilateral retinoblastoma patients in groups B, C, and D (11, 15, 35). Notably, IAC leads to 70% 5-year ocular survival for eyes with advanced retinoblastoma (36). Moreover, it has been reported that IAC is also feasible with low toxicity (37). IVitC is currently applied for refractory or recurrent vitreous

seeds succeeding IAC or IVC (38, 39). A study revealed that intravitreal melphalan achieved 69.2% effectiveness in eyes with vitreous disease (40). A subsequent study demonstrated IVitC as a promising method for the treatment of vitreous seeds (41). Recently, it has been reported that intravitreal chemotherapy combined with endoresection seems to be safe and effective in globe-salvaging for eyes with refractory group D (42). In addition, with the increasing attention having been paid to the clinical use of anti-VEGF (vascular endothelial growth factor) agents in the patients with eye disease (43), a retrospective review suggested that intravitreal anti-VEGF contributed to a globe salvage rate of 51%, indicating the potential of intravitreal anti-VEGF in the conservative treatment of retinoblastoma (44). Despite a few studies on multiple types of chemotherapy, IVitC, IAC, and IVC are still focused on the field of retinoblastoma research, and optimal indications are explored to improve the global salvage and quality of life of retinoblastoma patients.

Recent years have witnessed a research focus on migration and cell-proliferation have become research focus in the field, indicating that the mechanisms concerning the development of retinoblastoma by regulating the migration and proliferation of retinoblastoma cells are still worth exploring. Emerging evidence has suggested a critical role of non-coding RNAs in the pathogenesis and progression of retinoblastoma. LncRNA SNHG14 was reported to be function as a competing endogenous RNA (ceRNA) of miR-124, upregulating signal transducer and activator of transcription 3 (STAT3); consequently, SNHG14 silencing inhibited cell proliferation, migration and invasion as well as promoted apoptosis in retinoblastoma cells (45). Similarly, the knockdown of LINC00324 decreased retinoblastoma cell proliferation, colony formation, migration, and invasion, and promoted apoptosis and cell cycle arrest with respect to the mechanism by which LINC00324 acted as a ceRNA for miR-769-5p which directly targeted STAT3 (46). Furthermore, circular RNAs (circRNAs) can also serve as ceRNAs to regulate the proliferation and migration of retinoblastoma cells, such as the circDHDDS/miR-361-3p/WNT3A axis and Circ_0000034/miR-361-3p/ADAM19 axis (47, 48). In addition to non-coding RNAs, cyclin-dependent kinase regulatory subunit 1B (CKS1B) downregulation hinders the proliferation, migration, and angiogenesis of retinoblastoma cells through the MEK/ ERK signaling pathway, and an anti-oncogene scavenger receptor class A member 5 (SCARA5) was reported to prevent the proliferation and migration of retinoblastoma cell lines by suppressing the PI3K/AKT signaling pathway (49, 50). Studies revealing the mechanisms of the pathogenesis and evolution of retinoblastoma will provide a promising theoretical basis for clinical therapy.

Strengths and Limitations

Publications on retinoblastoma extracted from the WOS database were evaluated and analyzed comprehensively and objectively. However, there are still some inevitable limitations. For example, only publications in English were enrolled in the study; therefore, it is unavoidable that some important research in languages other than English were omitted. Moreover, the latest publications were not incorporated, which may in part affect our conclusions since they lack enough time to have accumulated considerable citations. Future investigations performing more complete search strategies and involving the latest and non-English language studies are expected. Of note, it is possible to mislabel document types by the literature database. As is reported that the

WOS database has more improved accuracy in document type assignment than Scopus, we employed the WOS database to minimize the influence of mislabeling (51).

CONCLUSIONS

The study has demonstrated global trends in retinoblastoma research. The United States has been at the cutting edge of the field based on its role as the lead contributor. Despite the considerable number of publications in China, the quality of the publications requires further improvement. Novel progress can be uncovered in the *British Journal of Ophthalmology* and *Ophthalmology*. Abramson DH and Shields CL are regarded as excellent candidates for academic collaboration in the field. Chemotherapy-related research has received the most attention previously and currently; furthermore, it may still be considered in the near future as the latest hotspot.

AUTHOR CONTRIBUTIONS

RJ and SG provided direction and guidance throughout the preparation of this manuscript. XG collected and interpreted the studies and was a major contributor to the writing and editing of the manuscript. MX reviewed and made significant revisions to the manuscript. All authors read and approved the final manuscript.

REFERENCES

1. Dimaras H, Kimani K, Dimba EA, Gronsdahl P, White A, Chan HS, et al. Retinoblastoma. *Lancet.* (2012) 379:1436–46. doi: 10.1016/S0140-6736(11)61137-9
2. Kivelä T. The epidemiological challenge of the most frequent eye cancer: retinoblastoma, an issue of birth and death. *Br J Ophthalmol.* (2009) 93:1129–31. doi: 10.1136/bjo.2008.150292
3. Jain M, Rojanaporn D, Chawla B, Sundar G, Gopal L, Khetan V. Retinoblastoma in Asia. *Eye.* (2019) 33:87–96. doi: 10.1038/s41433-018-0244-7
4. MacCarthy A, Draper GJ, Steliarova-Foucher E, Kingston JE. Retinoblastoma incidence and survival in European children (1978-1997). Report from the Automated Childhood Cancer Information System project. *Eur J Cancer.* (2006) 42:2092–102. doi: 10.1016/j.ejca.2006.06.003
5. National Retinoblastoma Strategy Canadian Guidelines for Care: Stratégie thérapeutique du rétinoblastome guide clinique canadien. *Can J Ophthalmol.* (2009) 44 Suppl 2: S1–88. doi: 10.1016/S0008-4182(09)80180-4
6. Abramson DH, Frank CM, Susman M, Whalen MP, Dunkel IJ, Boyd NW III. Presenting signs of retinoblastoma. *J Pediatr.* (1998) 132:505–8. doi: 10.1016/S0022-3476(98)70028-9
7. Rao R, Honavar SG. Retinoblastoma. *Indian J Pediatr.* (2017) 84:937–44. doi: 10.1007/s12098-017-2395-0

8. de Jong MC, de Graaf P, Noij DP, Göricke S, Maeder P, Galluzzi P, et al. Diagnostic performance of magnetic resonance imaging and computed tomography for advanced retinoblastoma: a systematic review and meta-analysis. *Ophthalmology.* (2014) 121:1109–18. doi: 10.1016/j.ophtha.2013.11.021
9. Karcioglu ZA. Fine needle aspiration biopsy (FNAB) for retinoblastoma. *Retina.* (2002) 22:707–10. doi: 10.1097/00006982-200212000-00004
10. Wilson MW, Qaddoumi I, Billups C, Haik BG, Rodriguez-Galindo C. A clinicopathological correlation of 67 eyes primarily enucleated for advanced intraocular retinoblastoma. *Br J Ophthalmol.* (2011) 95:553–8. doi: 10.1136/bjo.2009.177444
11. Fabian ID, Onadim Z, Karaa E, Duncan C, Chowdhury T, Scheimberg I, et al. The management of retinoblastoma. *Oncogene.* (2018) 37:1551–60. doi: 10.1038/s41388-017-0050-x
12. Shields CL, Mashayekhi A, Au AK, Czyz C, Leahey A, Meadows AT, et al. The International Classification of Retinoblastoma predicts chemoreduction success. *Ophthalmology.* (2006) 113:2276–80. doi: 10.1016/j.ophtha.2006.06.018
13. Yamane T, Kaneko A, Mohri M. The technique of ophthalmic arterial infusion therapy for patients with intraocular retinoblastoma. *Int J Clin Oncol.* (2004) 9:69–73. doi: 10.1007/s10147-004-0392-6
14. Shields CL, Douglass AM, Beggache M, Say EA, Shields JA. Intravitreous chemotherapy for active vitreous seeding from retinoblastoma:

outcomes after 192 consecutive injections. The 2015 Howard Naquin Lecture. *Retina.* (2016) 36:1184–90. doi: 10.1097/IAE.0000000000000903

15. Abramson DH, Daniels AB, Marr BP, Francis JH, Brodie SE, Dunkel IJ, et al. Intra-arterial chemotherapy (ophthalmic artery chemosurgery) for group D retinoblastoma. *PLoS ONE.* (2016) 11:e0146582. doi: 10.1371/journal.pone.0146582

16. Zhao Y, Zhang X, Song Z, Wei D, Wang H, Chen W, et al. Bibliometric analysis of ATAC-Seq and its use in cancer biology via nucleic acid detection. *Front Med.* (2020) 7:584728. doi: 10.3389/fmed.2020.584728

17. Tao Z, Zhou S, Yao R, Wen K, Da W, Meng Y, et al. COVID-19 will stimulate a new coronavirus research breakthrough: a 20-year bibliometric analysis. *Ann Transl Med.* (2020) 8:528. doi: 10.21037/atm.2020.04.26

18. Li Y, Wang X, Thomsen JB, Nahabedian MY, Ishii N, Rozen WM, et al. Research trends and performances of breast reconstruction: a bibliometric analysis. *Ann Transl Med.* (2020) 8:1529. doi: 10.21037/atm-20-3476

19. Stout NL, Alfano CM, Belter CW, Nitkin R, Cernich A, Lohmann Siegel K, et al. A bibliometric analysis of the landscape of cancer rehabilitation research (1992-2016). *J Natl Cancer Inst.* (2018) 110:815–24. doi: 10.1093/jnci/djy108

20. Xie M, Wu Q, Wang Y, Ge S, Fan X. Publication trends of research on uveal melanoma during 2000-2020: a 20-year bibliometric study. *Ann Transl Med.* (2020) 8:1463. doi: 10.21037/atm-20-3700

21. Yao RQ, Ren C, Wang JN, Wu GS, Zhu XM, Xia ZF, et al. Publication trends of research on sepsis and host immune response during 1999-2019: a 20-year bibliometric analysis. *Int J Biol Sci.* (2020) 16:27–37. doi: 10.7150/ijbs.37496

22. Ma C, Su H, Li H. Global research trends on prostate diseases and erectile dysfunction: a bibliometric and visualized study. *Front Oncol.* (2020) 10:627891. doi: 10.3389/fonc.2020.627891

23. Qu Y, Zhang C, Hu Z, Li S, Kong C, Ning Y, et al. The 100 most influential publications in asthma from 1960 to 2017: a bibliometric analysis. *Respir Med.* (2018) 137:206–12. doi: 10.1016/j.rmed.2018.03.014

24. Wang Y, Zhai X, Liu C, Wang N, Wang Y. Trends of triple negative breast cancer research (2007-2015): a bibliometric study. *Medicine.* (2016) 95:e5427. doi: 10.1097/MD.0000000000005427

25. Zhao J, Yu G, Cai M, Lei X, Yang Y, Wang Q, et al. Bibliometric analysis of global scientific activity on umbilical cord mesenchymal stem cells: a swiftly expanding and shifting focus. *Stem Cell Res Ther.* (2018) 9:32. doi: 10.1186/s13287-018-0785-5

26. Mendoza PR, Grossniklaus HE. The biology of retinoblastoma. *Prog Mol Biol Transl Sci.* (2015) 134:503–16. doi: 10.1016/bs.pmbts.2015.06.012

27. Dimaras H. Retinoblastoma genetics in India: from research to implementation. *Indian J Ophthalmol.* (2015) 63:219–26. doi: 10.4103/0301-4738.156917

28. Abramson DH, Dunkel IJ, Brodie SE, Kim JW, Gobin YP. A phase I/II study of direct intraarterial (ophthalmic artery) chemotherapy with melphalan for intraocular retinoblastoma initial results. *Ophthalmology.* (2008) 115:1398–404. doi: 10.1016/j.ophtha.2007.12.014

29. Gobin YP, Dunkel IJ, Marr BP, Brodie SE, Abramson DH. Intra-arterial chemotherapy for the management of retinoblastoma: four-year experience. *Arch Ophthalmol.* (2011) 129:732–7. doi: 10.1001/archophthalmol.2011.5

30. Abramson DH, Shields CL, Munier FL, Chantada GL. Treatment of retinoblastoma in 2015: agreement and disagreement. *JAMA Ophthalmol.* (2015) 133:1341–7. doi: 10.1001/jamaophthalmol.2015.3108

31. Laurie NA, Donovan SL, Shih CS, Zhang J, Mills N, Fuller C, et al. Inactivation of the p53 pathway in retinoblastoma. *Nature.* (2006) 444:61–6. doi: 10.1038/nature05194

32. Chen D, Livne-bar I, Vanderluit JL, Slack RS, Agochiya M, Bremner R. Cell-specific effects of RB or RB/p107 loss on retinal development implicate an intrinsically death-resistant cell-of-origin in retinoblastoma. *Cancer Cell.* (2004) 5:539–51. doi: 10.1016/j.ccr.2004.05.025

33. Zhang J, Benavente CA, McEvoy J, Flores-Otero J, Ding L, Chen X, et al. A novel retinoblastoma therapy from genomic and epigenetic analyses. *Nature.* (2012) 481:329–34. doi: 10.1038/nature10733

34. Ancona-Lezama D, Dalvin LA, Shields CL. Modern treatment of retinoblastoma: A 2020 review. *Indian J Ophthalmol.* (2020) 68:2356–65. doi: 10.4103/ijo.IJO_721_20

35. Munier FL, Mosimann P, Puccinelli F, Gaillard MC, Stathopoulos C, Houghton S, et al. First-line intra-arterial versus intravenous chemotherapy in unilateral sporadic group D retinoblastoma: evidence of better visual outcomes, ocular survival and shorter time to success with intra-arterial delivery from retrospective review of 20 years of treatment. *Br J Ophthalmol.* (2017) 101:1086–93. doi: 10.1136/bjophthalmol-2016-309298

36. Abramson DH, Fabius AW, Francis JH, Marr BP, Dunkel IJ, Brodie SE, et al. Ophthalmic artery chemosurgery for eyes with advanced retinoblastoma. *Ophthalmic Genet.* (2017) 38:16–21. doi: 10.1080/13816810.2016.1244695

37. Funes S, Sampor C, Villasante F, Fandiño A, Manzitti J, Sgroi M, et al. Feasibility and results of an intraarterial chemotherapy program for the conservative treatment of retinoblastoma in Argentina. *Pediatr Blood Cancer.* (2018) 65:e27086. doi: 10.1002/pbc.27086

38. Dimaras H, Corson TW, Cobrinik D, White A, Zhao J, Munier FL, et al. Retinoblastoma. *Nat Rev Dis Primers.* (2015) 1:15021. doi: 10.1038/nrdp.2015.62

39. Munier FL, Beck-Popovic M, Chantada GL, Cobrinik D, Kivelä TT, Lohmann D, et al. Conservative management of retinoblastoma: Challenging orthodoxy without compromising the state of metastatic grace. "Alive, with good vision and no comorbidity". *Prog Retin Eye Res.* (2019) 73:100764. doi: 10.1016/j.preteyeres.2019.05.005

40. Kiratli H, Koç I, Varan A, Akyüz C. Intravitreal chemotherapy in the management of vitreous disease in retinoblastoma. *Eur J Ophthalmol.* (2017) 27:423–7. doi: 10.5301/ejo.5000921

41. Yousef YA, Noureldin AM, Sultan I, Deebajah R, Al-Hussaini M, Shawagfeh M, et al. Intravitreal melphalan chemotherapy for vitreous seeds in retinoblastoma. *J Ophthalmol.* (2020) 2020:8628525. doi: 10.1155/2020/8628525

42. Yu X, Li X, Xing Y, Lu S, Tanumiharjo S, Ma J. Effectiveness of intravitreal chemotherapy-assisted endoresection in monocular patients with group D retinoblastoma. *BMC Cancer.* (2020) 20:808. doi: 10.1186/s12885-020-07314-1

43. Yeung AWK, Abdel-Daim MM, Abushouk AI, Kadonosono K. A literature analysis on anti-vascular endothelial growth factor therapy (anti-VEGF) using a bibliometric approach. *Naunyn Schmiedebergs Arch Pharmacol.* (2019) 392:393–403. doi: 10.1007/s00210-019-01629-y

44. Stathopoulos C, Gaillard MC, Moulin A, Puccinelli F, Beck-Popovic M, Munier FL. Intravitreal anti-vascular endothelial growth factor for the management of neovascularization in retinoblastoma after intravenous and/or intraarterial chemotherapY: long-term outcomes in a series of 35 eyes. *Retina.* (2019) 39:2273–82. doi: 10.1097/IAE.0000000000002339

45. Sun X, Shen H, Liu S, Gao J, Zhang S. Long noncoding RNA SNHG14 promotes the aggressiveness of retinoblastoma by sponging microRNA-124 and thereby upregulating STAT3. *Int J Mol Med.* (2020) 45:1685–96. doi: 10.3892/ijmm.2020.4547

46. Dong Y, Wan G, Yan P, Qian C, Li F, Peng G. Long noncoding RNA LINC00324 promotes retinoblastoma progression by acting as a competing endogenous RNA for microRNA-769-5p, thereby increasing STAT3 expression. *Aging.* (2020) 12:7729–46. doi: 10.18632/aging.103075

47. Wang H, Li M, Cui H, Song X, Sha Q. CircDHDDS/miR-361-3p/WNT3A axis promotes the development of retinoblastoma by regulating proliferation, cell cycle, migration, and invasion of retinoblastoma cells. *Neurochem Res.* (2020) 45:2691–702. doi: 10.1007/s11064-020-03112-0

48. Jiang Y, Xiao F, Wang L, Wang T, Chen L. Circular RNA has_circ_0000034 accelerates retinoblastoma advancement through the miR-361-3p/ADAM19 axis. *Mol Cell Biochem.* (2021) 476:69–80. doi: 10.1007/s11010-020-03886-5

49. Zeng Z, Gao ZL, Zhang ZP, Jiang HB, Yang CQ, Yang J, et al. Downregulation of CKS1B restrains the proliferation, migration, invasion and angiogenesis of retinoblastoma cells through the MEK/ERK signaling

pathway. *Int J Mol Med.* (2019) 44:103–14. doi: 10.3892/ijmm.2019.
4183

50. Wang J, Wang S, Chen L, Tan J. SCARA5 suppresses the proliferation and migration, and promotes the apoptosis of human retinoblastoma cells by inhibiting the PI3K/AKT pathway. *Mol Med Rep.* (2021) 23:11841. doi: 10.3892/mmr.2021.11841

51. Yeung AWK. Comparison between Scopus, Web of Science, PubMed and publishers for mislabelled review papers. *Curr Sci.* (2019) 116:1909–4. doi: 10.18520/cs/v116/i11/1909-1914

12

A Review of the Diagnosis and Treatment of Limbal Stem Cell Deficiency

Anahita Kate[1] and Sayan Basu[2,3]*

[1] The Cornea Institute, KVC Campus, LV Prasad Eye Institute, Vijayawada, India, [2] The Cornea Institute, KAR Campus, LV Prasad Eye Institute, Hyderabad, India, [3] Prof. Brien Holden Eye Research Centre (BHERC), LV Prasad Eye Institute, Hyderabad, Telangana, India

*Correspondence:
Sayan Basu
sayanbasu@lvpei.org

Limbal stem cell deficiency (LSCD) can cause significant corneal vascularization and scarring and often results in serious visual morbidity. An early and accurate diagnosis can help prevent the same with a timely and appropriate intervention. This review aims to provide an understanding of the different diagnostic tools and presents an algorithmic approach to the management based on a comprehensive clinical examination. Although the diagnosis of LSCD usually relies on the clinical findings, they can be subjective and non-specific. In such cases, using an investigative modality offers an objective method of confirming the diagnosis. Several diagnostic tools have been described in literature, each having its own advantages and limitations. Impression cytology and *in vivo* confocal microscopy (IVCM) aid in the diagnosis of LSCD by detecting the presence of goblet cells. With immunohistochemistry, impression cytology can help in confirming the corneal or conjunctival source of epithelium. Both IVCM and anterior segment optical coherence tomography can help supplement the diagnosis of LSCD by characterizing the corneal and limbal epithelial changes. Once the diagnosis is established, one of various surgical techniques can be adopted for the treatment of LSCD. These surgeries aim to provide a new source of corneal epithelial stem cells and help in restoring the stability of the ocular surface. The choice of procedure depends on several factors including the involvement of the ocular adnexa, presence of systemic co-morbidities, status of the fellow eye and the comfort level of the surgeon. In LSCD with wet ocular surfaces, autologous and allogeneic limbal stem cell transplantation is preferred in unilateral and bilateral cases, respectively. Another approach in bilateral LSCD with wet ocular surfaces is the use of an autologous stem cell source of a different epithelial lineage, like oral or nasal mucosa. In eyes with bilateral LSCD with significant adnexal issues, a keratoprosthesis is the only viable option. This review provides an overview on the diagnosis and treatment of LSCD, which will help the clinician choose the best option amongst all the therapeutic modalities currently available and gives a clinical perspective on customizing the treatment for each individual case.

Keywords: Limbal stem cell deficiency (LSCD), simple limbal epithelial transplantation (SLET), limbal stem cell transplantation (LSCT), Keratoprosthesis (KPro), Anterior segment optical coherence tomography (AS-OCT), impression cytology (IC), confocal microscopy, cultivated limbal epithelial transplantation (CLET)

INTRODUCTION

The corneal epithelium is essential for the maintenance of the anatomic integrity and physiological functioning of the transparent cornea. The maintenance of the corneal surface is ensured by the constant turnover of the corneal epithelium from the limbal epithelial stem cells (LESC) (1, 2). These LESC straddle the junction between the cornea and the conjunctiva and reside in the basal epithelial layer of the limbus. The microenvironment surrounding the LESC within the palisades of Vogt, is responsible for ensuring the viability and efficacy of the stem cells. The LESC prevent the migration of the conjunctival epithelial cells over the corneal surface and in the presence of a dysfunction of the LESC themselves or the surrounding niche, there occurs conjunctivalization of the cornea.

Limbal stem cell deficiency (LSCD) can stem from numerous etiologies, resulting in serious visual morbidity (3, 4). And so, early diagnosis of this entity is essential in order to institute the appropriate therapy in a timely manner. Also, the need for diagnosing LSCD is even more essential when a keratoplasty is planned as the graft is unlikely to fair well if the LSCD is not corrected in advance. Although the diagnosis of LSCD is still primarily a clinical one, there are several diseases that can mimic its clinical picture (5, 6). In such scenarios, the clinician can choose from an array of diagnostic tests aimed at detecting LSCD. Similarly, numerous therapeutic options are available in management of LSCD and the choice of one intervention over the other depends upon the severity of ocular and adnexal involvement. This review aims to provide an understanding of the various tools in the diagnostic armamentarium of LSCD in the context of their advantages and limitations. It also endeavors to crystallize the clinical approach to a case of LSCD based on the laterality, severity, and resources available.

ETIOLOGY

Pathologies that affect the LESC or their supporting niche can cause LSCD (3). These can be classified as per **Table 1**. Understanding the underlying primary disease process often provides an added perspective into the management of LSCD. Several conditions such as chemical or thermal ocular burns, Stevens-Johnson syndrome (SJS), etc. are one-time insults and usually the treatment approaches are limited to the sequalae that ensue (7). On the other hand, in autoimmune disorders such as mucous membrane pemphigoid (MMP), there is a constant disruption of the systemic and ocular milieu occurring via inflammatory mediators (8). In such cases, addressing the LSCD in isolation invariably has very poor outcomes and so it must be done in conjunction with the management of the systemic pathology. Furthermore, in case of congenital causes of LSCD, treatment options include specific gene targeted therapy which is possible only if a particular type of limbal stem cell transplant (LSCT) is performed. Therefore, it is essential for the treating physician to know the primary disease process in order to make an informed decision and choose the appropriate therapeutic modality on a case-to-case basis.

TABLE 1 | Causes of limbal stem cell deficiency.

Congenital
  Congenital aniridia
  Multiple endocrine deficiency
  Ectodermal dysplasia
  Epidermolysis bullosa
  Xeroderma pigmentosum
Traumatic/Acquired
  Ocular burns (Chemical/thermal)
  Post-surgical
  Contact lens wear
  Radiation
  Drug Induced
Autoimmune
  Stevens-Johnson syndrome
  Mucous membrane pemphigoid
  Sjogren's syndrome (Primary and Secondary)
  Vernal keratoconjunctivitis
  Graft-vs. host disease
Idiopathic

CLINICAL FEATURES

Symptoms

Patients with LSCD present with non-specific symptoms such as ocular redness, discomfort, pain, watering, and photophobia. When the disease is severe enough to involve the visual axis, the complaints extend to blurring or decreased vision (2, 7).

Signs

The diagnosis of LSCD is primarily clinical but needs to be confirmed by one or more objective methods. The clinical findings vary depending upon the severity of the disease. In early cases of LSCD, there may be focal areas of the corneal epithelium which take up the characteristic stippled staining pattern (7). There is loss of clarity within the epithelium, creating a lackluster appearance. The limbal palisades of Vogt, which are usually most easily visible superiorly and inferiorly, may be difficult to discern or may become flattened (**Figure 1**). With the progression of the disease there occurs conjunctivalization of the cornea and superficial corneal vascularization (**Figure 2**) (7, 8). Due to patches of irregular epithelial thinning, a whorl pattern is noted which is better picked up as areas of pooling up of fluorescein(**Figure 3**). These zones also exhibit late staining (7, 8). A sharp demarcation between the abnormal and normal corneal epithelium may also be seen in cases of sectoral involvement (7–9). Epithelial instability is a hallmark of the disease process which manifests as repeated breakdown of the epithelium and in advanced cases this can progress to form a persistent epithelial defect (PED) (7). Recurrent episodes of PEDs can affect the underlying stroma leading to scarring or sterile melts in non-resolving cases (7).

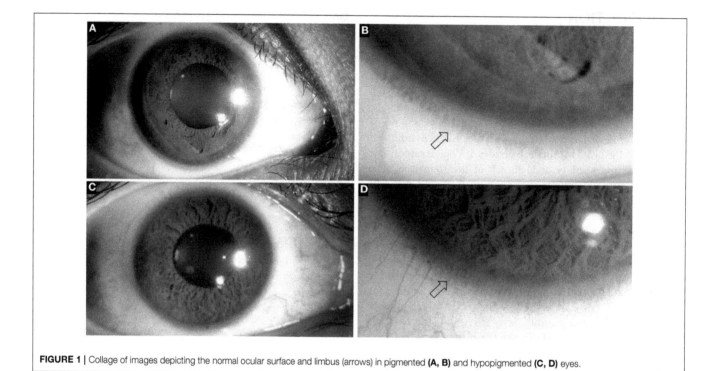

FIGURE 1 | Collage of images depicting the normal ocular surface and limbus (arrows) in pigmented **(A, B)** and hypopigmented **(C, D)** eyes.

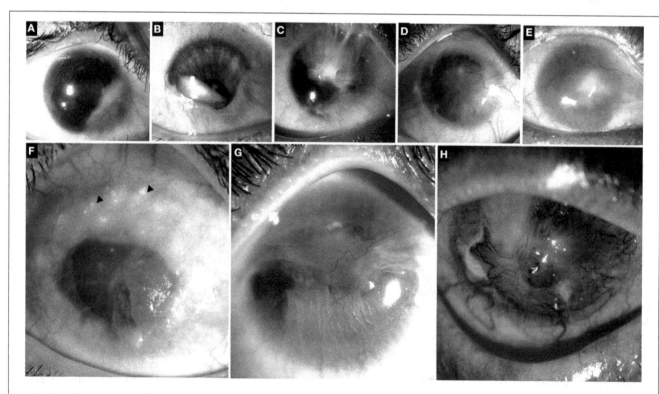

FIGURE 2 | Collage of images illustrating different grades and etiologies of limbal stem cell deficiency (LSCD). Top row: LSCD due to chemical injury which is partial and sparing the visual axis **(A)**, involving the visual axis **(B,C)**. **(D,E)** Total LSCD in chemical injury. **(F)** LSCD in chronic vernal keratoconjunctivitis. Superior cornea shows Horner-Trantas dots (black arrowheads). **(G)** LSCD in Epidermolysis Bullosa **(H)** LSCD in mucous membrane pemphigoid.

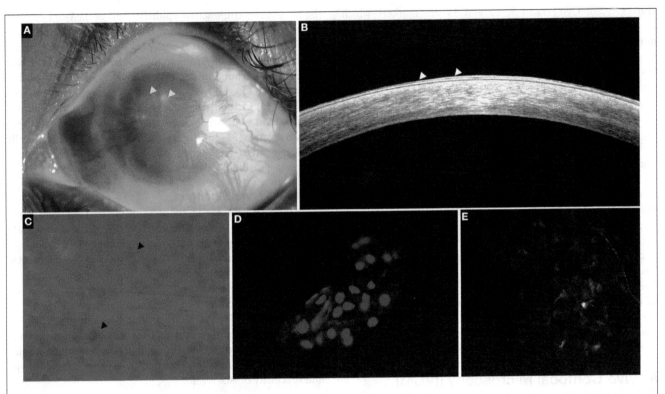

FIGURE 3 | A representative collage of various diagnostic modalities in limbal stem cell deficiency (LSCD). **(A)** Fluorescein-stained image showing characteristic stippled staining (yellow arrowheads). **(B)** Optical coherence tomography line scan showing hyperreflective epithelium indicative of LSCD (white arrowheads). **(C)** Impression cytology depicting Periodic acid-Schiff positive goblet cells (black arrowheads) and CK19 positive cells on immunohistochemistry **(D,E)** *in vivo* confocal microscopy showing decreased sub-basal nerve density.

DIAGNOSTIC INVESTIGATIONS

In cases of severe ocular burns or advanced cicatricial conjunctivitis following SJS, the diagnosis of LSCD can be straightforward. However, in several cases the clinical presentation is subtle and establishing the diagnosis may be challenging. In such cases the ancillary tests mentioned below help supplementing the diagnosis. In addition to confirming the diagnosis, these tests may facilitate the quantification of the disease and provide an understanding of its progression. They also help to confirm the epithelial phenotype following a stem cell transplant and in monitoring the postoperative recovery (10–13).

Impression Cytology

This test involves sampling of the superficial epithelial cells of the ocular surface and subjecting them to histopathological and immunohistochemistry tests. The sample can be obtained from the cornea or the conjunctiva and is usually acquired using a nitrocellulose or cellulose acetate filter paper (14). Although the test typically acquires the superficial corneal and conjunctival cells, repeated sampling in a particular area will facilitate access to the deeper layers as well (14). Following a standardized sampling technique is recommended as this will affect the quantity and quality of tissue obtained (7, 9, 14). Ensuring that the ocular surface is not too wet and that the pore size of the paper is adequate to collect the epithelial cells will also help in improving the yield (9, 15).

Histopathology

The cytology specimen procured undergoes histopathological processing with various stains such as hematoxylin and eosin (H&E), Giemsa, Periodic acid-Schiff, etc (14). These stains detect the presence of goblets cells which indicates the invasion of conjunctival epithelial cells over the surface of the cornea (14). Although the detection of goblet cells is considered the sine qua non of LSCD (**Figure 3**), its absence does not imply a healthy limbus. Also, there may be a decrease in the concentration of goblet cells due to the underlying disease process itself as is the case in SJS (16, 17). As mentioned earlier the sensitivity of the test is largely dependent on the sampling procedure. And so, assessment of the epithelial cells which are also concurrently sampled can enhance the detection rate of LSCD. However, the differentiation of corneal from conjunctival epithelial cells is not possible with the routine stains used and requires immunohistochemistry.

Immunohistochemistry

Several markers have been investigated and of these cytokeratin 12 has been found to be specific for the mature corneal epithelium (7, 18). Although cytokeratin 3 was also considered to be cornea specific, recent studies have found this marker in the conjunctiva also (19, 20). Cytokeratin 7, 13 and 19 are markers which are specifically expressed in conjunctival epithelial cells while mucin 5AC(MUC5AC) is used for the detection of goblet cells (**Figure 3**) (18, 20–22). However, negative MUC5AC staining has been noted despite positive conjunctival marker staining, signifying the low sensitivity of this marker (18). This fallacy has been subverted with the use of reverse transcriptase polymerase chain reaction test for the detection of MUC5AC which increases the test sensitivity to 98% (23).

Obtaining normal corneal cells through impression cytology is challenging because of the inherent adherence of the cells to each other and the underlying basement membrane. This is in contrast to the conjunctival cells which freely desquamate and so, the presence of an abundance of cellularity can itself indicate the presence of conjunctival cells (18, 20) Since conjunctivalization of the cornea is considered a hallmark of LSCD, the confirmation of conjunctival epithelial cells from a corneal cytology specimen has been deemed sufficient to diagnosis LSCD (**Figure 3**) (20). The subsequent presence of the cytokeratin 12 marker is used to quantify the disease which is considered mild or partial if the corneal marker can still be detected (20). The degree of the fluorescence exhibited by these markers has also been used to quantify the severity of the disease (19, 24).

In-Vivo Confocal Microscopy (IVCM)

IVCM is a non-invasive tool that provides an *in vivo* picture of the microstructures within the cornea. Of the various parameters measured by the device, presence of goblet cells, the basal epithelial measurements of the cornea and limbus along with the changes of the sub-basal nerve plexus are used in the diagnosis of LSCD (**Figure 3**).

Goblet Cells

The presence of goblet cells in a corneal IVCM scan is confirmatory of the diagnosis of LSCD. The detection rate of goblet cells with IVCM closely correlates with that of impression cytology (25). However, as mentioned previously, several factors may affect the detection of goblet cells in a case of LSCD and with an IVCM this is further confounded by the small area that is scanned. Also, the described morphology of a goblet cell is variable with descriptions of both a hypo and hyper-reflective cytoplasm (26–28). Thus, although the detection of goblet cells is feasible with an IVCM, the test has low sensitivity.

Corneal and Limbal Epithelial Changes

A decrease in basal cell density (BCD) with an increase in the size of the cells is noted in patients with LSCD (29–31). This decrease corresponds with the severity of the disease and in advanced cases, there is significant alteration in the morphology of the cells with an increased number of visible hyperreflective cell nuclei (31, 32). Deng et al. found that a BCD value of <7930 cells/mm^2 for basal cell density diagnosed LSCD with a 95.5% sensitivity and 100% specificity (31). In cases of partial LSCD, the epithelium in the clinically normal areas maintains the normal pattern on IVCM although there is often an increase in the number of dendritic cells in the underlying stroma (25, 33, 34). A clear demarcation is noted at the junction between

the corneal and conjunctival epithelial cells as the two have very distinct morphological features on IVCM (33). Corneal basal cells have a dark cytoplasm with well-defined borders and are much smaller than the conjunctival cells. Intraepithelial cystic lesions with surrounding goblet cells have also been described in cases of LSCD (33). Overall thinning of the epithelium is seen in LSCD (35). A similar pattern of change is noted in the limbal epithelium as well with a decreased BCD which correlates with disease severity (34–36). In cases of partial LSCD, the clinically unaffected areas also exhibit the same changes indicating a pre-clinical method of detection of LSCD (34, 36).

Corneal Nerves Changes

A progressive decrease in the density of the sub-basal plexus of nerves is noted with increasing severity of the disease until a complete nerve drop out occurs (**Figure 3**) (29, 34, 37). Additionally, several other changes have also been reported which include decreased branch length, increased angulation of branching, increased tortuosity, etc (31, 37). A cut off for sub-basal nerve density of 53 nerves/mm^2 resulted in an 87% sensitivity and 91.7% specificity for the diagnosis of LSCD (31). Caro-Magdaleno et al. found that the sub basal nerve density had an inverse association with conjunctivalization and a value of <17,215 μm/mm^2 diagnosed LSCD with a 95.5% sensitivity and specificity of 90.6% (38).

Anterior Segment Optical Coherence Tomography (AS-OCT)

AS-OCT is a non-invasive imaging tool that has low operator dependence and yields repeatable results. It has been used to augment the diagnosis of LSCD with its corneal and limbal epithelial measurements. Additionally, with the help of image processing software, the reflectivity from these measurements have been quantified. The role of the angiography feature of OCT for detecting LSCD has also been investigated.

Epithelial Changes

Similar to the IVCM findings, a decrease in both the corneal and limbal epithelial thickness has been observed with AS-OCT in eyes with LSCD (**Figure 3**) (30, 39). Although epithelial thinning is not specific to LSCD and is seen in disease entities such as keratoconus, dry eye, etc.; the degree to which the thinning occurs is different. A 20–30% thinning has been reported in eyes with LSCD, while in other disorders the thinning is <10% (35, 39, 40). Liang et al. proposed a new parameter measured as a mean of the central epithelial thickness and thickness measured at two points, 1 mm on either side of the central thickness (39). Values <46.6 μm for this parameter were considered diagnostic for LSCD with a sensitivity and specificity of 61.7% and 100% respectively (39).

In addition to measuring the limbal epithelium, the OCT can also provide an *in vivo* visualization of the palisades of Vogt. This is possible even in eyes where the palisades are not visualized clinically (41). Although the IVCM can also image the palisades, the image procurement takes time and requires a skilled and experienced operator whereas the process is much simpler in case of an OCT. Also, as seen with IVCM, in eyes with partial LSCD

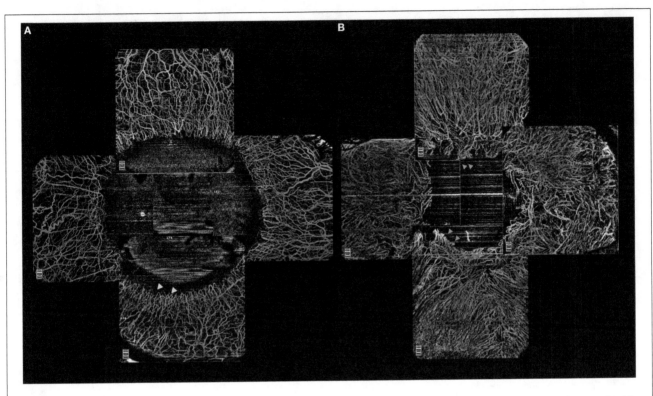

FIGURE 4 | (A) Optical coherence tomography-angiography (OCT-A) illustrating a normal limbal vasculature with hairpin looped limbal vessels (yellow arrowheads) and surrounding normal perilimbal conjunctival and episcleral vessels. (B) OCT-A in in limbal stem cell deficiency with vascular invasion of the peripheral corneal and distortion of the annular ring of hairpin looped limbal vessels (pink arrowheads).

the thinning of the limbal epithelium is similar in the affected and unaffected areas (39). This epithelial thickness correlates with the presence of the palisades with significant thinning manifesting when the palisades are absent (42). Volumetric scans of the limbus provide a three dimensional image which can further help quantify the severity of LSCD (43, 44).

Scans from an AS-OCT can be subjected to image processing and thus the epithelial and stromal reflectivity is derived. Varma et al. found the epithelial reflectivity value to be a better indicator of the presence of LSCD than stromal reflectivity (45). They also studied the ratio of these two reflectivities (ES ratio) and proposed a cut off 1.29 to be diagnostic of LSCD with good sensitivity and specificity. Furthermore, a reversal of this ratio following SLET was noted by Kate et al. (12). However the values at the end of one year follow up did not reach the ES ratio seen in normal eyes (12).

OCT Angiography (OCT-A)

The use of the angiography feature of the OCT has been explored in quantifying the changes seen in the limbal vasculature as well as in corneal neovascularization (**Figure 4**) (46, 47). A progressive increase in the density of vascularization and its extent into the cornea has been reported with increasing severity of LSCD (48). Also, OCT-A has been used to differentiate true LSCD from its mimickers which also have corneal vascularization. A significant reduction in vascular

density is noted after segmentation of the superficial layers in non-LSCD cases as in these eyes the vessels are usually located within the deep stromal layers (45). When this superficial vascular density values are >0.38, the diagnosis of LSCD can be confirmed with a sensitivity and specificity of 97.9% and 73.8% respectively (45).

CLASSIFICATION

Several classifications have been proposed to grade the severity of LSCD (1, 2, 31, 49). These are based on corneal epithelial thinning, fluorescein staining patterns, presence of neovascularization, fibrovascular pannus, etc. The grading proposed by the Limbal Stem Cell Working Group has divided the corneal involvement into three groups depending on involvement of the central 5 mm of the cornea and these groups have further been subcategorized based on the percentage of limbal involvement (7). These gradations which are based on corneal findings help understand disease severity and assess progression. This is particularly helpful for uniform and standardized documentation for research and monitoring progression or response to therapy. However, the classification does not include adnexal involvement, and this is vital in the decision-making process for the management of these eyes. Hence, classification systems that incorporate the eyelid and conjunctival changes in addition to the corneal ones may better

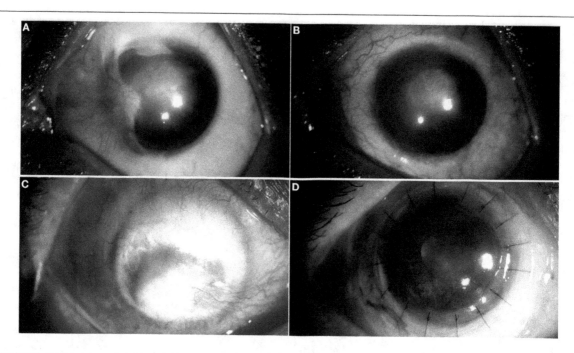

FIGURE 5 | (A) Partial limbal stem cell deficiency (LSCD) following chemical injury managed with conjunctival limbal autograft (CLAu). **(B)** Restoration of a stable ocular surface is noted. **(C)** Total LSCD with leucomatous corneal scarring. **(D)** Reestablishment of an optically clear visual axis and a stable corneal epithelium with deep anterior lamellar keratoplasty and CLAu.

help in delivering appropriate therapy based on the composite disease severity (50).

MANAGEMENT

The management of LSCD includes several surgical and non-surgical options and for each patient the treatment plan has to be tailored to suit the involved eye. However, LSCD rarely occurs in isolation and so the concurrent management of the systemic and ocular comorbidities is vital and often has to precede the surgical management of the disease. This includes systemic immunosuppression in cases of MMP, ocular anti-inflammatory therapy in cases of vernal keratoconjunctivitis, SJS, etc. A component of aqueous deficiency dry eye (ADDE) is usually present in most of these eyes and addressing the same with preservative free lubricants, punctal occlusion, etc. will aid in stabilizing the tear film prior to the surgical intervention.

Several of the comorbidities present with LSCD also require surgical intervention and the sequence of these surgeries often determines the final functional outcome. Ideally, lid and other adnexal issues are addressed prior to the stem cell deficiency. In the presence of significant corneal scarring there is often need for a keratoplasty for visual rehabilitation (**Figure 5**). Although LSCT contributes to stromal remodeling and eventually a decrease in the density of the scar is noted, the degree to which this happens may vary. And so, several of these cases ultimately require a partial or full thickness corneal transplantation to restore an optically clear visual axis.

The management of LSCD can be surgical or non-surgical depending upon the severity of damage to the LESC and the underlying pathology. Based on the clinical presentation, an algorithmic approach can be considered in most of the cases of LSCD (**Figure 6**).

Partial LSCD

In cases of partial LSCD, the decision of surgical intervention is dictated by the involvement of the visual axis (**Figures 2A-C**). If the visual axis is affected, a surgical therapy is required is most cases. However, if the axis is clear, the patient can be followed up at regular intervals to determine if the disease is progressive or stationary. In case of the former, again the eye will require a surgical procedure while in case of the latter the same can be deferred.

Non-surgical Intervention

Eyes with partial LSCD with sparing of the visual axis and documented non-progression of the disease can be observed with regular follow ups. These cases can be visually rehabilitated with glasses or with rigid contact lenses when significant irregular astigmatism is present. Scleral lenses with large vaults are particularly beneficial in such eyes as they provide a fluid layer which addresses the dry eye component in addition to improving the visual acuity (51–53). Lenses which vault over the limbus are preferred as mechanical compression and trauma to the limbal epithelium is prevented (53). Optimizing the fit of the lenses in eyes with LSCD is vital as the resultant hypoxia in eyes with a compromised fit can exacerbate the severity of the LSCD (54).

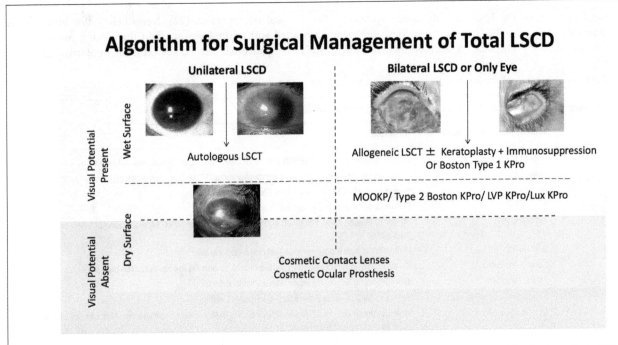

FIGURE 6 | Algorithmic approach of management of limbal stem cell deficiency (LSCD). LSCT: limbal stem cell transplantation, KPro: keratoprosthesis, MOOKP: modified osteo-odontokeratoprosthesis.

Surgical Intervention

When partial LSCD is progressive or involving the visual axis, a surgical procedure is usually carried out to correct the same. The choice of procedure depends upon the involvement of the fellow eye. In unilateral cases an autologous LSCT is preferred where the LESC can be harvested from the contralateral eye or from the uninvolved areas of the same eye. In a comparative series with 70 patients, the outcome in eyes where the LESC were harvested from the same eye was similar to the outcome of eyes with stem cells from the contralateral eye (55). In bilateral cases also an autologous LSCT can be considered if the involved areas are limited to 3-4 clock hours in both eyes (56). Several studies have described the use of an amniotic membrane (AM) alone in the treatment of partial LSCD (57–62). Most of these reports have combined a superficial keratectomy to remove the conjunctival epithelium prior to placing the AM. Although the initial corneal epithelialization rates are good, the ability of the AM to maintain a stable epithelial surface in the long run is poor (58–61, 63). And so, an AM can be used for the temporary restoration of the ocular surface, until a LSCT can be performed. The use of only conjunctival autografts (CAG) has also been described in the treatment of partial LSCD. Shanbhag et al. found a better anatomical success rate with CAG when compared to LSCT in eyes with partial unilateral LSCD (64). Following the treatment of the LSCD, these patients may eventually require rigid contact lenses for visual rehabilitation.

Total LSCD

In eyes with total LSCD, the initial step to determine the therapeutic approach would be to assess the presence of visual potential (**Figure 6**). In eyes with no visual potential, no further intervention is carried out unless there is a need to restore cosmesis in which case a contact lens trial is given, or an ocular prosthesis is implanted. In the presence of visual potential, the status of the fellow eye determines the next course of treatment.

Unilateral Total LSCD

In unilateral cases, if the surrounding adnexa is relatively uninvolved and the ocular surface is wet with a fairly clear corneal stroma, an autologous LSCT is performed. If there are significant cicatricial changes of the conjunctiva, a combined or staged procedure with a conjunctival autograft (in unilateral cases) or mucous membrane graft (in bilateral cases) can be planned (65). Similarly if a lamellar or penetrating keratoplasty (LK or PK) is planned for visual rehabilitation, it can carried out as a one or two step procedure (66–69). Although the grafts maintain clarity in the initial postoperative period after a combined procedure, the rate of rejection is usually higher in these cases and so a staged procedure is preferred (67–70). Whenever possible a LK is favored over a PK as the former lacks a transplanted endothelium and so is associated with lower rates of rejection.

Bilateral Total LSCD

The treatment algorithm for bilateral cases is similar to that of unilateral cases (71). If no dry eye is detected and the conjunctiva and lids are relatively uninvolved, then an allogeneic LSCT is the chosen procedure. In the presence of significant symblephara with adnexal pathologies the choice of LSCT over keratoprosthesis (KPro) depends upon the surgeon's preference.

The former will require multiple procedures to correct the co-morbid pathologies before the LSCD is addressed. Systemic immunosuppression will also be necessary in view of the allogeneic nature of the transplant. A keratoprosthesis will circumvent these issues and offers a one-step procedure with early visual rehabilitation (72). Nevertheless, this technique is associated with several serious sight threatening complications such as glaucoma, retinal detachment, implant extrusion,

TABLE 2 | Brief description of various KPros employed in the management of limbal stem cell deficiency.

	Type of Keratoprosthesis	Structure
Biocompatible KPro	Boston KPro 1 (77)	PMMA optical cylinder fitted with a titanium back plate. Complex is secured with a titanium locking ring
	Boston KPro 2 (78)	Similar to Boston KPro 1-has an additional anterior PPMA segment which projects through the lids
	Auro KPro (79)	Similar to Boston KPro 1 but with a PMMA backplate
	LUX (80)	PMMA optic, titanium backplate and a titanium sleeve
	LVP KPro (81)	Similar to Boston KPro 1 but with a longer optical cylinder which allows tucking of MMG beneath the front plate
	S-KPro (82, 83)	PMMA optic with a polyurethane and polypropylene skirt.
	Lucia KPro (84)	Boston KPro with reduced manufacturing cost by altering the design of the backplate
	Filatov KPro (85)	Titanium frame with two flanges with a PMMA cylinder
	Fyodorov–Zuev KPro (86)	Similar to MICOF KPro but implanted in a single sitting
	MICOF KPro (87)	Titanium frame with two flanges within which a PMMA cylinder is threaded. Auricular cartilage is also used to supplement the implant
Bio-integrable KPro	Pintucci KPro (88)	Central PMMA optic with a peripheral Dacron skirt
	AlphaCor (Chirila KPro) (89)	Made of poly-2-hydroxyethyl methacrylate with different water content in the central clear optical zone and peripheral bio-integrable skirt
	Legeais BioKPro-III	Polytetrafluoroethylene skirt and polyvinylpyrrolidone-coated polydimethylsiloxane optic
Biological KPro	MOOKP (90)	Optical cylinder is embedded in the canine tooth and implanted in a bed of MMG over the ocular surface
	Osteo-KPro (91)	Similar to MOOKP-tibia is used instead of a tooth

KPro, keratoprosthesis; MOOKP, Modified osteo-odonto keratoprosthesis; S-KPro, Seoul keratoprosthesis; MICOF, Moscow Eye Microsurgery Complex in Russia; LVP KPro, LV Prasad Keratoprosthesis.

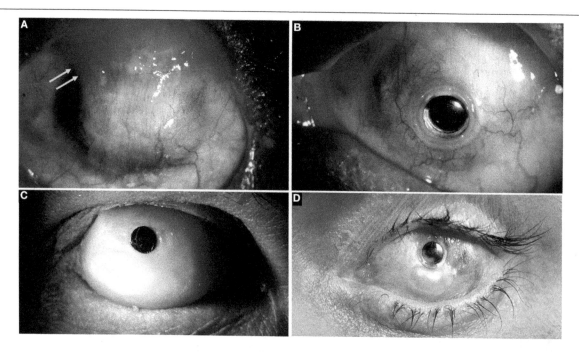

FIGURE 7 | (A) Left eye in a case of bilateral total limbal stem cell deficiency (LSCD) with a wet surface due to Stevens-Johnson syndrome (SJS). A superior conjunctival hooding (yellow arrows) was carried out previously for microbial keratitis with a corneal perforation. **(B)** A Boston keratoprosthesis in the same eye. **(C)** Modified osteo-odontokeratoprosthesis in an eye with total LSCD and a dry ocular surface. **(D)** LVP KPro in an eye with SJS.

TABLE 3 | Comparison of the most commonly used keratoprosthesis in the management of limbal stem cell deficiency.

KPro	Prerequisite*	Number of surgeries required	Outcomes**		
			Follow up years	*Retention rate %*	*Visual Recovery %*
Boston KPro Type 1 (95)	Wet ocular surface	1	5	74	51
AuroKPro (96)	Wet ocular surface	1	5	43	35
Boston KPro Type 2 (78)	Intact lids	1	5.9	50	38
LVP KPro (100)	-	2	2.5	76	36
MOOKP (99, 101)	Adults, healthy oral cavity	2	1	96–100	45–83#

*Prerequisites in addition to being suitable for a KPro.
**Visual recovery is proportion of eyes with vision better than 20/200.
#Proportion of eyes with vision better than 20/60.
KPro, keratoprosthesis.

endophthalmitis, etc (73–75). Thus, KPros are usually reserved for eyes with end stage corneal pathologies or in eyes where prior LSCTs have failed (76).

There are different types of KPros and the choice of one KPro over the other is determined by the presence or absence of ADDE. **Table 2** lists different types of KPros that have been utilized in the management of LSCD. If the surface is wet, a Boston KPro type 1 or Aurolab KPro (auroKPro) is carried out and if the eye has ADDE, then a Boston KPro type 2, LV Prasad KPro (LVP KPro) or modified osteo-odontokeratoprosthesis (MOOKP) is performed (**Figure 7**). The Boston KPro type 1 is the most commonly used prosthesis and has an optical cylinder with a skirt of donor cornea (**Figures 7A,B**). It has good visual outcomes and retention rates especially in eyes with non-autoimmune underlying diseases (74, 75, 77, 92–94) Since the cost of the device is a major inhibitory factor for its use, the auroKPro, its cheaper alternative is a more viable option in low resource settings. Both prosthesis have similar outcomes in terms of visual function, retention rates, and other secondary complications (95, 96).

In case of dry eyes or dermalised ocular surfaces with lid changes, both Boston KPro type 2 and the MOOKP have good functional and anatomical outcomes (90, 97–99). The former is similar to its type 1 counterpart and has a longer cylinder which is exteriorized through lid while the latter has a cylinder embedded in an osteo-dental lamina (**Figure 7C**). However, the surgical procedure for both devices is cumbersome, time consuming and has a steep learning curve. The LVP KPro, which is similar to the Boston KPro with a longer optical cylinder, is implanted as a two staged procedure under a mucous membrane graft used to reconstruct the ocular surface (**Figure 7D**) (78, 100). Its anatomical outcomes are better than those of Boston KPro type 2 but they are not superior than those of MOOKP (78). **Table 3** compares the outcomes of the most commonly used KPros in LSCD.

Transplantation of cultivated oral mucosal epithelium (COMET) is another alternative in eyes with bilateral LSCD where labial or buccal epithelial cells are cultured on an AM and transplanted over the cornea. Studies have reported a stable ocular surface following the procedure however there is a higher risk of persistent epithelial defects, corneal neovascularization

and graft rejection when compared to LSCT (81, 102–104). And so, an allogeneic LSCT is considered superior to and is favored over COMET despite the latter being an autologous transplant with no requirement for systemic immunosuppression (104). In a series comparing the outcomes of cell based therapies (CLET, CLAL, COMET) vs. Boston KPro type 1 in cases of bilateral LSCD without ADDE, the KPro group was found to have the best functional outcome at the end of five years (68, 71). However, a recent meta-analysis revealed that in patients undergoing LSCT, nearly 61% maintained a vision of at least 20/200 at end of 2.5 years which is similar to the 64% of patients who had the same vision in the KPro group (105).

Various modifications of the COMET procedure have been proposed which alter the type of carriers used to transfer the cultivated cells. These include the AM, fibrin glue and temperature sensitive polymers. In case of the latter, the polymer is stable at 37°C, however when the temperature drops to 30°C, the cultivated epithelial sheet detaches spontaneously (106, 107). This is in contrast to traditional methods where a carrier or enzymatic detachment is required. Furthermore, biomaterial free sheets have also been used, wherein the cultivated sheet is directly transplanted from the culture plate onto the eye without a carrier for the cells (108, 109). Establishment of a well epithelialized surface have been reported with the use of the same and these outcomes were found to be better than those of COMET with the use of AM as a substrate (108, 109).

As an alternative to cultivation of oral mucosal epithelial cells, which requires the necessary infrastructure, direct transplantation of the oral mucosa has also been described for the management of LSCD (110, 111). The graft is transplanted directly over the limbal area and can re-establish a stable surface and cause regression of neovascularization (110, 111). An additional benefit that the mucosal graft has over conventional LSCT is that adnexal pathologies such as lid margin keratinization or symblephara can be addressed with the same harvested tissue. As the procedure is autologous, no systemic immunosuppression is required. A similar approach has also been reported with the use of nasal mucosal grafts which primarily aim to replenish the goblet cells in the ocular surface (112).

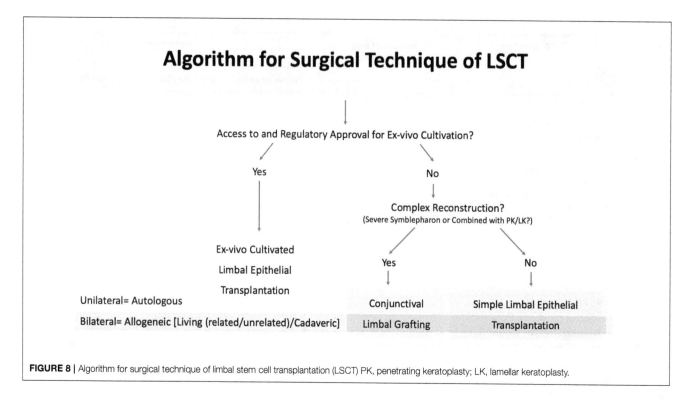

FIGURE 8 | Algorithm for surgical technique of limbal stem cell transplantation (LSCT) PK, penetrating keratoplasty; LK, lamellar keratoplasty.

Technique of LSCT

Types

There are two chief types of LSCT: allogeneic and autologous. These can be further divided into different types based on the anatomical source of the graft which includes conjunctival limbal auto or allograft (CLAu and CLAL), allogeneic keratolimbal allograft (KLAL) or pure limbal tissues as in cases of auto and allogeneic cultivated or simple limbal epithelial transplants (CLET and SLET). In cases of allogeneic LSCT, the donor can be a cadaveric or a living related donor. In pure limbal transplants, once the limbal lenticule is harvested it can be directly transplanted as in SLET where the proliferation of epithelial cells occurs *in vivo* over the corneal surface. Alternatively, the biopsied tissue can be cultivated *in vitro* and then transplanted as a sheet of epithelium as in case of CLET.

Choice of Procedure

As mentioned previously autologous procedures are performed in unilateral cases while allogeneic transplants are reserved for bilateral LSCD (**Figure 8**). The major difference between the two lies in the need for long term systemic immunosuppression for allogeneic LSCT. A combination of corticosteroids and steroid sparing agents are usually given initially, and the patients are then maintained only on the steroid sparing immunosuppressive agent (113, 114) Most of these medications are both expensive and associated with a side effect profile necessitating regular systemic monitoring (113, 114).

The choice of procedure is often determined by the extent of involvement of the surrounding adnexa. A limbal transplant (SLET/CLET for autologous cases, SLET/CLET/KLAL for allogeneic cases) is preferred for LSCD in wet eyes

without significant adnexal involvement (**Figure 9**). Access to a laboratory facility with regulatory approval is required for the practice of cultivated stem cells. CLAu or CLAL is preferred in cases where concurrent correction of cicatricial conjunctival changes is also required as seen in eyes with significant symblephara adjacent to a partial LSCD (**Figure 5**). The graft can be harvested from the same eye or fellow eye, depending upon the amount of healthy residual limbus. In the traditional CLAu, a large limbal graft is usually harvested (4-6 clock hours) which can result in an iatrogenic LSCD. To avoid this complication, a mini-CLAu with only 1-2 clock hours of limbal tissue is a viable substitute (66, 115). Alternatively conjunctival tissue can be harvested separately as a CAG along with a pure limbal transplant (CLET/SLET). This combination is usually adopted in eyes with total LSCD and symblephara. **Tables 4, 5** detail the relative advantages and disadvantages of each of the LSCT procedures.

Comparison of Outcomes

In a systematic review of 1023 eyes, SLET and CLAu were found to have better outcomes than CLET in cases of unilateral LSCD (116). A similar result was seen in a recent meta-analysis where SLET was found to have better functional outcomes when compared to CLET (117). The overall performance of autologous procedures has been deemed to be better than that of allogeneic procedures with the latter having a failure rate of up to 40% (105). The former group of procedures also have a higher percentage of patients with a 2 line improvement in visual acuity following surgery (105).

Ganger et al. found CLET and KLAL to have similar anatomical outcomes, but KLAL fared better than CLET in terms of functional outcomes (117). The cumulative success of KLAL

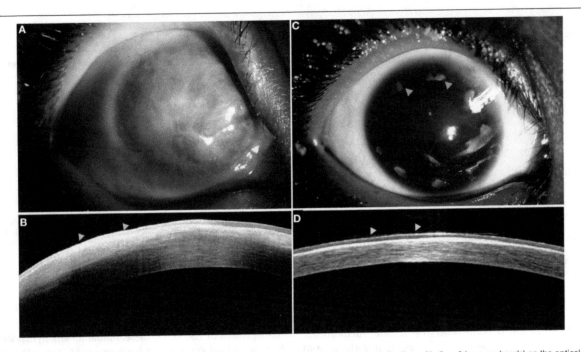

FIGURE 9 | (A) Total LSCD with a thick pannus in a case of chronic vernal keratoconjunctivitis with hyperreflective epithelium (blue arrowheads) on the optical coherence tomography (OCT) line scan **(B)**. **(C)** A stable ocular surface is observed following allogeneic simple epithelial limbal transplantation. The intact limbal tissues are also visible (pink arrowheads). **(D)** Restoration of epithelium with a normal reflectivity is noted on the OCT scan (yellow arrowheads).

TABLE 4 | Comparison of different autologous Limbal stem cell transplantation procedures.

Procedure	Regulatory approval	Laboratory set up	Risk of iatrogenic LSCD in donor eye	Feasibility of a repeat procedure	Number of procedures required
SLET	Not required	Not required	No	Yes	1
CLET	Required	Required	No	Yes	2
CLAu	Not required	Not required	Yes	No	1
Mini-CLAu	Not required	Not required	No	Yes	1

TABLE 5 | Comparison of different allogeneic Limbal stem cell transplantation procedures.

Procedure	Regulatory approval	Laboratory set up	Need for immunosuppression	Feasibility of a repeat procedure	Number of procedures required
SLET	Not required	Not required	Yes	Yes	1
CLET	Required	Required	Yes	Yes	2
CLAL	Not required	Not required	Yes	No	2
KLAL	Not required	Not required	Yes	Yes	1

SLET, simple limbal epithelial transplant; CLET, cultivated limbal epithelial transplant; CLAu, conjunctival limbal autograft; CLAL, conjunctival limbal allograft; KLAL, keratolimbal allograft.

from a systematic review was found to be 63% with 69% of cases having vision better than 20/200 (118). A recent series on allogeneic SLET reported a success rate of 83% and more than 60% of the cases had an improvement in vision which was >20/60 (119). And so, in the context of the expensive nature of CLET with its need for a laboratory set up, KLAL and allogeneic SLET are perhaps the more feasible options in cases of bilateral LSCD. However more studies are required on the long-term outcomes of allogeneic SLET to determine its benefits

over other allogeneic procedures. **Table 6** compares the outcomes of different modalities of stem cell transplants.

Recent Advances

The search for new therapies for LSCD is always ongoing because of the need for treatment modalities that do not have the risk of rejection, require immunosuppression, etc. And the epitome of such endeavors would be to arrive at a medical therapy for LSCD. One such intervention was identified serendipitously

TABLE 6 | Comparison of indications and outcomes of different surgical modalities of management of limbal stem cell deficiency.

Surgical Procedure	Tissue transplanted	Indication	Outcomes*	
			Anatomical %	Functional %
SLET (120)	LESC	Autologous, Allogeneic LSCD	78, 83	69, 60
CLAu (117)	Conjunctiva+LESC	Autologous LSCD	81	74.4
CLAL/KLAL (118)	Conjunctiva+LESC	Allogeneic LSCD	68	51
CLET (106)	Limbus	Autologous, Allogeneic LSCD	71, 52	65, 65
COMET (102)	Oral mucosal epithelium	Allogeneic LSCD	71	64
Oral mucosa transplantation (112)	Oral mucosa	Allogeneic LSCD	86	71
Nasal mucosa transplantation (113)	Nasal mucosa	Allogeneic LSCD	NA	18

SLET, simple limbal epithelial transplantation; CLET, Cultivated epithelial limbal transplantation; COMET, Cultivated oral mucosal epithelial transplantation; LSCD, limbal stem cell deficiency.

Anatomical outcomes: defined as a stable, avascular surface.

Functional outcome: proportion of eyes with vision better than 20/200.

during the treatment of patients with ocular surface neoplasia with interferon α-2b and retinoic acid (120). These cases had partial LSCD which responded to the topical medications. The rationale proposed for the same was that retinoic acid improves corneal wound healing and promotes proliferation of transient amplifying cells while interferon α-2b mediates the healing through its anti-inflammatory function, specifically on macrophages (120).

Another novel technique in the treatment of total LSCD is the amnion-assisted conjunctival epithelial redirection (ACER) which involves the placement of an amniotic membrane over the cornea and limbal explants. The edges of the membrane are tucked under the free edges of the recessed conjunctiva and as a result of this, the conjunctival cells migrate over the membrane (121). This allows the limbal explants under the membrane to proliferate over the surface of the cornea unhindered. Establishment of a stable ocular surface has been reported following this procedure. The use of a modified version of this procedure has also been described for partial LSCD with good outcomes (122).

Novel prosthetic devices such as the Lux and CorNeat keratoprosthesis are being developed as alternatives to LSCT. The former is similar to a traditional Boston KPro with a polymethylmethacrylate cylinder and a titanium backplate (123). This prothesis does not rely on the presence of intact lids which is required for Boston KPro type 2 and has better cosmesis than a MOOKP. Thus the Lux KPro is a viable option for eyes with dry ocular surfaces and LSCD, with good functional vision and retention rates (123). The long term outcomes with this device are awaited. The CorNeat is a true corneal prosthetic device and is structurally different from other KPros. This synthetic cornea has a central PMMA optic and a surrounding porous skirt made of polyurethane fibers (80). The skirt is implanted beneath the conjunctiva where it integrates with the surrounding tissue. Animal models with the CorNeat KPro have shown good retention of the implant while results of human trials are awaited (80).

The use of stems cells obtained from sources other than the LESC is another interesting avenue being explored in the management of LSCD. Of these, limbal mesenchymal stem cells have been best studied and have an established role in corneal wound healing, scar remodeling and angiogenesis (124–127). Its role as a therapeutic option for LSCD is being investigated with a recent clinical trial suggesting that they are as efficacious as CLET in restoring a stable ocular surface (128). Other stem cells that are being studied include those from hair follicles, dental pulp, embryonic stem cells, etc (129–133). Their exact utility and efficacy in LSCD is yet to be determined.

SUMMARY

This review presents an overview of the different diagnostic tests and management modalities in LSCD in order to provide a clinical perspective which will help the physician determine the best course of therapy in cases with LSCD. An in-depth write-up on the pathophysiology of stem cell deficiency is beyond the scope of this review. The diagnosis of limbal stem cell deficiency is often made based on clinical features but can be supplemented by several investigative tools especially when faced with challenging case scenarios. Although both impression cytology and IVCM can confirm the diagnosis of LSCD the expense of the equipment involved, and the skilled personnel required often restrict their use. AS-OCT is a more commonly available device and has several measurable parameters which can be used in the diagnosis of LSCD. However more studies are required to determine the exact diagnostic cut offs. The interpretation of the results of any of these tests must be made in the context of the clinical picture to arrive at the correct diagnosis. Additionally, these investigative modalities have also been used to monitor the response to LSCT and to confirm the restoration of a corneal epithelial phenotype (10, 134–136). Using a combination of clinical and one or more diagnostic tests, a standardized method of validating the outcomes of LSCT can be established.

A comprehensive approach is usually required for the management of LSCD with simultaneous treatment of comorbid ocular and systemic pathologies. Autologous LSCT for unilateral LSCD and allogeneic LSCT for bilateral cases, in the absence of dry eye, are the preferred modalities of therapy which render a stable ocular surface and good visual outcomes. A KPro is favored in more complex cases and provides a rapid visual recovery. The exact choice of procedure is ultimately dependent upon the status of the adnexa, the resources available and the expertise of the surgeon.

AUTHOR CONTRIBUTIONS

AK contributed to the collection of resources, original draft preparation, and revisions of the manuscript. SB contributed to the conceptualization, methodology, supervision, revision, and editing of the manuscript. Both authors contributed to the article and approved the submitted version.

REFERENCES

1. Dua HS, Joseph A, Shanmuganathan VA, Jones RE. Stem cell differentiation and the effects of deficiency. *Eye (Lond)*. (2003) 17:877–85. doi: 10.1038/sj.eye.6700573

2. Sacchetti M, Lambiase A, Cortes M, Sgrulletta R, Bonini S, Merlo D, et al. Clinical and cytological findings in limbal stem cell deficiency. *Graefes Arch Clin Exp Ophthalmol*. (2005) 243:870–6. doi: 10.1007/s00417-005-1159-0

3. Vazirani J, Nair D, Shanbhag S, Wurity S, Ranjan A, Sangwan V. Limbal stem cell deficiency-demography and underlying causes. *Am J Ophthalmol*. (2018) 188:99–103. doi: 10.1016/j.ajo.2018.01.020

4. Rama P, Matuska S, Paganoni G, Spinelli A, De Luca M, Pellegrini G. Limbal stem-cell therapy and long-term corneal regeneration. *N Engl J Med*. (2010) 363:147–55. doi: 10.1056/NEJMoa0905955

5. Le Q, Samson CM, Deng SX. A case of corneal neovascularization misdiagnosed as total limbal stem cell deficiency. *Cornea*. (2018) 37:1067–70. doi: 10.1097/ICO.0000000000001631

6. Chan E, Le Q, Codriansky A, Hong J, Xu J, Deng SX. Existence of normal limbal epithelium in eyes with clinical signs of total limbal stem cell deficiency. *Cornea*. (2016) 35:1483–7. doi: 10.1097/ICO.0000000000000914

7. Deng SX, Borderie V, Chan CC, Dana R, Figueiredo FC, Gomes JAP, et al. Global consensus on the definition, classification, diagnosis and staging of limbal stem cell deficiency. *Cornea*. (2019) 38:364–75. doi: 10.1097/ICO.0000000000001820

8. Taurone S, Spoletini M, Ralli M, Gobbi P, Artico M, Imre L, et al. Ocular mucous membrane pemphigoid: a review. *Immunol Res*. (2019) 67:280–9. doi: 10.1007/s12026-019-09087-7

9. Sejpal K, Bakhtiari P, Deng SX. Presentation, diagnosis and management of limbal stem cell deficiency. *Middle East Afr J Ophthalmol*. (2013) 20:5–10. doi: 10.4103/0974-9233.106381

10. Le Q, Xu J, Deng SX. The diagnosis of limbal stem cell deficiency. *Ocul Surf*. (2018) 16:58–69. doi: 10.1016/j.jtos.2017.11.002

11. Prabhasawat P, Chirapapaisan C, Ngowyutagon P, Ekpo P, Tangpagasit W, Lekhanont K, et al. Efficacy and outcome of simple limbal epithelial transplantation for limbal stem cell deficiency verified by epithelial phenotypes integrated with clinical evaluation. *Ocul Surf*. (2021) 22:27–37. doi: 10.1016/j.jtos.2021.06.012

12. Pauklin M, Kakkassery V, Steuhl K-P, Meller D. Expression of membrane-associated mucins in limbal stem cell deficiency and after transplantation of cultivated limbal epithelium. *Curr Eye Res*. (2009) 34:221–30. doi: 10.1080/02713680802699408

13. Kate A, Mudgil T, Basu S. Longitudinal changes in corneal epithelial thickness and reflectivity following simple limbal epithelial transplantation: an optical coherence tomography-based study. *Curr Eye Res*. (2022) 47:336–42. doi: 10.1080/02713683.2021.1988985

14. Pauklin M, Steuhl K-P, Meller D. Characterization of the corneal surface in limbal stem cell deficiency and after transplantation of cultivated limbal epithelium. *Ophthalmology*. (2009) 116:1048–56. doi: 10.1016/j.ophtha.2009.01.005

15. Singh R, Joseph A, Umapathy T, Tint NL, Dua HS. Impression cytology of the ocular surface. *Br J Ophthalmol*. (2005) 89:1655–9. doi: 10.1136/bjo.2005.073916

16. Vadrevu VL, Fullard RJ. Enhancements to the conjunctival impression cytology technique and examples of applications in a clinico-biochemical study of dry eye. *CLAO J*. (1994) 20:59–63.

17. Kinoshita S, Kiorpes TC, Friend J, Thoft RA. Goblet cell density in ocular surface disease. a better indicator than tear mucin. *Arch Ophthalmol*. (1983) 101:1284–7. doi: 10.1001/archopht.1983.01040020286025

18. Rivas L, Oroza MA, Perez-Esteban A. Murube-del-Castillo J. Morphological changes in ocular surface in dry eyes and other disorders by impression cytology. *Graefes Arch Clin Exp Ophthalmol*. (1992) 230:329–34. doi: 10.1007/BF00165940

19. Poli M, Burillon C, Auxenfans C, Rovere M-R, Damour O. Immunocytochemical diagnosis of limbal stem cell deficiency: comparative analysis of current corneal and conjunctival biomarkers. *Cornea*. (2015) 34:817–23. doi: 10.1097/ICO.0000000000000457

20. Barbaro V, Ferrari S, Fasolo A, Pedrotti E, Marchini G, Sbabo A, et al. Evaluation of ocular surface disorders: a new diagnostic tool based on impression cytology and confocal laser scanning microscopy. *Br J Ophthalmol*. (2010) 94:926–32. doi: 10.1136/bjo.2009.164152

21. Poli M, Janin H, Justin V, Auxenfans C, Burillon C, Damour O. Keratin 13 immunostaining in corneal impression cytology for the diagnosis of limbal stem cell deficiency. *Invest Ophthalmol Vis Sci*. (2011) 52:9411–5. doi: 10.1167/iovs.10-7049

22. Ramirez-Miranda A, Nakatsu MN, Zarei-Ghanavati S, Nguyen CV, Deng SX. Keratin 13 is a more specific marker of conjunctival epithelium than keratin 19. *Mol Vis*. (2011) 17:1652–61.

23. Liang Q, Le Q, Wang L, Cordova D, Baclagon E, Garrido SG, et al. Cytokeratin 13 is a new biomarker for the diagnosis of limbal stem cell deficiency. *Cornea*. (in press) doi: 10.1097/ICO.0000000000002903

24. García I, Etxebarria J, Merayo-Lloves J, Torras J. Boto-de-Los-Bueis A, Díaz-Valle D, et al. Novel molecular diagnostic system of limbal stem cell deficiency based on MUC5AC transcript detection in corneal epithelium by PCR-reverse dot blot. *Invest Ophthalmol Vis Sci*. (2013) 54:5643–52. doi: 10.1167/iovs.13-11933

25. Pisella PJ, Brignole F, Debbasch C, Lozato PA, Creuzot-Garcher C, Bara J, et al. Flow cytometric analysis of conjunctival epithelium in ocular rosacea and keratoconjunctivitis sicca. *Ophthalmology*. (2000) 107:1841–9. doi: 10.1016/s0161-6420(00)00347-x

26. Araújo AL de, Ricardo JR da S, Sakai VN, Barros JN de, Gomes JÁP. Impression cytology and *in vivo* confocal microscopy in corneas with total limbal stem cell deficiency. *Arq Bras Oftalmol*. (2013) 76:305–8. doi: 10.1590/s0004-27492013000500011

27. Efron N, Al-Dossari M, Pritchard N. *In vivo* confocal microscopy of the bulbar conjunctiva. *Clin Exp Ophthalmol*. (2009) 37:335–44. doi: 10.1111/j.1442-9071.2009.02065.x

28. Hong J, Zhu W, Zhuang H, Xu J, Sun X, Le Q, et al. *In vivo* confocal microscopy of conjunctival goblet cells in patients with Sjogren's syndrome dry eye. *Br J Ophthalmol*. (2010) 94:1454–8. doi: 10.1136/bjo.2009.161059

29. Zhu W, Hong J, Zheng T, Le Q, Xu J, Sun X. Age-Related changes of human conjunctiva on in vivo confocal microscopy. *Br J Ophthalmol*. (2010) 94:1448–53. doi: 10.1136/bjo.2008.155820

30. Bhattacharya P, Edwards K, Harkin D, Schmid KL. Central corneal basal cell density and nerve parameters in ocular surface disease and limbal stem cell deficiency: a review and meta-analysis. *Br J Ophthalmol.* (2020) 104:1633–9. doi: 10.1136/bjophthalmol-2019-315231

31. Banayan N, Georgeon C, Grieve K, Ghoubay D, Baudouin F, Borderie V. *In vivo* confocal microscopy and optical coherence tomography as innovative tools for the diagnosis of limbal stem cell deficiency. *J Fr Ophtalmol.* (2018) 41:e395–406. doi: 10.1016/j.jfo.2018.09.003

32. Deng SX, Sejpal KD, Tang Q, Aldave AJ, Lee OL Yu F. Characterization of limbal stem cell deficiency by *in vivo* laser scanning confocal microscopy: a microstructural approach. *Arch Ophthalmol.* (2012) 130:440–5. doi: 10.1001/archophthalmol.2011.378

33. Nubile M, Lanzini M, Miri A, Pocobelli A, Calienno R, Curcio C, et al. *In vivo* confocal microscopy in diagnosis of limbal stem cell deficiency. *Am J Ophthalmol.* (2013) 155:220–32. doi: 10.1016/j.ajo.2012.08.017

34. Miri A, Alomar T, Nubile M, Al-Aqaba M, Lanzini M, Fares U, et al. *In vivo* confocal microscopic findings in patients with limbal stem cell deficiency. *Br J Ophthalmol.* (2012) 96:523–9. doi: 10.1136/bjophthalmol-2011-300551

35. Chidambaranathan GP, Mathews S, Panigrahi AK, Mascarenhas J, Prajna NV, Muthukkaruppan V. *In vivo* confocal microscopic analysis of limbal stroma in patients with limbal stem cell Ddficiency. *Cornea.* (2015) 34:1478–86. doi: 10.1097/ICO.0000000000000593

36. Chan EH, Chen L, Yu F, Deng SX. Epithelial thinning in limbal stem cell deficiency. *Am J Ophthalmol.* (2015) 160:669–77.e4. doi: 10.1016/j.ajo.2015.06.029

37. Chan EH, Chen L, Rao JY, Yu F, Deng SX. Limbal basal cell density decreases in limbal stem cell deficiency. *Am J Ophthalmol.* (2015) 160:678–684.e4. doi: 10.1016/j.ajo.2015.06.026

38. Chuephanich P, Supiyaphun C, Aravena C, Bozkurt TK Yu F, Deng SX. Characterization of corneal subbasal nerve plexus in limbal stem cell deficiency. *Cornea.* (2017) 36:347–52. doi: 10.1097/ICO.0000000000001092

39. Caro-Magdaleno M, Alfaro-Juárez A, Montero-Iruzubieta J, Fernández-Palacín A, Muñoz-Morales A, Castilla-Martino MA, et al. *In vivo* confocal microscopy indicates an inverse relationship between the sub-basal corneal plexus and the conjunctivalisation in patients with limbal stem cell deficiency. *Br J Ophthalmol.* (2019) 103:327–31. doi: 10.1136/bjophthalmol-2017-311693

40. Liang Q, Le Q, Cordova DW, Tseng C-H, Deng SX. Corneal epithelial thickness measured using AS-OCT as a diagnostic parameter for limbal stem cell deficiency. *Am J Ophthalmol.* (2020) 216:132–9. doi: 10.1016/j.ajo.2020.04.006

41. Mehtani A, Agarwal MC, Sharma S, Chaudhary S. Diagnosis of limbal stem cell deficiency based on corneal epithelial thickness measured on anterior segment optical coherence tomography. *Indian J Ophthalmol.* (2017) 65:1120–6. doi: 10.4103/ijo.IJO_218_17

42. Haagdorens M, Behaegel J, Rozema J, Van Gerwen V, Michiels S, Ní Dhubhghaill S, et al. method for quantifying limbal stem cell niches using OCT imaging. *Br J Ophthalmol.* (2017) 101:1250–5. doi: 10.1136/bjophthalmol-2016-309549

43. Le Q, Yang Y, Deng SX, Xu J. Correlation between the existence of the palisades of Vogt and limbal epithelial thickness in limbal stem cell deficiency. *Clin Exp Ophthalmol.* (2017) 45:224–31. doi: 10.1111/ceo.12832

44. Grieve K, Ghoubay D, Georgeon C, Thouvenin O, Bouheraoua N, Paques M, et al. Three-Dimensional structure of the mammalian limbal stem cell niche. *Exp Eye Res.* (2015) 140:75–84. doi: 10.1016/j.exer.2015.08.003

45. Bizheva K, Hutchings N, Sorbara L, Moayed AA, Simpson T. *In vivo* volumetric imaging of the human corneo-scleral limbus with spectral domain OCT. *Biomed Opt Express.* (2011) 2:1794–1702. doi: 10.1364/BOE.2.001794

46. Varma S, Shanbhag SS, Donthineni PR, Mishra DK, Singh V, Basu S. High-Resolution optical coherence tomography angiography characteristics of limbal stem cell deficiency. *Diagnostics (Basel).* (2021) 11:1130. doi: 10.3390/diagnostics11061130

47. Patel CN, Antony AK, Kommula H, Shah S, Singh V, Basu S. Optical coherence tomography angiography of perilimbal vasculature: validation of a standardised imaging algorithm. *Br J Ophthalmol.* (2020) 104:404–9. doi: 10.1136/bjophthalmol-2019-314030

48. Oie Y, Nishida K. Evaluation of corneal neovascularization using optical coherence tomography angiography in patients with limbal stem cell deficiency. *Cornea.* (2017) 36 Suppl 1:S72–5. doi: 10.1097/ICO.0000000000001382

49. Binotti WW, Nosé RM, Koseoglu ND, Dieckmann GM, Kenyon K, Hamrah P. The utility of anterior segment optical coherence tomography angiography for the assessment of limbal stem cell deficiency. *Ocul Surf.* (2021) 19:94–103. doi: 10.1016/j.jtos.2020.04.007

50. Shortt AJ, Bunce C, Levis HJ, Blows P, Doré CJ, Vernon A, et al. Three-year outcomes of cultured limbal epithelial allografts in aniridia and Stevens-Johnson syndrome evaluated using the clinical outcome assessment in surgical trials assessment tool. *Stem Cells Transl Med.* (2014) 3:265–75. doi: 10.5966/sctm.2013-0025

51. Sotozono C, Ang LPK, Koizumi N, Higashihara H, Ueta M, Inatomi T, et al. New grading system for the evaluation of chronic ocular manifestations in patients with Stevens-Johnson syndrome. *Ophthalmology.* (2007) 114:1294–302. doi: 10.1016/j.ophtha.2006.10.029

52. Parra AS, Roth BM, Nguyen TM, Wang L, Pflugfelder SC, Al-Mohtaseb Z. Assessment of the Prosthetic Replacement of Ocular Surface Ecosystem (PROSE) scleral lens on visual acuity for corneal irregularity and ocular surface disease. *Ocul Surf.* (2018) 16:254–8. doi: 10.1016/j.jtos.2018.01.003

53. Wong BM, Garg A, Trinh T, Mimouni M, Ramdass S, Liao J, et al. Diagnoses and outcomes of prosthetic replacement of the ocular surface ecosystem treatment-a Canadian experience. *Eye Contact Lens.* (2021) 47:394–400. doi: 10.1097/ICL.0000000000000779

54. Harthan JS, Shorter E. Therapeutic uses of scleral contact lenses for ocular surface disease: patient selection and special considerations. *OPTO.* (2018) 10:65–74. doi: 10.2147/OPTO.S144357

55. Bonnet C, Lee A, Shibayama VP, Tseng C-H, Deng SX. Clinical outcomes and complications of fluid-filled scleral lens devices for the management of limbal stem cell deficiency. *Cont Lens Anterior Eye.* (in press) 101528. doi: 10.1016/j.clae.2021.101528

56. Vazirani J, Basu S, Kenia H, Ali MH, Kacham S, Mariappan I, et al. Unilateral partial limbal stem cell deficiency: contralateral versus ipsilateral autologous cultivated limbal epithelial transplantation. *Am J Ophthalmol.* (2014) 157:584–90.e1–2. doi: 10.1016/j.ajo.2013.11.011

57. Sangwan VS, Vemuganti GK, Iftekhar G, Bansal AK, Rao GN. Use of autologous cultured limbal and conjunctival epithelium in a patient with severe bilateral ocular surface disease induced by acid injury: a case report of unique application. *Cornea.* (2003) 22:478–81. doi: 10.1097/00003226-200307000-00016

58. Anderson DF, Ellies P, Pires RT, Tseng SC. Amniotic membrane transplantation for partial limbal stem cell deficiency. *Br J Ophthalmol.* (2001) 85:567–75. doi: 10.1136/bjo.85.5.567

59. Gomes JAP, dos Santos MS, Cunha MC, Mascaro VLD, Barros J de N, de Sousa LB. Amniotic membrane transplantation for partial and total limbal stem cell deficiency secondary to chemical burn. *Ophthalmology.* (2003) 110:466–73. doi: 10.1016/s0161-6420(02)01888-2

60. Kheirkhah A, Casas V, Raju VK, Tseng SCG. Sutureless amniotic membrane transplantation for partial limbal stem cell deficiency. *Am J Ophthalmol.* (2008) 145:787–94. doi: 10.1016/j.ajo.2008.01.009

61. Konomi K, Satake Y, Shimmura S, Tsubota K, Shimazaki J. Long-Term results of amniotic membrane transplantation for partial limbal deficiency. *Cornea.* (2013) 32:1110–5. doi: 10.1097/ICO.0b013e31828d06d2

62. Le Q, Deng SX. The application of human amniotic membrane in the surgical management of limbal stem cell deficiency. *Ocul Surf.* (2019) 17:221–9. doi: 10.1016/j.jtos.2019.01.003

63. Sangwan VS, Matalia HP, Vemuganti GK, Rao GN. Amniotic membrane transplantation for reconstruction of corneal epithelial surface in cases of partial limbal stem cell deficiency. *Indian J Ophthalmol.* (2004) 52:281–5.

64. Sharma N, Mohanty S, Jhanji V, Vajpayee RB. Amniotic membrane transplantation with or without autologous cultivated limbal stem cell transplantation for the management of partial limbal stem cell deficiency. *Clin Ophthalmol.* (2018) 12:2103–6. doi: 10.2147/OPTH.S181035

65. Shanbhag SS, Chanda S, Donthineni PR, Basu S. Surgical management of unilateral partial limbal stem cell deficiency: conjunctival autografts vs. simple limbal epithelial transplantation. *Clin Ophthalmol.* (2021) 15:4389–97. doi: 10.2147/OPTH.S338894

66. Shanbhag SS, Tarini S, Kunapuli A, Basu S. Simultaneous surgical management of unilateral limbal stem cell deficiency and symblepharon post chemical burn. BMJ Case Rep. (2020) 13:e237234. doi: 10.1136/bcr-2020-237234

67. Kate A, Basu S. Mini-conjunctival autograft combined with deep anterior lamellar keratoplasty for chronic sequelae of severe unilateral chemical burn: a case report. Int J Surg Case Rep. (2021) 88:106508. doi: 10.1016/j.ijscr.2021.106508

68. Fogla R, Padmanabhan P. Deep anterior lamellar keratoplasty combined with autologous limbal stem cell transplantation in unilateral severe chemical injury. Cornea. (2005) 24:421–5. doi: 10.1097/01.ico.0000151550.51556.2d

69. Deng SX, Kruse F, Gomes JAP, Chan CC, Daya S, Dana R, et al. Global consensus on the management of limbal stem cell deficiency. Cornea. (2020) 39:1291–302. doi: 10.1097/ICO.0000000000002358

70. Omoto M, Shimmura S, Hatou S, Ichihashi Y, Kawakita T, Tsubota K. Simultaneous deep anterior lamellar keratoplasty and limbal allograft in bilateral limbal stem cell deficiency. Jpn J Ophthalmol. (2010) 54:537–43. doi: 10.1007/s10384-010-0879-9

71. Basu S, Mohamed A, Chaurasia S, Sejpal K, Vemuganti GK, Sangwan VS. Clinical outcomes of penetrating keratoplasty after autologous cultivated limbal epithelial transplantation for ocular surface burns. Am J Ophthalmol. (2011) 152:917–24.e1. doi: 10.1016/j.ajo.2011.05.019

72. Vazirani J, Mariappan I, Ramamurthy S, Fatima S, Basu S, Sangwan VS. Surgical management of bilateral limbal stem cell deficiency. Ocul Surf. (2016) 14:350–64. doi: 10.1016/j.jtos.2016.02.006

73. Atallah MR, Palioura S, Perez VL, Amescua G. Limbal stem cell transplantation: current perspectives. Clin Ophthalmol. (2016) 10:593–602. doi: 10.2147/OPTH.S83676

74. Goldman DR, Hubschman J-P, Aldave AJ, Chiang A, Huang JS, Bourges J-L, et al. Postoperative posterior segment complications in eyes treated with the Boston type I keratoprosthesis. Retina. (2013) 33:532–41. doi: 10.1097/IAE.0b013e3182641848

75. Lee WB, Shtein RM, Kaufman SC, Deng SX, Rosenblatt MI. Boston keratoprosthesis: outcomes and complications: a report by the American academy of ophthalmology. Ophthalmology. (2015) 122:1504–11. doi: 10.1016/j.ophtha.2015.03.025

76. Greiner MA, Li JY, Mannis MJ. Longer-term vision outcomes and complications with the Boston type 1 keratoprosthesis at the university of California, Davis. Ophthalmology. (2011) 118:1543–50. doi: 10.1016/j.ophtha.2010.12.032

77. Shanbhag SS, Saeed HN, Paschalis EI, Chodosh J. Boston keratoprosthesis type 1 for limbal stem cell deficiency after severe chemical corneal injury: a systematic review. Ocul Surf. (2018) 16:272–81. doi: 10.1016/j.jtos.2018.03.007

78. Lee R, Khoueir Z, Tsikata E, Chodosh J, Dohlman CH, Chen TC. Long-Term visual outcomes and complications of Boston keratoprosthesis type II implantation. Ophthalmology. (2017) 124:27–35. doi: 10.1016/j.ophtha.2016.07.011

79. Sharma N, Falera R, Arora T, Agarwal T, Bandivadekar P, Vajpayee RB. Evaluation of a low-cost design keratoprosthesis in end-stage corneal disease: a preliminary study. Br J Ophthalmol. (2016) 100:323–7. doi: 10.1136/bjophthalmol-2015-306982

80. Bakshi SK, Graney J, Paschalis EI, Agarwal S, Basu S, Iyer G, et al. Design and outcomes of a novel keratoprosthesis: addressing unmet needs in end-stage cicatricial corneal blindness. Cornea. (2020) 39:484–90. doi: 10.1097/ICO.0000000000002207

81. Basu S, Sureka S, Shukla R, Sangwan V. Boston type 1 based keratoprosthesis (Auro Kpro) and its modification (LVP Kpro) in chronic Stevens Johnson syndrome. BMJ Case Rep. (2014) 2014:bcr2013202756. doi: 10.1136/bcr-2013-202756

82. Lee JH, Wee WR, Chung ES, Kim HY, Park SH, Kim YH. Development of a newly designed double-fixed Seoul-type keratoprosthesis. Arch Ophthalmol. (2000) 118:1673–8. doi: 10.1001/archopht.118.12.1673

83. Kim MK, Lee SM, Lee JL, Chung TY, Kim YH, Wee WR, et al. Long-Term outcome in ocular intractable surface disease with Seoul-type keratoprosthesis. Cornea. (2007) 26:546–51. doi: 10.1097/ICO.0b013e3180415d35

84. Bakshi SK, Paschalis EI, Graney J, Chodosh J. Lucia and beyond: development of an Affordable Keratoprosthesis. Cornea. (2019) 38:492–7. doi: 10.1097/ICO.0000000000001880

85. Iakymenko S. Forty-five years of keratoprosthesis study and application at the Filatov Institute: a retrospective analysis of 1 060 cases. Int J Ophthalmol. (2013) 6:375–80. doi: 10.3980/j.issn.2222-3959.2013.03.22

86. Ghaffariyeh A, Honarpisheh N, Karkhaneh A, Abudi R, Moroz ZI, Peyman A, et al. Fyodorov-Zuev keratoprosthesis implantation: long-term results in patients with multiple failed corneal grafts. Graefes Arch Clin Exp Ophthalmol. (2011) 249:93–101. doi: 10.1007/s00417-010-1493-8

87. Huang Y, Yu J, Liu L, Du G, Song J, Guo H. Moscow eye microsurgery complex in Russia keratoprosthesis in Beijing. Ophthalmology. (2011) 118:41–6. doi: 10.1016/j.ophtha.2010.05.019

88. Pintucci S, Pintucci F, Cecconi M, Caiazza S. New dacron tissue colonisable keratoprosthesis: clinical experience. Br J Ophthalmol. (1995) 79:825–9. doi: 10.1136/bjo.79.9.825

89. Hicks CR, Crawford GJ, Dart JKG, Grabner G, Holland EJ, Stulting RD, et al. AlphaCor: clinical outcomes. Cornea. (2006) 25:1034–42. doi: 10.1097/01.ico.0000229982.23334.6b

90. Falcinelli G, Falsini B, Taloni M, Colliardo P, Falcinelli G. Modified osteo-odonto-keratoprosthesis for treatment of corneal blindness: long-term anatomical and functional outcomes in 181 cases. Arch Ophthalmol. (2005) 123:1319–29. doi: 10.1001/archopht.123.10.1319

91. Iyer G, Srinivasan B, Agarwal S, Talele D, Rishi E, Rishi P, et al. Keratoprosthesis: current global scenario and a broad Indian perspective. Indian J Ophthalmol. (2018) 66:620–9. doi: 10.4103/ijo.IJO_22_18

92. Hou JH. de la Cruz J, Djalilian AR. Outcomes of Boston keratoprosthesis implantation for failed keratoplasty after keratolimbal allograft. Cornea. (2012) 31:1432–5. doi: 10.1097/ICO.0b013e31823e2ac6

93. Ciolino JB, Belin MW, Todani A, Al-Arfaj K, Rudnisky CJ. Boston keratoprosthesis type 1 study group. retention of the Boston keratoprosthesis type 1: multicenter study results. Ophthalmology. (2013) 120:1195–200. doi: 10.1016/j.ophtha.2012.11.025

94. Sejpal K, Yu F, Aldave AJ. The Boston keratoprosthesis in the management of corneal limbal stem cell deficiency. Cornea. (2011) 30:1187–94. doi: 10.1097/ICO.0b013e3182114467

95. Priddy J, Bardan AS, Tawfik HS, Liu C. Systematic review and meta-analysis of the medium- and long-term outcomes of the boston type 1 keratoprosthesis. Cornea. (2019) 38:1465–73. doi: 10.1097/ICO.0000000000002098

96. Shanbhag SS, Senthil S, Mohamed A, Basu S. Outcomes of the Boston type 1 and the aurolab keratoprosthesis in eyes with limbal stem cell deficiency. Br J Ophthalmol. (2021) 105:473–8. doi: 10.1136/bjophthalmol-2020-316369

97. Basu S, Serna-Ojeda JC, Senthil S, Pappuru RR, Bagga B, Sangwan V. The aurolab Keratoprosthesis (KPro) vs. the Boston type I Kpro: 5-year clinical outcomes in 134 cases of bilateral corneal blindness. Am J Ophthalmol. (2019) 205:175–83. doi: 10.1016/j.ajo.2019.03.016

98. Pujari S, Siddique SS, Dohlman CH, Chodosh J. The Boston keratoprosthesis type II: the Massachusetts eye and ear infirmary experience. Cornea. (2011) 30:1298–303. doi: 10.1097/ICO.0b013e318215207c

99. Iyer G, Pillai VS, Srinivasan B, Falcinelli G, Padmanabhan P, Guruswami S, et al. Modified osteo-odonto keratoprosthesis–the Indian experience–results of the first 50 cases. Cornea. (2010) 29:771–6. doi: 10.1097/ICO.0b013e3181ca31fc

100. Basu S, Nagpal R, Serna-Ojeda JC, Bhalekar S, Bagga B, Sangwan V. LVP keratoprosthesis: anatomical and functional outcomes in bilateral end-stage corneal blindness. Br J Ophthalmol. (2018) 103:592–98. doi: 10.1136/bjophthalmol-2017-311649

101. Basu S, Pillai VS, Sangwan VS. Mucosal complications of modified osteo-odonto keratoprosthesis in chronic Stevens-Johnson syndrome. Am J Ophthalmol. (2013) 156:867–73.e2. doi: 10.1016/j.ajo.2013.06.012

102. Cabral JV, Jackson CJ, Utheim TP, Jirsova K. Ex vivo cultivated oral mucosal epithelial cell transplantation for limbal stem cell deficiency: a review. Stem Cell Res Ther. (2020) 11:301. doi: 10.1186/s13287-020-01783-8

103. Satake Y, Dogru M, Yamane G-Y, Kinoshita S, Tsubota K, Shimazaki J. Barrier function and cytologic features of the ocular surface epithelium after autologous cultivated oral mucosal epithelial transplantation. *Arch Ophthalmol.* (2008) 126:23–8. doi: 10.1001/archopht.126.1.23

104. Ma DH-K, Kuo M-T, Tsai Y-J, Chen H-CJ, Chen X-L, Wang S-F, et al. Transplantation of cultivated oral mucosal epithelial cells for severe corneal burn. *Eye (Lond).* (2009) 23:1442–50. doi: 10.1038/eye.2009.60

105. Wang J, Qi X, Dong Y, Cheng J, Zhai H, Zhou Q, et al. Comparison of the efficacy of different cell sources for transplantation in total limbal stem cell deficiency. *Graefes Arch Clin Exp Ophthalmol.* (2019) 257:1253–63. doi: 10.1007/s00417-019-04316-z

106. Le Q, Chauhan T, Yung M, Tseng C-H, Deng SX. Outcomes of limbal stem cell transplant: a meta-analysis. *JAMA Ophthalmol.* (2020) 138:660–70. doi: 10.1001/jamaophthalmol.2020.1120

107. Nishida K, Yamato M, Hayashida Y, Watanabe K, Yamamoto K, Adachi E, et al. Corneal reconstruction with tissue-engineered cell sheets composed of autologous oral mucosal epithelium. *N Engl J Med.* (2004) 351:1187–96. doi: 10.1056/NEJMoa040455

108. Burillon C, Huot L, Justin V, Nataf S, Chapuis F, Decullier E, et al. Cultured autologous oral mucosal epithelial cell sheet (CAOMECS) transplantation for the treatment of corneal limbal epithelial stem cell deficiency. *Invest Ophthalmol Vis Sci.* (2012) 53:1325–31. doi: 10.1167/iovs.11-7744

109. Kim YJ, Lee HJ Ryu JS, Kim YH, Jeon S, Oh JY, Choung HK, et al. Prospective clinical trial of corneal reconstruction with biomaterial-free cultured oral mucosal epithelial cell sheets. *Cornea.* (2018) 37:76–83. doi: 10.1097/ICO.0000000000001409

110. Hirayama M, Satake Y, Higa K, Yamaguchi T, Shimazaki J. Transplantation of cultivated oral mucosal epithelium prepared in fibrin-coated culture dishes. *Invest Ophthalmol Vis Sci.* (2012) 53:1602–9. doi: 10.1167/iovs.11-7847

111. Liu J, Sheha H, Fu Y, Giegengack M, Tseng SC. Oral mucosal graft with amniotic membrane transplantation for total limbal stem cell deficiency. *Am J Ophthalmol.* (2011) 152:739-47.e1. doi: 10.1016/j.ajo.2011.03.037

112. Choe HR, Yoon CH, Kim MK. Ocular surface reconstruction using circumferentially trephined autologous oral mucosal graft transplantation in limbal stem cell deficiency. *Korean J Ophthalmol.* (2019) 33:16–25. doi: 10.3341/kjo.2018.0111

113. Wenkel H, Rummelt V, Naumann GOH. Long term results after autologous nasal mucosal transplantation in severe mucus deficiency syndromes. *Br J Ophthalmol.* (2000) 84:279–84. doi: 10.1136/bjo.84.3.279

114. Kate A, Basu S. Systemic immunosuppression in Cornea and ocular surface disorders: a ready reckoner for ophthalmologists. *Semin Ophthalmol.* (2022) 37:330–44. doi: 10.1080/08820538.2021.1966059

115. Serna-Ojeda JC, Basu S, Vazirani J, Garfias Y, Sangwan VS. Systemic immunosuppression for limbal allograft and allogenic limbal epithelial cell transplantation. *Med Hypothesis Discov Innov Ophthalmol.* (2020) 9:23–32.

116. Kheirkhah A, Raju VK, Tseng SCG. Minimal conjunctival limbal autograft for total limbal stem cell deficiency. *Cornea.* (2008) 27:730–3. doi: 10.1097/QAI.0b013e31815cea8b

117. Shanbhag SS, Nikpoor N, Rao Donthineni P, Singh V, Chodosh J, Basu S. Autologous limbal stem cell transplantation: a systematic review of clinical outcomes with different surgical techniques. *Br J Ophthalmol.* (2020) 104:247–53. doi: 10.1136/bjophthalmol-2019-314081

118. Ganger A, Singh A, Kalaivani M, Gupta N, Vanathi M, Mohanty S, et al. Outcomes of surgical interventions for the treatment of limbal stem cell deficiency. *Indian J Med Res.* (2021) 154:51–61. doi: 10.4103/ijmr.IJMR_1139_18

119. Shanbhag SS, Saeed HN, Paschalis EI, Chodosh J. Keratolimbal allograft for limbal stem cell deficiency after severe corneal chemical injury: a systematic review. *Br J Ophthalmol.* (2018) 102:1114–21. doi: 10.1136/bjophthalmol-2017-311249

120. Shanbhag SS, Patel CN, Goyal R, Donthineni PR, Singh V, Basu S. Simple limbal epithelial transplantation (SLET): review of indications, surgical technique, mechanism, outcomes, limitations, and impact. *Indian J Ophthalmol.* (2019) 67:1265–77. doi: 10.4103/ijo.IJO_117_19

121. Tan JC, Tat LT, Coroneo MT. Treatment of partial limbal stem cell deficiency with topical interferon α-2b and retinoic acid. *Br J Ophthalmol.* (2016) 100:944–8. doi: 10.1136/bjophthalmol-2015-307411

122. Dua HS, Miri A, Elalfy MS, Lencova A, Said DG. Amnion-Assisted conjunctival epithelial redirection in limbal stem cell grafting. *Br J Ophthalmol.* (2017) 101:913–9. doi: 10.1136/bjophthalmol-2015-307935

123. Han SB, Ibrahim FNIM, Liu Y-C, Mehta JS. Efficacy of modified Amnion-Assisted Conjunctival Epithelial Redirection (ACER) for partial limbal stem cell deficiency. *Medicina (Kaunas).* (2021) 57:369. doi: 10.3390/medicina57040369

124. Litvin G, Klein I, Litvin Y, Klaiman G, Nyska A. CorNeat KPro: ocular implantation study in rabbits. *Cornea.* (2021) 40:1165–74. doi: 10.1097/ICO.0000000000002798

125. Al-Jaibaji O, Swioklo S, Connon CJ. Mesenchymal stromal cells for ocular surface repair. *Expert Opin Biol Ther.* (2019) 19:643–53. doi: 10.1080/14712598.2019.1607836

126. Demirayak B, Yüksel N, Çelik OS, Subaşi C, Duruksu G, Unal ZS, et al. Effect of bone marrow and adipose tissue-derived mesenchymal stem cells on the natural course of corneal scarring after penetrating injury. *Exp Eye Res.* (2016) 151:227–35. doi: 10.1016/j.exer.2016.08.011

127. Basu S, Hertsenberg AJ, Funderburgh ML, Burrow MK, Mann MM, Du Y, et al. Human limbal biopsy-derived stromal stem cells prevent corneal scarring. *Sci Transl Med.* (2014) 6:266ra172. doi: 10.1126/scitranslmed.3009644

128. Alio del Barrio JL, Chiesa M, Garagorri N, Garcia-Urquia N, Fernandez-Delgado J, Bataille L, et al. Acellular human corneal matrix sheets seeded with human adipose-derived mesenchymal stem cells integrate functionally in an experimental animal model. *Exp Eye Res.* (2015) 132:91–100. doi: 10.1016/j.exer.2015.01.020

129. Calonge M, Pérez I, Galindo S, Nieto-Miguel T, López-Paniagua M, Fernández I, et al. proof-of-concept clinical trial using mesenchymal stem cells for the treatment of corneal epithelial stem cell deficiency. *Transl Res.* (2019) 206:18–40. doi: 10.1016/j.trsl.2018.11.003

130. Meyer-Blazejewska EA, Call MK, Yamanaka O, Liu H, Schlötzer-Schrehardt U, Kruse FE, et al. From hair to cornea: toward the therapeutic use of hair follicle-derived stem cells in the treatment of limbal stem cell deficiency. *Stem Cells.* (2011) 29:57–66. doi: 10.1002/stem.550

131. Gomes JAP, Geraldes Monteiro B, Melo GB, Smith RL, Cavenaghi Pereira da. Silva M, et al. Corneal reconstruction with tissue-engineered cell sheets composed of human immature dental pulp stem cells. *Invest Ophthalmol Vis Sci.* (2010) 51:1408–14. doi: 10.1167/iovs.09-4029

132. Kushnerev E, Shawcross SG, Sothirachagan S, Carley F, Brahma A, Yates JM, et al. Regeneration of corneal epithelium with dental pulp stem cells using a contact lens delivery system. *Invest Ophthalmol Vis Sci.* (2016) 57:5192–9. doi: 10.1167/iovs.15-17953

133. Kumagai Y, Kurokawa MS, Ueno H, Kayama M, Tsubota K, Nakatsuji N, et al. Induction of corneal epithelium-like cells from cynomolgus monkey embryonic stem cells and their experimental transplantation to damaged cornea. *Cornea.* (2010) 29:432–8. doi: 10.1097/ICO.0b013e3181b9ffcc

134. Ueno H, Kurokawa MS, Kayama M, Homma R, Kumagai Y, Masuda C, et al. Experimental transplantation of corneal epithelium-like cells induced by Pax6 gene transfection of mouse embryonic stem cells. *Cornea.* (2007) 26:1220–7. doi: 10.1097/ICO.0b013e31814fa814

135. Prabhasawat P, Chirapapaisan C, Jiravarnsirikul A, Ekpo P, Uiprasertkul M, Thamphithak R, et al. Phenotypic characterization of corneal epithelium in long-term follow-up of patients post-autologous cultivated oral mucosal epithelial transplantation. *Cornea.* (2021) 40:842–50. doi: 10.1097/ICO.0000000000002498

136. Prabhasawat P, Luangaram A, Ekpo P, Lekhanont K, Tangpagasit W, Boonwong C, et al. Epithelial analysis of simple limbal epithelial transplantation in limbal stem cell deficiency by in vivo confocal microscopy and impression cytology. *Cell Tissue Bank.* (2019) 20:95–108. doi: 10.1007/s10561-018-09746-3

13

The Ethical and Societal Considerations for the Rise of Artificial Intelligence and Big Data in Ophthalmology

T. Y. Alvin Liu[1]* and Jo-Hsuan Wu[2]

[1] Wilmer Eye Institute, Johns Hopkins University, Baltimore, MD, United States, [2] Shiley Eye Institute and Viterbi Family Department of Ophthalmology, University of California, San Diego, La Jolla, CA, United States

Medical specialties with access to a large amount of imaging data, such as ophthalmology, have been at the forefront of the artificial intelligence (AI) revolution in medicine, driven by deep learning (DL) and big data. With the rise of AI and big data, there has also been increasing concern on the issues of bias and privacy, which can be partially addressed by low-shot learning, generative DL, federated learning and a "model-to-data" approach, as demonstrated by various groups of investigators in ophthalmology. However, to adequately tackle the ethical and societal challenges associated with the rise of AI in ophthalmology, a more comprehensive approach is preferable. Specifically, AI should be viewed as sociotechnical, meaning this technology shapes, and is shaped by social phenomena.

Keywords: ethics, bias, artificial intelligence, fairness, privacy

*Correspondence:
T. Y. Alvin Liu
tliu25@jhmi.edu

INTRODUCTION

The rise of artificial intelligence (AI) and big data has been hailed as the 4th Industrial Revolution. Recent advancement in AI, in the form of deep learning (DL) which is a subtype of machine learning (ML), and improvement in hardware such as graphic processing units (GPU), have propelled medical AI applications to the forefront of the public discourse. This is because DL has been shown to be on par with human experts in analyzing medical images across different specialties, especially in medical specialties that interact with and have access to a large number of images, such as dermatology, radiology, and ophthalmology (1–10). In addition, "super-human" feats achieved by DL, such as the robust prediction of age, gender, blood pressure and smoking status of a person from a color fundus photograph alone (11), have captured the public's imagination and sparked a debate on the role and impact of AI on medicine.

Ophthalmology, being at the forefront of this AI revolution in medicine, is well-positioned to actively participate in and be a thought-leader on the societal implications for the rise of AI and big data in medicine. In the following perspective piece, we will highlight the ethical controversies and considerations from an ophthalmological perspective. The two major concerns regarding the rise of AI in medicine and ophthalmology center on bias and privacy.

DISCUSSION

Bias and Fairness

AI has the potential to entrench, or even exacerbate, existing biases in the healthcare system *via* unfair recommendations or decision-making. Fairness can be defined as "the absence of any prejudice or favoritism toward an individual or a group based on their inherent or acquired characteristics" (12). A prominent example of a medical AI algorithm providing unfair recommendations and exacerbating biases was highlighted by a study by Obermeyer at al. (13) showing that an AI algorithm systematically biased against Black patients, by erroneously using previous health costs as a proxy for predicting health needs and illness severity.

Bias in the training data is one of the most common reasons for a ML algorithm to produce unfair downstream predictions or recommendations. Many types of bias in ML exist. A comprehensive discussion of the different kinds of bias is beyond the scope of the current paper, but is nicely summarized here (14, 15). Specifically, within the context of ophthalmology DL studies, imbalance in training images is a common, yet addressable, reason that can lead to biases against a patient subgroup, such as patients of a certain race. For example, the AREDS image dataset (16), generated from a landmark longitudinal clinical trial and used in numerous important ophthalmology DL studies, was derived primarily from Caucasian patients (about 96% of participants). While age-related macular degeneration (AMD) is more prevalent in Caucasian patients (prevalence of 5.4% vs. 4.2% in Hispanic, 2.4% in Black and 4.6% in Asian) (17–19), the difference in prevalence on a population level does not explain fully the extreme imbalance in the AREDS dataset. Additional factors, such as unequal access to or interest in participating in clinical trials, likely also played a role.

However, such imbalance in training data can be addressed in three different ways. First, patient recruitment in prospective studies can be planned to ensure equal enrollment numbers for different pre-specified patient subgroups, e.g., based on sex, age, race, ethnicity, socioeconomic status and disease severity, etc. Second, if the recruitment of a certain patient subgroup is limited by practicality or natural prevalence of the disease, e.g., Black patients with AMD, then low-shot DL can be attempted. Low-shot DL, in contrast to traditional DL which requires a large amount of data for training, can be trained with relatively few samples (20), and can outperform traditional DL approaches when the available training dataset is small (5). Third, the patient subgroup that is under-represented in the training samples can be augmented by generative DL, a DL technique that can generate synthetic data. It has been shown that retinal images, created by generative DL, can be used to train a robust DL system for AMD classification (21). Specifically, in the context of DL-based detection of referable diabetic retinopathy, generative DL has been used to increase the training image samples of an under-represented patient subgroup and has been shown to decrease the bias against that particular under-represented patient subgroup during testing (22).

In addition to addressing the data distribution, the model itself can be fine-tuned to improve fairness. For example, instead of minimizing the average error across all statistics, we could aim to minimize the maximum error of a subset of statistics as evaluated across different demographic groups of interest.

A recent scoping review on digital health solutions (23) found that AI health applications generally lacked vigorous pragmatic prospective real-world validations. Addressing training data imbalance during model development should produce more generalizable ophthalmic AI applications that perform more robustly in real-world validations.

Privacy

DL models typically require a large amount of data for training, and the rise of DL in ophthalmology coincided with the rise of big data, both in the form of images and tabular data. The training and testing of DL models often involve combining ophthalmic images from different sources, and there is increasing concern that such transfer of data represents an unacceptable risk of privacy breach, especially since fundus images are now considered protected health information.

Such concerns can be addressed in two ways: federated learning and differential privacy. The training of DL models can be facilitated by federated learning, which allows model training in a decentralized fashion, takes advantage of the data heterogeneity from disparate sources, and does not require actual transfer of data between the sources (24). This approach has been successfully implemented in the context of retinal microvasculature segmentation and referable diabetic retinopathy detection on optical coherence tomography (OCT) and OCT angiography images. The authors demonstrated that a federated learning approach achieved similar results as a traditional centralized learning approach (25). Similarly, instead of transferring data to train a DL model, the model itself can be "brought" to the data for retraining. This concept has been successfully demonstrated in the context of DL-based intraretinal fluid segmentation on OCT images, in which the parameters of a pre-trained DL model were frozen, transferred to and retrained at a different institution. The authors showed that such a "model-to-data" work flow could update a model and improve the model's performance, without the transfer of actual data (26).

Besides image databases, ophthalmology is also at the forefront of establishing massive tabular databases. The Intelligent Research in Sight (IRIS) Registry, spearheaded by the American Academy of Ophthalmology, is the largest specialty database in all of medicine in the world. The data collected to date has been invaluable, and led to numerous new insights and publications. Without a question, the IRIS Registry will be indispensable in developing the next-generation predictive ML algorithms. The data collected in IRIS is first de-identified, before being distributed to researchers. Traditional data de-identification methods include complete removal of all unique identifiers or coarsening of the original dataset. Data coarsening is achieved by providing the exact values of only a subset of the original sample and thus creating an incomplete dataset (27, 28). What remains to be seen is whether traditional data de-identification methods will be sufficient for protecting the privacy of data in the IRIS registry or similar tabular databases. Traditional de-identification methods are vulnerable to linkage and other re-identification attacks, in which third parties correlate the supposedly anonymized data with unanticipated sources of auxiliary information to learn sensitive information about data participants. Examples of de-identification failure include the re-identification of "anonymized" hospital records released by Massachusetts' Group Insurance Commission and the re-identification of Netflix users' movie reviews from a dataset released as part of a ML challenge that Netflix hosted in 2006. A promising avenue of research is the application of differential privacy to large ophthalmic databases, such as IRIS.

Differential privacy is the only principled solution for releasing aggregate information about a statistical database, with provable guarantees that no information attributable to any individual in the dataset will be revealed. Briefly, differential privacy employs randomization to guarantee that the log odds ratio of any output of the analysis is bounded by and compared to a counterfactual world, in which any given participant has been entirely removed from the dataset, thereby formally limiting what inferences an arbitrarily well-informed observer can make about the data of any single participant (29). By definition, differential privacy prevents membership inference attacks as discussed above and provides a general umbrella of protection. However, the exact methods to create a differentially private dataset of unstructured data, e.g., ophthalmic images, are not currently available. This a major limitation of differential privacy as most recent advances in ML applications to ophthalmology have been in DL applications to ophthalmic images.

Finally, next-generation data infrastructure, specifically geared toward big data, ML and data privacy, is being developed, and a cutting-edge example is swarm learning. Swarm learning (30) is a decentralized data infrastructure that uses blockchain technology to ensure peer-to-peer data security. In contrast to federated learning which still requires a central parameter server, swarm learning is completely decentralized and, in addition, could inherit and be compatible with aforementioned differential privacy algorithms.

CONCLUSION

We are in the midst of the 4th Industrial Revolution, and ophthalmology has been at the forefront of the rise in AI/ML/DL and big data in medicine, and encountered various ethical and societal implications of this trend. While the concerns surrounding bias, fairness and privacy can be partially addressed by the strategies outlined above, a more comprehensive approach is preferable. This shift in mentality is best demonstrated by a recently announced special funding opportunity that was offered by the National Institute of Health as part of the Bridge2AI Common Fund[1]. The funding opportunity aims to produce Data Generation Projects that prospectively curate AI/ML ready data based on ethical principles. Multi-disciplinary teams, comprised of physicians, computer scientists and ethicists, are expected to promote a culture of ethical inquiry and consider ethical issues throughout the entire lifecycle of the project. Such an approach is grounded in the emerging view that AI is a sociotechnical issue: that is, AI shapes, and is shaped by social phenomena. The acknowledgment that the successful application of AI to medicine hinges on the holistic tackling of the associated ethical and societal implications is indeed a huge step forward, and we predict ophthalmologists in particular will play an important role in this regard in the years to come.

AUTHOR CONTRIBUTIONS

All authors listed have made a substantial, direct, and intellectual contribution to the work and approved it for publication.

[1]https://commonfund.nih.gov/bridge2ai

REFERENCES

1. Bridge J, Harding S, Zheng Y. Development and validation of a novel prognostic model for predicting AMD progression using longitudinal fundus images. *BMJ Open Ophthalmol.* (2020) 5:e000569. doi: 10.1136/bmjophth-2020-000569

2. Peng Y, Keenan TD, Chen Q, et al. Predicting risk of late age-related macular degeneration using deep learning. *NPJ Digit Med.* (2020) 3:111. doi: 10.1038/s41746-020-00317-z

3. Bhuiyan A, Wong TY, Ting DSW, Govindaiah A, Souied EH, Smith RT. Artificial intelligence to stratify severity of Age-Related Macular Degeneration (AMD) and predict risk of progression to late AMD. *Transl Vis Sci Technol.* (2020) 9:25. doi: 10.1167/tvst.9.2.25

4. Ludwig CA, Perera C, Myung D, Greven MA, Smith SJ, Chang RT, et al. Automatic identification of referral-warranted diabetic retinopathy using deep learning on mobile phone images. *Transl Vis Sci Technol.* (2020) 9:60. doi: 10.1167/tvst.9.2.60

5. Burlina P, Paul W, Mathew P, Joshi N, Pacheco KD, Bressler NM. Low-shot deep learning of diabetic retinopathy with potential applications to address artificial intelligence bias in retinal diagnostics

and rare ophthalmic diseases. *JAMA Ophthalmol.* (2020) 138:1070-7. doi: 10.1001/jamaophthalmol.2020.3269

6. Ting DSW, Cheung CY, Lim G, Tan GSW, Quang ND, Gan A, et al. Development and validation of a deep learning system for diabetic retinopathy and related eye diseases using retinal images from multiethnic populations with diabetes. *JAMA.* (2017) 318:2211-23. doi: 10.1001/jama.2017.18152

7. Brown JM, Campbell JP, Beers A, Chang K, Ostmo S, Chan RVP, et al. Automated diagnosis of plus disease in retinopathy of prematurity using deep convolutional neural networks. *JAMA Ophthalmol.* (2018) 136:803-10. doi: 10.1001/jamaophthalmol.2018.1934

8. Campbell JP, Kim SJ, Brown JM, Ostmo S, Chan RVP, Kalpathy-Cramer J, et al. Evaluation of a deep learning-derived quantitative retinopathy of prematurity severity scale. *Ophthalmology.* (2020) 128:1070-6. doi: 10.1016/j.ophtha.2020.10.025

9. Liu TYA, Wei J, Zhu H, Subramanian PS, Myung D, Yi PH, et al. Detection of optic disc abnormalities in color fundus photographs using deep learning. *J Neuroophthalmol.* (2021) 41:368-74. doi: 10.1097/WNO.00000000000 01358

10. Liu TYA, Zhu H, Chen H, Arevalo JF, Hui FK, Yi PH, et al. Gene expression profile prediction in uveal melanoma using deep learning: a pilot study for

the development of an alternative survival prediction tool. *Ophthalmol Retina.* (2020) 4:1213–5. doi: 10.1016/j.oret.2020.06.023

11. Poplin R, Varadarajan AV, Blumer K, Liu Y, McConnell MV, Corrado GS, et al. Prediction of cardiovascular risk factors from retinal fundus photographs via deep learning. *Nat Biomed Eng.* (2018) 2:158–64. doi: 10.1038/s41551-018-0195-0

12. Mehrabi N, Morstatter F, Saxena N, Lerman K, Galstyan A. A survey on bias and fairness in machine learning. *arXiv:1908.09635v3.* (2019). doi: 10.48550/arXiv.1908.09635

13. Obermeyer Z, Powers B, Vogeli C, Mullainathan S. Dissecting racial bias in an algorithm used to manage the health of populations. *Science.* (2019) 366:447–53. doi: 10.1126/science.aax2342

14. Olteanu A, Castillo C, Diaz F, Kiciman E. Social data: Biases, methodological pitfalls, and ethical boundaries. (2016) 2:13. doi: 10.2139/ssrn.28 86526

15. Suresh H, Guttag J. A framework for understanding sources of harm throughout the machine learning life cycle. In: *Equity and Access in Algorithms, Mechanisms, and Optimization (EAAMO '21).* New York, NY: Association for Computing Machinery (2021). p. 1–9. doi: 10.1145/3465416.3483305

16. Age-Related Eye Disease Study Research Group. The Age-Related Eye Disease Study (AREDS): design implications. AREDS report no 1. *Control Clin Trials.* (1999) 20:573–600. doi: 10.1016/S0197-2456(99)00031-8

17. Klein R, Klein BE, Knudtson MD, Wong TY, Cotch MF, Liu K, et al. Prevalence of age-related macular degeneration in 4 racial/ethnic groups in the multi-ethnic study of atherosclerosis. *Ophthalmology.* (2006) 113:373–80. doi: 10.1016/j.ophtha.2005.12.013

18. Friedman DS, Katz J, Bressler NM, Rahmani B, Tielsch JM. Racial differences in the prevalence of age-related macular degeneration: the Baltimore Eye Survey. *Ophthalmology.* (1999) 106:1049–55. doi: 10.1016/S0161-6420(99)90267-1

19. Zhou M, Duan P-C, Liang J-H, Zhang X-F, Pan C-W. Geographic distributions of age-related macular degeneration incidence: a systematic review and meta-analysis. *Br J Ophthalmol.* (2021) 105:1427–34. doi: 10.1136/bjophthalmol-2020-316820

20. Wang Y, Yao Q, Kwok J, Ni LM. Generalizing from a few examples: a survey on few-shot learning. *arXiv:1904.05046v3* (2020).

21. Burlina PM, Joshi N, Pacheco KD, Liu TYA, Bressler NM. Assessment of deep generative models for high-resolution synthetic retinal image generation of age-related macular degeneration. *JAMA Ophthalmol.* (2019) 137:258–64. doi: 10.1001/jamaophthalmol.2018.6156

22. Burlina P, Joshi N, Paul W, Pacheco KD, Bressler NM. Addressing artificial intelligence bias in retinal diagnostics. *Transl Vis Sci Technol.* (2021) 10:13. doi: 10.1167/tvst.10.2.13

23. Gunasekeran DV, Tseng RMWW, Tham Y-C, Wong TY. Applications of digital health for public health responses to COVID-19: a systematic scoping review of artificial intelligence, telehealth and related technologies. *NPJ Digital Med.* (2021) 4:40. doi: 10.1038/s41746-021-00412-9

24. Sheller MJ, Edwards B, Reina GA, Martin J, Pati S, Kotrotsou A, et al. Federated learning in medicine: facilitating multi-institutional collaborations without sharing patient data. *Sci Rep.* (2020) 10:12598. doi: 10.1038/s41598-020-69250-1

25. Lo J, Timothy TY, Ma D, Zang P, Owen JP, Zhang Q, et al. Federated learning for microvasculature segmentation and diabetic retinopathy classification of OCT data. *Ophthalm Sci.* (2021) 1:100069. doi: 10.1016/j.xops.2021.100069

26. Mehta N, Lee CS, Mendonça LSM, Raza K, Braun PX, Duker JS, et al. Model-to-data approach for deep learning in optical coherence tomography intraretinal fluid segmentation. *JAMA Ophthalmol.* (2020) 138:1017–24. doi: 10.1001/jamaophthalmol.2020.2769

27. Heitjan DF. Ignorability and coarse data: some biomedical examples. *Biometrics.* (1993) 49:1099–109. doi: 10.2307/2532251

28. Shardell M, El-Kamary SS. Sensitivity analysis of informatively coarsened data using pattern mixture models. *J Biopharm Stat.* (2009) 19:1018–38. doi: 10.1080/10543400903242779

29. Dwork C, Roth A. The algorithmic foundations of differential privacy. *Found Trends Theor Comput Sci.* (2013) 9:211–407. doi: 10.1561/9781601988195

30. Warnat-Herresthal S, Schultze H, Shastry KL, Manamohan S, Mukherjee S, Garg V, et al. Swarm learning for decentralized and confidential clinical machine learning. *Nature.* (2021) 594, 265–270. doi: 10.1038/s41586-021-03583-3

14

Do Ocular Fluids Represent a Transmission Route of SARS-CoV-2 Infection?

Giulio Petronio Petronio, Roberto Di Marco* and Ciro Costagliola

Department of Medicine and Health Science "V. Tiberio", Università degli Studi del Molise, Campobasso, Italy

*Correspondence:
Roberto Di Marco
roberto.dimarco@unimol.it

The spread of the new SARS-CoV-2 is marked by a short timeline. In this scenario, explaining or excluding the possible transmission routes is mandatory to contain and manage the spread of the disease in the community. In the recent pandemic, it is still unclear how coronavirus can end up in ocular fluids. Nevertheless, eye redness and irritation in COVID-19 patients have been reported, suggesting that a possible ocular manifestation of SARS-CoV-2 infection may be conjunctivitis. On the basis of epidemiological data provided by previous SARS-Cove infection, numerous theories have been proposed: (1) conjunctiva as the site of direct inoculation by infected droplets; (2) the nasolacrimal duct as a migration route of the virus to the upper respiratory tract, or (3) haematogenic infection of the tear gland. The demand for further investigations to verify ocular involvement in COVID-19 infection came out from the results of recent meta-analysis studies, so the eye cannot be completely excluded as a transmission route of the infection. Thus, healthcare personnel and all the people that enter in contact with infected or suspected patients must always use the prescribed protective equipment.

Keywords: COVID-19, ocular fluids, transmission route, SARS-CoV-2, healthcare protection

INTRODUCTION

The first cases of Severe Acute Respiratory Syndrome Coronavirus 2 (SARS-CoV-2) were directly linked to an animal market in Wuhan, China. To date, the virus disease clinical evidence such as symptoms and pathogenesis, as well as the systemic inflammatory response have been widely investigated by the scientific community (1).

Despite this, studies of the specific viral pathogenetic mechanisms in different human tissues are still a very broad subject that demands further considerations. In this regard, scientific evidence about the role of conjunctiva and ocular fluids as possible routes of transmission is still few and not conclusive.

For these reasons, the aim of this narrative review was to explore the role of conjunctiva and ocular fluids in the transmission of SARS-CoV-2 infection by a literature research focused on the most recent and relevant scientific publications.

The Epidemiological Data: The Italian Experience

On 30th Jan 2020, the WHO declared the coronavirus epidemic, and on 28th Feb, it raised the threat to the coronavirus epidemic to a "very high" level worldwide. On 11th Mar, WHO Director-General, on evidence that the SARS-CoV-2 was not confined to some geographical regions, stated the pandemic spread throughout the planet. On 13th Mar, Europe was becoming the new epicenter of the pandemic.

The first cases of SARS-CoV-2 reported in Europe date back to 30th Jan at the Spallanzani Institute (Rome, Italy). The first case of secondary transmission also occurred in Italy, in Codogno, Municipality of Lombardy in the province of Lodi, on 18th Feb. In a period of more than 3 months (from 13th May to 29th November), Italy ranked from 3th to 7th for the number of COVID-19 cases worldwide (2) with 1,585,178 cases reported, with 54,904 deceased, 734,503 dismissed/healed and 795,771 positives. According to the Italian Ministry of Health, COVID-19 percentage case fatality rate (CFR) by age group are: age group 0–9, 0% CFR; age group 10–19, 0% CFR; age group 20–29, 0.01% CFR; age group 30–39, 0.06% CFR; age group 40–49, 0.19% CFR; age group 50–59, 0.64% CFR; age group 60–69, 3% CFR; age group 70–79, 28% CFR; age group 80–89 18.86% CFR; age group ≥90 22.37% CFR (data available for 1,545,752 cases). The highest CFR % value was found in the over-90s age group (22.37%), this figure is significantly higher than the median age of cases (48 years) and the presence of comorbidity (3).

Based on available data on November 25th 2020 from Italian Ministry of Health, the most frequently observed symptoms before hospitalization in deceased patients are: fever 71%, dyspnoea 73%, cough 34%, diarrhea 6%, and hemoptysis 1%. Patients with 3 or more pre-existing pathologies are 65.7%, followed by 2 pre-existing pathologies (18.5%) and 1 pre-existing pathology (12.6%). The percentage of patients without pre-existing pathologies is very low (3.2%), demonstrating that the presence of comorbidities strongly influences the infection *exitus* (4).

The deaths in Milan, during the period January/March was of 3,888 people in 2019, whereas it has reached the number of 4,459 people during the same period of 2020, with a rise of 14.7%. Data becomes even more appalling if one considers the period March 1st–31st, with an increase of 76,1% compared to the same period of 2019. The higher mortality rate recorded in Italy over other countries can be explained, in part, by the older age distribution of the infected patients (5). These epidemiological data, together with those coming from other EU countries and United Kingdom, have allowed the formulation of the Risk Assessment by the European Center for Disease Prevention and Control (ECDC), that pointed out how the risk of severe disease associated with SARS-CoV-2 infection for people in Europe is mild for the population and high for the seniors and those with chronic illnesses (6).

Transmission Route

Looking at what is happening worldwide, it has been realized that the spread of the new SARS-CoV-2 is marked by a short timeline. In this scenario, explaining or excluding the possible transmission routes is mandatory to contain and manage the spread of the disease in the community. Until now, not all the transmission routes of SARS-CoV-2 are known. Nevertheless, the primary mode of infection for SARS CoV-2 is the human-to-human transmission by droplets and direct contacts, as previously recognized for CoVs infections, such as SARS Cove and MERS Cove (7). Beyond this modality, recent studies conducted on specimens from multiple sites of 205 patients with SARS-CoV-2, detected the live virus in feces, implying

that SARS-CoV-2 may also be transmitted through the fecal route (8). Furthermore, a possible systemic involvement has been suggested, given the presence of a small percentage of blood samples with positive results (9). In one case, the passage of the virus into the peritoneal cavity and fluids was also reported. This discovery raised concerns about the risks of exposure and contagion for the entire surgical staff, since all patients potentially, even those with mild respiratory symptoms, could present a viral load in the peritoneal fluid (10). A further hypothesis involves vectors such as domestic animals, flies, mosquitoes, or *Demodex folliculorum* in skin-to-skin transmission, as well as the direct human-to-human transmission (11). Thus, it would be helpful to cut nails as short as possible, to cut hair or to keep them tied back, and to shave beards, taking into account that sebum secretion too can be contaminated by the virus. In this context, disinfection of all instruments used for personal hygiene before and after use is strictly necessary and should not be shared to limit the spread of the virus (11).

Ocular Fluids

To date, it is still unclear how coronavirus can end up in ocular fluids, although feline and murine models have been used to record clinical manifestations such as conjunctivitis, anterior uveitis, retinitis, and optic neuritis (12). In the recent pandemic, a hypothesis about humans conjunctivitis as a possible ocular manifestation of SARS-CoV-2 infection was also made. This finding is partly supported by numerous clinical evidence, such as redness and eye irritation in patients with COVID-19. On the basis on epidemiological data provided by previous SARS-CoV infection, numerous theories have been proposed: (1) conjunctiva as the site of direct inoculation by infected droplets; (2) the nasolacrimal duct as a migration route of the virus to the upper respiratory tract; or (3) haematogenic infection of the tear gland (13).

New evidence about the novel coronavirus SARS-CoV-2 affecting the human eye has been reported. The main receptor of COVID-19 host cells that plays a crucial role in the entry of the virus into the cell to cause the final infection is the angiotensin 2 conversion enzyme (ACE2) (14). The expression of ACE2 in the conjunctiva (together with the epithelial cells of the lung, intestines, kidney, blood vessels), could indicate a potential infection route of the virus via these tissues (15). The presence of ACE2 receptors in human ocular tissue and CD147 in ocular fluids strongly suggests a role toward SARS-CoV-2 at the ocular level, consisting in the facilitation of virus entry inside the cell, followed by its replication and release (16).

Despite the presence of these facilitating mechanisms, ocular manifestations of COVID-19 are overall rare in the published literature. According to a study published on 30th Apr 2020, by Guan et al. (17) <1% of patients across 30 provinces in China (out of 33 of the total) were reported to have a conjunctiva involvement.

The demand for further investigations to verify ocular involvement in COVID-19 infection came out from the results of five reviews conducted by Sarma et al. (18), Loffredo et al. (19), Siedlecki et al. (20), Emparan et al. (21), and Torres-Costa

(22) that aimed to demonstrate a correlation between the manifestation of ocular symptoms and the occurrence of systemic ones.

On 20th Mar 2020, Sarma et al. screened 5 different literature databases (PubMed, Google Scholar, EMBASE, Medrixv, and BioRixv). In their systematic review and meta-Analysis, authors included studies about the ocular manifestation of SARS-COV-2 patients were without language restriction. It is interesting to highlight how the authors applied two different eligibility criteria, depending on the type of study conducted. Indeed, for systematic review, different types of study (i.e., case report, case series) were included along with observations and any other type of study design that reported an ocular manifestation or its possible complication due to viral infection. On the other hand, for the meta-analysis study, only observational studies that included patients with Novel Coronavirus Pneumonia (confirmed by clinical or laboratory tests or both) were reported.

Loffredo et al. evaluated the frequency of conjunctivitis in patients affected by severe and non-severe COVID-19 infection according to the PRISMA (Preferred Reporting Items for Systematic Reviews and Meta-Analysis) only on clinical studies identified by searching Pubmed, ISI Web of Science, SCOPUS, and Cochrane electronic databases. On 5th Apr 2020, authors included 1,167 COVID-19 patients in their meta-analysis (19).

Siedlecki et al. used the PubMed.gov for searching relevant articles. On 16th Apr 2020, authors identified more than 20 articles on the ophthalmological aspects of COVID-19, of these, close to 60% were from Asia, around 30% were from the USA, and <15% were from Europe. The authors have analyzed different types of scientific articles, including original studies, letters, case studies, and reviews (20).

On 29th May 2020, Emparan et al. published a structured review on COVID-19 and ophthalmology using PubMed, ScienceDirect, LILACS, SciELO, the Cochrane Library, and Google Scholar as electronic databases. The Oxford Center for Evidence-Based Medicine 2011 Levels of Evidence worksheet was employed by authors for quality assessments. More than 1,000 manuscripts were identified in the research; only 26 records were included in the qualitative synthesis and of these only 17 were classified as level 5 within the classification system of the Oxford CBME methodology, the rest were level 4 (21).

Lastly, on 16th Jun 2020, Torres-Costa et al. reviewed the most relevant articles together with the official recommendations of ophthalmological societies by literature search on PubMed electronic database.

Despite the different research strategies and bibliographic analysis methods used by the authors, all the studies concluded that keratoconjunctivitis is the most representative ocular finding and that there is a correlation between the severity of the infection and eye involvement. The eye can be both an active (through tears) and passive (via the nasolacrimal duct) infection pathway. Tear film represents a natural defensive barrier against pathogens, thanks to the presence of antimicrobial proteins (such as lactoferrin, lysozyme, lipocalin, and beta-lysine) and immunoglobulins (23). Specifically, lactoferrin inhibits the virus binding protein by preventing the attachment of SARS-CoV to heparan sulfate proteoglycans (24). In addition, the possibility of foreign particles adhering and potentially invading epithelial cells is significantly reduced by the continuous rinsing of tears from the anterior surface of the eye to the nasolacrimal system together with the thick layer of mucin above the epithelium (25). Lastly, the outer lipid layer of tear film also enhances the resistance to the pathogen invasion. The lack of this layer in the mucosal membrane of the nasal and respiratory tract might explain the high affinity of Covid-19 for respiratory tract compared to that observed for the anterior ocular surface. Contrarily, a degraded anterior ocular surface, like in dry eye, could facilitate the viral infection into ocular and nasopharyngeal tissues (26). Indeed, dry eye is characterized by an abnormal tear film, through a broad spectrum of anomalies which varies from tear deficiency to atypical tear composition. The final result consists of a disruption of the tear film homeostasis that adversely affects the ability both to perform essential physiologic functions and to prevent microbial invasion (27). Especially the anatomical and physiological properties of the eyes may explain the discrepancy between the theoretically expected high rate of eye surface inflammation due to viral infection and the relatively low clinical incidence observed. Among these, the role played by the electrical standing potential of the eye in repelling aerosol particles (microdroplets) from the ocular surface should also be considered in terms of prevention of ocular infections (28).

On 17th Apr 2020, Colavita et al. (29) observed an early ocular involvement of SARS-CoV-2 in the COVID-19 course of a patient with prolonged viral RNA detection. This important finding is not representative of the general population since the patient was a 65-year-old woman, and it is well-known that: (1) women are more likely to report frequent symptoms of dry eye; (2) the prevalence of dry eye is relatively higher in Chinese population than that reported for white, and lastly (3) age over 60 has significantly higher prevalence rates (30).

A more recent study cohort conducted by Valente et al. on pediatric patients with confirmed COVID-19 infection hospitalized from 16th Mar to 15th Apr 2020, at the Bambino Gesù Children's Hospital concluded that the ocular manifestations associated with the viral infection appear to have had a milder clinical course in pediatric patients than in adult patients showing the same symptoms (31).

Taken together, both clinical evidence and laboratory test findings suggest that the conjunctiva is rarely involved in SARS-CoV-2 infection since it is naturally protected, so conjunctiva is neither a tissue of choice for SARS-CoV-2 infection and is not a preferential route of entry for the virus to infect the respiratory tract.

These findings are supported by Kumar et al., who performed a study on 45 infected patients. Although the study results showed that SARS-CoV-2 could be detected in conjunctival swabs, the rate of positive detection of SARS-CoV-2 in conjunctival swabs is much lower when compared to nasal ones (32).

A second report on 43 patients with severe COVID-19 published by Karimi et al. (33) on 18th May 2020 demonstrated that ocular manifestation was rare also in patients with severe COVID-19 (7%).

Another study on 36 SARS-CoV-2 patients divided into two groups (18 with conjunctivitis and 18 without) published by Güemes-Villahoz et al. (34) on 24th Jun 2020 concluded that the clinical course was the same regardless of the onset of conjunctivitis.

All these results taken together, suggest that conjunctivitis is not a conditioning factor for SARS-CoV-2 detection in ocular fluids.

DISCUSSION

Detection of SARS-CoV-2

In this scenario, although the early detection of infectious SARS-CoV-2 from ocular fluids may represent an important diagnostic advancement useful to counteract the spread of the virus in the community, the mechanisms of virus ocular tropism and how human eye cells could support viral replication is yet to be clarified (35). One of the factors that could explain the very low positive rate of SARS-CoV-2 confirmed by RT-PCR in tears and conjunctival secretions in patients with COVID-19 can be attributed to the low sensitivity of the RT-PCR test currently used for SARS-CoV-2 RNA. The sampling time can also be a determining factor since the virus, and its genetic material may be present in ocular fluids for a short period of the disease. Finally, the low amount of collected tears and conjunctival secretions may also be responsible for PCR negativity (36). On the other hand, the amount of virus or receptor expression necessary to cause infection is not known; however, currently, the eye is not considered to be a high-risk tissue due to the low ACE2 and TMPRSS2 expression (37).

Although ocular manifestations of COVID-19 are currently thought to be self-limited, the necessary condition for the SARS-CoV-2 to be transmitted through the conjunctival epithelial tissue is the ability to replicate in conjunctival cells, inducing cytopathic changes necessary for its identification (38) thus the eye cannot be completely excluded as a transmission route of the infection.

Healthcare Prevention and Protection

Healthcare personnel and all the people that enter in contact with infected or suspected patient must always use the approved personal protective equipment (PPE). In Italy, a high number of medical doctors and other healthcare professionals have died of COVID-19; this list includes mainly general practitioners but also several dentists and one ophthalmologist. The dramatic situation in which the medical community finds itself mirrors what was reported for the overall deaths related to COVID-19 in Italy. Indeed most of the dead doctors were male. The high rate of infection among nurses and healthcare staff is due to the lack of an adequate number or even the absence of PPE in some hospitals. Besides, very often, nurses and doctors are forced to wear masks inappropriately, thus reducing their effectiveness in containing the spread of the disease.

It is unacceptable to work without sufficient protection, and governments must ensure an adequate and constant supply for all health facilities involved. In this context, already in February 2020, the Italian Ministry of Health had issued the "ASSISTENTIAL ADDRESS LINES OF THE CRITICAL PATIENT AFFECTED BY COVID-19" (39). This document stressed the importance of prescribed PPE such as masks, overalls, long gloves and visors to protect the ocular mucous membranes from the moment the patient is admitted and during all those procedures that could generate aerosols (i.e., endotracheal aspiration, intubation, tracheostomy, bronchoscopy, central venous catheter placement in the jugular, subclavian or femoral vein or during cardiopulmonary resuscitation). Lastly, taking into account the proximity to patients during eye examination make ophthalmologists at risk for droplet transmission; moreover, the unavoidable physical contact they have with patients' eyes, results in increased susceptibility through direct contact (40). For these reasons strict hand hygiene and PPE are highly recommended for health care workers to avoid hospital-related viral transmission during ophthalmic practice.

AUTHOR CONTRIBUTIONS

GPP conceptualized and wrote the manuscript. RDM edited the microbiological findings and CC edited the ophthalmological implications.

REFERENCES

1. Bellinvia S, Edwards CJ, Schisano M, Banfi P, Fallico M, Murabito P. The unleashing of the immune system in COVID-19 and sepsis: the calm before the storm? *Inflamm Res.* (2020) 69:757–63. doi: 10.1007/s00011-020-01366-6

2. Dong E, Du H, Gardner L. An interactive web-based dashboard to track COVID-19 in real time. *Lancet Infect Dis.* (2020) 20:533–4. doi: 10.1016/S1473-3099(20)30120-1

3. Health IMO. *COVID-19 Italy Situation.* (2020). Available online at: http://www.salute.gov.it/portale/nuovocoronavirus/homeNuovoCoronavirus.jsp?lingua=english (accessed November 30, 2020).

4. Health IMO. *COVID-19 Integrated Surveillance Data in Italy.* (2020). Available online at: https://www.epicentro.iss.it/en/coronavirus/sars-cov-2-dashboard (accessed November 30, 2020).

5. Onder G, Rezza G, Brusaferro S. Case-fatality rate and characteristics of patients dying in relation to COVID-19 in Italy. *JAMA.* (2020) 23:1775–6. doi: 10.1001/jama.2020.4683

6. Team EE. Updated rapid risk assessment from ECDC on the novel coronavirus disease 2019 (COVID-19) pandemic: increased transmission in the EU/EEA and the UK. *Euro Surveill.* (2020) 25:2003121. doi: 10.2807/1560-7917.ES.2020.25.10.2003121

7. Meo S, Alhowikan A, Al-Khlaiwi T, Meo I, Halepoto D, Iqbal M, et al. Novel coronavirus 2019-nCoV: prevalence, biological and clinical characteristics comparison with SARS-CoV and MERS-CoV. *Eur Rev Med Pharmacol Sci.* (2020) 24:2012–9. doi: 10.26355/eurrev_202002_20379

8. Hindson J. COVID-19: faecal–oral transmission? *Nat Rev Gastroenterol Hepatol.* (2020) 17:259. doi: 10.1038/s41575-020-0295-7

9. Bulut C, Kato Y. Epidemiology of COVID-19. *Turkish J Med Sci.* (2020) 50:563–70. doi: 10.3906/sag-2004-172

10. Coccolini F, Tartaglia D, Puglisi A, Lodato M, Chiarugi M. SARS-CoV-2 is present in peritoneal fluid in COVID-19 patients. *Ann Surg.* (2020) 272:e240–2. doi: 10.1097/SLA.0000000000004030

11. Tatu A, Nadasdy T, Nwabudike L. Observations about sexual and other routes of SARS-CoV-2 (COVID-19) transmission and its prevention. *Clin Exp Dermatol.* (2020) 45:761–2. doi: 10.1111/ced.14274

12. Jun ISY, Anderson DE, Kang AEZ, Wang L-F, Rao P, Young BE, et al. Assessing viral shedding and infectivity of tears in coronavirus disease 2019 (COVID-19) patients. *Ophthalmology.* (2020) 127:977–9. doi: 10.1016/j.ophtha.2020.03.026

13. Seah I, Agrawal R. Can the coronavirus disease 2019 (COVID-19) affect the eyes? A review of coronaviruses and ocular implications in humans and animals. *Ocul Immunol Inflamm.* (2020) 28:1–5. doi: 10.1080/09273948.2020.1738501

14. Lu R, Zhao X, Li J, Niu P, Yang B, Wu H, et al. Genomic characterisation and epidemiology of 2019 novel coronavirus: implications for virus origins and receptor binding. *Lancet.* (2020) 395:565–74. doi: 10.1016/S0140-6736(20)30251-8

15. Xu H, Zhong L, Deng J, Peng J, Dan H, Zeng X, et al. High expression of ACE2 receptor of 2019-nCoV on the epithelial cells of oral mucosa. *Int J Oral Sci.* (2020) 12:1–5. doi: 10.1038/s41368-020-0074-x

16. Belser JA, Rota PA, Tumpey TM. Ocular tropism of respiratory viruses. *Microbiol Mol Biol Rev.* (2013) 77:144–56. doi: 10.1128/MMBR.00058-12

17. Guan W-J, Ni Z-Y, Hu Y, Liang W-H, Ou C-Q, He J-X, et al. Clinical characteristics of coronavirus disease 2019 in China. *N Engl J Med.* (2020) 382:1708–20. doi: 10.1056/NEJMoa2002032

18. Sarma P, Kaur H, Kaur H, Bhattacharyya J, Prajapat M, Shekhar N, et al. *Ocular Manifestations and Tear or Conjunctival Swab PCR Positivity for 2019-nCoV in Patients With COVID-19: A Systematic Review and Meta-Analysis.* (2020). Available online at: https://ssrn.com/abstract=3566161.

19. Loffredo L, Pacella F, Pacella E, Tiscione G, Oliva A, Violi F. Conjunctivitis and COVID-19: a meta-analysis. *J Med Virol.* (2020) 92:1413–4. doi: 10.1002/jmv.25938

20. Siedlecki J, Brantl V, Schworm B, Mayer WJ, Gerhardt M, Michalakis S, et al. COVID-19: ophthalmological aspects of the SARS-CoV 2 global pandemic. *Klin Monbl Augenheilkd.* (2020) 237:675–80. doi: 10.1055/a-1164-9381

21. Emparan JPO, Sardi-Correa C, López-Ulloa JA, Viteri-Soria J, Penniecook JA, Jimenez-Román J, et al. COVID-19 and the eye: how much do we really know? A best evidence review. *Arq Bras Oftalmol.* (2020) 83:250–61. doi: 10.5935/0004-2749.20200067

22. Torres-Costa S, Lima-Fontes M, Falcão-Reis F, Falcão M. SARS-COV-2 in ophthalmology: current evidence and standards for clinical practice. *Acta Méd Port.* (2020) 33:593–600. doi: 10.20344/amp.14118

23. Mannis M, Smolin G. Natural defense mechanisms of the ocular surface. In: Pepose JS, Holland GN, Wilhelmus KR, editors. *Ocular Infection and Immunity.* St. Louis, MO: Mosby (1996). p. 185–90.

24. Lang J, Yang N, Deng J, Liu K, Yang P, Zhang G, et al. Inhibition of SARS pseudovirus cell entry by lactoferrin binding to heparan sulfate proteoglycans. *PLoS ONE.* (2011) 6:e23710. doi: 10.1371/journal.pone.0023710

25. Akpek EK, Gottsch JD. Immune defense at the ocular surface. *Eye.* (2003) 17:949–56. doi: 10.1038/sj.eye.6700617

26. Hong N, Yu W, Xia J, Shen Y, Yap M, Han W. Evaluation of ocular symptoms and tropism of SARS-CoV-2 in patients confirmed with COVID-19. *Acta Ophthalmol.* (2020) 98:e649–55. doi: 10.1111/aos.14445

27. Johnson ME, Murphy PJ. Changes in the tear film and ocular surface from dry eye syndrome. *Progr Retinal Eye Res.* (2004) 23:449–74. doi: 10.1016/j.preteyeres.2004.04.003

28. Zimmerman K, Kearns F, Tzekov R. Natural protection of ocular surface from viral infections–a hypothesis. *Med Hypoth.* (2020) 143:110082. doi: 10.1016/j.mehy.2020.110082

29. Colavita F, Lapa D, Carletti F, Lalle E, Bordi L, Marsella P, et al. SARS-CoV-2 isolation from ocular secretions of a patient with COVID-19 in Italy with prolonged viral RNA detection. *Ann Intern Med.* (2020) 17:M20-1176. doi: 10.7326/M20-1176

30. Pei-Yu L, Su-Ying T, Ching-Yu C, Jorn-Hon L, Pesus C, Wen-Ming H. Prevalence of dry eye among an elderly Chinese population in Taiwan. *Ophthalmology.* (2003) 110:1096–101. doi: 10.1016/S0161-6420(03)00262-8

31. Valente P, Iarossi G, Federici M, Petroni S, Palma P, Cotugno N, et al. Ocular manifestations and viral shedding in tears of pediatric patients with coronavirus disease 2019: a preliminary report. *J Am Assoc Pediatric Ophthalmol Strabismus.* (2020) 24:212–5. doi: 10.1016/j.jaapos.2020.05.002

32. Kumar K, Prakash AA, Gangasagara SB, Rathod SB, Ravi K, Rangaiah A, et al. Presence of viral RNA of SARS-CoV-2 in conjunctival swab specimens of COVID-19 patients. *Indian J Ophthalmol.* (2020) 68:1015–7. doi: 10.4103/ijo.IJO_1287_20

33. Karimi S, Arabi A, Shahraki T, Safi S. Detection of severe acute respiratory syndrome coronavirus-2 in the tears of patients with coronavirus disease 2019. *Eye.* (2020) 34:1220–3. doi: 10.1038/s41433-020-0965-2

34. Güemes-Villahoz N, Burgos-Blasco B, Vilela AA, Arriola-Villalobos P, Luna CMR, Sardiña RC, et al. Detecting SARS-CoV-2 RNA in conjunctival secretions: is it a valuable diagnostic method of COVID-19? *J. Med. Virol.* (2020). doi: 10.1002/jmv.26219. [Epub ahead of print].

35. Al-Sharif E, Strianese D, AlMadhi NH, D'Aponte A, dell'Omo R, Di Benedetto R, et al. Ocular tropism of coronavirus (CoVs): a comparison of the interaction between the animal-to-human transmitted coronaviruses (SARS-CoV-1, SARS-CoV-2, MERS-CoV, CoV-229E, NL63, OC43, HKU1) and the eye. *Int. Ophthalmol.* (2020) 1–14. doi: 10.1007/s10792-020-01575-2

36. Sun C-B, Wang Y-Y, Liu G-H, Liu Z. Role of the eye in transmitting human coronavirus: what we know and what we do not know. *Front Public Health.* (2020) 8:155. doi: 10.3389/fpubh.2020.00155

37. Schnichels S, Rohrbach JM, Bayyoud T, Thaler S, Ziemssen F, Hurst J. Kann SARS-CoV-2 das auge infizieren?–ein überblick über den Rezeptorstatus in okularem Gewebe. *Ophthalmologe.* (2020) 24:1–4. doi: 10.1007/s00347-020-01160-z

38. Peng Y, Zhou YH. Is novel coronavirus disease (COVID-19) transmitted through conjunctiva? *J Med Virol.* (2020) 92:1408–9. doi: 10.1002/jmv.25753

39. Salute MD. *Linee di Indirizzo Assistenziali Del Paziente Critico Affetto da Covid-19.* Rome: Gazzetta Ufficiale Italiana (2020).

40. Galiero R, Pafundi PC, Nevola R, Rinaldi L, Acierno C, Caturano A, et al. The importance of telemedicine during COVID-19 pandemic: a focus on diabetic retinopathy. *J Diabetes Res.* (2020) 2020:9036847. doi: 10.1155/2020/9036847

15

Host Defense Peptides at the Ocular Surface: Roles in Health and Major Diseases and Therapeutic Potentials

Darren Shu Jeng Ting[1,2,3], Imran Mohammed[1], Rajamani Lakshminarayanan[3], Roger W. Beuerman[3] and Harminder S. Dua[1,2]*

[1] Academic Ophthalmology, School of Medicine, University of Nottingham, Nottingham, United Kingdom, [2] Department of Ophthalmology, Queen's Medical Centre, Nottingham, United Kingdom, [3] Anti-Infectives Research Group, Singapore Eye Research Institute, Singapore, Singapore

Correspondence:
Darren Shu Jeng Ting
ting.darren@gmail.com

Sight is arguably the most important sense in human. Being constantly exposed to the environmental stress, irritants and pathogens, the ocular surface – a specialized functional and anatomical unit composed of tear film, conjunctival and corneal epithelium, lacrimal glands, meibomian glands, and nasolacrimal drainage apparatus – serves as a crucial front-line defense of the eye. Host defense peptides (HDPs), also known as antimicrobial peptides, are evolutionarily conserved molecular components of innate immunity that are found in all classes of life. Since the first discovery of lysozyme in 1922, a wide range of HDPs have been identified at the ocular surface. In addition to their antimicrobial activity, HDPs are increasingly recognized for their wide array of biological functions, including anti-biofilm, immunomodulation, wound healing, and anti-cancer properties. In this review, we provide an updated review on: (1) spectrum and expression of HDPs at the ocular surface; (2) participation of HDPs in ocular surface diseases/conditions such as infectious keratitis, conjunctivitis, dry eye disease, keratoconus, allergic eye disease, rosacea keratitis, and post-ocular surgery; (3) HDPs that are currently in the development pipeline for treatment of ocular diseases and infections; and (4) future potential of HDP-based clinical pharmacotherapy for ocular diseases.

Keywords: antimicrobial peptide, cathelicidin, defensin, dry eye, host defense peptide, infection, keratitis, ocular surface

INTRODUCTION

The ocular surface (OS) is a specialized anatomical and functional system composed of various structures and components, including the tear film, conjunctival and corneal epithelium, lacrimal glands, meibomian glands, and nasolacrimal drainage apparatus. Originating embryologically from the surface ectoderm, all these OS structures are linked anatomically *via* the epithelium and functionally *via* the regulation of neuronal, vascular, endocrinological, and immunological systems (1). Together, they maintain the homeostasis of the OS which has critical roles in the optical quality of the eye to focus light at the retina and serving as the most front-line defense system of the eye against a wide array of pathogens as well as physical and chemical insults (2). In addition, the periocular skin, which is in close vicinity to the eye, has important influences on the health of OS. Inflammatory diseases of the periocular skin such as atopic dermatitis and rosacea often result in the manifestation of OS damage (3–5).

Being constantly exposed to pathogens, environmental irritants and stress, the OS relies on a highly functional innate immunity. Innate immunity mechanisms for the OS are composed of three major components, including the physical barrier (e.g., epithelial layers of conjunctiva and cornea), chemical barriers (e.g., tears), and cellular responses (e.g., macrophages, neutrophils, and others), for which the host defense peptides (HDPs) play important roles in the latter two.

Antimicrobial peptides (AMPs) are a group of evolutionarily conserved molecules of the innate immunity (6). To better capture the increasingly recognized multi-faceted roles of AMPs, a broader term "host defense peptides (HDPs)" has been subsequently introduced (7). They are ubiquitously expressed at epithelial surfaces (e.g., eye, skin, respiratory, gastrointestinal linings, etc.) and secreted by immune cells (e.g., polymorphonuclear leukocytes and macrophages) (8, 9). So far more than 3,000 naturally occurring and synthetic HDPs have been discovered across six life kingdoms (10, 11). These HDPs are usually cationic (due to the relative excess of arginine, lysine and/or histidine residues) and amphiphilic, with 30%−50% hydrophobicity (12). They exhibit high structural plasticity and can exist in the form of alpha-helical, beta-sheet, linear extension or mixed a-helical and beta-sheet structures (**Figure 1**) (13). They have recently shown promise as potential therapeutic agents due to their broad-spectrum antimicrobial properties against a wide array of infection, including drug-resistant bacteria, fungi, acanthamoeba, and viruses, with minimal risk of inducing antimicrobial resistance (11). In principle, HDPs are shown to primarily exert their broad-spectrum and rapid antimicrobial action through three main mechanisms of action, namely the barrel-stave, toroidal pore, and carpet models (**Figure 2**) (14, 15). The positively charged amino acid residues are responsible for the adsorption of AMPs onto the anionic bacterial membrane (*via* electrostatic interaction) and the hydrophobic residues interact with the lipid tail region of the membrane, culminating in membrane permeation, leakage of fluid into the bacterial cytoplasm and subsequent bacterial cell death (14). In addition to the membrane-targeting action, emerging evidence has highlighted that HDPs can kill microorganisms through several non-membrane perturbing mechanisms, such as biosynthesis of disorganized bacterial membranes and direct intercalation into the membrane, interfering with the intracellular DNA and RNA molecules, and others (7). HDPs are also shown to participate in chemotaxis, immunomodulation, wound healing, anti-biofilm and anti-cancer activities (16–19), offering a wide range of potential therapeutic applications.

The history of HDPs (or AMPs) dates back to 1922 when lysozyme was first discovered in various human tissues and body secretions, including the tear fluids (20). Since then, a wide spectrum of human HDPs have been identified and reported at the OS. These include lactoferrin, alpha- and beta-defensins, cathelicidin (LL-37), ribonuclease, psoriasin and dermcidin, amongst others (9, 21, 22). The expressions and actions of HDPs in several OS diseases have been previously summarized by Kolar and McDermott (23). Since then, there is a growing body of evidence underlining the roles and therapeutic potential of HDPs at the OS, ranging from novel observations at the molecular level

(e.g., upregulation of defensins and LL-37 in ocular rosacea) (24) to the advancement of designed HDPs toward human clinical trials (e.g., development of Mel4 as an antimicrobial coating for contact lens) (25). In view of the rapid evolution of this field, this review article aimed to provide an up-to-date, focused review of the spectrum and expression of HDPs at the OS, the roles in major OS diseases, and the therapeutic potential for OS diseases.

METHOD OF LITERATURE SEARCH

Electronic databases, including MEDLINE and EMBASE, were searched to identify relevant studies on HDPs at the OS. Only English articles were included in this review article. Key words used were "antimicrobial peptide," "defense peptide," "ocular surface," "tear fluid," "defensins," "cathelicidin," "keratitis," "dry eye," "atopic keratoconjunctivitis/atopic dermatitis," "ocular rosacea." The bibliographies of included articles were manually screened to identify further relevant studies. The final search was last updated in November 2021.

SPECTRUM AND CHARACTERISTICS OF HDPs AT OCULAR SURFACE

A wide array of HDPs have been identified and reported at the OS. In this section, we summarize the sources, characteristics, and functions of important HDPs, including lysozyme, lactoferrin, alpha- and beta-defensins, cathelicidin, ribonucleases, psoriasin, dermcidin, and histatin (**Table 1**).

Lysozyme

In 1922, lysozyme was discovered by Sir Alexander Fleming during the investigation of his patient with acute coryza. The nasal secretion of the patient was found to completely inhibit the growth of *Micrococcus* spp. (a Gram-positive bacteria). This striking observation prompted a series of experiments, which led to the discovery of lysozyme in various human tissues and body secretions, including tear fluids, saliva, blood, semen, respiratory tract linings, and connective tissues, amongst others (20). Interestingly, the antibacterial potency of lysozyme was influenced by the location of the tissues and types of microbes (e.g., lysozyme in tears was very active against micrococci, but was much less effective against other cocci in other parts of the body), highlighting the specific adaptation of the human immune system against specific pathogens at defined sties (20).

Lysozyme is primarily secreted in the tear fluid by the tubuloacinar cells of the main and accessory lacrimal glands (82) and, to a lesser extent, expressed by corneal epithelium and meibomian glands (83). It constitutes around 20%−30% of the total protein in tear fluids (82). Lysozyme exhibits its broad-spectrum antimicrobial activity *via* dual mechanisms of action (26). First, it hydrolyzes the bacterial cell wall by breaking down the β-1,4 glycosidic linkages between the disaccharides, *N*-acetylmuramic acid (NAM) and *N*-acetylglucosamine (NAG), which forms the backbone of peptidoglycan in the bacterial membrane. Second, the cationic property of lysozyme enables pore formation in the anionic bacterial membrane, which is

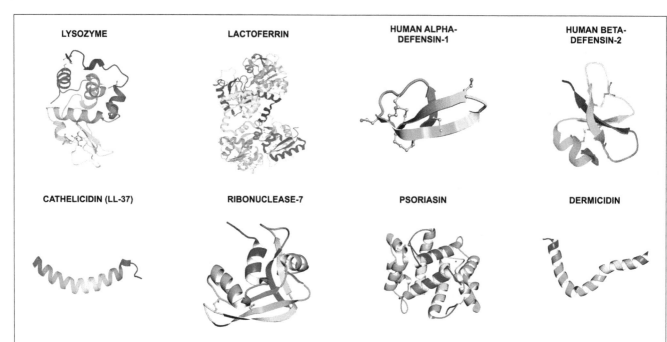

FIGURE 1 | Illustrations of the 3-dimensional secondary structures of the important host defense peptides (HDPs) at the ocular surface. The structures are obtained from the RCSB Protein Data Bank. Cathelicidin, psoriasin, and dermcidin are primarily made of alpha-helical helixes whereas human alpha- and beta-defensins are composed of triple beta-sheets. Lysozyme, lactoferrin and ribonuclease-7 (or RNase-7) are made of mixed alpha-helixes and beta-sheets.

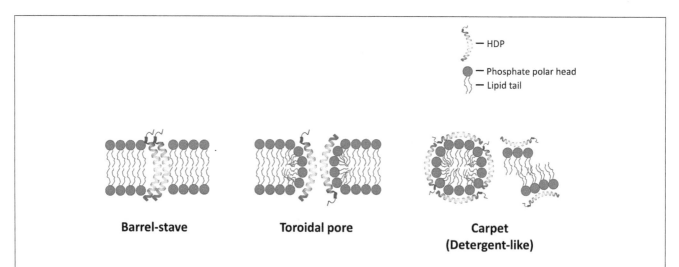

FIGURE 2 | Illustrations of the common membrane-permeabilizing mechanisms of host defense peptides (HDPs) against bacteria (and other microbes), namely: (1) barrel-stave; (2) toroidal pore; and (3) carpet (detergent-like) mechanisms. In the barrel-stave model, the HDPs act as a stave and penetrate vertically into the negatively charged, lipid bilayer bacterial membrane, creating permanent "barrel-shaped" pores. In the toroidal pore model, the HDPs interact with the negatively charged phosphate head groups electrostatically, distort the arrangement of the lipid bilayer, and create a transient membrane pore, with HDPs lining and stabilizing the internal part of the pore. In the carpet (detergent-like) model, the HDPs interact with the bacterial membrane electrostatically, and, upon reaching the critical concentration on the bacterial membrane, they result in membrane fragmentation / aggregation. These mechanisms result in destabilization of the membrane integrity, which leads to influx of fluid and efflux of intracellular content, culminating in cell lysis. Although less common (not shown in this figure), HDPs may also exert their antimicrobial action *via* binding to microbial intracellular targets (i.e., non-membrane-permeabilizing mechanisms), inhibiting DNA/RNA synthesis, protein synthesis and protein folding.

responsible for its rapid and broad-spectrum antimicrobial activity against a wide range of organisms.

In addition to its antimicrobial activity, lysozyme plays an important immunomodulatory role in host defense. Particularly, it activates lysozyme-dependent degradation of the engulfed bacteria within the phagolysosomes of macrophages and releases pathogen associated molecular patterns (PAMPs) from the lysed bacteria, resulting in a pro-inflammatory response *via* interaction with various pattern recognition receptors (PRRs) such as Toll-like receptors (TLRs), nucleotide-binding oligomerization

TABLE 1 | Characteristics and functions of common HDPs at the ocular surface (OS).

Type	Source	Functions
Lysozyme	- Tear fluid (secreted by tubuloacinar cells of lacrimal glands) - Corneal epithelium - Meibomian glands	- Antimicrobial property (*via* hydrolysis and pore formation of cell wall) (20, 26) - Immunomodulatory function *via* interaction with various pattern recognition receptors (26, 27)
Lactoferrin	- Tear fluid (secreted by acinar cells of lacrimal glands) - Conjunctival epithelium - Corneal epithelium - Meibomian glands	- Antimicrobial activity (*via* binding to free iron and membrane permeabilization) (28–30) and anti-biofilm (31) - Immunomodulatory function (anti- and pro-inflammatory) (32, 33) - Antioxidant (*via* inhibition of iron-dependent formation of hydroxyl radicals) (34) - Wound healing (32, 33)
Human alpha-defensins (or HNP)-1 to−4	- Azurophil granules of neutrophils	- All: antimicrobial activity (*via* membrane perturbation) (35) - HNP-1 to−3: immunomodulatory (Pro-inflammatory and anti-inflammatory) (36–38) - HNP-1 to−3: anti-cancer (39, 40)
Human beta-defensins (HBD)-1 to−3	- Conjunctival and corneal epithelium	- All: antimicrobial activity (*via* membrane perturbation) (41, 42) - All: immunomodulatory function (pro-inflammatory and anti-inflammatory) (42, 43) - HBD-3: wound healing (44) - All: anti-cancer (45, 46)
Cathelicidin	- Conjunctival epithelium - Corneal epithelium	- Antimicrobial activity (*via* membrane perturbation) (47–52) and anti-biofilm (47, 53) - Immunomodulatory function (pro-inflammatory and anti-inflammatory) (54, 55) - Wound healing (48, 56) - Anti-cancer (40, 57)
Ribonucleases - (RNases)	- RNase-5: Tear fluid and corneal endothelium - RNase-7: Corneal epithelium and stroma	- Antimicrobial activity (*via* binding to bacterial membrane lipoprotein and membrane perturbation) (58–66) - Immunomodulatory function (activates adaptive immunity) (67, 68) - Angiogenic and neurogenic (69, 70) - Wound healing (71)
Psoriasin	- Conjunctiva - Cornea - Lacrimal gland - Nasolacrimal duct	- Antimicrobial activity (*via* zinc-dependent mechanism) (72, 73) - Immunomodulatory function (chemotaxis, activates adaptive immune system *via* CD4+) (74, 75)
Dermcidin	- Corneal epithelium - Tear fluid	- Antimicrobial activity (*via* zinc-dependent mechanism) (76)
Histatin	- Tear fluid	- Antimicrobial activity (*via* membrane perturbation) (77, 78) - Anti-inflammatory function (79) - Wound healing property (80, 81)

HNP, human neutrophil peptide/human alpha-defensin; HBD, human beta-defensins.

domain-like receptors (NLRs), and inflammasomes (26). Lysozyme may decrease systemic inflammation by restricting bacterial growth (27). In view of the ubiquitous presence and inherent antimicrobial and immunomodulatory activities of host lysozyme, bacteria have evolved several ingenious resistant mechanisms to survive against lysozyme. These include modification of membrane peptidoglycan, alteration of the membrane charges, and production of protein inhibitors against lysozyme (26). The understanding of the mechanisms of antimicrobial resistance (AMR) related to lysozyme (and potentially other naturally occurring HDPs) is unequivocally pivotal for development of the next generation of synthetic peptide-based therapeutics for tackling AMR.

Lactoferrin

Lactoferrin, belongs to the transferrin family, is an 80 kDa iron-sequestering HDP. It consists of a polypeptide chain that is folded into two highly symmetrical lobes (N- and C-lobes), which are capable of binding a variety of metal ions including ferric and ferrous ions (28). It is found abundantly in milk

and in many other body tissues and secretions, including tears, saliva, sweat, nasal secretion, bronchial mucus, hepatic bile and others (84). Similar to lysozyme, lactoferrin is also primarily synthesized by the acinar cells of the main and accessory lacrimal glands (85). Some evidence has suggested the expression of lactoferrin in meibomian glands (83) and epithelium of conjunctiva and cornea (83, 86). It constitutes around 25% of the total protein in tear fluids, with a concentration of ~2.2 mg/ml (29).

Lactoferrin has been shown to play multi-functional roles in host defense, armed with antimicrobial, anti-biofilm, anti-inflammatory, anti-cancer and anti-complement functions (28, 87). The antimicrobial activity of lactoferrin is attributed to its underlying dual mechanisms of action: (a) binding to free iron, an essential element for microbial growth; and (b) interaction and permeabilization of the anionic bacterial membrane through its positively charged N-terminal, which accounts for its rapid antimicrobial action (28). At the OS, it has been shown to exert broad-spectrum antimicrobial activity against Gram-positive and Gram-negative bacteria, fungi, and viruses (29). It has a strong affinity toward the lipopolysaccharides (LPS) of the Gram-negative bacterial membrane, resulting in increased permeability. Studies have also shown that lysozyme and lactoferrin work in synergy where lactoferrin binds to the lipotechoic acid (LTA) of staphylococcal membrane and enables a greater access of lysozyme to the peptidoglycan (30). Another recent study by Avery et al. (31) showed that lactoferrin exhibits strong antimicrobial and antibiofilm activities against *Acinetobacter baumannii*, which is an important member of the ESKAPE pathogens commonly responsible for multidrug resistance in clinical setting. Interestingly, lactoferrin is ineffective against *Acanthamoeba trophozoites* and this is attributed to the effect of proteases released by *Acanthamoeba* (88).

Lactoferrin has been shown to play an important role in corneal wound closure where it regulates the anti-inflammatory and pro-inflammatory responses (32, 89). Pattamatta et al. (32, 33) demonstrated that lactoferrin stimulates corneal wound healing *via* upregulation of plate-derived growth factor and IL-6, downregulation of IL-1, and reduction of infiltrating inflammatory cells. Lactoferrin also acts as an antioxidant *via* inhibition of iron-dependent formation of hydroxyl radicals, thereby protecting corneal epithelium from oxidation-mediated tissue injury (34). This may have an implication on the pathogenesis of keratoconus (refer to Section Keratoconus). Furthermore, reduced levels of lactoferrin have been associated with systemic mucosal immunity incompetence. Hanstock et al. (90) observed that patients affected by upper respiratory tract infection had a significantly lower concentration of tear lysozyme and/or lactoferrin compared to healthy volunteers, suggesting that lysozyme and lactoferrin may serve as clinically relevant biomarkers for mucosal immune competence.

Defensins

Defensins are a large family of cysteine-rich HDPs that consist of a predominantly triple-stranded beta-sheet core structure stabilized with three pairs of intramolecular disulfide bridges (91). Depending on the pattern of the disulfide linkage, human defensins can be broadly divided into two groups, namely the alpha- and beta-defensins. Alpha-defensins have a cysteine pairing motif of Cys1–Cys6, Cys2–Cys4, and Cys3–Cys5 whereas beta-defensins form disulfide bridges at Cys1–Cys5, Cys2–Cys4, and Cys3–Cys6 (35, 91). Interestingly, this evolutionarily conserved disulphide bridge motif is similarly observed in defensins found in plants and invertebrates (92, 93).

Human alpha-defensins, also known as human neutrophil peptide (HNP) due to their abundant presence in neutrophils, can be subclassified into 6 main subtypes (HNP-1 to–6). HNP-1 to–4 are found primarily in the azurophil granules of neutrophils (35). HNP-1 to–3 sequences are highly homologous with only difference in a single N-terminal residue; removal of the alanine (the first amino acid of HNP-1 at the N-terminal) gives rise to HNP-2 and substitution of the alanine with aspartic acid yields HNP-3. HNP-5 and–6 are primarily located in the epithelium of Paneth cells of small intestines (35). On the other hand, more than 30 types of human beta-defensins (HBDs) have been described in the literature (94). HBD are mainly synthesized by the epithelial cells, including the conjunctiva, cornea, skin, oral mucosa, lining of respiratory and gastrointestinal tracts, and others (95). As described by McIntosh et al. (96), about 28 novel beta defensins were identified in human genome using the hidden Markov model. Thus far, only few, namely the HBD-1 to–4 and HBD-9 were shown to be involved in host immunity at the OS.

In view of the diverse function of defensins, it is not surprising that a plethora of HNPs and HBDs are abundantly present at a variety of bodily surfaces. At the OS, HNP-1 to–3, but not HNP-4 to–6, have been identified in normal human tears, conjunctival and corneal epithelium, lacrimal gland, and inflamed conjunctiva (in relation to infiltrating polymorphonuclear cells) (22, 97, 98). Similarly, McIntosh et al. (96) discovered an array of HBDs, including HBD-1 to–4, at the corneal and conjunctival epithelium, though the level of HBD-4 was relatively low. Another novel HDP, HBD-9, was discovered at the ocular surface epithelia and corneal stroma by our research group (99, 100). Further studies from our group and others have also shown that the expressions of HBDs are modulated by various PRRs, including TLRs and NLRs (99, 101, 102).

Defensins have been shown to exhibit broad-spectrum antimicrobial activity against bacteria, fungi, enveloped viruses, and parasites (35, 41). Similar to most cationic HDPs, the defensins also perturb the microbial membrane through direct interaction with the anionic and lipid microbial membrane. The antimicrobial efficacy of defensins is likely related to their inherent physicochemical characteristics such as cationicity, hydrophobicity, and amphiphilicity (35). It has been shown that cationicity plays a more important role in Gram-negative infections, whereas increased hydrophobicity enhances the antimicrobial action against Gram-positive infections (103, 104). In addition, synergy between different families of HDPs have been reported; for instance, HBD-2 and LL-37 exhibit synergistic antimicrobial killing of *Staphylococcus aureus*, which is likely accountable for the minimal risk of *S. aureus* infection in inflamed psoriatic skin (105).

In addition to the antimicrobial function, defensins are endowed with a wide range of functions, including immunomodulatory (pro-inflammatory and anti-inflammatory), wound healing, maintenance of skin barrier, and anti-cancer (**Figure 3**) (17, 36, 39–41, 43–46, 106). HBD has been shown to orchestrate the cross-talk between innate and adaptive immunity by recruiting T cells and dendritic cells to the infection site through interaction with chemokine (CCR6) receptor (43). HNP-1 regulates inflammation by inhibiting macrophage mRNA translation and secretion of proinflammatory cytokines and nitric oxide, enabling clearance of pathogen and resolution of inflammation with minimal collateral tissue damage (37, 38). Moreover, HBD-3 has been shown to promote wound closure in *S. aureus* infected diabetic wounds (44).

To gain a better understanding of the structure-activity relationship, many research groups have investigated the functional role of the evolutionarily conserved cysteine disulfide bridge moiety of defensins. Although this moiety is widely observed in vertebrate and invertebrate defensins, Wu et al. (42)

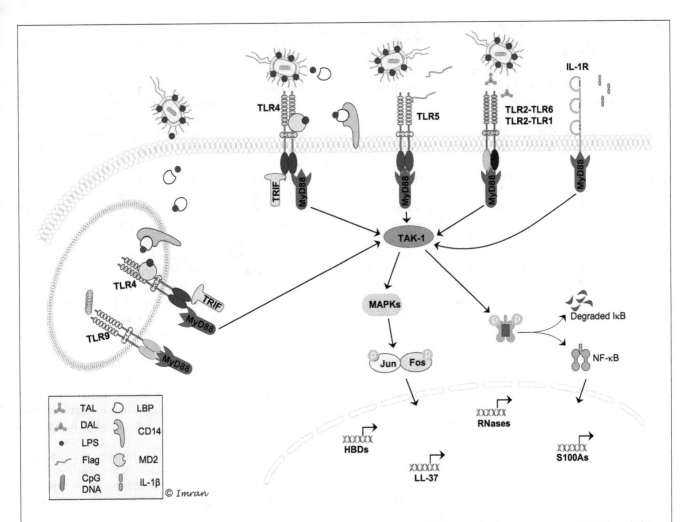

FIGURE 3 | Schematic representation of key signaling mechanisms involved in host defense peptides (HDPs) production in response to bacterial infection. Multiple intracellular signaling pathways are activated downstream of toll-like receptors (TLRs) in response to a variety of pathogen-associated molecular pattern (PAMPs), resulting in production of HDPs and cytokines/chemokines. TLR2/1 and TLR2/6 are shown to recognize diacylated (DAL) and triacylated (TAL) lipopeptides, respectively. TLR4 is present both on cell-surface and intracellularly on endosomes specifically recognizes lipopolysaccharide (LPS). LPS is recognized by LPS binding protein (LBP) and presented to CD14 (present in a soluble form in tear fluid), which transports LPS to myeloid differentiation-2 (MD-2)/TLR4 complex. Flagellin (Flag), a flagellar protein of Gram-negative bacteria, is recognized by TLR5. TLR9 present on endosomes recognizes CpG containing bacterial DNA; however, its role in production of HDPs and associated signaling mechanisms in corneal epithelial cells remain unclear. A pleiotropic cytokine, interleukin-1β (IL-1β) is recognized by IL-1R on cell surface. Activation of toll/IL-1-receptor (TIR) domain of both TLR and IL-1R triggers recruitment of the adaptor molecule myeloid differentiation primary response protein 88 (MyD88). TLR4 signaling can be activated via MyD88 and TIR-domain-containing adaptor protein inducing interferon-β (TRIF). Both MyD88 and TRIF initiate phosphorylation and ubiquitylation of several other molecules (not shown) leading to activation of transforming growth-factor-β activated kinase-1 (TAK1). In the cytosol, TAK-1 triggers activation of mitogen-activated protein kinases (MAPKs) and nuclear-factor-κ-B (NF-κB) pathways. This allows nuclear translocation of NF-κB and activator protein 1 (AP-1; complex of Jun and Fos protein) transcription factors and modulates expression of target HDPs. The scheme was adapted from Mohammed et al. paper (9).

demonstrated that removal of this structure has no influence on their inherent antibacterial activity against *Escherichia coli*. On the other hand, the chemotactic function (e.g., HBD-3) (42), anti-tumor necrosis factor (TNF)-alpha (e.g., HNP-1) (38), and antiviral activity (e.g., HNP-1 to−3) (107) are abolished when this disulfide moiety is destabilized or removed, suggesting that the disulfide bridges play important immunomodulatory and antiviral roles in innate immunity. These observations provide invaluable insight into the design and development of antimicrobial HDPs that are based on cysteine-rich native templates (108).

Cathelicidin

Cathelicidins are a large family of AMPs widely found in vertebrates (93, 109). The hallmark of cathelicidin is the presence of highly conserved cathelin domain, which was first identified in pig leukocytes as a cathepsin-L inhibitor and termed "cathelin" based on this property. Cathelicidin proteins comprised of a conserved 14 kDa cathelin domain flanked by a signal peptide (up to 30 residues) on N-terminus and an antimicrobial peptide region on its C-terminus. hCAP18, an 18 kDa preprotein, is the lone member of cathelicidin found in humans (110, 111). Its derivative, hCAP18(104−140), was shown to neutralize lipopolysaccharide (LPS) activity both *in vitro* and *in vivo* (112). Proteinase-3, a proteolytic enzyme in human neutrophils can cleave hCAP18 into an active 37 amino-acid AMP, known as LL-37 (110, 113, 114). Moreover, another serum protease, gastricsin, at low vaginal pH was shown to cleave hCAP18 into a slightly longer active peptide, termed ALL-38 (115).

Since its first discovery in 1988 (116), cathelicidin is the most studied cationic HDP due to its wide-spectrum of activity, including anti-infective, anti-biofilm, anti-cancer, immunomodulatory, chemotactic, and wound healing properties (47, 53, 54, 57, 104, 117–120). The protective function of LL-37 against OS has been widely established (48, 49, 121, 122). LL-37 is constitutively expressed in OS epithelial specimens from healthy living patients and donor cadaveric tissues, including conjunctival and corneal epithelium (96, 123). It has been shown to play an important role in corneal wound healing and protection against various types of microbes at the OS (48, 123). In addition to its antimicrobial activity, Torres-Juarez et al. (55) demonstrated the immunomodulatory effects of LL-37 during mycobacterial infection, including reduction of tumor necrosis factor (TNF)-alpha and IL-17, and promoting the production of transforming growth factor (TGF-beta) and anti-inflammatory IL-10. Furthermore, LL-37 promotes wound healing *via* keratinocyte migration, which occurs *via* epidermal growth factor receptor transactivation (56).

Biochemical studies have elegantly demonstrated that smaller synthetic fragments derived from the parent LL-37 sequence were as effective as the full-length LL-37 (124–128). Studies have revealed that the middle region of LL-37$_{17-29}$ (i.e., FK13) and/or LL-37$_{18-29}$ (i.e., KR12) is largely responsible for the antimicrobial activity of LL-37 and has the ability to form amphipathic helix rich in positive charge, which enables effective interaction with the anionic membrane and subsequent microbial killing (126, 127, 129). In view of its therapeutic promise, a variety of strategies have been adopted to enhance the safety and efficacy of LL-37 and its derivatives (104, 130). Similar to LL-37, its smaller derivatives have shown considerable activity against a range of pathogens, including ESKAPE bacteria, fungi and viruses (47, 50–52). Our group has recently demonstrated that LL-37$_{17-32}$ (FK16 peptide with free N- and C-termini) could also be utilized to improve the activity of conventional antibiotics such as vancomycin against *Pseudomonas aeruginosa*, as a strategy to repurpose the antibiotics and tackle AMR (131).

Ribonucleases (RNases)

Human ribonucleases (RNases) have an inherent ability to hydrolyze polymeric RNA and share a unique structural similarity to bovine pancreatic RNase A, therefore, also referred to as RNase A superfamily (132, 133). Similar to defensins, members of RNase A superfamily are comprised of six to eight conserved cysteine residues forming disulfide bridges. Genes encoding for human RNases 1 to 13 are clustered on chromosome 14q11.2 (133, 134). RNases are highly cationic and exhibit strong cytotoxic and microbicidal properties. Human RNase-2 (eosinophil derived neurotoxin) and RNase-3 (eosinophil cationic protein) are the first members of RNase A superfamily to show a strong role in host defense against an RNA virus,

respiratory syncytial virus (RSV) (58, 59). Further studies have demonstrated that RNase-2 and−3 also have an ability to activate adaptive immunity (67, 68) and possess potent bactericidal and anti-helminthic properties (60–63). RNase-4 and−5 are shown to display potent angiogenic and neurogenic properties (69, 70). RNase-5, also known as angiogenin, has been widely studied due to its immunomodulatory properties. It is shown to be produced by skin keratinocytes and mast cells and has been detected in lacrimal secretions. RNase-5 has been shown to promote corneal endothelial wound healing *via* activation of PI3-kinase/Akt pathway (71), highlighting its therapeutic potential for corneal endothelial diseases. RNase-6 is ubiquitously expressed in immune cells including neutrophils and monocytes. Similar to RNase-3, it also exhibits bactericidal effect through agglutination and membrane disruption (64). Against *Mycobacterium* spp., it has been shown to induce autophagy in the infected macrophages leading to intracellular growth inhibition (135).

RNase-7 and−8 despite being structurally similar, their expression in different bodily tissues is greatly varied. On the OS, RNase-7 is constitutively expressed in healthy corneal epithelium and stroma (65). Further studies have demonstrated elevated levels of RNase-7 in samples collected from patients with bacterial, viral and Acanthamoeba keratitis as well as in CECs treated with cytokines, live bacteria and different pathogenic proteins that activates innate immune receptor signaling (65, 66). Specifically, the signaling mechanisms that are involved in elevation of RNase-7 levels in CECs in response to activation of interleukin 1β (IL-1β)/IL-1 receptor (IL-1R) axis was mapped by our group (65). Notably, the canonical nuclear factor κB (NFκB) transcription factor which mediates transcription of most HDPs in OS epithelium was found to be non-redundant in regulation of RNase-7. It was shown that IL-1b/IL-1R triggered mitogen activated protein kinases (MAPKs) signaling was responsible for RNase-7 regulation in CECs. Further analysis showed that the transcription factors, c-JUN and ATF, are involved in transcription of RNase-7 in CECs. This suggested that a biomarker or protein that directly activates these transcription factors could elicit HDPs in CECs during infection.

Psoriasin

Psoriasin, or S100A7, represents one of the main members of the S100 family of calcium-binding proteins (136). It is a low molecular weight protein (~11 kDa) which consists of five alpha-helices and the structure relies on the binding of calcium (137). The term "psoriasin" was first coined in 1991 by Madsen et al. (138), who observed the upregulation of this novel HDP in psoriatic skin. Subsequently, its immunomodulatory role in psoriasis was shown to be related to the downstream stimulation of interleukin-1a (IL-1a) expression in human epidermal keratinocytes *via* the receptor for advanced glycation endproducts (RAGE)-p38 MAPK and calpain-1 pathways (139). At the OS, psoriasin was also found to be constitutively present various structures, including the conjunctiva, cornea, lacrimal gland and nasolacrimal ducts (72, 140), highlighting its protective role at the OS.

Psoriasin has been shown to exhibit strong antimicrobial activity against *E. coli* and *S. aureus*, likely *via* a zinc-dependent mechanism (72, 73). The upregulation of psoriasin against *E. coli* was found to be mediated *via* TLR5 (141). Interestingly, studies have shown that the antibacterial efficacy of psoriasin is likely conferred by the central region of the protein (amino acids at 35–80) (73). In addition to its antimicrobial activity, psoriasin has been shown to play essential important immunomodulatory roles, including chemotaxis for CD4$^+$ and neutrophils, production of cytokines and chemokines by neutrophils, generation of reactive oxygen species, and release of HNP-1 to−3 (74, 75).

Dermcidin

Dermcidin (DCD) is an important 110-residue HDP that is constitutively present in the golgi complex and the secretory granules of eccrine sweat. After being proteolytically processed, it is secreted into the sweat and transported onto the epidermal surface of skin as DCD-1L (which constitutes the N-terminal 48 residues of DCD) (76, 142, 143). It has been shown to adopt a unique high-conductance transmembrane hexameric channel architecture comprising trimers of antiparallel helical pairs, which is responsible for its membrane-disruptive antimicrobial mechanism (144).

The presence of DCD was first discovered in 2001 by Schittek et al. (145) and was found to possess broad-spectrum antimicrobial activity that is maintained over a broad pH range and in high salt concentrations, which resembles the human sweat. At the OS, McIntosh et al. (96) observed that dermcidin may be present at the corneal epithelium but this was only detected in one of the nine corneal samples. The presence of dermcidin in tear fluid was further confirmed by You et al. (146). Unlike most HDPs (which are cationic and kill bacteria *via* pore formation), dermcidin is an anionic peptide (147). It exerts its antimicrobial killing through interaction with the anionic bacterial phospholipids with subsequent zinc-dependent formation of oligomeric complexes in the bacterial membrane, resulting in formation of ion channels, membrane depolarization and cell death (76).

Histatin

Histatin belongs to a family of histidine-rich, cationic HDPs that are produced by the salivary gland into the saliva. They were first identified in 1988 by Oppenheim et al. (77) in human parotid secretion. Within the family, histatin-1,−3 and−5 are the major and most widely studied members and have been shown to exhibit antibacterial, antifungal and wound healing properties (77, 78). Histatin-1 and−3 are encoded by HTN1 and HTN3 genes, respectively, and histatin-5 is a proteolytic product of histatin-3 (148).

The first evidence of the presence of histatin at the ocular surface was demonstrated by Kalmodia et al. (149) in 2019. Histatin-1 was found to be present in normal human tears and reduced in aqueous-deficient dry eye disease by around 10-fold, suggesting the potential diagnostic value in evaluating dry eye disease. Based on *in vitro* studies, histatin-1 has been shown to enhance human corneal epithelial wound healing (80). In addition, histatin-1 can significantly reduce lipopolysaccharide-induced inflammatory signaling and production of nitric oxide and inflammatory cytokines *via* the JNK and NF-kB pathways in RAW264.7 macrophages (79). The multi-faceted properties of histatin, including antimicrobial, anti-inflammatory and wound healing properties, are particularly attractive for ocular surface diseases, especially infectious keratitis where inflammation overdrive and persistent epithelial wound are common sequelae of the infection (81, 150, 151).

ROLES OF HDPs IN MAJOR OCULAR SURFACE DISEASES

It is evident that HDPs play important roles in innate immunity and crosstalk between innate and adaptive immunity. In this section, we aim to provide a concise overview of the roles of HDPs in major OS diseases.

Infectious Keratitis

Infectious keratitis (IK) represents a major cause of corneal blindness worldwide (152). It has been estimated to cause 1.5–2 million new cases of monocular blindness every year, highlighting its significant burden on human health, healthcare resources and economy (152–154). Subject to geographical, temporal and seasonal variations, bacteria and fungi are the most common culprits for IK globally (150, 155–161). Broad-spectrum topical antimicrobials are currently the mainstay of treatment for IK but adjuvant therapy such as amniotic membrane transplant, therapeutic corneal cross-linking treatment (i.e., PACK-CXL) and therapeutic keratoplasty are often required to manage refractory cases of IK (162–166).

The pivotal roles of HDPs in IK are supported by a number of *in vitro* and *in vivo* observations and experiments (9). McIntosh et al. (96) investigated differential gene expression of HDPs in non-infected and infected eyes and demonstrated that some HDPs, notably HBD-3 and LL-37, were significantly elevated during OS infection. In addition, HBD-2 and−3, LL-37, MIP-3α, and thymosin β-4 were shown to exhibit moderate to strong *in vitro* antimicrobial activity against a range of ocular pathogens, including *S. aureus*, *P. aeruginosa*, adenovirus and HSV-1 (49, 123). Furthermore, cathelicidin-deficient/knockout mice were found to be more susceptible to *P. aeruginosa* corneal infection when compared to the wild type mice, underlining the antimicrobial function of cathelicidin at the OS (122). Synergistic antimicrobial action among different HDPs has also been reported in several studies (167, 168). For instance, Chen et al. (167) demonstrated that various combinations of HDPs, including HBD-1 to−3, LL-37 and lysozyme, exhibited synergistic or additive antimicrobial effect against *S. aureus* and *E. coli*.

The role of HDPs has also been implicated in other types of IK such as fungal and Acanthamoeba keratitis (9). Our recent study demonstrated that a range of HDPs, including HBD-1,−2,−3 and−9, LL-37 and S100A7, were upregulated during the active phase of fungal keratitis and returned to the baseline level upon resolution of the infection (169). Interestingly, there was a preferential increase in mRNA expression of different types of HDPs, with HBD-1 and−2 being most commonly upregulated (90% of the cases) and LL-37 being least commonly upregulated (35% of the cases), highlighting the pathogen-specificity of HDPs. Similarly in Acanthamoeba keratitis, a wide range of HDPs such as HBD-2 and−3, LL-37, LEAP-1 and−2, and RNase-7 (but not HBD-1), were shown to be upregulated (66). Interestingly, HBD-1 and HBD-9 were significantly downregulated in Acanthamoeba keratitis (66, 170). Taken together, it is evident that HDPs serve as an integral component of the innate immunity of the OS, *via* their broad-spectrum and rapid antimicrobial activity against a wide range of ocular pathogens. These unique characteristics also render HDPs (usually those that are membrane-active) an attractive class of antimicrobial agent for managing IK, particularly in the face of polymicrobial keratitis and emerging antimicrobial resistance (152, 158, 171, 172).

Dry Eye Disease and Sjogren's Syndrome

Dry eye disease (DED) is one of the most common ocular surface morbidities with severe impact on vision and quality of life of affected individuals (173, 174). According to the recent TFOS DEWS II report, DED is defined as "a multifactorial disease of the ocular surface characterized by a loss of homeostasis of the tear film, and accompanied by ocular symptoms, in which tear film instability and hyperosmolarity, ocular surface inflammation and damage, and neurosensory abnormalities play etiological roles" (173). Sjogren's syndrome is a systemic autoimmune disease that primarily affects the lacrimal and salivary exocrine glands, leading to dry eyes and dry mouth (175). It is caused by lymphocytic infiltration of the exocrine glands secondary to the abnormal B- and T-cell autoimmune response against the auto-antigens, particularly SSA and SSB (175).

Several studies have demonstrated the dysregulation of HDPs in the DED. A range of HDPs, particularly lysozyme and/or lactoferrin, have been shown to be reduced in various types of DED, including SS and non-SS-related DED (176), evaporative DED (177), graft versus host disease (GvHD)-related DED (178), and others. Furthermore, HBD-2 and HBD-9 are found to be upregulated and downregulated, respectively, whereas HBD-1 and−3 remain unchanged in DED (100, 179). In addition, tear HDPs may also serve as useful biomarkers in DED. Studies have shown that tear lactoferrin was significantly reduced in various types of DED, including SS-related and non-SS-related DED, Steven–Johnson syndrome and evaporative DED secondary to meibomian gland dysfunction (177, 180). Sonobe et al. (176) recently demonstrated an inverse correlation between reduced lactoferrin concentration in tears and increased severity of DED using a novel and innovative microfluidic paper-based analytical device (μPAD). It has been shown that reduced level of lactoferrin serves as a good biomarker for distinguishing SS-related DED from non-SS-related DED (181), and for diagnosing DED in postmenopausal patients (182). The reduction of these tear HDPs in DED, in addition to the breakdown of corneal epithelium and increased bacterial load associated with DED, may potentially account for the increased risk of IK (though lack of strong evidence) (183, 184).

Keratoconus

Keratoconus is a bilateral, non-inflammatory corneal condition characterized by progressive corneal thinning and protrusion with resultant myopia and irregular astigmatism. It is the most common corneal ectatic disorder with an estimated prevalence of 1:2,000 to 1:400 people (185, 186). Depending on the severity and stability of keratoconus, it can be managed with glasses, soft and rigid contact lens, corneal cross-linking, intrastromal corneal ring segments, and corneal transplantation if all other measures fail (187–189). Although uncommon, keratoconus still remains a leading indication for corneal transplantation in many countries (190, 191).

The pathogenesis of keratoconus is likely to be multifactorial, contributed by genetic predisposition, environmental factors, proteolytic degradation of collagen, and mechanical trauma such as eye rubbing (192). Several molecular and proteomics studies (193–196) have also demonstrated the upregulation of certain tear proteins and inflammatory molecules in keratoconus, including interleukin-6, TNF-alpha, matrix metalloproteinases (MMP)-1,−3,−7,−9, and−13, lipocalin-1, neutrophil-defensin 1 precursor, mammaglobulin-B precursor, and keratin types 1 and 2, suggesting that inflammation plays a role in the pathogenesis of keratoconus. A recent proteomic study by Yam et al. (197) demonstrated that the epithelial and stromal proteins in keratoconic corneas were altered. The proteomic changes were primarily related to developmental and metabolic disorders (particularly in relation to mitochondria), cellular assembly, tissue organization and connective tissue disorders (particularly in relation to endoplasmic reticulum protein folding). Interestingly, the changes were not limited to the "cone area" but also involved the peripheral non-cone region of the keratoconic corneas. In addition, patients with keratoconus were found to have a significantly lower level of tear lactoferrin and the amount of reduction correlated with the severity of keratoconus (198). It is postulated that reduced lactoferrin results in accumulation of free iron in the tear fluids and iron deposition on the cornea ("Fleischer's ring"), thereby increasing cytotoxicity to the corneal epithelial cells (199). Based on these observations, Pastori et al. (199) have demonstrated that the oxidative stress induced by the tears in keratoconic patients, due to increased free iron, may be dampened by lactoferrin-loaded contact lens, potentially deterring the progression of keratoconus.

Pterygium

Pterygium is a common inflammatory ocular surface disease that is commonly encountered in tropical countries, with an estimated prevalence of 12% (200). It is characterized by fibrovascular growth of the conjunctiva into the cornea, resulting in ocular surface discomfort, pain, visual disturbance and impairment (if visual axis is encroached upon) (201). The pathogenesis of pterygium is likely attributed to a number of factors, including chronic ultraviolet radiation, human papillomavirus infection, oxidative stress, and genetic predisposition (202). So far, few groups have examined the role of HDPs in patients with pterygium. Ikeda et al. (98) observed the presence of HBD-2 in one of two conjunctival tissues of pterygium but in none of all eight normal conjunctival samples.

In addition, Zhou et al. (203) reported an upregulated expression of HNP-1 to—3, and calcium-binding proteins S100A8 and S100A9 in the tear fluids of eyes affected with pterygium. Another demonstrated the upregulation of HBD-1 and—2 along with a downregulation of HBD-9 in pterygium (204). These observations may be related to the underlying fibrovascular proliferative changes or inflammation. It was also suggested that the dysregulation of these HDPs may play an important contributory role to the pathogenesis of pterygium and may serve as useful biomarkers for predicting the recurrence of pterygium (203).

Post-ocular Surface Surgery and Wound Healing

The integrity of corneal epithelium is of utmost importance for ocular surface defense. Corneal wound healing relies on the regenerative capability of limbal stem cells and involves a complex process of cell death, migration, proliferation, differentiation, and remodeling of extracellular matrix (205). The integral role of HDPs for ocular surface wound healing has been evidently demonstrated in many studies. Zhou et al. (206) observed that the level of HNP-1 to—3 in tear fluids increased significantly after surgical removal of ocular surface neoplasm and returned to the baseline level after complete healing. Moreover, the concentration of HNP-1 and—2 reached a therapeutic level at day 3 postoperative (206). In addition, upregulation of HBD-2 mRNA expression was observed during the phase of corneal re-epithelialization (207).

Similarly, Huang et al. (48) previously demonstrated that LL-37 was increased in injured corneal epithelial cells (CEC), and recombinant LL-37 was capable of increasing the pro-inflammatory cytokines from CECs through the activation of G-protein coupled receptors (i.e., formyl peptide receptor-like 1). Application of vitamin D on wounded mouse corneas was shown to delay the normal wound healing process and increase the production of cathelin-related antimicrobial peptide (CRAMP) (208). However, the cause-effect relationship between CRAMP and corneal wound healing remains unknown but it was suggested that the increase levels of HDPs during epithelial defect would protect the cornea from infection during the healing phase. Recent studies have demonstrated that a deficiency of vitamin D receptors significantly delays the corneal wound healing and decreases the nerve density (209, 210). These findings suggest that HDPs play a crucial role in wound healing and protection against ocular surface infection.

Atopic Dermatitis and Allergic Keratoconjunctivitis

Atopic dermatitis (AD) is the most common inflammatory skin condition characterized by intense pruritus and chronic, relapsing eczematous lesions (211). The lifetime prevalence has been estimated at 20% (211). The pathogenesis of AD is multifactorial, with loss-of-function of the filaggrin gene (which regulates the epidermal barrier function), overgrowth of S. aureus (which may be caused by the dysregulation of HBD), IgE-mediated sensitization, and neuroinflammation

playing important contributory roles (105, 211). Patients with AD may also suffer concurrently from atopic keratoconjunctivitis (AKC), which is a potentially sight-threatening ocular surface disease. Vernal keratoconjunctivitis (VKC) is another severe form of allergic eye disease that primarily affects the children and young adults (212).

Several studies have implicated the roles of HDPs in AD, AKC and VKC. Both HBD-2 and LL-37 are known to possess good antimicrobial activity against S. aureus and they work in synergy (105). Patients with AD are found to have substantially lower expressions of HBD-2 and—3, LL-37, and dermcidin, which may explain their increased susceptibility to staphylococcal skin infection compared to patients with psoriasis (105, 213). Similarly, patients with AKC are at risk of developing staphylococcal and herpetic infectious keratitis (214), which may be linked to the downregulation of mBD-2 mRNA at the ocular surface based on in vivo murine allergic eye conjunctivitis studies (215). Hida et al. (216) observed significantly higher levels of HNP-1 to—3 in the tears of patients with AKC complicated by allergic corneal epithelial disease compared to healthy patients or AKC patients with no corneal disease, suggesting a potentially protective role of HDP in corneal complications related to allergic eye disease. In addition, tear lactoferrin is reduced in VKC and the underlying mechanism is likely not related to lacrimal gland dysfunction but other factors since the level of tear lysozyme is unaffected (217).

Rosacea

Rosacea is a chronic, relapsing inflammatory skin disease that affects around 5% of the population (218). The risk of ocular surface involvement may develop in up to 70% of the rosacea patients and may occur with or without concurrent facial/skin rosacea (3). It can result in a wide array of ocular symptoms and signs, ranging from grittiness, visual blurring, and pain to sight-threatening complications such as corneal infection and perforation. The pathogenesis of rosacea remains to be fully elucidated; however dysregulation of the innate immunity (e.g., dysfunctional expression of HDPs) has been implicated, in addition to a number of environmental factors, genetic predisposition, and neurovascular dysregulation (219). The level of LL-37 is significantly increased in the skin epidermis in rosacea, which promotes skin inflammation via leukocyte chemotaxis and angiogenesis (220, 221). Gokcinar et al. (24) recently examined the role of HDPs in ocular rosacea and observed that the gene expressions of a wide range of HDPs, including tear HNP-1 to—3 and HBD-2, and conjunctival LL-37, were upregulated. On the other hand, tear lactoferrin was found to be reduced in rosacea (222).

THERAPEUTIC POTENTIALS OF HDPs FOR OCULAR SURFACE DISEASES

Despite their promising potential as effective antimicrobial and immunomodulatory therapies, several issues have impeded the successful translation of HDPs into clinical use. Complex structure-activity relationship, susceptibility to

TABLE 2 | A summary of host defense peptide (HDP)-based molecules that are in the development pipeline for ocular surface diseases.

Molecules (sequence)	Primary sources	Current development stage	Activities
B2088* ([RGRKVVRR]₂KK)	HBD-3 (C-terminal)	Pre-clinical stage	- Good activity against PA (108, 226) - Synergism with gatifloxacin and tobramycin (108)
Esculentin1–21(NH2) (GIFSK LAGKK IKNLL ISGLK G-NH₂)	Esculentin (N-terminal)	Pre-clinical stage	- Good activity against SA and PA (227, 228) - Good anti-biofilm activity against PA (228, 229)
RP444 (FAOOF AOOFO OFAOO FAOFA FAF)	Cecropin and magainins	Pre-clinical stage	- Good activity against Gram-positive and Gram-negative bacteria (230)
Melimine/Mel4 (KNKRK RRRRR RGGRR RR)	Melittin and protamine	Pre-clinical stage + phase 3	- Good activity against Gram-positive and Gram-negative bacteria (231, 232) - Reduces risk of CL-related infection (if CL coated with Mel4) (233)
MEL-4** (GIGAV L*K*VLT TGLPA LISWI *K*RKRQ Q)	Melittin (full-length)	Pre-clinical stage	- Good activity against Gram-positive and Gram-negative bacteria and fungi (234)
CaD23 (KRIVQ RIKDW LRKLC KKW)	Cathelicidin and HBD-2	Pre-clinical stage	- Good activity against SA, MRSA and PA (104) - Strong additive effect when used with levofloxacin or amikacin (235)
Histatin-5 (DSHAK RHHGY KRKFH EKHHS HRGY)	Histatin-5	Pre-clinical stage	- Promote corneal wound healing (81)

HBD, human beta-defensin; SA, Staphylococcus aureus; MRSA, methicillin-resistant S. aureus; PA, Pseudomonas aeruginosa; CL, contact lens.
*This is a branched peptide. The duplicating residues are in bracket.
**The italicized "K" residue refers to epsilon-lysylated lysine residue. This MEL-4 molecule is different from the other Mel4 molecule.

host/bacterial proteases and physiological conditions, pro-inflammatory properties, discrepancy between *in vitro* and *in vivo* efficacies, and toxicity to the host tissues are the main barriers (14, 23, 223, 224)Furthermore the lack of interest and investment from the pharmaceutical companies, stemming from limited life-span of antimicrobial therapy and low profits, poses another significant hurdle for the development of new antimicrobial agents (225). Herein, we present some of the key HDP-based molecules that have completed *in vivo* animal studies and are in the developmental pipeline for treating ocular surface diseases. These include B2088 branched peptide, Esculentin1–21(NH2), RP444, melimine/Mel4 antimicrobial coating for contact lens, epsilon-lysylated melittin (MEL-4), CaD23, histatin-5, and endogenous LL-37 (**Table 2**).

B2088 Branched Peptide

B2088 is a covalent dimeric peptide that is derived from the C-terminal of HBD-3 [peptide sequence: (RGRKVVRR)₂KK] (226). The development of this branched peptide was started in 2007 where Liu et al. (236) demonstrated that the linear form of HBD3 maintained similar antimicrobial efficacy and exhibited lower cytotoxicity and haemolytic activity compared to the native form of HBD3, after refining the hydrophobicity and substituting the cysteine residues with various amino acids. Such properties were postulated to be related to the removal of the disulfide bridges and the loss of secondary structure. Bai et al. (237) further enhanced the antimicrobial activity and reduced the host toxicity of linear HBD3 analogs by shortening the HBD3 to 10 amino acids from the C-terminal end. Taking it further, the antimicrobial efficacy of the truncated HBD3 was further optimized *via* dimerization at the lysine, which yielded the final lead compound of B2088 (108, 226).

B2088 has been shown to demonstrate strong antimicrobial activity against Gram-negative bacteria, particularly *P. aeruginosa* (108, 226). It exerts its bacterial killing through the binding of lipid A and disruption of supramolecular organization of lipopolysaccharides, a major component of the outer membrane of Gram-negative bacteria. In addition, B2088 strong synergism with various antibiotics through time-kill and checkerboard assays. This was further validated in an *in vivo* murine *P. aeruginosa* keratitis study where B2088 0.05%-gatifloxacin 0.15% combination treatment reduced the bacterial burden of corneal infection by an additional 1 LogCFU compared to gatifloxacin 0.3% alone (108).

Esculentin-1a(1–21)NH₂

The skin of amphibians contains a rich source of HDPs (238). Esculentin-1a is a type of frog-derived HDP isolated from the skin of *Rana esculenta*, or now known as *Pelophylax lessonae/ridibundus*. The modified version, Esculentin-1a(1–21)NH₂, is composed of the first 20 amino acids of esculentin-1a with a glycinamide residue at the C-terminal end (peptide sequence: GIFSKLAGKKIKNLLISGLKG-NH₂) (227). It has been shown to demonstrate strong *in vitro* antimicrobial activity against various *P. aeruginosa* laboratory strains (both invasive and cytotoxic strains) and clinical strains (isolated from eyes with keratitis and conjunctivitis), and *Staphylococci species* (with a MIC range of 1–16 μM) (227). In an *in vivo* murine bacterial IK model infected with cytotoxic *P. aeruginosa* strain, topical treatment of esculentin-1a(1–21)NH₂ significantly reduces the bacterial load, clinical severity and recruitment of inflammatory cells to the infected corneas measured by the relative myeloperoxidase activity (227). In addition, it was shown to exhibit anti-biofilm activity against *P. aeruginosa* (228, 229) and prolong the survival of PAO1-infected mice in both sepsis and pneumonia models (228). The potent activity against both planktonic and sessile forms of *P. aeruginosa* was ascribed to its underlying membrane perturbation activity (228).

RP444

The development of RP444 was inspired by the "freedom from infection" observed in Cecropia moth and African clawed frog, which is attributed to the cecropins and magainins peptides, respectively (113). RP444 is a 23-amino acid designed HDP primarily composed of phenylalanine, alanine and ornithine, which is an unnatural amino acid used to replace lysine residue to enhance antimicrobial activity and proteolytic stability (peptide sequence: FAOOFAOOFOOFAOOFAOFAFAF) (230). This designed HDP possesses a broad-spectrum antimicrobial activity against a range of Gram-positive and Gram-negative bacteria (MIC ranges between 4 and 64 μg/ml) and anti-biofilm efficacy. Similar to other natural and synthetic HDPs, RP444 exhibits rapid bacterial killing within 30–60 min with no risk of developing resistance. Further *in vivo* murine bacterial keratitis study showed that RP444 was able to significantly reduce the bacterial load and clinical severity of *P. aeruginosa* keratitis and reduce inflammatory cell infiltration toward the infected site (230).

Melimine and Mel4 Antimicrobial Coating for Contact Lenses

Melimine is a 29-amino acid cationic synthetic HDP derived from melittin (from honeybee venom) and protamine (from salmon sperm) (239). This hybrid HDP combines the C-terminals of both melittin and protamine, yielding a total cationic charge of +14 (peptide sequence: TLISWIKNKRKQRPRVSRRRRRRGGRRRR). When attached to contact lenses, either through adsorption or covalent binding, melimine demonstrates higher antimicrobial activities against both Gram-positive and Gram-negative bacteria than melittin or protamine alone (239). In addition, the hemolytic activity of melimine is significantly lower than melittin. Furthermore, *in vivo* rabbit models successfully showed that melimine-coated lenses were safe to wear and they prevented bacterial growth on contact lenses, which consequently reduced the rate and severity of adverse reactions such as contact lens-induced acute red eye (CLARE), contact lens-induced peripheral ulcers (CLPUs) and IK (240–242). This suggests that hybridization of two different HDPs serves as a novel strategy to enhance antimicrobial efficacy and reduce toxicity.

However, when the melimine-coated contact lenses were tested in a human clinical trial, these lenses were paradoxically associated with significantly higher corneal staining compared to uncoated lenses at day 1 (241). To overcome this unforeseen corneal toxicity, the same research group has further refined the hybrid HDP, which has led to the creation of Mel4 – a truncated version of melimine with +14 net charge (peptide sequence: KNKRKRRRRRRGGRRRR) (231). This modified HDP exhibits modest antimicrobial activity against a broad range of Gram-positive and Gram-negative bacteria, with good *in vivo* safety

demonstrated in rabbit and human trials (231). The mechanism of action of Mel4 against *P. aeruginosa* was found to be related to the neutralization of lipopolysaccharide and disruption of cytoplasmic membrane whereas its action against *S. aureus* was likely attributed to the release of autolysins with resultant cell death instead of pore formation (232, 243). A recent randomized controlled trial demonstrated that Mel4-coated antimicrobial contact lens was able to reduce corneal infiltrative events by at least 50% when compared to uncoated control lens during extended wear over 3 months (233).

Epsilon Lysylated Melittin (MEL-4)

Being as one of the main basic and cationic amino acids, lysine serves as a major constituent of many naturally occurring and synthetic HDPs (244, 245). In addition to the L- and D-form, lysine can also exist in epsilon form (ε-) where the NH_2 group at the side chain of L-lysine is linked to the alpha-carbon. ε-Poly-L-lysine (EPL) is a basic polyamide consisting of 25–30 ε-lysine that is naturally produced by *Streptomycetaceae* and *Ergot* fungi (246). It is commonly used as a food preservative with strong antimicrobial activity (247, 248). Compared to alpha-poly-L-lysine, EPL exhibits enhanced antimicrobial efficacy against a range of Gram-positive and Gram-negative bacteria (248, 249). Employing the similar strategy, Mayandi et al. (234) explored the selective incorporation of ε-lysine in melittin, which is a potent yet toxic HDP that is found in honeybee venom. They showed that ε-lysylation of melittin, in particular MEL-4 (different from the Mel4 described in the above Pterygium Section), improved the cell selectivity of the synthetic HDP toward a range of Gram-positive and Gram-negative bacteria with reduced host cytotoxic and hemolytic activities, whilst maintaining the *in vivo* efficacy of melittin (234). This suggests that ε-lysylation may serve as a novel strategy for improving the cell selectivity in lysine-rich HDPs.

Hybridized LL-37 and HBD-2 (CaD23)

LL-37 and HBDs are major groups of HDP that have been shown to play vital roles in various ocular surface diseases, particularly infectious keratitis. Inspired by these observations, our group recently developed a novel molecule, CaD23, *via* rationale hybridization of LL-37 and HBD-2 (peptide sequence: KRIVQRIKDWLRKLCKKW), and demonstrated good antimicrobial activity against a range of organisms commonly responsible for infectious keratitis, including *S. aureus*, MRSA and *P. aeruginosa* (104). The therapeutic potential of CaD23 was further substantiated by the strong *in vivo* antimicrobial activity against *S. aureus* in a pre-clinical murine model with good safety profile.

In addition, CaD23 demonstrates eight times faster antimicrobial action when compared to amikacin, a commonly used antibiotics for infectious keratitis (104). CaD23 also demonstrates a strong additive effect when used in combination with amikacin and levofloxacin against *S. aureus* and MRSA, underscoring the translational potential of peptide-antibiotic combined therapy in clinic (235). More importantly, when *S. aureus* was exposed to 10 consecutive sub-lethal concentration of treatment, the bacteria did not develop any antimicrobial resistance against CaD23 whereas it developed significant antimicrobial resistance against amikacin by 32-fold (104). The rapid antimicrobial action (thence low risk of AMR) is likely attributed to its membrane-permeabilizing properties, evidenced by a combination of experimental and computational studies. Moreover, the molecular dynamics (MD) simulations study revealed the importance of alpha-helicity, cationicity, hydrophobicity and amphiphilicity in contributing to the antimicrobial action of CaD23 (235).

Histatin-5

Histatin peptides have been shown to demonstrate antimicrobial activity and wound healing properties. Based on a combination of *in vitro* and *in vivo* murine studies, Shah et al. (81) demonstrated that histatin-5 was able to promote corneal wound healing, and the effect pro-migratory effect was extracellular signal-regulated kinase 1/2 (ERK1/2) dependent. The authors were also able to determine that the C-terminal of histatin-5 (i.e., SHRGY) was the critical functional domain responsible for the wound healing property. These findings highlighting the potential of histatin-5 and/or the SHRGY pentapeptide for further development into clinical therapeutics for ocular surface diseases such as neurotrophic keratopathy or persistent corneal epithelial defect following infection or injury.

Endogenous LL-37 for Atopic Dermatitis

Understanding of the dysregulated expression of HDPs provides a unique opportunity to explore new therapeutic avenue in managing atopic dermatitis and potentially allergic eye diseases. As mentioned, a number of HDPs, including defensins and LL-37, are downregulated in the AD skin lesions (250). It has also been shown that the expression of LL-37 at the skin can be induced by the active 1,25 dihydroxy-vitamin D, which is regulated by the TLR-2 in keratinocytes and monocytes (251). In addition, the severity of AD is inversely proportionate to the level of LL-37 (252). Leveraging on these observations, several research groups have investigated and demonstrated that administration of oral vitamin D may improve the clinical severity of AD (253, 254), accompanied by an increased level of LL-37 (252). Similar strategy can potentially be employed for treating OS diseases, including allergic eye disease.

FUTURE DIRECTIONS

Currently there are a few clinical trials underway investigating the potential translation of HDPs from bench to clinics. Learning from the previous experience of other trials, particularly those that had reached but failed phase 3 trials (255, 256), it is important to select clinical areas and diseases that are likely to benefit from HDP treatment; for instance, comparing the efficacy between HDPs and antibiotic treatment for diseases

caused by multi-drug resistant infection instead of routine and mild infection (which can be simply managed by current antibiotic treatment) is more likely to yield significant and clinically relevant results (130). In addition, based on the synergistic effect and benefit of reducing dose-related toxicity and AMR, researchers are exploring the use of HDP as adjuvant therapy in addition to antibiotic instead of monotherapy (108, 235). Furthermore, the increasingly recognized multi-faceted biological functions of HDPs, including anti-biofilm, immunomodulatory, wound healing, and anti-cancer properties, have yet to be fully capitalized in the clinic. For instance, HDPs such as defensins and lactoferricin have been shown to exert strong anti-cancer activity against various types of cancer, including colorectal, bladder, neuroblastoma, melanoma, and cutaneous squamous cell carcinoma (257). Nonetheless, the effect of HDP on OS neoplasia (e.g., squamous cell papilloma / carcinoma) has never been investigated or reported, highlighting a potential area for future research.

As there is no one set rule or principle to predict the efficacy and toxicity of designed HDPs, the infinite chemical space renders the design of HDPs a formidable task (7). With the rapid advancement in bioinformatics study (including molecular dynamic simulation), artificial intelligence and drug delivery technologies, efficient design and development of more effective HDPs are more likely to be achieved (130, 258). Integrating synthetic HDPs with novel delivery systems (e.g., nanoparticles, liposomes) may serve as a useful strategy to enhance the proteolytic stability and reduce toxicity of HDPs in the future (130, 259). Stimulation of the production of endogenous HDP using FDA-approved drugs or supplements, for instance using 4-phenylbutyrate and/or vitamin D to increase the level of LL-37, may also serve as a useful strategy in exploiting the benefits of HDP (251, 260, 261). Such an approach helps overcome the significant hurdles encountered during the bench-to-bedside translational process, including the regulatory barriers, for synthetic HDP-based molecules. In addition, the advancement in proteomics and whole genome sequencing technologies could facilitate the mining of previously unknown and undetected natural gene-encoded HDP sequences (262, 263), which can be utilized for therapeutic use in the future.

AUTHOR CONTRIBUTIONS

Study design and conceptualization: DT. Literature review, data collection, and manuscript drafting: DT and IM. Data interpretation: DT, IM, RL, RB, and HD. Critical revision of manuscript: RL, RB, and HD. Approval of the final version of manuscript. All authors contributed to the article and approved the submitted version.

REFERENCES

1. Gipson IK. The ocular surface: the challenge to enable and protect vision: the Friedenwald lecture. *Invest Ophthalmol Vis Sci.* (2007) 48:4390; 1–8. doi: 10.1167/iovs.07-0770

2. Ueta M, Kinoshita S. Innate immunity of the ocular surface. *Brain Res Bull.* (2010) 81:219–28. doi: 10.1016/j.brainresbull.2009.10.001

3. Wladis EJ, Adam AP. Treatment of ocular rosacea. *Surv Ophthalmol.* (2018) 63:340–6. doi: 10.1016/j.survophthal.2017.07.005

4. Guglielmetti S, Dart JK, Calder V. Atopic keratoconjunctivitis and atopic dermatitis. *Curr Opin Allergy Clin Immunol.* (2010) 10:478–85. doi: 10.1097/ACI.0b013e32833e16e4

5. Ting DSJ, Bandyopadhyay J, Patel T. Microbial keratitis complicated by acute hydrops following corneal collagen cross-linking for keratoconus. *Clin Exp Optom.* (2019) 102:434–6. doi: 10.1111/cxo.12856

6. Hancock RE, Lehrer R. Cationic peptides: a new source of antibiotics. *Trends Biotechnol.* (1998) 16:82–8. doi: 10.1016/S0167-7799(97)01156-6

7. Haney EF, Straus SK, Hancock REW. Reassessing the host defense peptide landscape. *Front Chem.* (2019) 7:43. doi: 10.3389/fchem.2019.00043

8. Mansour SC, Pena OM, Hancock RE. Host defense peptides: front-line immunomodulators. *Trends Immunol.* (2014) 35:443–50. doi: 10.1016/j.it.2014.07.004

9. Mohammed I, Said DG, Dua HS. Human antimicrobial peptides in ocular surface defense. *Prog Retin Eye Res.* (2017) 61:1–22. doi: 10.1016/j.preteyeres.2017.03.004

10. Zhao X, Wu H, Lu H, Li G, Huang Q, LAMP. A database linking antimicrobial peptides. *PLoS ONE.* (2013) 8:e66557. doi: 10.1371/journal.pone.0066557

11. Wang G, Li X, Wang Z. APD3: the antimicrobial peptide database as a tool for research and education. *Nucleic Acids Res.* (2016) 44:D1087–93. doi: 10.1093/nar/gkv1278

12. Mookherjee N, Anderson MA, Haagsman HP, Davidson DJ. Antimicrobial host defence peptides: functions and clinical potential. *Nat Rev Drug Discov.* (2020) 19:311–32. doi: 10.1038/s41573-019-0058-8

13. Huan Y, Kong Q, Mou H, Yi H. Antimicrobial peptides: classification, design, application and research progress in multiple fields. *Front Microbiol.* (2020) 11:582779. doi: 10.3389/fmicb.2020.582779

14. Li J, Koh JJ, Liu S, Lakshminarayanan R, Verma CS, Beuerman RW. Membrane active antimicrobial peptides: translating mechanistic insights to design. *Front Neurosci.* (2017) 11:73. doi: 10.3389/fnins.2017.00073

15. Bechinger B. Insights into the mechanisms of action of host defence peptides from biophysical and structural investigations. *J Pept Sci.* (2011) 17:306–14. doi: 10.1002/psc.1343

16. Steinstraesser L, Koehler T, Jacobsen F, Daigeler A, Goertz O, Langer S, et al. Host defense peptides in wound healing. *Mol Med.* (2008) 14:528–37. doi: 10.2119/2008-00002.Steinstraesser

17. Hancock RE, Haney EF, Gill EE. The immunology of host defence peptides: beyond antimicrobial activity. *Nat Rev Immunol.* (2016) 16:321–34. doi: 10.1038/nri.2016.29

18. Pletzer D, Coleman SR, Hancock RE. Anti-biofilm peptides as a new weapon in antimicrobial warfare. *Curr Opin Microbiol.* (2016) 33:35–40. doi: 10.1016/j.mib.2016.05.016

19. Riedl S, Zweytick D, Lohner K. Membrane-active host defense peptides–challenges and perspectives for the development of novel anticancer drugs. *Chem Phys Lipids.* (2011) 164:766–81. doi: 10.1016/j.chemphyslip.2011.09.004

20. Fleming A. On a remarkable bacteriolytic element found in tissues and secretions. *Proc R Soc B.* (1922) 93:306–17. doi: 10.1098/rspb.1922.0023

21. Wang G. Human antimicrobial peptides and proteins. *Pharmaceuticals.* (2014) 7:545–94. doi: 10.3390/ph7050545

22. Haynes RJ, Tighe PJ, Dua HS. Innate defence of the eye by antimicrobial defensin peptides. *Lancet.* (1998) 352:451–2. doi: 10.1016/S0140-6736(05)79185-6

23. Kolar SS, McDermott AM. Role of host-defence peptides in eye diseases. *Cell Mol Life Sci.* (2011) 68:2201–13. doi: 10.1007/s00018-011-0713-7

24. Gokcinar NB, Karabulut AA, Onaran Z, Yumusak E, Budak Yildiran FA. Elevated tear human neutrophil peptides 1-3, human beta defensin-2 levels

and conjunctival cathelicidin LL-37 Gene expression in ocular rosacea. *Ocul Immunol Inflamm.* (2019) 27:1174–83. doi: 10.1080/09273948.2018.1504971

25. Willcox MD, Chen R, Kalaiselvan P, Yasir M, Rasul R, Kumar N, et al. The development of an antimicrobial contact lens - from the laboratory to the clinic. *Curr Protein Pept Sci.* (2020) 21:357–68. doi: 10.2174/1389203720666190820152508

26. Ragland SA, Criss AK. From bacterial killing to immune modulation: recent insights into the functions of lysozyme. *PLoS Pathog.* (2017) 13:e1006512. doi: 10.1371/journal.ppat.1006512

27. Ganz T, Gabayan V, Liao HI, Liu L, Oren A, Graf T, et al. Increased inflammation in lysozyme M-deficient mice in response to *Micrococcus luteus* and its peptidoglycan. *Blood.* (2003) 101:2388–92. doi: 10.1182/blood-2002-07-2319

28. Garcia-Montoya IA, Cendon TS, Arevalo-Gallegos S, Rascon-Cruz Q. Lactoferrin a multiple bioactive protein: an overview. *Biochim Biophys Acta.* (2012) 1820:226–36. doi: 10.1016/j.bbagen.2011.06.018

29. Flanagan JL, Willcox MD. Role of lactoferrin in the tear film. *Biochimie.* (2009) 91:35–43. doi: 10.1016/j.biochi.2008.07.007

30. Leitch EC, Willcox MD. Elucidation of the antistaphylococcal action of lactoferrin and lysozyme. *J Med Microbiol.* (1999) 48:867–71. doi: 10.1099/00222615-48-9-867

31. Avery TM, Boone RL, Lu J, Spicer SK, Guevara MA, Moore RE, et al. Analysis of antimicrobial and antibiofilm activity of human milk lactoferrin compared to bovine lactoferrin against multidrug resistant and susceptible *Acinetobacter baumannii* clinical isolates. *ACS Infect Dis.* (2021) 7:2116–26. doi: 10.1021/acsinfecdis.1c00087

32. Pattamatta U, Willcox M, Stapleton F, Cole N, Garrett Q. Bovine lactoferrin stimulates human corneal epithelial alkali wound healing *in vitro. Invest Ophthalmol Vis Sci.* (2009) 50:1636–43. doi: 10.1167/iovs.08-1882

33. Pattamatta U, Willcox M, Stapleton F, Garrett Q. Bovine lactoferrin promotes corneal wound healing and suppresses IL-1 expression in alkali wounded mouse cornea. *Curr Eye Res.* (2013) 38:1110–7. doi: 10.3109/02713683.2013.811259

34. Kijlstra A. The role of lactoferrin in the nonspecific immune response on the ocular surface. *Reg Immunol.* (1990) 3:193–7.

35. Lehrer RI, Lu W. Alpha-Defensins in human innate immunity. *Immunol Rev.* (2012) 245:84–112. doi: 10.1111/j.1600-065X.2011.01082.x

36. Grigat J, Soruri A, Forssmann U, Riggert J, Zwirner J. Chemoattraction of macrophages, T lymphocytes, and mast cells is evolutionarily conserved within the human alpha-defensin family. *J Immunol.* (2007) 179:3958–65. doi: 10.4049/jimmunol.179.6.3958

37. Brook M, Tomlinson GH, Miles K, Smith RW, Rossi AG, Hiemstra PS, et al. Neutrophil-derived alpha defensins control inflammation by inhibiting macrophage mRNA translation. *Proc Natl Acad Sci USA.* (2016) 113:4350–5. doi: 10.1073/pnas.1601831113

38. Miles K, Clarke DJ, Lu W, Sibinska Z, Beaumont PE, Davidson DJ, et al. Dying and necrotic neutrophils are anti-inflammatory secondary to the release of alpha-defensins. *J Immunol.* (2009) 183:2122–32. doi: 10.4049/jimmunol.0804187

39. Gaspar D, Freire JM, Pacheco TR, Barata JT, Castanho MA. Apoptotic human neutrophil peptide-1 anti-tumor activity revealed by cellular biomechanics. *Biochim Biophys Acta.* (2015) 1853:308–16. doi: 10.1016/j.bbamcr.2014.11.006

40. Ferdowsi S, Pourfathollah AA, Amiri F, Rafiee MH, Aghaei A. Evaluation of anticancer activity of α-defensins purified from neutrophils trapped in leukoreduction filters. *Life Sci.* (2019) 224:249–54. doi: 10.1016/j.lfs.2019.03.072

41. Semple F, Dorin JR. beta-Defensins: multifunctional modulators of infection, inflammation and more? *J Innate Immun.* (2012) 4:337–48. doi: 10.1159/000336619

42. Wu Z, Hoover DM, Yang D, Boulegue C, Santamaria F, Oppenheim JJ, et al. Engineering disulfide bridges to dissect antimicrobial and chemotactic activities of human beta-defensin 3. *Proc Natl Acad Sci USA.* (2003) 100:8880–5. doi: 10.1073/pnas.1533186100

43. Yang D, Chertov O, Bykovskaia SN, Chen Q, Buffo MJ, Shogan J, et al. Beta-defensins: linking innate and adaptive immunity through dendritic and T cell CCR6. *Science.* (1999) 286:525–8. doi: 10.1126/science.286.5439.525

44. Hirsch T, Spielmann M, Zuhaili B, Fossum M, Metzig M, Koehler T, et al. Human beta-defensin-3 promotes wound healing in infected diabetic wounds. *J Gene Med.* (2009) 11:220–8. doi: 10.1002/jgm.1287

45. Hanaoka Y, Yamaguchi Y, Yamamoto H, Ishii M, Nagase T, Kurihara H, et al. *In vitro* and *in vivo* anticancer activity of human β-defensin-3 and its mouse homolog. *Anticancer Res.* (2016) 36:5999–6004. doi: 10.21873/anticanres.11188

46. Ghosh SK, McCormick TS, Weinberg A. Human beta defensins and cancer: contradictions and common ground. *Front Oncol.* (2019) 9:341. doi: 10.3389/fonc.2019.00341

47. Luo Y, McLean DT, Linden GJ, McAuley DF, McMullan R, Lundy FT. The naturally occurring host defense peptide, LL-37, and its truncated mimetics KE-18 and KR-12 have selected biocidal and antibiofilm activities against *Candida albicans, Staphylococcus aureus,* and *Escherichia coli in vitro. Front Microbiol.* (2017) 8:544. doi: 10.3389/fmicb.2017.00544

48. Huang LC, Petkova TD, Reins RY, Proske RJ, McDermott AM. Multifunctional roles of human cathelicidin (LL-37) at the ocular surface. *Invest Ophthalmol Vis Sci.* (2006) 47:2369–80. doi: 10.1167/iovs.05-1649

49. Huang LC, Jean D, Proske RJ, Reins RY, McDermott AM. Ocular surface expression and *in vitro* activity of antimicrobial peptides. *Curr Eye Res.* (2007) 32:595–609. doi: 10.1080/02713680701446653

50. Yu Y, Cooper CL, Wang G, Morwitzer MJ, Kota K, Tran JP, et al. Engineered human cathelicidin antimicrobial peptides inhibit ebola virus infection. *iScience.* (2020) 23:100999. doi: 10.1016/j.isci.2020.100999

51. Narayana JL, Mishra B, Lushnikova T, Golla RM, Wang G. Modulation of antimicrobial potency of human cathelicidin peptides against the ESKAPE pathogens and *in vivo* efficacy in a murine catheter-associated biofilm model. *Biochim Biophys Acta Biomembr.* (2019) 1861:1592–602. doi: 10.1016/j.bbamem.2019.07.012

52. He M, Zhang H, Li Y, Wang G, Tang B, Zhao J, et al. Cathelicidin-derived antimicrobial peptides inhibit zika virus through direct inactivation and interferon pathway. *Front Immunol.* (2018) 9:722. doi: 10.3389/fimmu.2018.00722

53. Kanthawong S, Bolscher JG, Veerman EC, van Marle J, de Soet HJ, Nazmi K, et al. Antimicrobial and antibiofilm activity of LL-37 and its truncated variants against *Burkholderia pseudomallei. Int J Antimicrob Agents.* (2012) 39:39–44. doi: 10.1016/j.ijantimicag.2011.09.010

54. Chen X, Takai T, Xie Y, Niyonsaba F, Okumura K, Ogawa H. Human antimicrobial peptide LL-37 modulates proinflammatory responses induced by cytokine milieus and double-stranded RNA in human keratinocytes. *Biochem Biophys Res Commun.* (2013) 433:532–7. doi: 10.1016/j.bbrc.2013.03.024

55. Torres-Juarez F, Cardenas-Vargas A, Montoya-Rosales A, González-Curiel I, Garcia-Hernandez MH, Enciso-Moreno JA, et al. LL-37 immunomodulatory activity during Mycobacterium tuberculosis infection in macrophages. *Infect Immun.* (2015) 83:4495–503. doi: 10.1128/IAI.00936-15

56. Tokumaru S, Sayama K, Shirakata Y, Komatsuzawa H, Ouhara K, Hanakawa Y, et al. Induction of keratinocyte migration *via* transactivation of the epidermal growth factor receptor by the antimicrobial peptide LL-37. *J Immunol.* (2005) 175:4662–8. doi: 10.4049/jimmunol.175.7.4662

57. Wu WK, Sung JJ, To KF Yu L, Li HT Li ZJ, et al. The host defense peptide LL-37 activates the tumor-suppressing bone morphogenetic protein signaling *via* inhibition of proteasome in gastric cancer cells. *J Cell Physiol.* (2010) 223:178–86. doi: 10.1002/jcp.22026

58. Domachowske JB, Dyer KD, Bonville CA, Rosenberg HF. Recombinant human eosinophil-derived neurotoxin/RNase 2 functions as an effective antiviral agent against respiratory syncytial virus. *J Infect Dis.* (1998) 177:1458–64. doi: 10.1086/515322

59. Domachowske JB, Dyer KD, Adams AG, Leto TL, Rosenberg HF. Eosinophil cationic protein/RNase 3 is another RNase A-family ribonuclease with direct antiviral activity. *Nucleic Acids Res.* (1998) 26:3358–63. doi: 10.1093/nar/26.14.3358

60. Lehrer RI, Szklarek D, Barton A, Ganz T, Hamann KJ, Gleich GJ. Antibacterial properties of eosinophil major basic protein and eosinophil cationic protein. *J Immunol.* (1989) 142:4428–34.

61. Ackerman SJ, Loegering DA, Venge P, Olsson I, Harley JB, Fauci AS, et al. Distinctive cationic proteins of the human eosinophil granule: major basic protein, eosinophil cationic protein, and eosinophil-derived neurotoxin. *J Immunol.* (1983) 131:2977–82.

62. Ackerman SJ, Gleich GJ, Loegering DA, Richardson BA, Butterworth AE. Comparative toxicity of purified human eosinophil granule cationic proteins for schistosomula of Schistosoma mansoni. *Am J Trop Med Hyg.* (1985) 34:735–45. doi: 10.4269/ajtmh.1985.34.735

63. Molina HA, Kierszenbaum F, Hamann KJ, Gleich GJ. Toxic effects produced or mediated by human eosinophil granule components on *Trypanosoma cruzi. Am J Trop Med Hyg.* (1988) 38:327–34. doi: 10.4269/ajtmh.1988.38.327

64. Lu L, Li J, Moussaoui M, Boix E. Immune modulation by human secreted RNases at the extracellular space. *Front Immunol.* (2018) 9:1012. doi: 10.3389/fimmu.2018.01012

65. Mohammed I, Yeung A, Abedin A, Hopkinson A, Dua HS. Signalling pathways involved in ribonuclease-7 expression. *Cell Mol Life Sci.* (2011) 68:1941–52. doi: 10.1007/s00018-010-0540-2

66. Otri AM, Mohammed I, Abedin A, Cao Z, Hopkinson A, Panjwani N, et al. Antimicrobial peptides expression by ocular surface cells in response to *Acanthamoeba castellanii:* an *in vitro* study. *Br J Ophthalmol.* (2010) 94:1523–7. doi: 10.1136/bjo.2009.178236

67. Yang D, Chen Q, Rosenberg HF, Rybak SM, Newton DL, Wang ZY, et al. Human ribonuclease A superfamily members, eosinophil-derived neurotoxin and pancreatic ribonuclease, induce dendritic cell maturation and activation. *J Immunol.* (2004) 173:6134–42. doi: 10.4049/jimmunol.173.10.6134

68. Yang D, Rosenberg HF, Chen Q, Dyer KD, Kurosaka K, Oppenheim JJ. Eosinophil-derived neurotoxin (EDN), an antimicrobial protein with chemotactic activities for dendritic cells. *Blood.* (2003) 102:3396–403. doi: 10.1182/blood-2003-01-0151

69. Li S, Sheng J, Hu JK Yu W, Kishikawa H, Hu MG, et al. Ribonuclease 4 protects neuron degeneration by promoting angiogenesis, neurogenesis, and neuronal survival under stress. *Angiogenesis.* (2013) 16:387–404. doi: 10.1007/s10456-012-9322-9

70. Ferguson R, Subramanian V. The cellular uptake of angiogenin, an angiogenic and neurotrophic factor is through multiple pathways and largely dynamin independent. *PLoS ONE.* (2018) 13:e0193302. doi: 10.1371/journal.pone.0193302

71. Kim KW, Park SH, Lee SJ, Kim JC. Ribonuclease 5 facilitates corneal endothelial wound healing *via* activation of PI3-kinase/Akt pathway. *Sci Rep.* (2016) 6:31162. doi: 10.1038/srep31162

72. Gläser R, Harder J, Lange H, Bartels J, Christophers E, Schröder JM. Antimicrobial psoriasin (S100A7) protects human skin from *Escherichia coli* infection. *Nat Immunol.* (2005) 6:57–64. doi: 10.1038/ni1142

73. Lee KC, Eckert RL. S100A7 (Psoriasin)–mechanism of antibacterial action in wounds. *J Invest Dermatol.* (2007) 127:945–57. doi: 10.1038/sj.jid.5700663

74. Jinquan T, Vorum H, Larsen CG, Madsen P, Rasmussen HH, Gesser B, et al. Psoriasin: a novel chemotactic protein. *J Invest Dermatol.* (1996) 107:5–10. doi: 10.1111/1523-1747.ep12294284

75. Zheng Y, Niyonsaba F, Ushio H, Ikeda S, Nagaoka I, Okumura K, et al. Microbicidal protein psoriasin is a multifunctional modulator of neutrophil activation. *Immunology.* (2008) 124:357–67. doi: 10.1111/j.1365-2567.2007.02782.x

76. Burian M, Schittek B. The secrets of dermcidin action. *Int J Med Microbiol.* (2015) 305:283–6. doi: 10.1016/j.ijmm.2014.12.012

77. Oppenheim FG, Xu T, McMillian FM, Levitz SM, Diamond RD, Offner GD, et al. Histatins, a novel family of histidine-rich proteins in human parotid secretion. Isolation, characterization, primary structure, and fungistatic effects on *Candida albicans. J Biolo Chem.* (1988) 263:7472–7. doi: 10.1016/S0021-9258(18)68522-9

78. Zolin GVS, Fonseca FHD, Zambom CR, Garrido SS. Histatin 5 metallopeptides and their potential against *Candida albicans* pathogenicity and drug resistance. *Biomolecules.* (2021) 11:1209. doi: 10.3390/biom11081209

79. Lee SM, Son KN, Shah D, Ali M, Balasubramaniam A, Shukla D, et al. Histatin-1 attenuates LPS-induced inflammatory signaling in RAW264.7 macrophages. *Int J Mol Sci.* (2021) 22:7856. doi: 10.3390/ijms22157856

80. Shah D, Ali M, Shukla D, Jain S, Aakalu VK. Effects of histatin-1 peptide on human corneal epithelial cells. *PLoS ONE.* (2017) 12:e0178030. doi: 10.1371/journal.pone.0178030

81. Shah D, Son KN, Kalmodia S, Lee BS, Ali M, Balasubramaniam A, et al. Wound Healing properties of histatin-5 and identification of a functional domain required for histatin-5-induced cell migration. *Mol Ther Methods Clin Dev.* (2020) 17:709–16. doi: 10.1016/j.omtm.2020.03.027

82. McDermott AM. Antimicrobial compounds in tears. *Exp Eye Res.* (2013) 117:53–61. doi: 10.1016/j.exer.2013.07.014

83. Tsai PS, Evans JE, Green KM, Sullivan RM, Schaumberg DA, Richards SM, et al. Proteomic analysis of human meibomian gland secretions. *Br J Ophthalmol.* (2006) 90:372–7. doi: 10.1136/bjo.2005.080846

84. Hao L, Shan Q, Wei J, Ma F, Sun P. Lactoferrin: major physiological functions and applications. *Curr Protein Pept Sci.* (2019) 20:139–44. doi: 10.2174/1389203719666180514150921

85. Gillette TE, Allansmith MR. Lactoferrin in human ocular tissues. *Am J Ophthalmol.* (1980) 90:30–7. doi: 10.1016/S0002-9394(14)75074-3

86. Santagati MG, La Terra Mule S, Amico C, Pistone M, Rusciano D, Enea V. Lactoferrin expression by bovine ocular surface epithelia: a primary cell culture model to study lactoferrin gene promoter activity. *Ophthalmic Res.* (2005) 37:270–8. doi: 10.1159/000087372

87. Samuelsen O, Haukland HH, Ulvatne H, Vorland LH. Anti-complement effects of lactoferrin-derived peptides. *FEMS Immunol Med Microbiol.* (2004) 41:141–8. doi: 10.1016/j.femsim.2004.02.006

88. Ramirez-Rico G, Martinez-Castillo M. de la Garza M, Shibayama M, Serrano-Luna J. *Acanthamoeba castellanii* proteases are capable of degrading iron-binding proteins as a possible mechanism of pathogenicity. *J Eukaryot Microbiol.* (2015) 62:614–22. doi: 10.1111/jeu.12215

89. Ashby B, Garrett Q, Willcox M. Bovine lactoferrin structures promoting corneal epithelial wound healing *in vitro. Invest Ophthalmol Vis Sci.* (2011) 52:2719–26. doi: 10.1167/iovs.10-6352

90. Hanstock HG, Edwards JP, Walsh NP. Tear lactoferrin and lysozyme as clinically relevant biomarkers of mucosal immune competence. *Front Immunol.* (2019) 10:1178. doi: 10.3389/fimmu.2019.01178

91. Ganz T. Defensins: antimicrobial peptides of innate immunity. *Nat Rev Immunol.* (2003) 3:710–20. doi: 10.1038/nri1180

92. Stotz HU, Thomson JG, Wang Y. Plant defensins: defense, development and application. *Plant Signal Behav.* (2009) 4:1010–2. doi: 10.4161/psb.4.11.9755

93. Bulet P, Stöcklin R, Menin L. Anti-microbial peptides: from invertebrates to vertebrates. *Immunol Rev.* (2004) 198:169–84. doi: 10.1111/j.0105-2896.2004.0124.x

94. Pazgier M, Hoover DM, Yang D, Lu W, Lubkowski J. Human beta-defensins. *Cell Mol Life Sci.* (2006) 63:1294–313. doi: 10.1007/s00018-005-5540-2

95. Weinberg A, Jin G, Sieg S, McCormick TS. The yin and yang of human Beta-defensins in health and disease. *Front Immunol.* (2012) 3:294. doi: 10.3389/fimmu.2012.00294

96. McIntosh RS, Cade JE, Al-Abed M, Shanmuganathan V, Gupta R, Bhan A, et al. The spectrum of antimicrobial peptide expression at the ocular surface. *Invest Ophthalmol Vis Sci.* (2005) 46:1379–85. doi: 10.1167/iovs.04-0607

97. Haynes RJ, Tighe PJ, Dua HS. Antimicrobial defensin peptides of the human ocular surface. *Br J Ophthalmol.* (1999) 83:737–41. doi: 10.1136/bjo.83.6.737

98. Ikeda A, Sakimoto T, Shoji J, Sawa M. Expression of alpha- and beta-defensins in human ocular surface tissue. *Jpn J Ophthalmol.* (2005) 49:73–8. doi: 10.1007/s10384-004-0163-y

99. Mohammed I, Suleman H, Otri AM, Kulkarni BB, Chen P, Hopkinson A, et al. Localization and gene expression of human beta-defensin 9 at the human ocular surface epithelium. *Invest Ophthalmol Vis Sci.* (2010) 51:4677–82. doi: 10.1167/iovs.10-5334

100. Abedin A, Mohammed I, Hopkinson A, Dua HS, A. novel antimicrobial peptide on the ocular surface shows decreased expression in inflammation and infection. *Invest Ophthalmol Vis Sci.* (2008) 49:28–33. doi: 10.1167/iovs.07-0645

101. Redfern RL, Reins RY, McDermott AM. Toll-like receptor activation modulates antimicrobial peptide expression by ocular surface cells. *Exp Eye Res.* (2011) 92:209–20. doi: 10.1016/j.exer.2010.12.005

102. Redfern RL, McDermott AM. Toll-like receptors in ocular surface disease. *Exp Eye Res.* (2010) 90:679–87. doi: 10.1016/j.exer.2010.03.012

103. Jiang Z, Mant CT, Vasil M, Hodges RS. Role of positively charged residues on the polar and non-polar faces of amphipathic alpha-helical antimicrobial peptides on specificity and selectivity for Gram-negative pathogens. *Chem Biol Drug Des.* (2018) 91:75–92. doi: 10.1111/cbdd.13058

104. Ting DSJ, Goh ETL, Mayandi V, Busoy JMF, Aung TT, Periayah MH, et al. Hybrid derivative of cathelicidin and human beta defensin-2 against Gram-positive bacteria: a novel approach for the treatment of bacterial keratitis. *Sci Rep.* (2021) 11:18304. doi: 10.1038/s41598-021-97821-3

105. Ong PY, Ohtake T, Brandt C, Strickland I, Boguniewicz M, Ganz T, et al. Endogenous antimicrobial peptides and skin infections in atopic dermatitis. *N Engl J Med.* (2002) 347:1151–60. doi: 10.1056/NEJMoa021481

106. Kiatsurayanon C, Ogawa H, Niyonsaba F. The role of host defense peptide human beta-defensins in the maintenance of skin barriers. *Curr Pharm Des.* (2018) 24:1092–9. doi: 10.2174/1381612824666180327164445

107. Daher KA, Selsted ME, Lehrer RI. Direct inactivation of viruses by human granulocyte defensins. *J Virol.* (1986) 60:1068–74. doi: 10.1128/jvi.60.3.1068-1074.1986

108. Lakshminarayanan R, Tan WX, Aung TT, Goh ET, Muruganantham N, Li J, et al. Branched peptide, B2088, disrupts the supramolecular organization of lipopolysaccharides and sensitizes the gram-negative bacteria. *Sci Rep.* (2016) 6:25905. doi: 10.1038/srep25905

109. Coorens M, Scheenstra MR, Veldhuizen EJ, Haagsman HP. Interspecies cathelicidin comparison reveals divergence in antimicrobial activity, TLR modulation, chemokine induction and regulation of phagocytosis. *Sci Rep.* (2017) 7:40874. doi: 10.1038/srep40874

110. Zanetti M, Gennaro R, Skerlavaj B, Tomasinsig L, Circo R. Cathelicidin peptides as candidates for a novel class of antimicrobials. *Curr Pharm Des.* (2002) 8:779–93. doi: 10.2174/1381612023395457

111. Cowland JB, Johnsen AH, Borregaard N. hCAP-18, a cathelin/pro-bactenecin-like protein of human neutrophil specific granules. *FEBS Lett.* (1995) 368:173–6. doi: 10.1016/0014-5793(95)00634-L

112. Larrick JW, Hirata M, Balint RF, Lee J, Zhong J, Wright SC. Human CAP18: a novel antimicrobial lipopolysaccharide-binding protein. *Infect Immun.* (1995) 63:1291–7. doi: 10.1128/iai.63.4.1291-1297.1995

113. Zasloff M. Antimicrobial peptides of multicellular organisms: my perspective. *Adv Exp Med Biol.* (2019) 1117:3–6. doi: 10.1007/978-981-13-3588-4_1

114. Gudmundsson GH, Agerberth B, Odeberg J, Bergman T, Olsson B, Salcedo R. The human gene FALL39 and processing of the cathelin precursor to the antibacterial peptide LL-37 in granulocytes. *Eur J Biochem.* (1996) 238:325–32. doi: 10.1111/j.1432-1033.1996.0325z.x

115. Sørensen OE, Gram L, Johnsen AH, Andersson E, Bangsbøll S, Tjabringa GS, et al. Processing of seminal plasma hCAP-18 to ALL-38 by gastricsin: a novel mechanism of generating antimicrobial peptides in vagina. *J Biol Chem.* (2003) 278:28540–6. doi: 10.1074/jbc.M301608200

116. Romeo D, Skerlavaj B, Bolognesi M, Gennaro R. Structure and bactericidal activity of an antibiotic dodecapeptide purified from bovine neutrophils. *J Biol Chem.* (1988) 263:9573–5. doi: 10.1016/S0021-9258(19)81553-3

117. Mookherjee N, Hancock RE. Cationic host defence peptides: innate immune regulatory peptides as a novel approach for treating infections. *Cell Mol Life Sci.* (2007) 64:922–33. doi: 10.1007/s00018-007-6475-6

118. Scheenstra MR, van Harten RM, Veldhuizen EJA, Haagsman HP, Coorens M. Cathelicidins modulate TLR-activation and inflammation. *Front Immunol.* (2020) 11:1137. doi: 10.3389/fimmu.2020.01137

119. Ren SX, Shen J, Cheng AS, Lu L, Chan RL Li ZJ, et al. FK-16 derived from the anticancer peptide LL-37 induces caspase-independent apoptosis and autophagic cell death in colon cancer cells. *PLoS ONE.* (2013) 8:e63641. doi: 10.1371/journal.pone.0063641

120. Ren SX, Cheng AS, To KF, Tong JH Li MS, Shen J, et al. Host immune defense peptide LL-37 activates caspase-independent apoptosis and suppresses colon cancer. *Cancer Res.* (2012) 72:6512–23. doi: 10.1158/0008-5472.CAN-12-2359

121. Lee PH, Ohtake T, Zaiou M, Murakami M, Rudisill JA, Lin KH, et al. Expression of an additional cathelicidin antimicrobial peptide protects against bacterial skin infection. *Proc Natl Acad Sci USA.* (2005) 102:3750–5. doi: 10.1073/pnas.0500268102

122. Huang LC, Reins RY, Gallo RL, McDermott AM. Cathelicidin-deficient (Cnlp -/-) mice show increased susceptibility to *Pseudomonas aeruginosa* keratitis. *Invest Ophthalmol Vis Sci.* (2007) 48:4498–508. doi: 10.1167/iovs.07-0274

123. Gordon YJ, Huang LC, Romanowski EG, Yates KA, Proske RJ, McDermott AM. Human cathelicidin (LL-37), a multifunctional peptide, is expressed by

ocular surface epithelia and has potent antibacterial and antiviral activity. *Curr Eye Res.* (2005) 30:385–94. doi: 10.1080/02713680590934111

124. Li X, Li Y, Han H, Miller DW, Wang G. Solution structures of human LL-37 fragments and NMR-based identification of a minimal membrane-targeting antimicrobial and anticancer region. *J Am Chem Soc.* (2006) 128:5776–85. doi: 10.1021/ja0584875

125. Wang G, Mishra B, Epand RF, Epand RM. High-quality 3D structures shine light on antibacterial, anti-biofilm and antiviral activities of human cathelicidin LL-37 and its fragments. *Biochim Biophys Acta.* (2014) 1838:2160–72. doi: 10.1016/j.bbamem.2014.01.016

126. Engelberg Y, Landau M. The human LL-37(17-29) antimicrobial peptide reveals a functional supramolecular structure. *Nat Commun.* (2020) 11:3894. doi: 10.1038/s41467-020-17736-x

127. Wang G. Structures of human host defense cathelicidin LL-37 and its smallest antimicrobial peptide KR-12 in lipid micelles. *J Biol Chem.* (2008) 283:32637–43. doi: 10.1074/jbc.M805533200

128. Wang G, Epand RF, Mishra B, Lushnikova T, Thomas VC, Bayles KW, et al. Decoding the functional roles of cationic side chains of the major antimicrobial region of human cathelicidin LL-37. *Antimicrob Agents Chemother.* (2012) 56:845–56. doi: 10.1128/AAC.05637-11

129. Rajasekaran G, Kim EY, Shin SY. LL-37-derived membrane-active FK-13 analogs possessing cell selectivity, anti-biofilm activity and synergy with chloramphenicol and anti-inflammatory activity. *Biochim Biophys Acta Biomembr.* (2017) 1859:722–33. doi: 10.1016/j.bbamem.2017.01.037

130. Ting DSJ, Beuerman RW, Dua HS, Lakshminarayanan R, Mohammed I. Strategies in translating the therapeutic potentials of host defense peptides. *Front Immunol.* (2020) 11:983. doi: 10.3389/fimmu.2020.00983

131. Mohammed I, Said DG, Nubile M, Mastropasqua L, Dua HS. Cathelicidin-derived synthetic peptide improves therapeutic potential of vancomycin against *Pseudomonas aeruginosa. Front Microbiol.* (2019) 10:2190. doi: 10.3389/fmicb.2019.02190

132. Rosenberg HF. RNase A ribonucleases and host defense: an evolving story. *J Leukoc Biol.* (2008) 83:1079–87. doi: 10.1189/jlb.1107725

133. Beintema JJ, Wietzes P, Weickmann JL, Glitz DG. The amino acid sequence of human pancreatic ribonuclease. *Anal Biochem.* (1984) 136:48–64. doi: 10.1016/0003-2697(84)90306-3

134. Raines RT. Ribonuclease A. *Chem Rev.* (1998) 98:1045–66. doi: 10.1021/cr960427h

135. Lu L, Arranz-Trullén J, Prats-Ejarque G, Pulido D, Bhakta S, Boix E. Human antimicrobial RNases inhibit intracellular bacterial growth and induce autophagy in mycobacteria-infected macrophages. *Front Immunol.* (2019) 10:1500. doi: 10.3389/fimmu.2019.01500

136. Donato R. Functional roles of S100 proteins, calcium-binding proteins of the EF-hand type. *Biochim Biophys Acta.* (1999) 1450:191–231. doi: 10.1016/S0167-4889(99)00058-0

137. Brodersen DE, Etzerodt M, Madsen P, Celis JE, Thøgersen HC, Nyborg J, et al. EF-hands at atomic resolution: the structure of human psoriasin (S100A7) solved by MAD phasing. *Structure.* (1998) 6:477–89. doi: 10.1016/S0969-2126(98)00049-5

138. Madsen P, Rasmussen HH, Leffers H, Honoré B, Dejgaard K, Olsen E, et al. Molecular cloning, occurrence, and expression of a novel partially secreted protein "psoriasin" that is highly up-regulated in psoriatic skin. *J Invest Dermatol.* (1991) 97:701–12. doi: 10.1111/1523-1747.ep12484041

139. Lei H, Li X, Jing B, Xu H, Wu Y. Human S100A7 induces mature interleukin1α expression by RAGE-p38 MAPK-CALPAIN1 PATHWAY IN PSORIASIS. *PLoS ONE.* (2017) 12:e0169788. doi: 10.1371/journal.pone.0169788

140. Garreis F, Gottschalt M, Schlorf T, Gläser R, Harder J, Worlitzsch D, et al. Expression and regulation of antimicrobial peptide psoriasin (S100A7) at the ocular surface and in the lacrimal apparatus. *Invest Ophthalmol Vis Sci.* (2011) 52:4914–22. doi: 10.1167/iovs.10-6598

141. Abtin A, Eckhart L, Mildner M, Gruber F, Schröder JM, Tschachler E. Flagellin is the principal inducer of the antimicrobial peptide S100A7c (psoriasin) in human epidermal keratinocytes exposed to *Escherichia coli. FASEB J.* (2008) 22:2168–76. doi: 10.1096/fj.07-104117

142. Murakami M, Ohtake T, Dorschner RA, Schittek B, Garbe C, Gallo RL. Cathelicidin anti-microbial peptide expression in sweat, an innate defense system for the skin. *J Invest Dermatol.* (2002) 119:1090–5. doi: 10.1046/j.1523-1747.2002.19507.x

143. Flad T, Bogumil R, Tolson J, Schittek B, Garbe C, Deeg M, et al. Detection of dermcidin-derived peptides in sweat by ProteinChip technology. *J Immunol Methods.* (2002) 270:53–62. doi: 10.1016/S0022-1759(02)00229-6

144. Song C, Weichbrodt C, Salnikov ES, Dynowski M, Forsberg BO, Bechinger B, et al. Crystal structure and functional mechanism of a human antimicrobial membrane channel. *Proc Natl Acad Sci USA.* (2013) 110:4586–91. doi: 10.1073/pnas.1214739110

145. Schittek B, Hipfel R, Sauer B, Bauer J, Kalbacher H, Stevanovic S, et al. Dermcidin: a novel human antibiotic peptide secreted by sweat glands. *Nat Immunol.* (2001) 2:1133–7. doi: 10.1038/ni732

146. You J, Fitzgerald A, Cozzi PJ, Zhao Z, Graham P, Russell PJ, et al. Post-translation modification of proteins in tears. *Electrophoresis.* (2010) 31:1853–61. doi: 10.1002/elps.200900755

147. Steffen H, Rieg S, Wiedemann I, Kalbacher H, Deeg M, Sahl HG, et al. Naturally processed dermcidin-derived peptides do not permeabilize bacterial membranes and kill microorganisms irrespective of their charge. *Antimicrob Agents Chemother.* (2006) 50:2608–20. doi: 10.1128/AAC.00181-06

148. Khurshid Z, Najeeb S, Mali M, Moin SF, Raza SQ, Zohaib S, et al. Histatin peptides: pharmacological functions and their applications in dentistry. *Saudi Pharm J.* (2017) 25:25–31. doi: 10.1016/j.jsps.2016.04.027

149. Kalmodia S, Son KN, Cao D, Lee BS, Surenkhuu B, Shah D, et al. Presence of histatin-1 in human tears and association with aqueous deficient dry eye diagnosis: a preliminary study. *Sci Rep.* (2019) 9:10304. doi: 10.1038/s41598-019-46623-9

150. Ting DSJ, Cairns J, Gopal BP, Ho CS, Krstic L, Elsahn A, et al. Risk factors, clinical outcomes, and prognostic factors of bacterial keratitis: the Nottingham Infectious Keratitis Study. *Front Med.* (2021) 8:715118. doi: 10.3389/fmed.2021.715118

151. Ung L, Chodosh J. Foundational concepts in the biology of bacterial keratitis. *Exp Eye Res.* (2021) 209:108647. doi: 10.1016/j.exer.2021.108647

152. Ting DSJ, Ho CS, Deshmukh R, Said DG, Dua HS. Infectious keratitis: an update on epidemiology, causative microorganisms, risk factors, and antimicrobial resistance. *Eye.* (2021) 35:1084–101. doi: 10.1038/s41433-020-01339-3

153. Collier SA, Gronostaj MP, MacGurn AK, Cope JR, Awsumb KL, Yoder JS, et al. Estimated burden of keratitis–United States, 2010. *MMWR Morb Mortal Wkly Rep.* (2014) 63:1027–30.

154. Song X, Xie L, Tan X, Wang Z, Yang Y, Yuan Y, et al. A multi-center, cross-sectional study on the burden of infectious keratitis in China. *PLoS ONE.* (2014) 9:e113843. doi: 10.1371/journal.pone.0113843

155. Ting DSJ, Settle C, Morgan SJ, Baylis O, Ghosh S. A 10-year analysis of microbiological profiles of microbial keratitis: the North East England Study. *Eye.* (2018) 32:1416–7. doi: 10.1038/s41433-018-0085-4

156. Khor WB, Prajna VN, Garg P, Mehta JS, Xie L, Liu Z, et al. The Asia Cornea Society Infectious Keratitis Study: a prospective multicenter study of infectious keratitis in Asia. *Am J Ophthalmol.* (2018) 195:161–70. doi: 10.1016/j.ajo.2018.07.040

157. Ung L, Bispo PJM, Shanbhag SS, Gilmore MS, Chodosh J. The persistent dilemma of microbial keratitis: global burden, diagnosis, and antimicrobial resistance. *Surv Ophthalmol.* (2019) 64:255–71. doi: 10.1016/j.survophthal.2018.12.003

158. Ting DSJ, Ho CS, Cairns J, Elsahn A, Al-Aqaba M, Boswell T, et al. 12-year analysis of incidence, microbiological profiles and *in vitro* antimicrobial susceptibility of infectious keratitis: the Nottingham Infectious Keratitis Study. *Br J Ophthalmol.* (2021) 105:328–33. doi: 10.1136/bjophthalmol-2020-316128

159. Ting DSJ, Ho CS, Cairns J, Gopal BP, Elsahn A, Al-Aqaba MA, et al. Seasonal patterns of incidence, demographic factors, and microbiological profiles of infectious keratitis: the Nottingham Infectious Keratitis Study. *Eye.* (2021) 35:2543–9. doi: 10.1038/s41433-020-01272-5

160. Ting DSJ, Galal M, Kulkarni B, Elalfy MS, Lake D, Hamada S, et al. Clinical characteristics and outcomes of fungal keratitis in the United Kingdom 2011-2020: a 10-year study. *J Fungi.* (2021) 7:966. doi: 10.20944/preprints202110.0104.v1

161. Brown L, Leck AK, Gichangi M, Burton MJ, Denning DW. The global incidence and diagnosis of fungal keratitis. *Lancet Infect Dis.* (2021) 21:e49–57. doi: 10.1016/S1473-3099(20)30448-5

162. Ting DSJ, Henein C, Said DG, Dua HS. Photoactivated chromophore for infectious keratitis - corneal cross-linking (PACK-CXL): a systematic review and meta-analysis. *Ocul Surf.* (2019) 17:624–34. doi: 10.1016/j.jtos.2019.08.006

163. Ting DSJ, McKenna M, Sadiq SN, Martin J, Mudhar HS, Meeney A, et al. Arthrographis kalrae keratitis complicated by endophthalmitis: a case report with literature review. *Eye Contact Lens.* (2020) 46:e59–65. doi: 10.1097/ICL.0000000000000713

164. Anshu A, Parthasarathy A, Mehta JS, Htoon HM, Tan DT. Outcomes of therapeutic deep lamellar keratoplasty and penetrating keratoplasty for advanced infectious keratitis: a comparative study. *Ophthalmology.* (2009) 116:615–23. doi: 10.1016/j.ophtha.2008.12.043

165. Ting DSJ, Henein C, Said DG, Dua HS. Amniotic membrane transplantation for infectious keratitis: a systematic review and meta-analysis. *Sci Rep.* (2021) 11:13007. doi: 10.1038/s41598-021-92366-x

166. Said DG, Rallis KI, Al-Aqaba MA, Ting DSJ, Dua HS. Surgical management of infectious keratitis. *Ocul Surf.* (2021). doi: 10.1016/j.jtos.2021.09.005. [Epub ahead of print].

167. Chen X, Niyonsaba F, Ushio H, Okuda D, Nagaoka I, Ikeda S, et al. Synergistic effect of antibacterial agents human beta-defensins, cathelicidin LL-37 and lysozyme against *Staphylococcus aureus* and *Escherichia coli*. *J Dermatol Sci.* (2005) 40:123–32. doi: 10.1016/j.jdermsci.2005.03.014

168. Singh PK, Tack BF, McCray PB Jr., Welsh MJ. Synergistic and additive killing by antimicrobial factors found in human airway surface liquid. *Am J Physiol Lung Cell Mol Physiol.* (2000) 279:L799–805. doi: 10.1152/ajplung.2000.279.5.L799

169. Mohammed I, Mohanty D, Said DG, Barik MR, Reddy MM, Alsaadi A, et al. Antimicrobial peptides in human corneal tissue of patients with fungal keratitis. *Br J Ophthalmol.* (2021) 105:1172–7. doi: 10.1136/bjophthalmol-2020-316329

170. Otri AM, Mohammed I, Al-Aqaba MA, Fares U, Peng C, Hopkinson A, et al. Variable expression of human Beta defensins 3 and 9 at the human ocular surface in infectious keratitis. *Invest Ophthalmol Vis Sci.* (2012) 53:757–61. doi: 10.1167/iovs.11-8467

171. Ting DSJ, Bignardi G, Koerner R, Irion LD, Johnson E, Morgan SJ, et al. Polymicrobial keratitis with *Cryptococcus curvatus, Candida parapsilosis,* and *Stenotrophomonas maltophilia* after penetrating keratoplasty: a rare case report with literature review. *Eye Contact Lens.* (2019) 45:e5–10. doi: 10.1097/ICL.0000000000000517

172. Asbell PA, Sanfilippo CM, Sahm DF, DeCory HH. Trends in antibiotic resistance among ocular microorganisms in the United States from 2009 to 2018. *JAMA Ophthalmol.* (2020) 138:439–50. doi: 10.1001/jamaophthalmol.2020.0155

173. Craig JP, Nichols KK, Akpek EK, Caffery B, Dua HS, Joo CK, et al. TFOS DEWS II definition and classification report. *Ocul Surf.* (2017) 15:276–83. doi: 10.1016/j.jtos.2017.05.008

174. Ting DSJ, Ghosh S. Acute corneal perforation 1 week following uncomplicated cataract surgery: the implication of undiagnosed dry eye disease and topical NSAIDs. *Ther Adv Ophthalmol.* (2019) 11:2515841419869508. doi: 10.1177/2515841419869508

175. Brito-Zerón P, Baldini C, Bootsma H, Bowman SJ, Jonsson R, Mariette X, et al. Sjögren syndrome. *Nat Rev Dis Primers.* (2016) 2:16047. doi: 10.1038/nrdp.2016.47

176. Sonobe H, Ogawa Y, Yamada K, Shimizu E, Uchino Y, Kamoi M, et al. A novel and innovative paper-based analytical device for assessing tear lactoferrin of dry eye patients. *Ocul Surf.* (2019) 17:160–6. doi: 10.1016/j.jtos.2018.11.001

177. Chao C, Tong L. Tear lactoferrin and features of ocular allergy in different severities of meibomian gland dysfunction. *Optom Vis Sci.* (2018) 95:930–6. doi: 10.1097/OPX.0000000000001285

178. Gerber-Hollbach N, Plattner K, O'Leary OE, Jenoe P, Moes S, Drexler B, et al. Tear film proteomics reveal important differences between patients with and without ocular GvHD after allogeneic hematopoietic cell transplantation. *Invest Ophthalmol Vis Sci.* (2018) 59:3521–30. doi: 10.1167/iovs.18-24433

179. Narayanan S, Miller WL, McDermott AM. Expression of human beta-defensins in conjunctival epithelium: relevance to dry eye disease. *Invest Ophthalmol Vis Sci.* (2003) 44:3795–801. doi: 10.1167/iovs.02-1301

180. Ohashi Y, Ishida R, Kojima T, Goto E, Matsumoto Y, Watanabe K, et al. Abnormal protein profiles in tears with dry eye syndrome. *Am J Ophthalmol.* (2003) 136:291–9. doi: 10.1016/S0002-9394(03)00203-4

181. Kuo MT, Fang PC, Chao TL, Chen A, Lai YH, Huang YT, et al. Tear proteomics approach to monitoring Sjögren syndrome or dry eye disease. *Int J Mol Sci.* (2019) 20:1932. doi: 10.3390/ijms20081932

182. Careba I, Chiva A, Totir M, Ungureanu E, Gradinaru S. Tear lipocalin, lysozyme and lactoferrin concentrations in postmenopausal women. *J Med Life.* (2015) 8(Spec Issue):94–8.

183. Narayanan S, Redfern RL, Miller WL, Nichols KK, McDermott AM. Dry eye disease and microbial keratitis: is there a connection? *Ocul Surf.* (2013) 11:75–92. doi: 10.1016/j.jtos.2012.12.002

184. Khoo P, Cabrera-Aguas M, Robaei D, Lahra MM, Watson S. Microbial keratitis and ocular surface disease: a 5-year study of the microbiology, risk factors and clinical outcomes in Sydney, Australia. *Curr Eye Res.* (2019) 44:1195–202. doi: 10.1080/02713683.2019.1631852

185. Godefrooij DA, de Wit GA, Uiterwaal CS, Imhof SM, Wisse RP. Age-specific incidence and prevalence of keratoconus: a Nationwide Registration Study. *Am J Ophthalmol.* (2017) 175:169–72. doi: 10.1016/j.ajo.2016.12.015

186. Kennedy RH, Bourne WM, Dyer JA. A 48-year clinical and epidemiologic study of keratoconus. *Am J Ophthalmol.* (1986) 101:267–73. doi: 10.1016/0002-9394(86)90817-2

187. Andreanos KD, Hashemi K, Petrelli M, Droutsas K, Georgalas I, Kymionis GD. Keratoconus treatment algorithm. *Ophthalmol Ther.* (2017) 6:245–62. doi: 10.1007/s40123-017-0099-1

188. Mohammadpour M, Heidari Z, Hashemi H. Updates on managements for keratoconus. *J Curr Ophthalmol.* (2018) 30:110–24. doi: 10.1016/j.joco.2017.11.002

189. Ting DSJ, Rana-Rahman R, Chen Y, Bell D, Danjoux JP, Morgan SJ, et al. Effectiveness and safety of accelerated (9 mW/cm) corneal collagen cross-linking for progressive keratoconus: a 24-month follow-up. *Eye.* (2019) 33:812–8. doi: 10.1038/s41433-018-0323-9

190. Ting DS, Sau CY, Srinivasan S, Ramaesh K, Mantry S, Roberts F. Changing trends in keratoplasty in the West of Scotland: a 10-year review. *Br J Ophthalmol.* (2012) 96:405–8. doi: 10.1136/bjophthalmol-2011-300244

191. Fasolo A, Frigo AC, Bohm E, Genisi C, Rama P, Spadea L, et al. The CORTES study: corneal transplant indications and graft survival in an Italian cohort of patients. *Cornea.* (2006) 25:507–15. doi: 10.1097/01.ico.0000214211.60317.1f

192. Mas Tur V, MacGregor C, Jayaswal R, O'Brart D, Maycock N. A review of keratoconus: diagnosis, pathophysiology, and genetics. *Surv Ophthalmol.* (2017) 62:770–83. doi: 10.1016/j.survophthal.2017.06.009

193. Pannebaker C, Chandler HL, Nichols JJ. Tear proteomics in keratoconus. *Mol Vis.* (2010) 16:1949–57.

194. Lema I, Duran JA. Inflammatory molecules in the tears of patients with keratoconus. *Ophthalmology.* (2005) 112:654–9. doi: 10.1016/j.ophtha.2004.11.050

195. Galvis V, Sherwin T, Tello A, Merayo J, Barrera R, Acera A. Keratoconus: an inflammatory disorder? *Eye.* (2015) 29:843–59. doi: 10.1038/eye.2015.63

196. Balasubramanian SA, Mohan S, Pye DC, Willcox MD. Proteases, proteolysis and inflammatory molecules in the tears of people with keratoconus. *Acta Ophthalmol.* (2012) 90:e303–9. doi: 10.1111/j.1755-3768.2011.02369.x

197. Yam GH, Fuest M, Zhou L, Liu YC, Deng L, Chan AS, et al. Differential epithelial and stromal protein profiles in cone and non-cone regions of keratoconus corneas. *Sci Rep.* (2019) 9:2965. doi: 10.1038/s41598-019-39182-6

198. Balasubramanian SA, Pye DC, Willcox MD. Levels of lactoferrin, secretory IgA and serum albumin in the tear film of people with keratoconus. *Exp Eye Res.* (2012) 96:132–7. doi: 10.1016/j.exer.2011.12.010

199. Pastori V, Tavazzi S, Lecchi M. Lactoferrin-loaded contact lenses counteract cytotoxicity caused *in vitro* by keratoconic tears. *Cont Lens Anterior Eye.* (2019) 42:253–7. doi: 10.1016/j.clae.2018.12.004

200. Rezvan F, Khabazkhoob M, Hooshmand E, Yekta A, Saatchi M, Hashemi H. Prevalence and risk factors of pterygium: a systematic review and meta-analysis. *Surv Ophthalmol.* (2018) 63:719–35. doi: 10.1016/j.survophthal.2018.03.001

201. Ting DSJ, Liu YC, Patil M, Ji AJS, Fang XL, Tham YC, et al. Proposal and validation of a new grading system for pterygium (SLIT2). *Br J Ophthalmol.* (2021) 105:921–4. doi: 10.1136/bjophthalmol-2020-315831

202. Liu T, Liu Y, Xie L, He X, Bai J. Progress in the pathogenesis of pterygium. *Curr Eye Res.* (2013) 38:1191–7. doi: 10.3109/02713683.2013.823212

203. Zhou L, Beuerman RW, Ang LP, Chan CM Li SF, Chew FT, et al. Elevation of human alpha-defensins and S100 calcium-binding proteins A8 and A9 in tear fluid of patients with pterygium. *Invest Ophthalmol Vis Sci.* (2009) 50:2077–86. doi: 10.1167/iovs.08-2604

204. Abubakar SA, Isa MM, Omar N, Tan SW. Relative quantification of human β-defensins gene expression in pterygium and normal conjunctiva samples. *Mol Med Rep.* (2020) 22:4931–7. doi: 10.3892/mmr.2020.11560

205. Ljubimov AV, Saghizadeh M. Progress in corneal wound healing. *Prog Retin Eye Res.* (2015) 49:17–45. doi: 10.1016/j.preteyeres.2015.07.002

206. Zhou L, Huang LQ, Beuerman RW, Grigg ME Li SF, Chew FT, et al. Proteomic analysis of human tears: defensin expression after ocular surface surgery. *J Proteome Res.* (2004) 3:410–6. doi: 10.1021/pr034065n

207. McDermott AM, Redfern RL, Zhang B. Human beta-defensin 2 is upregulated during re-epithelialization of the cornea. *Curr Eye Res.* (2001) 22:64–7. doi: 10.1076/ceyr.22.1.64.6978

208. Reins RY, Hanlon SD, Magadi S, McDermott AM. Effects of topically applied vitamin d during corneal wound healing. *PLoS ONE.* (2016) 11:e0152889. doi: 10.1371/journal.pone.0152889

209. Lu X, Vick S, Chen Z, Chen J, Watsky MA. Effects of vitamin D receptor knockout and vitamin D deficiency on corneal epithelial wound healing and nerve density in diabetic mice. *Diabetes.* (2020) 69:1042–51. doi: 10.2337/db19-1051

210. Elizondo RA, Yin Z, Lu X, Watsky MA. Effect of vitamin D receptor knockout on cornea epithelium wound healing and tight junctions. *Invest Ophthalmol Vis Sci.* (2014) 55:5245–51. doi: 10.1167/iovs.13-13553

211. Weidinger S, Beck LA, Bieber T, Kabashima K, Irvine AD. Atopic dermatitis. *Nat Rev Dis Primers.* (2018) 4:1. doi: 10.1038/s41572-018-0001-z

212. Kumar S. Vernal keratoconjunctivitis: a major review. *Acta Ophthalmol.* (2009) 87:133–47. doi: 10.1111/j.1755-3768.2008.01347.x

213. Takahashi T, Gallo RL. The critical and multifunctional roles of antimicrobial peptides in dermatology. *Dermatol Clin.* (2017) 35:39–50. doi: 10.1016/j.det.2016.07.006

214. Chen JJ, Applebaum DS, Sun GS, Pflugfelder SC. Atopic keratoconjunctivitis: a review. *J Am Acad Dermatol.* (2014) 70:569–75. doi: 10.1016/j.jaad.2013.10.036

215. Ikeda A, Nakanishi Y, Sakimoto T, Shoji J, Sawa M, Nemoto N. Expression of beta defensins in ocular surface tissue of experimentally developed allergic conjunctivitis mouse model. *Jpn J Ophthalmol.* (2006) 50:1–6. doi: 10.1007/s10384-005-0262-4

216. Hida RY, Ohashi Y, Takano Y, Dogru M, Goto E, Fujishima H, et al. Elevated levels of human alpha -defensin in tears of patients with allergic conjunctival disease complicated by corneal lesions: detection by SELDI ProteinChip system and quantification. *Curr Eye Res.* (2005) 30:723–30. doi: 10.1080/02713680591005986

217. Rapacz P, Tedesco J, Donshik PC, Ballow M. Tear lysozyme and lactoferrin levels in giant papillary conjunctivitis and vernal conjunctivitis. *CLAO J.* (1988) 14:207–9.

218. Gether L, Overgaard LK, Egeberg A, Thyssen JP. Incidence and prevalence of rosacea: a systematic review and meta-analysis. *Br J Dermatol.* (2018) 179:282–9. doi: 10.1111/bjd.16481

219. Rainer BM, Kang S, Chien AL. Rosacea: epidemiology, pathogenesis, and treatment. *Dermatoendocrinol.* (2017) 9:e1361574. doi: 10.1080/19381980.2017.1361574

220. Yamasaki K, Di Nardo A, Bardan A, Murakami M, Ohtake T, Coda A, et al. Increased serine protease activity and cathelicidin promotes skin inflammation in rosacea. *Nat Med.* (2007) 13:975–80. doi: 10.1038/nm1616

221. Koczulla R, von Degenfeld G, Kupatt C, Krotz F, Zahler S, Gloe T, et al. An angiogenic role for the human peptide antibiotic LL-37/hCAP-18. *J Clin Invest.* (2003) 111:1665–72. doi: 10.1172/JCI17545

222. Kiratli H, Irkec M, Orhan M. Tear lactoferrin levels in chronic meibomitis associated with acne rosacea. *Eur J Ophthalmol.* (2000) 10:11–4.

223. Hancock RE, Sahl HG. Antimicrobial and host-defense peptides as new anti-infective therapeutic strategies. *Nat Biotechnol.* (2006) 24:1551–7. doi: 10.1038/nbt1267

224. Fjell CD, Hiss JA, Hancock RE, Schneider G. Designing antimicrobial peptides: form follows function. *Nat Rev Drug Discov.* (2011) 11:37–51. doi: 10.1038/nrd3591

225. Christoffersen RE. Antibiotics–an investment worth making? *Nat Biotechnol.* (2006) 24:1512–4. doi: 10.1038/nbt1206-1512

226. Zhou L, Liu SP, Chen LY Li J, Ong LB, Guo L, et al. The structural parameters for antimicrobial activity, human epithelial cell cytotoxicity and killing mechanism of synthetic monomer and dimer analogues derived from hBD3 C-terminal region. *Amino Acids.* (2011) 40:123–33. doi: 10.1007/s00726-010-0565-8

227. Kolar SSN, Luca V, Baidouri H, Mannino G, McDermott AM, Mangoni ML. Esculentin-1a(1-21)NH2: a frog skin-derived peptide for microbial keratitis. *Cell Mol Life Sci.* (2015) 72:617–27. doi: 10.1007/s00018-014-1694-0

228. Luca V, Stringaro A, Colone M, Pini A, Mangoni ML. Esculentin(1-21), an amphibian skin membrane-active peptide with potent activity on both planktonic and biofilm cells of the bacterial pathogen *Pseudomonas aeruginosa. Cell Mol Life Sci.* (2013) 70:2773–86. doi: 10.1007/s00018-013-1291-7

229. Casciaro B, Dutta D, Loffredo MR, Marcheggiani S, McDermott AM, Willcox MD, et al. Esculentin-1a derived peptides kill *Pseudomonas aeruginosa* biofilm on soft contact lenses and retain antibacterial activity upon immobilization to the lens surface. *Biopolymers.* (2017) 110:e23074. doi: 10.1002/bip.23074

230. Clemens LE, Jaynes J, Lim E, Kolar SS, Reins RY, Baidouri H, et al. Designed host defense peptides for the treatment of bacterial keratitis. *Invest Ophthalmol Vis Sci.* (2017) 58:6273–81. doi: 10.1167/iovs.17-22243

231. Dutta D, Zhao T, Cheah KB, Holmlund L, Willcox MDP. Activity of a melimine derived peptide Mel4 against *Stenotrophomonas, Delftia, Elizabethkingia, Burkholderia* and biocompatibility as a contact lens coating. *Cont Lens Anterior Eye.* (2017) 40:175–83. doi: 10.1016/j.clae.2017.01.002

232. Yasir M, Dutta D, Willcox MDP. Mode of action of the antimicrobial peptide Mel4 is independent of *Staphylococcus aureus* cell membrane permeability. *PLoS ONE.* (2019) 14:e0215703. doi: 10.1371/journal.pone.0215703

233. Kalaiselvan P, Konda N, Pampi N, Vaddavalli PK, Sharma S, Stapleton F, et al. Effect of antimicrobial contact lenses on corneal infiltrative events: a randomized clinical trial. *Transl Vis Sci Technol.* (2021) 10:32. doi: 10.1167/tvst.10.7.32

234. Mayandi V, Xi Q, Leng Goh ET, Koh SK, Jie Toh TY, Barathi VA, et al. Rational substitution of ε-lysine for α-lysine enhances the cell and membrane selectivity of pore-forming melittin. *J Med Chem.* (2020) 63:3522–37. doi: 10.1021/acs.jmedchem.9b01846

235. Ting DSJ Li J, Verma CS, Goh ETL, Nubile M, Mastropasqua L, et al. Evaluation of host defense peptide (CaD23)-antibiotic interaction and mechanism of action: insights from experimental and molecular dynamics simulations studies. *Front Pharmacol.* (2021) 12:731499. doi: 10.3389/fphar.2021.731499

236. Liu S, Zhou L, Li J, Suresh A, Verma C, Foo YH, et al. Linear analogues of human beta-defensin 3: concepts for design of antimicrobial peptides with reduced cytotoxicity to mammalian cells. *Chembiochem.* (2008) 9:964–73. doi: 10.1002/cbic.200700560

237. Bai Y, Liu S, Jiang P, Zhou L, Li J, Tang C, et al. Structure-dependent charge density as a determinant of antimicrobial activity of peptide analogues of defensin. *Biochemistry.* (2009) 48:7229–39. doi: 10.1021/bi900670d

238. Ladram A, Nicolas P. Antimicrobial peptides from frog skin: biodiversity and therapeutic promises. *Front Biosci.* (2016) 21:1341–71. doi: 10.2741/4461

239. Willcox MD, Hume EB, Aliwarga Y, Kumar N, Cole N, A. novel cationic-peptide coating for the prevention of microbial colonization on contact lenses. *J Appl Microbiol.* (2008) 105:1817–25. doi: 10.1111/j.1365-2672.2008.03942.x

240. Cole N, Hume EB, Vijay AK, Sankaridurg P, Kumar N, Willcox MD. *In vivo* performance of melimine as an antimicrobial coating for contact lenses in models of CLARE and CLPU. *Invest Ophthalmol Vis Sci.* (2010) 51:390–5. doi: 10.1167/iovs.09-4068

241. Dutta D, Ozkan J, Willcox MD. Biocompatibility of antimicrobial melimine lenses: rabbit and human studies. *Optom Vis Sci.* (2014) 91:570–81. doi: 10.1097/OPX.0000000000000232

242. Dutta D, Vijay AK, Kumar N, Willcox MD. Melimine-coated antimicrobial contact lenses reduce microbial keratitis in an animal model. *Invest Ophthalmol Vis Sci.* (2016) 57:5616–24. doi: 10.1167/iovs.16-19882

243. Yasir M, Dutta D, Willcox MDP. Comparative mode of action of the antimicrobial peptide melimine and its derivative Mel4 against *Pseudomonas aeruginosa. Sci Rep.* (2019) 9:7063. doi: 10.1038/s41598-019-42440-2

244. Jin L, Bai X, Luan N, Yao H, Zhang Z, Liu W, et al. A designed tryptophan- and lysine/arginine-rich antimicrobial peptide with therapeutic potential for clinical antibiotic-resistant *Candida albicans* vaginitis. *J Med Chem.* (2016) 59:1791–9. doi: 10.1021/acs.jmedchem.5b01264

245. Mishra B, Wang G. The importance of amino acid composition in natural AMPs: an evolutional, structural, and functional perspective. *Front Immunol.* (2012) 3:221. doi: 10.3389/fimmu.2012.00221

246. Shukla SC, Singh A, Pandey AK, Mishra A. Review on production and medical applications of ε-polylysine. *Biochem Eng J.* (2012) 65:70–81. doi: 10.1016/j.bej.2012.04.001

247. Geornaras I, Yoon Y, Belk KE, Smith GC, Sofos JN. Antimicrobial activity of epsilon-polylysine against *Escherichia coli* O157:H7, *Salmonella* Typhimurium, and *Listeria monocytogenes* in various food extracts. *J Food Sci.* (2007) 72:M330–4. doi: 10.1111/j.1750-3841.2007.00510.x

248. Shima S, Matsuoka H, Iwamoto T, Sakai H. Antimicrobial action of epsilon-poly-L-lysine. *J Antibiot.* (1984) 37:1449–55. doi: 10.7164/antibiotics.37.1449

249. Venkatesh M, Barathi VA, Goh ETL, Anggara R, Fazil M, Ng AJY, et al. Antimicrobial activity and cell selectivity of synthetic and biosynthetic cationic polymers. *Antimicrob Agents Chemother.* (2017) 61:e00469-17. doi: 10.1128/AAC.00469-17

250. Clausen ML, Slotved HC, Krogfelt KA, Andersen PS, Agner T. *In vivo* expression of antimicrobial peptides in atopic dermatitis. *Exp Dermatol.* (2016) 25:3–9. doi: 10.1111/exd.12831

251. Liu PT, Stenger S, Li H, Wenzel L, Tan BH, Krutzik SR, et al. Toll-like receptor triggering of a vitamin D-mediated human antimicrobial response. *Science.* (2006) 311:1770–3. doi: 10.1126/science.1123933

252. Albenali LH, Danby S, Moustafa M, Brown K, Chittock J, Shackley F, et al. Vitamin D and antimicrobial peptide levels in patients with atopic dermatitis and atopic dermatitis complicated by eczema herpeticum: a pilot study. *J Allergy Clin Immunol.* (2016) 138:1715–9.e4. doi: 10.1016/j.jaci.2016.05.039

253. Javanbakht MH, Keshavarz SA, Djalali M, Siassi F, Eshraghian MR, Firooz A, et al. Randomized controlled trial using vitamins E and D supplementation in atopic dermatitis. *J Dermatolog Treat.* (2011) 22:144–50. doi: 10.3109/09546630903578566

254. Amestejani M, Salehi BS, Vasigh M, Sobhkhiz A, Karami M, Alinia H, et al. Vitamin D supplementation in the treatment of atopic dermatitis: a clinical trial study. *J Drugs Dermatol.* (2012) 11:327–30.

255. https://clinicaltrials.gov/ct2/show/results/NCT01590758 (accessed November 02, 2021).

256. https://www.fiercebiotech.com/biotech/dipexium-plummets-total-phiii-failure (accessed November 02, 2021).

257. Roudi R, Syn NL, Roudbary M. Antimicrobial peptides as biologic and immunotherapeutic agents against cancer: a comprehensive overview. *Front Immunol.* (2017) 8:1320. doi: 10.3389/fimmu.2017.01320

258. Das P, Sercu T, Wadhawan K, Padhi I, Gehrmann S, Cipcigan F, et al. Accelerated antimicrobial discovery *via* deep generative models and molecular dynamics simulations. *Nat Biomed Eng.* (2021) 5:613–23. doi: 10.1038/s41551-021-00689-x

259. Biswaro LS, da Costa Sousa MG, Rezende TMB, Dias SC, Franco OL. Antimicrobial peptides and nanotechnology, recent advances and challenges. *Front Microbiol.* (2018) 9:855. doi: 10.3389/fmicb.2018.00855

260. Tangpricha V, Judd SE, Ziegler TR, Hao L, Alvarez JA, Fitzpatrick AM, et al. LL-37 concentrations and the relationship to vitamin D, immune status, and inflammation in HIV-infected children and young adults. *AIDS Res Hum Retroviruses.* (2014) 30:670–6. doi: 10.1089/aid.2013.0279

261. Mily A, Rekha RS, Kamal SM, Akhtar E, Sarker P, Rahim Z, et al. Oral intake of phenylbutyrate with or without vitamin D3 upregulates the cathelicidin LL-37 in human macrophages: a dose finding study for treatment of tuberculosis. *BMC Pulm Med.* (2013) 13:23. doi: 10.1186/1471-2466-13-23

262. Yeung ATY, Choi YH, Lee AHY, Hale C, Ponstingl H, Pickard D, et al. A genome-wide knockout screen in human macrophages identified host factors modulating *Salmonella* infection. *mBio.* (2019) 10:e02169-19. doi: 10.1128/mBio.02169-19

263. Pajor M, Sogin J, Worobo RW, Szweda P. Draft genome sequence of antimicrobial producing *Paenibacillus alvei* strain MP1 reveals putative novel antimicrobials. *BMC Res Notes.* (2020) 13:280. doi: 10.1186/s13104-020-05124-z

16

Machine Learning to Analyze Factors Associated with Ten-Year Graft Survival of Keratoplasty for Cornea Endothelial Disease

Marcus Ang[1,2,3]*, Feng He[2], Stephanie Lang[1], Charumathi Sabanayagam[2,3], Ching-Yu Cheng[2,3], Anshu Arundhati[1,2,3] and Jodhbir S. Mehta[1,2,3]

[1] Singapore National Eye Centre, Singapore, Singapore, [2] Singapore Eye Research Institute, Singapore, Singapore,
[3] Department of Ophthalmology and Visual Sciences, Duke-NUS Medical School, Singapore, Singapore

Correspondence:
Marcus Ang
marcus.ang@snec.com.sg

Purpose: Machine learning analysis of factors associated with 10-year graft survival of Descemet stripping automated endothelial keratoplasty (DSAEK) and penetrating keratoplasty (PK) in Asian eyes.

Methods: Prospective study of donor characteristics, clinical outcomes and complications from consecutive patients ($n = 1,335$) who underwent DSAEK (946 eyes) or PK (389 eyes) for Fuchs' endothelial dystrophy (FED) or bullous keratopathy (BK) were analyzed. Random survival forests (RSF) analysis using the highest variable importance (VIMP) factors were determined to develop the optimal Cox proportional hazards regression model. Main outcome measure was 10-year graft survival with RSF analysis of factors associated with graft failure.

Results: Mean age was 68 ± 11 years, 47.6% male, in our predominantly Chinese (76.6%) Asian cohort, with more BK compared to FED (62.2 vs. 37.8%, $P < 0.001$). Overall 10-year survival for DSAEK was superior to PK (73.6 vs. 50.9%, log-rank $P < 0.001$). RSF based on VIMP (best Harrell C statistic: 0.701) with multivariable modeling revealed that BK (HR:2.84, 95%CI:1.89–4.26; $P < 0.001$), PK (HR: 1.64, 95%CI:1.19–2.27; $P = 0.002$), male recipients (HR:1.75, 95%CI:1.31–2.34; $P < 0.001$) and poor pre-operative visual acuity (HR: 1.60, 95%CI:1.15–2.22, $P = 0.005$) were associated with graft failure. Ten-year cumulative incidence of complications such as immune-mediated graft rejection ($P < 0.001$), epitheliopathy ($P < 0.001$), and wound dehiscence ($P = 0.002$) were greater in the PK compared to the DSAEK group.

Conclusion: In our study, RSF combined with Cox regression was superior to traditional regression techniques alone in analyzing a large number of high-dimensional factors associated with 10-year corneal graft survival in Asian eyes with cornea endothelial disease.

Keywords: machine learning, keratoplasty, graft survival, endothelial (dys)function, penetrating keratoplasty

INTRODUCTION

Corneal transplantation is currently the most frequently performed type of transplant worldwide (1), with corneal endothelial diseases as the leading surgical indication (2). Today, endothelial keratoplasty (EK) has replaced penetrating keratoplasty (PK) as the corneal transplantation of choice for endothelial disease in the United States (3), and increasingly in the rest of the world (4). Currently, Descemet stripping automated endothelial keratoplasty (DSAEK) is the most popular EK technique, supported by eye banks providing pre-cut donor tissue (5). The short-term advantages of DSAEK over PK are related to its minimally invasive approach—avoiding a full-thickness wound that requires sutures, thereby reducing the risk of intraoperative sight-threatening complications, suture-related problems, graft rejection and potential wound dehiscence (6). Thus, faster visual rehabilitation can be achieved, with reduced post-operative corneal astigmatism and potentially superior visual outcomes (7).

However, long-term outcomes of DSAEK compared to the traditional PK in terms of graft survival and complications such as graft rejection still vary in the published literature. Long-term studies from the Asia-Pacific (8, 9) and Europe (10) support the advantages of DSAEK over PK, but national registries in the United Kingdom (11) and Australia (12), have suggested poorer survival outcomes for DSAEK compared to PK for the same indications. While registries reflect "real-world" data from multiple centers with varying surgical techniques and surgeon experience (12), outcomes from such studies are often confounded by differences in donor characteristics or recipient populations, which may be not well delineated (13). Thus, there is an unmet need for long-term studies that directly compare DSAEK and PK outcomes from a variety of populations (14).

A randomized controlled trial is not always feasible to compare DSAEK and PK, and outcomes from registry studies are valuable in providing representative results by including a large number of cases performed by several surgeons (14). However, cornea graft registries often collect a large number of variables generating enormous datasets over time, which can be difficult to analyze using traditional statistical techniques such as Kaplan-Meier survival and Cox proportional hazards regression analyses. Random forests is a machine-learning technique that is gaining popularity to analyze large datasets with less restrictive assumptions, and random survival forests (RSF) can be used to analyze high-dimensional graft survival data (15, 16). This potentially allows us to study a larger number of factors that influence graft survival outcomes with comparable or even better prediction measures. Thus, we used this machine learning method to examine the large database of outcomes prospectively collected from the Singapore Cornea Transplant Registry over 10 years, to examine factors associated with graft failure comparing PK and DSAEK for corneal endothelial diseases.

MATERIALS AND METHODS

We collated all the data from our ongoing prospective Singapore Corneal Transplant Study (SCTS) cohort, which tracks all patients who have underwent a cornea transplant through an annual audit (17). Our inclusion and exclusion criteria have been previously described (18), and in this study we included all consecutive patients with either FED or BK who underwent either a primary DSAEK or PK for optical indications, excluding re-grafts and patients requiring systemic immunosuppresion (19). All corneal surgeons from the Singapore National Eye Center performed all surgeries over the same time period (1999–2011), which included cases performed or partially performed by numerous local or international corneal fellows in training under direct supervision. All data collected in this registry audit include patient demographics, diagnosis, details of surgeries including intra-operative complications, pre- and post-operative best-corrected LogMar visual acuity (BCVA), clinical outcomes and post-operative complications (18).

Our main outcome measure was graft survival, where graft failure was defined as irreversible loss of optical clarity, sufficient to compromise vision for a minimum of three consecutive months (20). Complications were monitored and recorded such as primary graft failure, graft rejection, and graft-related infections as previously defined (21). Graft rejection was defined as presence of an endothelial rejection line or inflammation (keratic precipitates, cells in the stroma, or an increase in aqueous cells from a previous visit, with or without any clinically apparent change in recipient stromal thickness or clarity) in the absence of an endothelial rejection line in a previously clear graft. Endothelial cell counts were performed by certified ophthalmic technicians using a non-contact specular microscope (Konan Medical Corp, Hyogo, Japan) as previously decribed (22). Our study followed the principles of the Declaration of Helsinki, with ethics approval obtained from our local Institutional Review Board (SingHealth Centralized IRB, R847/42/2011).

Surgical Technique

Essentially, PK surgeries were performed using a standard technique previously described (18), with a Hanna vacuum trephine system (Moria Inc, Antony, France). Briefly, the recipient cornea was first excised using the Hanna trephine system. A 0.25- to 0.50-mm oversized donor cornea then was punched out endothelial side up and sutured on to

TABLE 1 | Baseline characteristics of study cohort comparing penetrating keratoplasty (PK) and Descemet stripping automated endothelial keratoplasty (DSAEK) from the Singapore Cornea Transplant Registry.

Characteristics		Corneal Graft		P value*
	Total (*n* = 1,335)	PK (*n* = 389)	DSAEK (*n* = 946)	
Mean age, years (± SD)	68.3 ± 11.4	67.4 ± 12.0	68.7 ± 11.1	0.212
Gender (%)				
Male	635 (47.6)	191 (49.1)	444 (46.9)	0.509
Female	700 (52.4)	198 (50.9)	502 (53.1)	
Race (%)				
Chinese	1,023 (76.6)	306 (78.7)	717 (75.8)	0.515
Malay	63 (4.7)	20 (5.1)	43 (4.5)	
Indian	70 (5.2)	18 (4.6)	52 (5.5)	
Others	179 (13.4)	45 (11.6)	134 (14.2)	
Surgical indication				
Fuchs Dystrophy (FED)	504 (37.8)	93 (23.9)	411 (43.4)	<0.001
Bullous Keratopathy (BK)	831 (62.2)	296 (76.1)	535 (56.6)	
Baseline/preoperative				
Visual Acuity (logMAR) (mean, SD)	1.24 ± 0.58	1.57 ± 0.45	1.10 ± 0.57	<0.001
Endothelial cell counts (cells/mm^2, SD)	2,819 ± 281	2,704 ± 340	2,865 ± 237	<0.001

PK, penetrating keratoplasty; DSAEK, Descemet's stripping automated endothelial keratoplasty; SD, standard deviation.
*P value from Mann–Whitney test or chi-square test as appropriate.

the recipient with 10-0 nylon, using either 8-bite, 10-0 nylon double continuous running suture or a combination of a single 8-bite 10-0 nylon continuous and 8 interrupted sutures. All DSAEK surgeries were performed using pull-through techniques as previously described (23). Donors were prepared by the surgeon or eye bank technician using an automated lamellar therapeutic keratoplasty system (ALTK, Moria SA, Antony, France). Essentially, after recipient Descemets membrane stripping, insertion of anterior chamber (AC) maintainer and preplaced venting incisions, a DSAEK forceps (ASICO, IL, United States) was used to pull the donor cornea through the scleral incision using a sheets glide (BD Visitec) (23), or a donor inserter device (Endoglide, Network Medical Products, North Yorkshire, United Kingdom) (24). An inferior peripheral iridectomy was performed through a limbal stab incision. Wounds were secured with 10/0 nylon interrupted sutures, and a full air tamponade under slight compression was achieved with a large bubble in the AC for varying periods of time, ranging from 2 to 8 min, while removing interface fluid from the venting incisions. For both PK and DSAEK surgeries a bandage contact lens was placed at the end, and dexamethasone (0.1%) (Merck & Co Inc, Rahway, NJ, United States), gentamicin (14 mg/ml, Schering AG, Berlin-Wedding, Germany), and cefazolin (50 mg/ml, GlaxoSmithKline,

NC, United States) was injected subconjunctivally after all surgeries. All PK and DSAEK patients received a standard post-operative regime: topical antibiotic (levofloxacin 0.5%, Santen, Osaka, Japan) and topical prednisolone acetate ophthalmic suspension 1% (Allergan, Marlow, United Kingdom) three hourly for a month, four times daily for 2 months, which was tapered by one drop per 3 month down to 1 drop per day dosing by one year, and thereafter continued indefinitely.

Statistical Analysis

For the current study, 49 variables from SCTS audit were identified by literature review for their potential relevance to the graft failure, including donor and recipient demographics, clinical data (visual acuity, ocular findings, etc.), and operative data (primary procedure, secondary procedure, donor/recipient sizes, surgical complications, etc.) (**Supplementary Table 1**). We used a RSF machine learning algorithm for multivariate survival analysis to detect important linear, non-linear, and interaction effects among variables (25). These variables were fed into a RSF model consisting of 10,000 trees, where each tree was grown using the log-rank splitting rule on a random sample of 63.2% of the original population by default, with additional RSF parameters (e.g., node size, number of variables to try at each potential split) tuned using a greedy approach to minimize the out-of-bag (OOB) error rate, that is, the error rate using the remaining data not used for model training (25). We then ranked top variables and pair-wise interactions according to their VIMP scores (larger VIMP indicates greater importance for a successful prediction model). Based on VIMP ranking, we then analyzed a sequence of nested Cox regression models using the top 15 variables, among which the model using best variables that achieved the best OOB Harrell C statistic (OOB C-index) will be used. Simply, the OOB C-index is a validation score that estimates the prediction error of random forests (25). Multivariate Cox proportional hazards regression analysis based on this model was used to describe the factors associated with graft failure represented using hazard ratios (HR) and its relative 95% confidence interval (95% CI). Proportional hazard assumption was validated using both individual and global Schoenfeld Test. We used penalized splines from R package survival to assess non-linearity for all continuous variables in the nested Cox regression models. Kaplan–Meier (KM) survival analysis was conducted to compare 10-year survival probabilities of PK and DSAEK groups. Complications were recorded prospectively in our Singapore Cornea Transplant Registry database and represented as a cumulative incidence rate during the follow-up period of 10 years (17). A P-value <0.05 was considered statistically significant. The analysis was conducted using R, version 4.0.2 (R Foundation for Statistical Computing) with the *randomForestSRC* package (26, 27).

RESULTS

We analyzed 1,335 consecutive patients who underwent either PK (389 eyes) or DSAEK (946 eyes) based on our inclusion criteria. Overall mean age was 68 ± 11 years, 47.6% male, in our predominantly Chinese (76.6%) Asian cohort with no significant

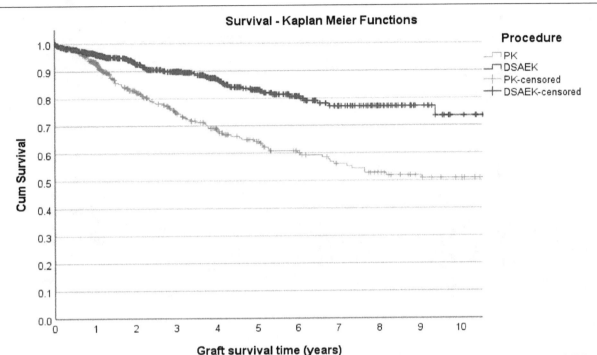

	PK		DSAEK	
Year	N	%	N	%
1	374	93.2%	920	96.2%
2	296	82.5%	700	92.4%
3	199	74.8%	412	89.7%
4	152	68.5%	323	87.0%
5	121	64.3%	224	83.1%
10	51	50.9%	27	73.6%
Kaplan Meier Survival comparing penetrating keratoplasty (PK) with Descemet stripping automated endothelial keratoplasty (DSAEK) log-rank P<0.001				

FIGURE 1 | Kaplan–Meier graft survival curves demonstrated superior 5- and 10-year graft survival comparing Descemet stropping automated endothelial keratoplasty (DSAEK) to penetrating keratoplasty (PK), N = number of grafts analyzed (log-rank P-value < 0.001).

differences in these baseline demographics in our PK and DSAEK groups (**Table 1**). We had a higher proportion of patients with BK compared to FED (62.2 vs. 37.8%, $P < 0.001$) in our study cohort (**Supplementary Table 2**). Five-year cumulative graft survival was superior for DSAEK compared to PK (83.1 vs. 64.3%)—log-rank P value < 0.001; while 10-year cumulative graft survival was superior for DSAEK compared to PK (73.6 vs. 50.9%)—log-rank P value < 0.001 in the remaining surviving grafts ($n = 78$) (**Figure 1**). Sub-group analysis also revealed significantly superior 10-year survival comparing DSAEK to PK in the BK (57.5 vs. 43.1%, $P < 0.001$) and FED (89.2 vs. 68.1%, $P < 0.001$) groups (**Figure 2**).

We ranked top variables and pair-wise interactions according to their VIMP scores (**Figure 3**) to develop a sequence of nested Cox regression models using the top 15 variables, among which we chose the model with the best variables (diagnosis, procedure, gender, pre-operative visual acuity, and donor endothelial cell count) that achieved the highest OOB C-index of 0.701 on 3,000 bootstrap samples. Using likelihood-ratio tests

for nested models, no significant improvement was observed on the model performance after including additional variables (**Supplementary Figure 1**). Multivariate Cox proportional hazards regression was performed for the top VIMP factors identified by the RSF model that achieved the best OOB Harrell C statistic, i.e., diagnosis (surgical indication, i.e., BK or FED), procedure (surgical technique, i.e., PK or DSAEK), gender, pre-operative visual acuity and donor endothelial cell count was performed (**Table 2**). We found that BK was a significant factor associated with graft failure (HR: 2.84 95%CI 1.89–4.26; $P < 0.001$) compared to FED and PK was a significant factor associated with graft failure more likely to fail compared to DSAEK (HR: 1.64 95%CI 1.19–2.27; $P = 0.002$).

Overall, we observed a greater 10-year cumulative incidence of complications in the PK compared to DSAEK group (**Table 3**). Five-year endothelial cell loss was greater in PK compared to DSAEK (67.6 ± 10.7% vs. 53.3 ± 21.0%, $P = 0.011$), as our study was not adequately powered to compare 10-year endothelial cell loss between groups. Complications such as graft rejection

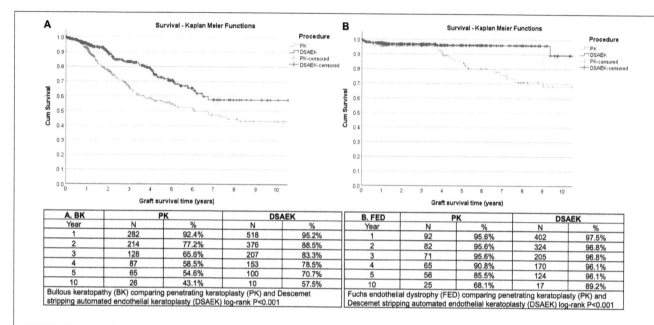

A. BK	PK		DSAEK	
Year	N	%	N	%
1	282	92.4%	518	95.2%
2	214	77.2%	376	88.5%
3	128	65.6%	207	83.3%
4	87	58.5%	153	78.5%
5	65	54.6%	100	70.7%
10	26	43.1%	10	57.5%

Bullous keratopathy (BK) comparing penetrating keratoplasty (PK) and Descemet stripping automated endothelial keratoplasty (DSAEK) log-rank P<0.001

B. FED	PK		DSAEK	
Year	N	%	N	%
1	92	95.6%	402	97.5%
2	82	95.6%	324	96.8%
3	71	95.6%	205	96.8%
4	65	90.8%	170	96.1%
5	56	85.5%	124	96.1%
10	25	68.1%	17	89.2%

Fuchs endothelial dystrophy (FED) comparing penetrating keratoplasty (PK) and Descemet stripping automated endothelial keratoplasty (DSAEK) log-rank P<0.001

FIGURE 2 | Kaplan Meier graft survival curves demonstrated superior 10-year graft survival comparing Descemet stropping automated endothelial keratoplasty (DSAEK) to penetrating keratoplasty (PK) in eyes (N = number of grafts analyzed) with (A) bullous keratopathy (BK, log-rank P < 0.001) and (B) Fuchs endothelial dystrophy (FED, log-rank P < 0.001).

(9.5 vs. 4.2%, $P < 0.001$) and corneal epitheliopathy (11.6 vs. 2.5%, $P < 0.001$) were significantly greater in PK compared to DSAEK. There was a greater incidence of transient intraocular pressure (IOP) elevation (as previously defined, i.e., short-term IOP readings > 21 mmHg with ≤ 3 months use of anti-glaucoma medications) comparing PK and DSAEK (26.0 vs. 20.8%, $P = 0.04$). Complications such as wound dehiscence was unique to PK ($P < 0.001$) and graft detachment was unique to DSAEK ($P < 0.001$).

DISCUSSION

The Singapore Cornea Transplant Registry prospectively collects a large database of variables and outcomes as an audit of multiple surgeons of various surgical experience, practicing with standardized surgical techniques and post-operative management (28). Traditionally, we have used statistical methods such as Kaplan-Meier survival with the log-rank test to analyze graft outcomes, which is only able to examine only one variable at a time (29). While Cox proportional hazards regression analysis can analyze multiple factors associated with graft survival, the various stepwise (e.g., backward or forward) variable selection methods often lead to well-described limitations (30). Random forests is gaining popularity as a machine learning technique that is able to handle big data with more flexibility in modeling non-linear effects with interactions, for regression and prediction tasks (15, 16). In this current study, we used a RSF model that enabled us to analyze a large number of variables to determine high-importance values, and derive a model with improved prediction performance (OOB C-index of 0.701, compared to traditional Cox regression modeling OOB

C-index of 0.576–0.686) (**Supplementary Figure 1**). However, the advantages of using a machine learning model may come at a cost when it comes to clinical interpretation, due to the complexity of the ensemble tree learning methods. Thus, we presented our results combining features of the robust decision tree ensemble from the random forest, with elements of a Cox proportional hazards regression to explain the factors associated with graft failure in our study (31).

Based on this RSF technique, we found that PK was almost twice as more likely to fail in 10 years compared to DSAEK in the treatment of corneal endothelial diseases, i.e., bullous keratopathy (BK) and Fuchs dystrophy (FED) in our study cohort. Similar to previous studies (32, 33), our 10-year graft survival was superior in DSAEK compared to PK in eyes with BK (57.5 vs. 43.1%, $P < 0.001$) and FED (89.2 vs. 68.1%, $P < 0.001$). These long-term graft survival results reflect the higher proportion of BK compared in FED in our Asian population, as BK was almost three times more likely to be associated with graft failure compared to FED, and BK has been shown to have poorer outcomes in both PK (34–36) and DSAEK (37–39). Another advantage of using the RSF is the ability to examine non-linear associations between various factors and graft failure. A Cox proportional hazards regression analysis assumes a linear relationship between any continuous predictors and an outcome, i.e., graft failure, and thus donor endothelial cell count was not a significant factor (HR: 1.0, $P = 0.171$) after adjusting for other variables. However, the RSF describes a closely associated but non-linear relationship between the donor endothelial cell count and 10-year graft survival in both PK and DSAEK (**Supplementary Figure 2**).

The RSF analysis also identified recipient gender as an important factor, with the multivariate Cox regression

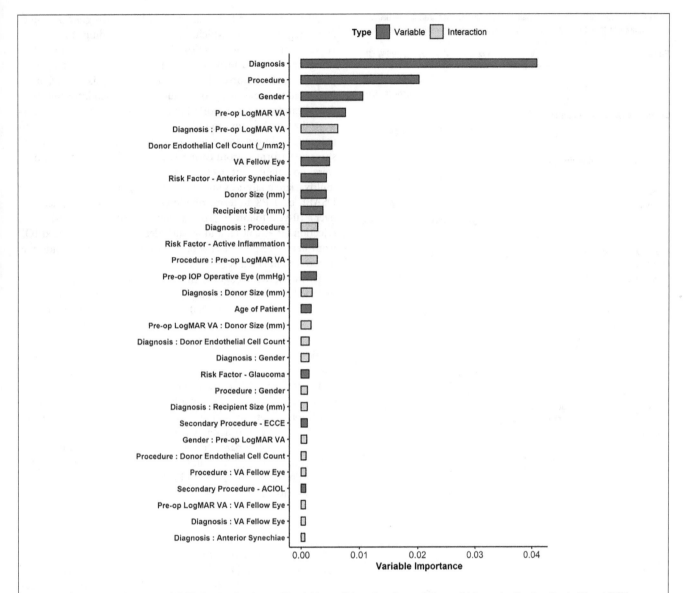

FIGURE 3 | The variable importance (VIMP) plot showing the top 30 variables and interactions for predicting graft failure using Random Survival Forest (RSF) machine learning algorithm. The VIMP score for each candidate variable calculates the difference between the original OOB error rate and the rate after permuting variable values, while VIMP for pair-wise interaction measures the difference between the sum of paired VIMP scores and the VIMP permuting two variables simultaneously. Top-ranked interactions highlight the association between variable pairs that is important for successful prediction in the model.

demonstrating that male recipients and those with poorer pre-operative visual acuity are associated with graft failure. A sub-group multivariate Cox regression analysis of our study cohort comparing gender-recipient matched and unmatched subjects revealed a higher risk of 10-year graft failure amongst the gender unmatched (HR: 1.57 95%CI 1.06–2.33, $P = 0.024$) in the PK group but not in the DSAEK group (HR: 0.82 95%CI 0.53–1.276, $P = 0.382$) (**Supplementary Table 3**). While this observation is consistent with previous large studies on gender matching in penetrating keratoplasty (40), we found male recipients to be still an independent factor associated with 10-year graft failure in the multivariate model, which requires further study. A poor pre-operative visual acuity may suggest

presence of more severe corneal decompensation with edema, or underlying factors such as glaucoma or inflammation that could lead to a higher risk of graft failure (41). Our RSF machine learning technique took into account these possible confounders to suggest that poor pre-operative visual acuity was an important, independent factor associated with graft failure. This has useful clinical implications as we may use this as a potential surrogate to counsel patients for risk of graft failure based on their pre-morbid visual acuity and ocular condition.

There are currently few studies that have reported 10-year outcomes of DSAEK, and to our knowledge, no reports that directly compare 10-year outcomes and complication rates of DSAEK to PK from the same study cohort. Moreover,

TABLE 2 | Hazard ratios for factors associated with 10-year graft failure using random survival forest to determine optimal multivariate regression model.

Factors	N* (n = 1,283)	Hazard ratio	P > |z|	95% CI Lower	95% CI Upper
Diagnosis/Surgical indication					
BK	791	2.838	<0.001	1.892	4.259
FED	492				
Procedure/surgical technique					
PK	368	1.643	0.002	1.192	2.265
DSAEK	915				
Gender					
Male	608	1.751	<0.001	1.308	2.344
Female	675				
Pre-operative visual acuity (logMAR)**	1,283	1.601	0.005	1.154	2.220
Donor endothelial cell count**	1,283	1.000	0.171	0.999	1.000

*N = 1283 after excluding 52 subjects who did not have pre-operative visual acuity data available.
**For continuous variables, but linear and non-linear associations were also assessed using penalized splines.
BK, bullous keratopathy; FED, Fuchs endothelial dystrophy; PK, penetrating keratoplasty; DSAEK, Descemet stripping automated endothelial keratoplasty.

TABLE 3 | Ten-year cumulative incidence of complications comparing Descemet stripping automated endothelial keratoplasty (DSAEK) and penetrating keratoplasty (PK) in our study cohort.

*Complications	Cumulative incidence (%) ± 95%CI PK	DSAEK	P value
Transient elevated IOP (>21 mmHg)	26.0 (21.7–30.6)	20.8 (18.3–23.6)	0.040
Late graft failure	12.3 (9.2–16.0)	4.5 (3.3–6.1)	<0.001
Epithelial problems	11.6 (8.6–15.2)	2.5 (1.6–3.8)	<0.001
Graft rejection episode	9.5 (6.8–12.9)	4.2 (3.0–5.7)	<0.001
Primary graft failure	2.3 (1.1–4.3)	1.8 (1.1–2.9)	0.535
Anterior synechiae	2.3 (1.1–4.3)	1.4 (0.7–2.3)	0.221
Microbial keratitis	2.1 (0.9–4.0)	1.3 (0.7–2.2)	0.281
Wound dehiscence	2.1 (0.9–4.0)	0 (0–0.4)	<0.001
Cytomegalovirus infection	1.3 (0.4–3.0)	1.4 (0.7–2.3)	0.898
Herpes simplex virus infection	1.0 (0.3–2.6)	0.8 (0.4–1.7)	0.754
Endophthalmitis	0.5 (0.1–1.8)	0.2 (0–0.8)	0.585
Graft detachment	0 (0–0.9)	3.5 (2.4–4.9)	<0.001

PK, penetrating keratoplasty; DSAEK, Descemet's stripping automated endothelial keratoplasty; SD, standard deviation; IOP, intraocular pressure.
*Complications as recorded in our prospective Singapore Corneal Transplant Registry database.

our study used a relatively novel machine learning analysis technique to study a large number of variables while accounting for interactions and non-linear associations with a better prediction compared to traditional model development methods.

Another strength is the availability of long-term graft outcomes from registry data, which can vary according to surgeon versus center experience as surgical outcomes are improved by using standardized techniques and post-operative management protocols (42). Compared to a *post hoc* re-analysis of the Cornea Preservation Time Study to specifically examined intra-operative complications, it was reported that surgeon and eye bank factors were the top 2 factors found to be important predictor of graft failure (16). In our study, we found that surgeon experience and surgery performed from earlier years (based on year performed) were not significant factors associated with graft failure on multivariate analysis. Our study also supports the advantages of DSAEK over PK in terms of a lower incidence of complications over a 10-year follow-up, such as epitheliopathy (P < 0.001), graft rejection (P < 0.001), and as such, less incidence of raised IOP from steroid response as the need for post-operative steroids may be reduced in DSAEK (P = 0.04).

However, we recognize the limitations of our study which included the transition of surgical techniques from PK to DSAEK that was introduced in 2006 onward, and the reduction in number of follow-ups at 10 years. We discussed the effect of surgical experience and patient selection in our previous studies, which was mitigated by our standardized protocols and surgical techniques. Thus, we only selected primary grafts for specific corneal endothelial diseases, i.e., Fuchs dystrophy or bullous keratopathy, and previously detailed the transition of proportion of PK toward DSAEK in our study cohort (8). We also acknowledge the differences in our study demographics compared to other reports, in our predominantly Asian population with shallow anterior chambers and a higher proportion of BK compared to FED (5). Despite these limitations common to most registry studies, we believe that our results provide additional evidence to support the trend toward selective lamellar keratoplasty for endothelial diseases. We also recognize the limitations of the RSF analysis used in our study—for example, potentially favoring continuous variables that have more split points (43). Nonetheless, our RSF model selected categorical variables, which further validated these factors' significance to graft failure. The use of other algorithms such as conditional inference forest may help generate more accurate VIMP scores (43); however, we highlight that the RSF analysis merely serves as a complementary technique to the traditional Cox regression model.

In summary, our study provides long-term graft survival outcomes and cumulative incidence of complications, highlighting the advantages of DSAEK over PK in the treatment of end-stage corneal endothelial decompensation in Asian eyes. We used machine learning techniques to analyze the large registry database collected over a 10-year audit to determine the most important factors associated with graft failure, and used these factors to derive the optimal model for multivariate analysis, which was superior to traditional techniques. A combination of predictive (machine learning) and explanatory (regression) modeling may be a useful way of analyzing large registry datasets to examine cornea graft survival and factors associated with graft failure in future studies, which may then be used to develop a risk prediction model.

AUTHOR CONTRIBUTIONS

All authors contributed significantly to the development of the study, analysis, and manuscript preparation.

SUPPLEMENTARY MATERIAL

Supplementary Figure 1 | Boxplot showing the out of bag (OOB) Harrell C Statistic (C-index) of nested models using top variables identified by VIMP.

Forward and backward step-wise multivariate Cox regression modeling only achieved OOB C-index of 0.576–0.686 (based on age, gender, race, diagnosis, surgery, glaucoma, donor age).

Supplementary Figure 2 | Partial dependence plot showing the adjusted non-linear association between donor endothelial cell count and 10-year graft survival comparing Descemet stripping automated endothelial keratoplasty (DSAEK) and penetrating keratoplasty (PK).

REFERENCES

1. Gain P, Jullienne R, He Z, Aldossary M, Acquart S, Cognasse F, et al. Global survey of corneal transplantation and eye banking. *JAMA Ophthalmol.* (2016) 134:167–73. doi: 10.1001/jamaophthalmol.2015.4776

2. Ong HS, Ang M, Mehta JS. Evolution of therapies for the corneal endothelium: past, present and future approaches. *Br J Ophthalmol.* (2020) 105:454–67. doi: 10.1136/bjophthalmol-2020-316149

3. Park CY, Lee JK, Gore PK, Lim CY, Chuck RS. Keratoplasty in the United States: a 10-year review from 2005 through 2014. *Ophthalmology.* (2015) 122:2432–42. doi: 10.1016/j.ophtha.2015.08.017

4. Mathews PM, Lindsley K, Aldave AJ, Akpek EK. Etiology of global corneal blindness and current practices of corneal transplantation: a focused review. *Cornea.* (2018) 37:1198–203. doi: 10.1097/ICO.0000000000001666

5. Bose S, Ang M, Mehta JS, Tan DT, Finkelstein E. Cost-effectiveness of Descemet's stripping endothelial keratoplasty versus penetrating keratoplasty. *Ophthalmology.* (2013) 120:464–70. doi: 10.1016/j.ophtha.2012.08.024

6. Lee WB, Jacobs DS, Musch DC, Kaufman SC, Reinhart WJ, Shtein RM. Descemet's stripping endothelial keratoplasty: safety and outcomes: a report by the American academy of ophthalmology. *Ophthalmology.* (2009) 116:1818–30. doi: 10.1016/j.ophtha.2009.06.021

7. Ang M, Lim F, Htoon HM, Tan D, Mehta JS. Visual acuity and contrast sensitivity following Descemet stripping automated endothelial keratoplasty. *Br J Ophthalmol.* (2016) 100:307–11. doi: 10.1136/bjophthalmol-2015-306975

8. Tan D, Ang M, Arundhati A, Khor WB. Development of selective lamellar keratoplasty within an Asian corneal transplant program: the Singapore corneal transplant study (an American ophthalmological society thesis). *Trans Am Ophthalmol Soc.* (2015) 113:T10.

9. Williams K, Keane M, Galettis R, Jones V, Mills R, Coster D. *The Australian Corneal Graft Registry – 2015 Report.* Adelaide, SA: Flinders University (2015).

10. Dickman MM, Peeters JM, van den Biggelaar FJ, Ambergen TA, van Dongen MC, Kruit PJ, et al. Changing practice patterns and long-term outcomes of endothelial versus penetrating keratoplasty: a prospective dutch registry study. *Am J Ophthalmol.* (2016) 170:133–42. doi: 10.1016/j.ajo.2016.07.024

11. Greenrod EB, Jones MN, Kaye S, Larkin DF, National Health Service Blood and Transplant Ocular Tissue Advisory Group and Contributing Ophthalmologists (Ocular Tissue Advisory Group Audit Study 16). Center and surgeon effect on outcomes of endothelial keratoplasty versus penetrating keratoplasty in the United Kingdom. *Am J Ophthalmol.* (2014) 158:957–66.

12. Coster DJ, Lowe MT, Keane MC, Williams KA, Australian Corneal Graft Registry Contributors. A comparison of lamellar and penetrating keratoplasty outcomes: a registry study. *Ophthalmology.* (2014) 121:979–87.

13. Fajgenbaum MA, Hollick EJ. Center and surgeon effect on outcomes of endothelial keratoplasty versus penetrating keratoplasty in the United Kingdom. *Am J Ophthalmol.* (2015) 160:392–3.

14. Patel SV, Armitage WJ, Claesson M. Keratoplasty outcomes: are we making advances? *Ophthalmology.* (2014) 121:977–8. doi: 10.1016/j.ophtha.2014.01.029

15. Hallak JA. A machine learning Model with survival statistics to identify predictors of Descemet stripping automated endothelial keratoplasty graft failure. *JAMA Ophthalmol.* (2021) 139:198–9. doi: 10.1001/jamaophthalmol.2020.5741

16. O'Brien RC, Ishwaran H, Szczotka-Flynn LB, Lass JH, Cornea Preservation Time Study (CPTS) Group. Random survival forests analysis of intraoperative complications as predictors of Descemet stripping automated endothelial keratoplasty graft failure in the cornea preservation time study. *JAMA Ophthalmol.* (2021) 139:191–7. doi: 10.1001/jamaophthalmol.2020.5743

17. Tan DT, Janardhanan P, Zhou H, Chan YH, Htoon HM, Ang LP, et al. Penetrating keratoplasty in Asian eyes: the Singapore corneal transplant study. *Ophthalmology.* (2008) 115:975–82.e1. doi: 10.1016/j.ophtha.2007.08.049

18. Ang M, Mehta JS, Lim F, Bose S, Htoon HM, Tan D. Endothelial cell loss and graft survival after Descemet's stripping automated endothelial keratoplasty and penetrating keratoplasty. *Ophthalmology.* (2012) 119:2239–44. doi: 10.1016/j.ophtha.2012.06.012

19. Ang M, Ho H, Wong C, Htoon HM, Mehta JS, Tan D. Endothelial keratoplasty after failed penetrating keratoplasty: an alternative to repeat penetrating keratoplasty. *Am J Ophthalmol.* (2014) 158:1221–7.e1. doi: 10.1016/j.ajo.2014.08.024

20. Ang M, Mehta JS, Sng CC, Htoon HM, Tan DT. Indications, outcomes, and risk factors for failure in tectonic keratoplasty. *Ophthalmology.* (2012) 119:1311–9. doi: 10.1016/j.ophtha.2012.01.021

21. Ang M, Htoon HM, Cajucom-Uy HY, Tan D, Mehta JS. Donor and surgical risk factors for primary graft failure following Descemet's stripping automated endothelial keratoplasty in Asian eyes. *Clin Ophthalmol.* (2011) 5:1503–8. doi: 10.2147/OPTH.S25973

22. Ang M, Mehta JS, Anshu A, Wong HK, Htoon HM, Tan D. Endothelial cell counts after Descemet's stripping automated endothelial keratoplasty versus penetrating keratoplasty in Asian eyes. *Clin Ophthalmol.* (2012) 6:537–44. doi: 10.2147/OPTH.S26343

23. Ang M, Saroj L, Htoon HM, Kiew S, Mehta JS, Tan D. Comparison of a donor insertion device to sheets glide in Descemet stripping endothelial keratoplasty: 3-year outcomes. *Am J Ophthalmol.* (2014) 157:1163–9.e3. doi: 10.1016/j.ajo.2014.02.049

24. Khor WB, Han SB, Mehta JS, Tan DT. Descemet stripping automated endothelial keratoplasty with a donor insertion device: clinical results and complications in 100 eyes. *Am J Ophthalmol.* (2013) 156:773–9. doi: 10.1016/j.ajo.2013.05.012

25. Ishwaran H, Kogalur UB, Blackstone EH, Lauer MS. Random survival forests. *Ann Appl Stat.* (2008) 2:841–60.

26. R Core Team. *R: A Language and Environment for Statistical Computing.* Vienna: R Foundation for Statistical Computing (2013).

27. Ishwaran H, Kogalur UB, Kogalur MUB. *Package 'randomForestSRC'.* (2021).

28. Woo JH, Ang M, Htoon HM, Tan D. Descemet membrane endothelial keratoplasty versus Descemet stripping automated endothelial keratoplasty and penetrating keratoplasty. *Am J Ophthalmol.* (2019) 207:288–303. doi: 10.1016/j.ajo.2019.06.012

29. Ang M, Soh Y, Htoon HM, Mehta JS, Tan D. Five-year graft survival comparing Descemet stripping automated endothelial keratoplasty and penetrating keratoplasty. *Ophthalmology.* (2016) 123:1646–52. doi: 10.1016/j.ophtha.2016.04.049

30. Wiegand RE. Performance of using multiple stepwise algorithms for variable selection. *Stat Med.* (2010) 29:1647–59.

31. Ishwaran H, Kogalur UB. Consistency of random survival forests. *Stat Probab Lett.* (2010) 80:1056–64. doi: 10.1016/j.spl.2010.02.020

32. Price MO, Fairchild KM, Price DA, Price FW Jr. Descemet's stripping endothelial keratoplasty five-year graft survival and endothelial cell loss. *Ophthalmology.* (2011) 118:725–9. doi: 10.1016/j.ophtha.2010.08.012

33. Writing Committee for the Cornea Donor Study Research Group, Mannis MJ, Holland EJ, Gal RL, Dontchev M, Kollman C, et al. The effect of donor age on penetrating keratoplasty for endothelial disease: graft survival after 10 years in the cornea donor study. *Ophthalmology.* (2013) 120:2419–27. doi: 10.1016/j.ophtha.2013.08.026

34. Writing Committee for the Cornea Donor Study Research Group, Sugar A, Gal RL, Kollman C, Raghinaru D, Dontchev M, et al. Factors associated with corneal graft survival in the cornea donor study. *JAMA Ophthalmol.* (2015) 133:246–54. doi: 10.1001/jamaophthalmol.2014.3923

35. Dandona L, Naduvilath TJ, Janarthanan M, Ragu K, Rao GN. Survival analysis and visual outcome in a large series of corneal transplants in India. *Br J Ophthalmol.* (1997) 81:726–31. doi: 10.1136/bjo.81.9.726

36. Anshu A, Li L, Htoon HM, de Benito-Llopis L, Shuang LS, Singh MJ, et al. Long-term review of penetrating keratoplasty: a 20-year review in Asian eyes. *Am J Ophthalmol.* (2021) 224:254–66. doi: 10.1016/j.ajo.2020.10.014

37. Price DA, Kelley M, Price FW Jr, Price MO. Five-year graft survival of Descemet membrane endothelial keratoplasty (EK) versus Descemet stripping EK and the effect of donor sex matching. *Ophthalmology.* (2018) 125:1508–14. doi: 10.1016/j.ophtha.2018.03.050

38. Wacker K, Baratz KH, Maguire LJ, McLaren JW, Patel SV. Descemet stripping endothelial keratoplasty for fuchs' endothelial corneal dystrophy: five-year results of a prospective study. *Ophthalmology.* (2016) 123:154–60. doi: 10.1016/j.ophtha.2015.09.023

39. Fajgenbaum MA, Hollick EJ. Modeling endothelial cell loss after Descemet stripping endothelial keratoplasty: data from 5 years of follow-up. *Cornea.* (2017) 36:553–60. doi: 10.1097/ICO.0000000000001177

40. Hopkinson CL, Romano V, Kaye RA, Steger B, Stewart RM, Tsagkataki M, et al. The influence of donor and recipient gender incompatibility on corneal transplant rejection and failure. *Am J Transplant.* (2017) 17:210–7. doi: 10.1111/ajt.13926

41. Fuest M, Ang M, Htoon HM, Tan D, Mehta JS. Long-term visual outcomes comparing Descemet stripping automated endothelial keratoplasty and penetrating keratoplasty. *Am J Ophthalmol.* (2017) 182:62–71. doi: 10.1016/j.ajo.2017.07.014

42. Baydoun L, Liarakos VS, Dapena I, Melles GR. Re: Coster et al.: a comparison of lamellar and penetrating keratoplasty outcomes (Ophthalmology 2014;121:979-87). *Ophthalmology.* (2014) 121:e61–2. doi: 10.1016/j.ophtha.2013.12.017

43. Nasejje JB, Mwambi H, Dheda K, Lesosky M. A comparison of the conditional inference survival forest model to random survival forests based on a simulation study as well as on two applications with time-to-event data. *BMC Med Res Methodol.* (2017) 17:115. doi: 10.1186/s12874-017-0383-8

17

Considerations for Polymers used in Ocular Drug Delivery

Megan M. Allyn[1], Richard H. Luo[2], Elle B. Hellwarth[2] and Katelyn E. Swindle-Reilly[1,2,3]*

[1] William G. Lowrie Department of Chemical and Biomolecular Engineering, The Ohio State University, Columbus, OH, United States, [2] Department of Biomedical Engineering, The Ohio State University, Columbus, OH, United States, [3] Department of Ophthalmology and Visual Sciences, The Ohio State University, Columbus, OH, United States

Purpose: Age-related eye diseases are becoming more prevalent. A notable increase has been seen in the most common causes including glaucoma, age-related macular degeneration (AMD), and cataract. Current clinical treatments vary from tissue replacement with polymers to topical eye drops and intravitreal injections. Research and development efforts have increased using polymers for sustained release to the eye to overcome treatment challenges, showing promise in improving drug release and delivery, patient experience, and treatment compliance. Polymers provide unique properties that allow for specific engineered devices to provide improved treatment options. Recent work has shown the utilization of synthetic and biopolymer derived biomaterials in various forms, with this review containing a focus on polymers Food and Drug Administration (FDA) approved for ocular use.

Methods: This provides an overview of some prevalent synthetic polymers and biopolymers used in ocular delivery and their benefits, brief discussion of the various types and synthesis methods used, and administration techniques. Polymers approved by the FDA for different applications in the eye are listed and compared to new polymers being explored in the literature. This article summarizes research findings using polymers for ocular drug delivery from various stages: laboratory, preclinical studies, clinical trials, and currently approved. This review also focuses on some of the challenges to bringing these new innovations to the clinic, including limited selection of approved polymers.

Results: Polymers help improve drug delivery by increasing solubility, controlling pharmacokinetics, and extending release. Several polymer classes including synthetic, biopolymer, and combinations were discussed along with the benefits and challenges of each class. The ways both polymer synthesis and processing techniques can influence drug release in the eye were discussed.

Conclusion: The use of biomaterials, specifically polymers, is a well-studied field for drug delivery, and polymers have been used as implants in the eye for over 75 years. Promising new ocular drug delivery systems are emerging using polymers an innovative option for treating ocular diseases because of their tunable properties. This review touches on important considerations and challenges of using polymers for sustained ocular drug delivery with the goal translating research to the clinic.

Keywords: drug delivery, polymer, hydrogel, ophthalmic delivery, ocular implants, controlled release, ocular biomaterials

Correspondence:
Katelyn E. Swindle-Reilly
reilly.198@osu.edu

INTRODUCTION

In 2020, the World Health Organization reported 196 million cases of age-related macular degeneration (AMD), 146 million cases of diabetic retinopathy (DR), 76 million cases of glaucoma, and 65 million cases of cataract globally (1). Nearly 44 million people in the United States (US) over the age of 40 are afflicted by some form of eye disease, with 2010 National Eye Institute statistics showing 24 million cataract cases, 11 million early and late stage AMD cases, 7 million DR cases, and 2 million glaucoma cases (2–4). While each disease has unique causes, symptoms, and treatments, all will result in complete vision loss if left untreated. Difficulties in ocular drug delivery stem from the complex anatomy of the eye, its compartmentalization, and its separation from the rest of the body.

Ocular anatomy is generally classified into two segments: the anterior segment comprised of the iris, cornea, lens, and surrounding aqueous humor; and the posterior segment including the vitreous humor, retina, macula, and optic nerve (5). Cataract and glaucoma impact the lens and fluid drainage pathways, respectively, in the anterior segment. The lens is responsible for accommodation, or fine focusing of light to produce vision. The proteins within the lens work to manage absorbed UV light to maintain the oxidative balance necessary for proper function. With age, the ability of the lens to mitigate oxidative damage and repair cellular damage diminishes, causing protein aggregation, lens opacities, and eventual vision loss due to cataract (6). Though not yet fully understood, it is believed that glaucoma develops when anterior fluid drainage systems based in the trabecular meshwork and uveoscleral outflow pathway become imbalanced (7). Impaired drainage causes an increase in intraocular pressure (IOP) that applies stress on anterior and posterior segments of the eye. Increased posterior IOP can subject the lamina cribrosa to conformational changes that inhibit axonal signal transportation to the optic nerve, resulting in retinal ganglion cell death and vision loss (7). This increased IOP has been theorized to also impact the cornea and corneal endothelium. In patients with angle-closure glaucoma, high IOP was found to cause up to an 11% decrease in endothelial cell density (8). Other common anterior segment disorders affecting the cornea include dry eye disease, corneal neovascularization, anterior uveitis, and keratitis.

Visual disorders affecting the posterior segment include retinal diseases such as AMD, non-proliferative and proliferative diabetic retinopathy (PDR), diabetic macular edema (DME), and posterior conjunctivitis. These present additional difficulties in treatment due to limited accessibility of disease sites and complexity of disease progression. In AMD, disease propagation occurs from an increased inflammatory environment caused by accumulation of reactive oxygen species (ROS) within the retina that leads to protein aggregation and drusen formation. This signals a local over-production of vascular endothelial growth factor (VEGF) that leads to abnormal blood vessel growth, permanently impacting the retinal pigment epithelium (RPE), leading to late stage "wet" AMD (9, 10). Posterior segment diseases resulting from diabetes stem from increased levels of glucose in the bloodstream that cause pericyte apoptosis,

outpouching of the capillaries, and the eventual development of microaneurysms. Hyperglycemic oxidative stress and chronic inflammation stimulate the expression of signaling cytokines that increase the permeability of the endothelium to VEGF, resulting in neovascularization, breakdown of the blood-retinal barrier (BRB), and neuronal degradation (11, 12).

Approved therapeutics for treatment of ocular diseases include steroids such as hydrocortisone, triamcinolone acetonide, fluocinolone, and dexamethasone; antibiotics such as fluoroquinolones, tetracyclines, and aminoglycosides; and biological pharmaceuticals such as anti-VEGFs. Experimental therapeutics currently being investigated include antioxidants such as glutathione and ascorbic acid, complement factor inhibitors such as avacincaptad pegol and APL-2, and novel therapeutic mechanisms such as mesenchymal stem cell extracellular vesicles, miotic based eye drops, viral vectors for gene therapy, and adenosine receptors (13–18).

Local delivery is often a necessity in the eye due to the BRB. However, direct administration through eye drops, subconjunctival injection, or intravitreal injection provide only short-term relief and require frequent administration, with outcomes heavily relying on patient compliance (19). Newly emerging ocular drug delivery technology has focused on the use of polymeric biomaterials to address the present obstacles within the field. Several current treatments rely on polymers to extend release duration in the eye, and extensive research is being conducted with current and investigational therapeutics to reduce application frequency.

In this review, a polymeric biomaterial is defined as large macromolecule composed of building blocks being applied in a biomedical application. These building blocks can be composed of synthetic monomers and/or natural components such as amino acids or sugars. These building blocks, in addition to polymer processing techniques, provide tunable chemical and physical characteristics to improve drug delivery and/or dosing of the therapeutic. Polymers are currently being used clinically to increase solubility of a drug in the target environment, control release rates of therapeutics, and improve drug retention within the eye (5, 20). The variety of polymers available to be used in drug delivery are vast but generally fall into two categories: synthetic polymers or biopolymers. The differences, benefits, and specific uses for both types are summarized below.

SYNTHETIC POLYMERIC BIOMATERIALS

Synthetic polymers are based on chemically derived monomers and provide a plethora of mechanical, chemical, and degradation options when utilized for ocular drug delivery applications. Notable synthetic polymers that are US Food and Drug Administration (FDA) approved for ocular applications and in clinical use include poly(ethylene glycol) (PEG), poly(vinyl alcohol) (PVA), poly(glycolic acid) (PGA), poly(lactic-co-glycolic acid) (PLGA), poly[2-(dimethylamino)ethyl methacrylate] (DMAEM), poly(caprolactone) (PCL), poly(acrylic acid) (PAA), and poly(amidoamine) (PAMAM), but many other polymers are available for experimental use or have been approved for use in different applications outside the eye. Monomers used to synthesize most of the synthetic polymers of interest are shown in **Figure 1**.

Polyethylene Oxides

PEG is a clear, colorless hydrophilic polymer based on ethylene oxide monomers that can increase the biocompatibility, solubility, and bioavailability of incorporated therapeutics. PEG is available in many forms (liquid, solid), molecular weights, configurations (e.g., linear vs. multi-armed), and activities (e.g., bioinert, tetrafunctional). It is generally regarded as safe (GRAS) by the FDA and is approved for many applications including ophthalmic use. Macugen® is a PEGylated oligoribonucleotide, approved for use in 2004, that possesses a high binding affinity for VEGFs and is an injectable treatment for late stage AMD (21, 22). Shorter term implants such as Dextenza®, a PEG-based cylindrical implant, utilize the controlled release properties of PEG by slowing hydrolytic erosion to provide 1 month of dexamethasone release for both inflammation and pain management after surgery. The device is implanted through intracanalicular insertion, has been FDA approved since 2018 for its indicated use, and is currently in phase 3 clinical trials for treatment of allergic conjunctivits (23). Additional products from Ocular Therapeutix, such as their dexamethasone intracanalicular ophthalmic insert (OTX-DED) and tyrosine kinase inhibitor (OTX-TKI), use PEG. OTX-DED is a smaller dose, shorter duration therapeutic based on the same PEG technology as Dextenza® for delivering dexamethasone (24). The implant is an intracanalicular insert that is currently in phase 2 clinical trials for treatment of dry eye disease (24). OTX-TKI is an *in situ* forming injectable PEG hydrogel for sustained release of axitinib for treatment of wet AMD. The implant was developed to provide therapeutic for up to 12 months and is currently in phase 1 clinical trials (25). Topically applied ReSure® sealant by Ocular Therapeutix is a *in situ* forming PEG hydrogel used to prevent wound leakage after cataract surgery (26). Experimental work done by Foroutan et al. (27) and Hussein et al. (28) confirms that incorporation of PEG units or PEGylation increases the bioavailability and corneal absorption of topically applied steroids by steric hinderance of hydrolytic enzymes and enhanced adherence to the subconjunctiva, reducing drug loss during tear clearance. In intravitreal injections, PEGylation has shown to improve the half-life of hydrophobic therapeutics in the vitreous, allowing for a longer, more effective targeting to the posterior of the eye (29). Further experimental work was completed by Lakhani et al. (30) and showed the incorporation of PEG in nanostructured lipid carriers helped to solubilize amphotericin B, an effective anti-mycotic compound for topical treatment of ocular fungal infections (30). PEG is currently used clinically, in clinical trials, and being investigated for both delivery systems and PEGylation of therapeutics.

Polyvinyl Alcohols

PVA is a water soluble, biodegradable polymer often used for solubilizing hydrophobic drugs, providing chemical resistivity and ease of processing (31). Variations in synthesis methods allow PVA to be obtained in a range of hydration states and

molecular weights (31). PVA's polymer structure provides tunable permeability for controlled release applications. It is on the FDA GRAS list and is currently employed in several nondegradable implants used in the eye, including Vitrasert®, Retisert®, and Iluvien®. Vitrasert® was the first FDA approved PVA and ethylene-vinyl acetate (EVA) copolymer implant for intravitreal treatment of cytomegalovirus retinitis, providing 6–8 months of therapeutic dosing through passive diffusive release from the implant (32). Retisert® is a multi-layered implant that uses a permeable PVA outer layer to provide controlled release of fluocinolone acetonide for up to 2.5 years for treatment of non-infectious posterior uveitis (32, 33). Iluvien® was recently FDA approved for treatment of DME, and the delivery technology is in clinical trials for treatment of additional ocular conditions such as wet AMD. The PVA-based implant provides controlled release of fluocinolone acetonide to the vitreous chamber for up to 36 months (34–36). While similar in composition and eluted therapeutic to Retisert®, implantation of Iluvien® can be completed in out-patient facilities due to its smaller size, reducing surgical risks (37). Yutiq® is another recently approved polyimide/PVA implant for controlled release of fluocinolone acetonide, improving not only on the administration method of both Retisert® and Iluvien®, but also on the ability to treat uveitis (38). PVA is also being evaluated for topical ocular drug delivery through wafers (39).

Polyesters

PGA, PLA, and PLGA are the most common synthetic polymers in drug delivery vehicles used to treat ocular diseases and are FDA approved for ocular use. These hydrophobic polyesters provide tunable *in vivo* biodegradation based on the monomer ratio incorporated in the polymer, and have seen usage as drug carriers for small molecules, proteins, and genes (40). PLA and PGA are composed of naturally sourced lactic acid and glycolic acid monomers; both are synthesized through ring-opening polymerization (41). Due to its susceptibility to hydrolysis, PGA has a faster degradation rate compared to PLA, which has an *in vivo* biodegradation rate of up to 2 years, but biodegradation of both polymers produces non-toxic byproducts (42). PLA has high thermal stability and can be formed by many methods, i.e., injection molding and extrusion (42). PGA is brittle and insoluble in common organic solvents, thus limiting its processing as a standalone polymer; however, it is often used in conjunction with other polymers. Utilization of PLA's slow biodegradation rate can be seen in Brimo DDS®, an intravitreal implant containing PLA for slow release of brimonidine for treatment of geographic atrophy which has completed phase 2 clinical trials (43).

PGA and PLA are often co-polymerized to produce PLGA, which offers tunable monomer ratios and end groups that alter biodegradation profiles. Implementation of PLGA for ocular drug delivery vehicles is aimed at controlling the release of therapeutic through tunable polymer properties and improving biocompatibility and bioavailability. Altering the ratios of PGA and PLA also allows for optimization of degradation time, degrees of crystallinity, and hydrophobicity (44). Incorporation of a hydrophobic polymer can allow for selective permeation across mucus membranes if applied

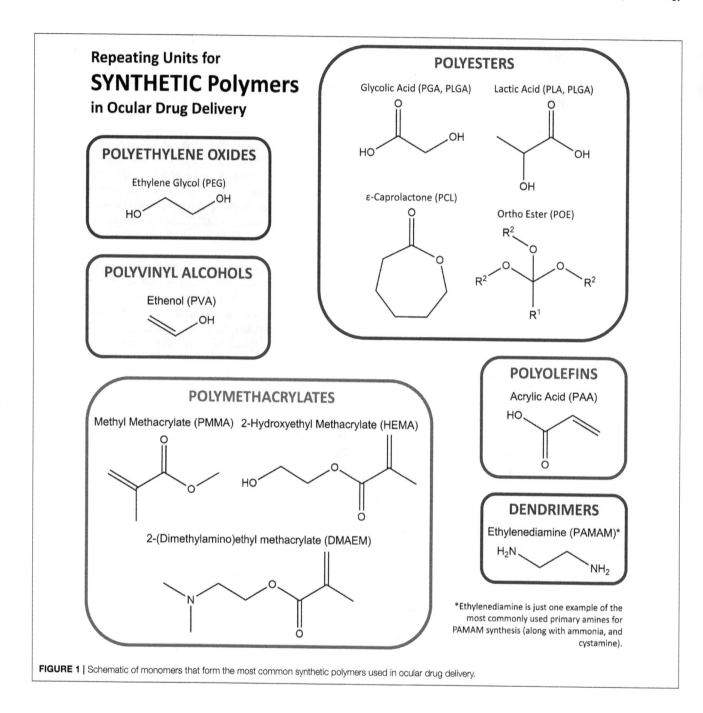

FIGURE 1 | Schematic of monomers that form the most common synthetic polymers used in ocular drug delivery.

topically, or, if administered intravitreally, can work to minimize diffusion of therapeutic away from the target region and slow release. These degradation characteristics make PLGA one of the most common biomaterials found in approved polymeric ocular drug delivery vehicles. However, there have been challenges with some PLGA-based systems due to acidic degradation byproducts (44, 45). Ozurdex® is an FDA approved PLGA-based intravitreal implant used for extended release of dexamethasone in treatment of retinal vein occlusion, non-infectious posterior uveitis, and DME. The implant is co-extruded with dexamethasone to provide controlled release for

4–6 months and degrades entirely *in vivo* (46, 47). PLGA-based implant Durysta® has been recently approved for controlling IOP in patients with open angle glaucoma. A schematic of the implant applicator and location shown in **Figure 2**. The implant provides controlled release of the prostaglandin analog bimatoprost, lowering IOP for 4–6 months (48). Beyond these biodegradable implants, PLGA is currently being investigated for use in hydrogel, microparticle, and nanoparticle delivery systems. There have been several promising preclinical studies evaluating an intravitreal biodegradable system with PLGA microspheres embedded in a hydrogel for delivery of biologics for treatment

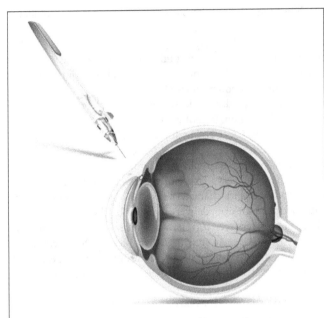

FIGURE 2 | Schematic of Durysta® intracameral implant and applicator. The PLGA-based insert allows extended release of bimatoprost for treatment of open-angle glaucoma, overcoming some of the challenges associated with frequent eyedrop administration.

of wet AMD (49–52). PLGA is a popular choice for ocular drug delivery due to its clinical acceptance and tunable properties, but is limited by a 6 month release duration.

PCL is composed of ε-caprolactone monomers and is formed through induced ring opening polymerization. It is a hydrophobic, semicrystalline polymer with a slow biodegradation rate, taking months to years depending on polymer molecular weight and implant size and location (53). PCL is a common choice for experimental drug delivery vehicles due to its low cost, ease of modification and copolymerization, and processability. While it has been FDA approved for other indications such as in sutures, it has not yet been approved for use in the eye (54). PCL's crystalline properties make it an excellent choice for thin films and cell delivery due to its ability to maintain structural integrity through late stages of degradation. Experimental work done by Shuamo et al. (55) and Samy (56) present PCL thin films capable of extended drug release with limited intraocular inflammation. Additionally, PCL has shown promise as an intraocular drug delivery vehicle, with recent experimental work focusing on embedding nanoparticles within contact lenses, injectable *in situ* forming hydrogels, nanoparticle emulsions and suspensions, microparticles, and capsules for treatment of several diseases including glaucoma and wet AMD (57–62).

Poly(ortho ester) (POE) is another notable polyester-based synthetic polymer that has seen use in ocular drug delivery vehicles. While POE has been FDA approved for drug delivery in other applications, it has not yet been approved for ocular drug delivery but shows potential as a promising candidate that relies on surface erosion for therapeutic release. A thermosetting

PEG-Polyacetal-POE hydrogel has been developed and patented for drug delivery (63). The use of POE as a therapeutic delivery system appears to hold significant untapped potential.

Polymethacrylates

Poly(methyl methacrylate) (PMMA) and other methacrylate-based polymer derivatives are acrylic, biocompatible thermoplastics that possess good optical clarity when processed, high mechanical strength, water transmissibility and thermal stability (64, 65). They are FDA approved for intraocular use, and were first used in ocular applications in contact lenses in 1936 (66). Methacrylate based polymeric biomaterials have expanded to include uses in nanoparticle and micelle delivery, ocular hydrogels for topical administration and intravitreal injection, and ocular implants. Notable methacrylate derivatives include poly(2-hydroxylethylmethacrylate) (HEMA) and poly(2-(dimethylamino)ethyl methacrylate) (DMAEM). Titanium-based intravitreal implant I-vation® utilized PMMA as a non-biodegradable polymer coating for sustained release of triamcinolone acetonide for patients with DME (32). The implant was successful through phase I clinical trials but was suspended in phase IIb (67). Drug eluting HEMA-based contact lenses are a growing focus in ocular drug delivery because of the large population of contact wearers. In particular, experimental work with Acuvue® HEMA-based soft contacts has shown their potential as drug delivery vehicles, capable of extended release of Ofloxacin after incorporation of a vitamin E release barrier (68). Work by Pereira-da-Mota et al. (69) utilizes HEMA and other methacrylates for experimental atorvastatin-eluting lenses for topical treatment of diabetes-related ocular diseases. The formed contacts were designed to contain molecules similar to natural cholesterol regulator 3-methylglutaryl-CoA to improve incorporation of lipophilic drugs into the polymer matrix. Experimental work with methacrylate-based polymers includes investigations into HEMA-based lenses for elution of olopatadine for allergic conjunctivitis, HEMA contact lenses with temperature triggered release for treatment of glaucoma, and DMAEM nanogel-based drug carriers to increase mucoadhesion in topically administered delivery vehicles (70–72).

Polyolefins

Poly(acrylic acid) (PAA), also known commercially as Carbopol®, is a synthetic polymer composed of acrylic acid monomers with high water solubility and viscosity enhancing properties (73). It is biodegradable, but the resultant acrylic acid byproducts can cause inflammation (74). PAA displays good mucoadhesive properties due to its charged state at physiological conditions and has found use in several experimental hydrogel applications for anterior ocular delivery including copolymerization with PNIPAAm for generation of thermally sensitive *in situ* forming hydrogels for controlled release of epinephrine for glaucoma (75, 76). PAA is FDA approved for many topical applications including ocular administration and is commercially available in several eye drops, including the drug eluting ophthalmic emulsion Restasis®. Restasis® is a carbomer copolymer type A-based emulsion for topical administration of cyclosporine for treatment of dry eye disease (77).

Dendrimers

Dendrimers are long branching chain polymers that have distinct physical and chemical properties depending on chain characteristics and branch functionalization. Dendrimers have found application in ocular drug delivery due to their biocompatibility, water solubility, drug entrapment capabilities, and the reactivity of terminal functional groups at the end of each branch (78). The variety of dendrimers, their ability to hold several surface charge groups, and the ease of drug entrapment make them a superior polymer system for drug delivery (79). Poly(amidoamine) (PAMAM) is a dendrimer with FDA approval for certain uses that has seen use as a tool for ocular drug delivery, but is not on the GRAS list due to toxicity concerns (80). Experimental work completed by Yavuz et al. (81). evaluated PAMAM conjugation with dexamethasone for posterior eye sustained drug release for AMD and DR while Iezzi et al. (82). investigated PAMAM conjugation with fluocinolone acetonide for treatment of retinal inflammation in AMD and retinitis pigmentosa. Both works showed successful conjugation of the therapeutic into the dendrimer and were administered *via* intravitreal injection into rats. Topical administration of PAMAM hydrogels has also been reported, with one publication presenting a crosslinked PAMAM-PEG hydrogel for controlled delivery of the anti-glaucoma drug brimonidine tartrate (83). The current regulatory status, advantages, and disadvantages of common synthetic polymers are listed in **Table 1**.

BIOPOLYMERS OR BIOLOGICALLY DERIVED POLYMERIC BIOMATERIALS

Biopolymers have become more widely used in polymeric applications as technology for production has improved and understanding of material properties increases. They are based on naturally derived monomers or building blocks (animal, plant, fungi, bacteria) and generally possess high biocompatibility, fast degradation in aqueous environments, and a broad range of viscoelastic properties with the potential to produce biomaterials for use in ocular drug delivery (84). Common biological polymers in use for ocular biomaterials and drug delivery systems include cellulose, chitosan, hyaluronic acid (HA), collagen, carboxymethyl cellulose (CMC), gelatin, dextran, guar gum, pullulan, and polydopamine. The monomers and repeating units that produce those biological polymers are displayed in **Figure 3**.

Polysaccharide Biopolymers

Cellulose is considered the most common biopolymer and is derived from plant cell walls. It contains a large number of hydroxyl units and is thus very hydrophilic. It is biocompatible, biodegradable through enzymatic reactions and hydrolysis, easily conjugated and reacted, FDA approved for ocular use, and relatively inexpensive. For ocular drug delivery, carboxymethylcellulose (CMC), an ether derivative of cellulose, is the most prominent version of the polysaccharide as the addition of carboxy groups to the biopolymer chains increases water

solubility (84). Due to its biocompatibility and hydrophilicity, CMC is often found in topically administered eye drops such as Refresh® or Optive® for treatment of dry eye, but many more brands and formulations are available (85). The linear nature of CMC provides an excellent framework for experimental biopolymer-based hydrogels and thin films for extended topical drug release and *in situ* forming gels for intravitreal injection. Recent work by Deng et al. (86) synthesized *in situ* forming CMC/HA hydrogels capable of releasing bovine serum albumin for up to 30 days. CMC based micro- and nano-carriers have also been produced for anterior and posterior ocular drug delivery. Experimental work from Yuan et al. (87) produced and characterized CMC-based nanowafers for extended anterior drug delivery of axitinib. The topically applied clear nanowafers contain nanoreservoirs of therapeutic for extended drug release and increased bioavailability compared to traditional eye drop delivery. Additionally, experimental CMC nanowafers for extended release of dexamethasone have been shown to effectively treat dry eye disease (88). The nanowafers contained a 500 nm array of drug reservoirs and showed successful drug release for 24 h. Another notable cellulose derivative, hydroxypropyl methylcellulose (HPMC), is commonly used in ocular drug delivery due to its viscosity enhancing properties and biocompatibility (89).

Chitosan is a polysaccharide comprised of glucosamine and N-acetyl-glucosamine monomers that possesses a strong positive charge due to primary amine groups along the backbone (90). The highly cationic nature of the polymer provides mucoadhesive benefits that have been employed for use in eye drops, to improve therapeutic bioavailability, and extended release gels for subconjunctival injection (91, 92). The amphiphilic nature of chitosan allows for improved solubility of hydrophobic drugs and increased penetration through the corneal membrane when compared to non-conjugated drug (93). Chitosan has limited FDA approval and is not currently approved for ocular applications; however, there are several publications demonstrating *in vitro* and *in vivo* efficacy (94). Technologies such as chitosan liposomes and micelles provide a high drug payload with longer drug release period that can be easily administered through intravitreal injection. Because of its cationic nature, chitosan is often employed as a polymer coating for less biocompatible anionic polymers, used in layer by layer assembly of core shell biomaterials, and used for delivery of anionic therapeutics and genetic material (60, 61, 95). Chitosan-based hydrogels have recently been investigated to increase bioavailability of the topically administered antibiotic, levofloxacin (96). Thermosensitive hexanoyl glycol chitosan hydrogels were shown to possess low ocular irritation and 1.92-fold greater bioavailability in the aqueous humor of rabbits when compared to traditional antibiotic suspension.

Like chitosan, hyaluronic acid (HA) is a hydrophilic polysaccharide made up of D-glucuronic and N-acetyl-glucosamine monomers. HA is endogenously found in many ocular tissues including the cornea, aqueous humor, vitreous humor, and retina, and fulfills a variety of important roles in the eye. HA's structure allows for high water content and potential swelling in aqueous environments and fast degradation

TABLE 1 | Summary of synthetic polymers, biomaterial uses, regulatory status, benefits, and disadvantages.

Polymer name	Experimental/Clinical/FDA approved biomaterial forms	GRAS	FDA approved indications	Approved for use in eye	Pros/Cons
Poly(ethylene glycol) (PEG)	Implants, hydrogels, nanoparticles	Yes	Yes: injectables, topicals, rectal and nasal	Yes	Pros: water soluble, biocompatible Cons: fast degradation compared to other synthetic polymers
Poly(vinyl alcohol) (PVA)	Implants, hydrogels, nanoparticles	Yes	Yes: coatings, food additives, food packaging	Yes	Pros: slow degradation rate Cons: synthesized with aggressive solvents
Poly(glycolic acid) (PGA)	Implants	Yes	Yes: absorbable sutures, medical devices	Yes	Pros: fast degradation rate Cons: weak mechanical properties, brittle
Poly(glycolic acid – co – lactic acid) (PLGA)	All types	Yes	Yes: implants, drug delivery, medical devices	Yes	Pros: tunable degradation rate, water soluble, most common polymer used in ocular drug delivery Cons: acidic degradation byproducts
Poly(lactic acid) (PLA)	All types	Yes	Yes: absorbable sutures, medical devices, food packaging	Yes	Pros: Synthesized from natural sources, easily processed Cons: slow degradation rate
Poly(caprolactone) (PCL)	Hydrogels, films, nanoparticles	No	Yes: implants, delivery devices	No	Pros: easily modified, inexpensive Cons: not FDA approved for ocular applications
Poly(orthoester) (POE)	Nanoparticles	No	Yes: drug delivery	No	Pros: degrades *via* surface erosion Con: not heavily investigated for drug delivery uses
Poly(methacrylates) and derivatives (PMMA)	Hydrogels, contact lenses	Yes (mostly)	Yes: coatings, ocular lens, dental fillers, bone cement	Yes	Pros: well established ocular polymer, inexpensive Cons: non-biodegradable
Poly(acrylic acid) PAA	Hydrogels, eye drops,	No	Yes: topicals,	Yes	Pros: highly water soluble, mucoadhesive Cons: biodegradation into acidic byproducts
Poly(amidoamine) (PAMAM)	Nanoparticles, hydrogels	No	Yes: topicals, drug delivery	No	Pros: easily functionalized, contains many reactive groups Cons: not FDA approved for ocular uses

via enzymatic pathways (97, 98). HA's biocompatibility, high degree of hydration, tunable water content, and viscoelastic properties have made it a popular choice for certain types of ocular drug delivery systems such as polymer gels. It has also been used as a biocompatible coating for delivery devices, and as an integral part of retinal cell based therapies (99). Work by Liu et al. (100) showed that delivery of retinal progenitor cells using a HA-based hydrogel was able to correctly transplant the cells into the sub-retinal area without disruption of function and that upon complete degradation of HA, the cells expressed mature photoreceptor markers (100). HA has also recently been applied as a self-sealing inner needle coating for intravitreal injection to minimize extraocular regurgitation of drugs (101). The most common application of HA has been as a lubricating agent in eyedrops for dry eye, with HA eyedrops serving as an

artificial tear layer in products such as Optive Fusion, Vismed Multi, DROPSTAR®, Hyalistil®, and Neop (85, 102). Other applications include the Solaraze™ gel, which uses HA gel to form a depot for controlled release of diclofenac for treatment of ocular inflammation and pain (102, 103). Future research is likely to explore this further, as HA presents an easily prepared and biodegradable polymer with significant potential for the formation of degradable reservoirs for controlled drug release in addition to hydration and healing properties.

Dextran is a polysaccharide biopolymer composed of D-glucose units and is synthesized by lactic acid bacteria. It is biocompatible, biodegradable, hydrophilic, and able to form hydrogels (104). Dextran is an FDA approved biopolymer found in ophthalmic eye drop solutions such as Tears Natural Forte® and Tears Natural II® for treatment of dry eye

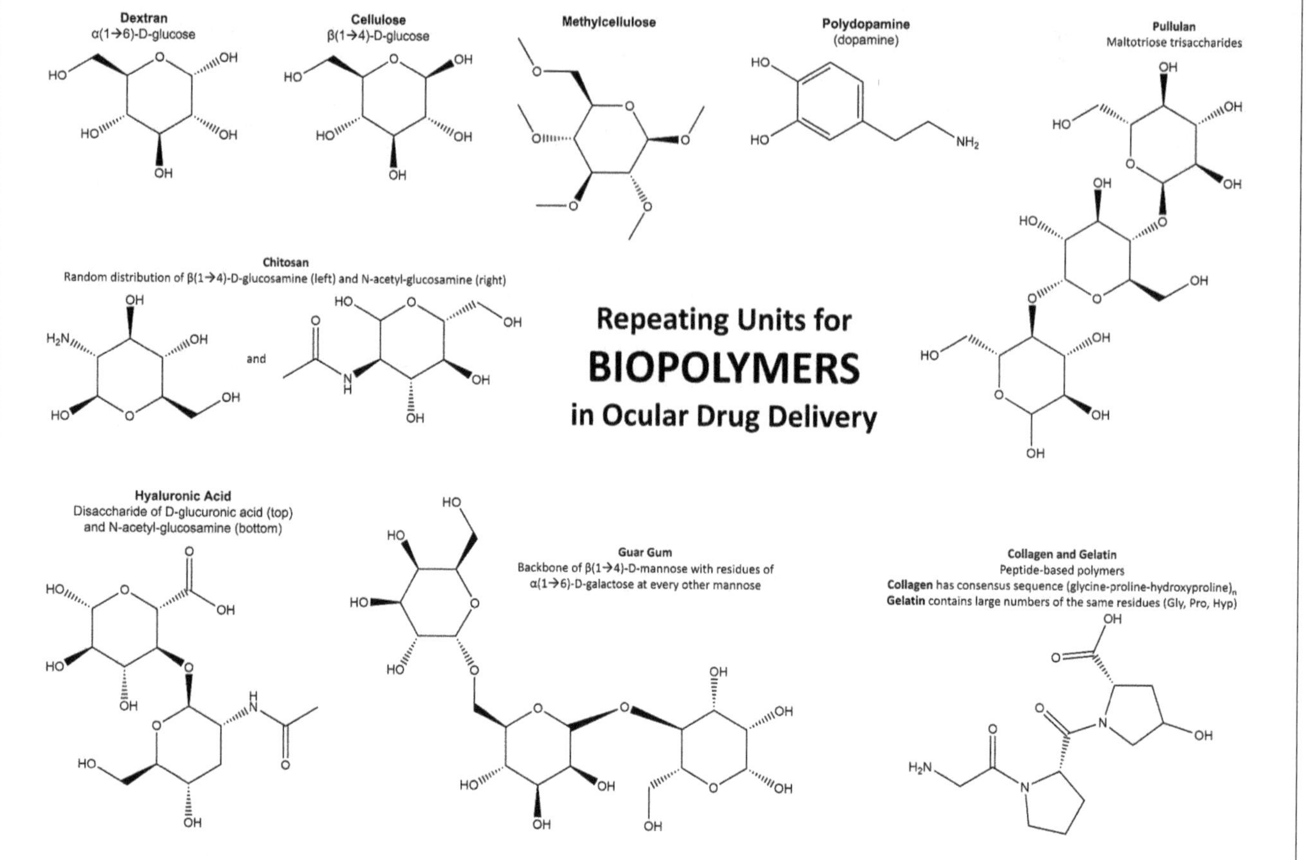

FIGURE 3 | Schematic of the repeating units that form the most noteworthy biopolymers used in ocular drug delivery.

syndrome (105). It is easily chemically crosslinked and has been experimentally investigated with chitosan, PLA/PLGA, and PEG for topical and intravitreal administration of ocular therapeutics (106). Recent experimental work has shown successful delivery of lutein, an antioxidant, from dextran-chitosan crosslinked nanoparticles for topical administration (106). Dextran is also capable of drug conjugation for ocular delivery. Low molecular weight dextran has seen experimental use as a cationic DNA carrier for targeted gene therapy to treat X-linked juvenile retinoschisis. Recent work showed successful *in vivo* transfection and expression of a dextran-protamine-DNA complex adsorbed onto the surface of solid-lipid nanoparticles after intravitreal injection into rats (107).

Guar gum is a seed-derived polysaccharide with linear backbone chains of β-d-mannose units and branch points of α-d-galactose units (108). As a biopolymer, guar gum is biocompatible, water soluble, a viscosity enhancer, capable of high degrees of swelling, mucoadhesive, non-ionic, and degradable by hydrolysis (109). The gelling ability of guar gum makes it beneficial as an additive to lubricating eye drops and is currently FDA approved for ocular use. Unfortunately, guar gum has limited solubility in alcohols and organic solvents and

is unstable in solution. Derivatives such as hydroxymethyl-guar gum, hydroxypropyl-guar gum, and o-carboxymethyl o-hydroxypropyl-guar gum have been synthesized to improve solubility and stability (109). Hydroxypropyl-guar gum is found in several lubricating eye drops (110). Guar gum has been experimentally investigated to increase the bioavailability of natamycin for treatment of ocular fungal infection by integration onto PEG nanolipid carriers for controlled release from a carboxyvinyl polymer-guar gum-borate gelling system (110). Guar gum grafted PCL micelles have also been investigated for prolonged release of ofloxacin. Experimental guar gum-PCL micelles conjugated with retinol, biotinylated glutathione, and cell specific targeting agents before incorporation of ofloxacin showed drug release for at least 8 h (111).

Pullulan is a polysaccharide derived from the yeast *Aureobasidium pullulans*, composed of maltotriose units joined by α-1,6 linkages (112). Pullulan is biocompatible, non-ionic, stable over a broad temperature and pH range, water soluble, insoluble in most organic solvents, easily processed, oxygen impermeable, viscosity enhancing, and biodegradable (112, 113). Pullulan has FDA GRAS status and has been used in many experimental biopolymer applications, including ocular drug delivery (114). The non-ionic nature of pullulan often requires derivation such as sulfation or amination to incorporate a charge for improved reactivity. Co-polymerization of pullulan with other biopolymers or synthetic polymers has shown promise for extending biodegradation rate compared to the polysaccharide alone. Examples include pullulan-gellan gum electrospun nanofibers for an *in situ* forming gel for extended topical therapeutic bioavailability (115). The gelation properties of pullulan in water make it popular for use in thin films and hydrogel inserts. Experimental work completed by Pai and Reddy (116). investigated the *in vitro* properties of a 10% pullulan gel insert intended for conjunctival drug delivery. The insert showed complete degradation *in vitro* and complete drug release within 3 h of application.

Protein Biopolymers

Collagen is a naturally occurring fibrous protein present in most connective tissue, including the cornea, sclera, lens capsule, and vitreous humor. Because it is naturally occurring, collagen is biocompatible, enzymatically degradable, can be relatively easily processed, and is widely available from primarily bovine and porcine sources. Recombinant collagen is also available, offering reduced dependence on animal sources through more consistent and safe production in plants and yeast cells (117). Collagen has a long established use in collagen shields for eye protection after ocular trauma or cataract surgery (118). More recent work utilizes collagen as a drug delivery device for encapsulated cell therapy *via* intravitreal injection, extended drug release *via* gels, or as a scaffold base for retinal tissue regeneration (119, 120). Current ocular drug delivery technologies that utilize collagen include Photrexa®, a collagen containing riboflavin ophthalmic suspension that when exposed to ultraviolet A light, crosslinks the biopolymer for treatment of progressive keratoconus (121).

Gelatin is a protein-based polymer formed from the irreversible hydrolysis of collagen. Like collagen, it is biocompatible, biodegradable, water soluble, gel forming and viscosity enhancing, readily available, and low cost, but shows advantages in lower gelation temperature and improved aqueous solubility (122, 123). It is derived from mammalian, avian, and ichthyoid collagen I sources, allowing for a broad range of available molecular weights, and is GRAS approved. Recombinant gelatin is also available to circumvent potential immunogenicity and provides access to specific gelatin molecular weights and isoelectric points (124). In ocular drug delivery, gelatin has seen applications in eye drops as a demulcent, in anteriorly and posteriorly applied hydrogels, nanoparticles for extended drug release, ocular tissue engineering, and siRNA carriers for gene therapy (105, 123, 125–127).

Other Biopolymers

Polydopamine is a relatively recently investigated biopolymer, formed through oxidative polymerization of dopamine, one of the body's major neurotransmitters (128). Its biocompatibility and low toxicity have led to significant interest in its use in drug delivery, with particular attention paid to the development of coatings and nanostructures (128). These two applications have seen recent investigation as a novel method of ocular

drug delivery. Liu et al. (129) developed an intraocular lens (IOL) with a self-polymerizing polydopamine coating capable of loading and eluting doxorubicin, preventing posterior capsule opacification (PCO) in rabbit models. Jiang et al. (130) developed polydopamine nanoparticles which showed effective loading and oxidative stress-dependent release of anti-VEGF *in vitro*. Recent findings that polydopamine coatings enhance nanoparticle mucopenetration may open the door to further applications of polydopamine in corneal drug delivery, especially as cellular uptake of these nanoparticles is also enhanced compared to uncoated nanoparticles (131). While polydopamine has only been under evaluation as a biomaterial since 2007, it has shown clear potential in ocular drug delivery, and will likely continue to mature with further research efforts (128). Several biopolymers used in ocular drug delivery are summarized in **Table 2**.

POLYMERIC BIOMATERIAL FORMS

Micro- and Nano-Scale Technologies

The versatility of biopolymers and synthetic polymers opens the door to many types and forms of biomaterials used as drug delivery vehicles to treat ocular diseases. Within the field of micro- and nanotechnology, there are a variety of drug delivery vehicles such as microparticles, nanoparticles, micelles, and liposomes. These drug delivery vehicles show significant promise in the eye due to their less invasive application approaches topically as well as ease of injection through small gauge needles (44, 142). These have also been explored for incorporation into drug-eluting contact lenses to facilitate topical delivery (143). **Figure 4** presents several ocular drug delivery forms that utilize nanotechnology.

Microparticles are small-scale particles generally in the size range of 1–1,000 μm. Microparticles have been evaluated for ocular drug delivery for decades, and typically demonstrate higher drug loading capacity and release duration than nanoparticles due to the larger size of the particles, but a balance between drug loading and size considerations for injectability must be established. Several articles have focused on microparticles in the range of 1–50 μm for intravitreal injection to balance these considerations (144). It has been recently proposed to use nanoparticles embedded in microparticles to overcome some of these challenges (145). Microparticles have also shown controlled variable monodispersity upon application, demonstrating versatility of this approach.

Nanoparticles are particles between 10 and 1,000 nm which can possess a surface charge, based on monomer properties, that allows for increased permeability or mucoadhesion of the therapeutic (146). Nanoparticles allow for drug delivery through encapsulation of the target therapeutic or surface loading through electrostatic interactions. Most of the biopolymers and synthetic polymers discussed in this review have been prepared as nanoparticles and extensively evaluated for drug delivery from contact lenses, intravitreal injection, topical, and suprachoroidal administration (144, 147, 148). Nanoparticles have the advantage of being small enough to penetrate cells, maximizing therapeutic efficacy through targeted therapeutic release. Their small size also facilitates overcoming many of the barriers to ocular delivery.

TABLE 2 | Summary of biopolymers used in ocular drug delivery and their properties.

Polymer name	Experimental/Clinical/FDA approved biomaterial uses	GRAS	FDA approved indications	Pros/Cons
Cellulose	Hydrogels, films, nanoparticles, inserts	Yes	Yes: food additive, topicals	Pros: Biocompatible, nontoxic, high molecular loading potential, nanomaterial fabrication possible (132) Cons: Low solubility (132)
Chitosan	Nanoparticles, hydrogels	No	Yes: food additive, wound dressing	Pros: Mucoadhesive, positively charged at physiologic pH (133) Cons: Insoluble in neutral or alkaline solutions, brittle in hydrogel form, strong electrostatic behavior (134)
Hyaluronic acid	Hydrogels, nanoparticles, films, tissue scaffolds	No: classified as medical device currently	Yes: cosmetic fillers, injectable for osteoarthritis, topicals	Pros: Biocompatible, mucoadhesive, good viscoelastic behavior (133), naturally occurring (135) Cons: Difficult to functionalize, challenging drug conjugation (136), effect of molecular weight unclear (137)
Collagen	Hydrogels, nanoparticles, contact lenses	Yes	Yes: food additive, cosmetic injectables, wound healing	Pros: Biodegradable, biocompatible, bioactive, significant existing use in medicine (118) Cons: Immunogenicity risks, variable quality, concerns about animal sources (117)
Carboxymethylcellulose	Hydrogels, eye drops, nanoparticles	Yes	Yes: disintegrant, dental devices	Pros: Biodegradable, biocompatible, capable of sustained release, pH-sensitive (132) Cons: Challenging to develop proper viscous solutions (133)
Gelatin	Hydrogels, nanoparticles, films, tissue engineering	Yes	Yes: medical devices, food additive	Pros: Easily derived, biocompatible, rich in ECM protein, less immunogenic, transparent, low cost (123) Cons: Strength depends on source and processing conditions, still immunogenic, challenging to safely crosslink (123)
Dextran	Hydrogels, films, nanoparticles	Yes	Yes: shock and other blood related indications, inhalant	Pros: Excellent biocompatibility (134) Cons: Difficult to functionalize (134)
Guar Gum	Hydrogels, films	Yes	Yes: food additive	Pros: Mucoadhesive, antioxidant, low antigenicity, biodegradable, low cost, stable and biocompatible (138) Cons: Brittle, high swelling, poor mechanical properties in hydrogel, low recoverability (138)
Pullulan	Hydrogels, nanoparticles, eye drops, fibers	Yes	Yes: food additives, tablet coatings, stabilizer, and thickener	Pros: Easily derived, stable, good film-forming properties, biodegradable (116), nontoxic (139) Cons: Unexpectedly slow diffusion (140), requires functionalization to load drugs (141)
Polydopamine	Nanoparticles, Intraocular Lenses	Not evaluated	No: Dopamine HCl indicated for correction of hemodynamic imbalances	Pros: Biocompatible, biodegradable, low toxicity, excellent adhesion Cons: Synthesis is challenging to control and poorly understood, need for investigation of toxicology, degradation, elimination

While there are many advantages to nanoparticles and there has been a significant shift to focus on nanoparticles for ocular drug delivery in recent years, a nanoparticle ocular drug delivery system has yet to be commercialized (149).

Experimental systems include GB-102®, a PLGA microparticle-based drug delivery vehicle designed by Graybug

Vision for treatment of wet AMD and macular edema. The injectable drug depot is currently in clinical trials and has shown controlled release of sunitinib malate for up to 6 months post injection (32). POE-based nanoparticles maintained vitreous localization in rabbits after intravitreal injection for up to 14 days with minimal increases in IOP (150). Work by Fu et al.

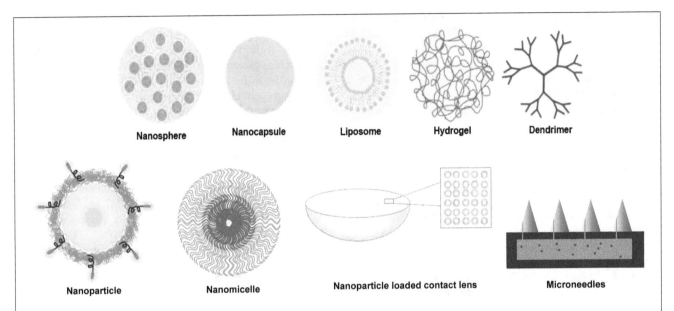

FIGURE 4 | Various polymer forms that have been applied to facilitate and modulate ocular drug delivery at the macroscale and nanoscale. Both synthetic and biopolymers can be formulated into nanospheres, nanocapsules, liposomes, hydrogels, dendrimers, nanoparticles, nanomicelles, and microneedles. Nanoscale polymers can be incorporated into composites, such as the hydrogel-based contact lens shown with nanoparticles.

(151) developed poly(ortho ester urethane) nanoparticles that showed pH-sensitive degradation properties and were efficient in delivering doxorubicin to *in vitro* tumor spheroids. Experimental work by Jiang et al. (60) utilized chitosan's cationic properties for intravitreal delivery of anti-VEGF bevacizumab through microparticles composed of a cationic chitosan core and PCL shell. Chitosan nanoparticles have also been evaluated for transscleral delivery of bevacizumab (152). Lu et al. reported bevacizumab-loaded chitosan nanoparticles for treating DR (153). Work by Dionisio et al. (154) modified pullulan through sulfation and amination to produce both negatively and positively charged pullulan-chitosan and pullulan-carrageenan nanoparticles for transmucosal drug delivery, while Garhwal et al. (155) integrated experimental pullulan-PCL nanospheres encapsulating ciprofloxacin into HEMA-based contact lenses for topical administration of antibiotics. Recent research on corneal applications of gelatin include positively charged gelatin nanoparticles for extended release of moxifloxacin (156). The particles showed *in vitro* drug release up to 12 h and showed *in vivo* antimicrobial properties superior to the market available product MoxiGram®.

Micelles are core/shell structures formed by amphiphilic block copolymers with hydrophobic and hydrophilic domains, and are often <100 nm in size. Polymeric micelles can enhance solubility of poorly soluble drugs and are being explored for use in promoting drug transport through the cornea and sclera (157). Micelles offer several advantages to enhance topical delivery, including thermodynamic stability, relative ease of preparation, high loading capacity, and lack of interference with optical properties of devices or solutions (143). These are likely to be adopted clinically due to relatively simple and inexpensive fabrication techniques (158). Micelles have been explored

for several classes of therapeutics including cyclosporine, anti-inflammatories, immunosuppressants, anti-glaucoma drugs, antifungals, antivirals, and experimental antioxidants (159). Several stimuli-responsive poloxamers have been evaluated, including PF-127 for topical delivery of a hydrophobic drug to the anterior segment for treatment of allergic conjunctivitis (160), PF-68 for delivery of ferulic acid (161) or enhancing solubility of gatifloxacin in contact lenses (162), and their combination for delivery of antifungals (163). Triamcinolone acetonide delivery with PEG-block-PCL and PEG-block-PLA micelles was also evaluated (164). Other types of polymeric micelles evaluated include amino-terminated PEG-block-PLA and HPMC for delivery of tacrolimus (165). Chitosan has even been explored for micellar delivery (166), including delivery of dexamethasone (167), and HA has been conjugated to peptides to enhance solubility through micelles (97). Challenges that remain include improving micelle stability for longer shelf-life and therapeutic delivery duration. These factors can be controlled by polymer molecular weight, hydrophobicity/hydrophilicity, and block arrangement, with promise demonstrated with pentablock copolymer micelles (168). Further, micelles can be assembled into larger hydrogels to extend delivery (58).

While liposomes are not polymers, they have been used with polymers for ocular drug delivery. Liposomes have a cell membrane-like structure made from one or more phospholipid layers, enabling adhesion to cell membranes. They can be complexed with polymers to facilitate ocular drug delivery by improving liposome stability (148). Liposome conjugates evaluated for ocular drug release have included chitosan, silk fibroin, and PEG (169, 170).

These small systems have several advantages, including ease of injection, extended topical release, and enhanced permeability.

Two key challenges are establishing long-term extended release and increasing drug loading efficiency. Other challenges include preserving therapeutic activity during preparation and loading of these delivery systems. That being said, injecting a micro- or nano-delivery system 2–3 times per year may still be a viable option for patients receiving more frequent intravitreal injections since injection would still be in office through a small gauge needle.

Hydrogels

Hydrogels consist of bound networks of synthetic and/or biologic hydrophilic polymers that absorb aqueous fluids. Many hydrogels exist specifically for intra- and extra-ocular applications ranging from contact lenses to vitreous substitutes. Hydrogels have also been used for drug delivery and/or cell encapsulation, and have been evaluated for use with optic nerve stabilization (171) and intraocular lens prosthetics (172). The large array of ocular applications may be attributed to both the hydrophilicity of hydrogels and the customizability of component polymers.

Hydrogels possess several modifiable and customizable properties such as degree of swelling, biodegradability/erosion, viscoelasticity, pore size, diffusion rate/flux, permeability, stimuli responsiveness, and drug/protein loading efficiency. Each of these characteristics may be directly or indirectly impacted by changing one or more of the following: degree of crosslinking (crosslinking density), monomer and polymer concentrations, and polymer type (atomic/molecular composition). The inherent hydrophilicity of hydrogels can provide systems with biological and mechanical stability in various ocular environments. A hydrogel's degree of crosslinking and hydrophilicity have a strong impact on the degree of swelling by their effect on variables such as pore size and diffusion rate/flux, which can be used to tune drug release. The aqueous environment in hydrogels allows investigators to mimic the extracellular matrix and tissues for cell delivery systems, may provide stability and improve cellular uptake for hydrophilic drugs, genes, and biologics. However, some therapeutics suffer reduced bioactivity in aqueous environments, and modifications may need to be made to incorporate hydrophobic drugs or prevent fast elution of hydrophilic drugs.

Due to the customizable nature of hydrogels and vast array of viable polymers, this area of research has potential for clinical translation and continued development. One specific area of recent growth for ocular applications is *in situ* hydrogel formation, where a hydrogel undergoes gelation (polymerization and/or crosslinking or self-assembly) in the ocular environment in response to specific stimuli (light, temperature, pH, oxygenation, etc.). From intraocular applications such as intravitreal injections to topical treatments with films and inserts, hydrogels formed *in situ* show promise as a major player in the future of ocular drug delivery. *In situ* forming gels enable injection through smaller gauge needles, facilitating intraocular delivery in an outpatient setting. Furthermore, *in situ* formation can enable conformal coating of curved surfaces like the cornea, enabling direct contact and more consistent drug delivery.

Xie et al. (173) developed a nanoparticle/hydrogel composite for the sustained release of an anti-tumor therapeutic to the posterior segment of the eye. The hydrogel, composed of collagen II and sodium hyaluronate, was formed *in situ* following injection in to the vitreous and in response to physiological temperature stimuli. Thermo-responsivity was attributed to a thermo-responsive crosslinking reaction at 37°C between amine groups of collagen and succinimidyl groups of the additive 8-arm PEG succinimidyl glutarate (tipentaerythritol). Another injectable hydrogel was presented by Osswald et al. (51) to deliver anti-VEGF to the choroid *via* intravitreal injection. This hydrogel consisted of poly(N-isopropylacrylamide) (PNIPAAm) and poly(ethylene glycol) diacrylate (PEGDA) and utilized the properties of PNIPAAm to create a thermo-responsive *in situ* forming hydrogel. In 2016, researchers developed a hydrogel that underwent gelation upon exposure to aqueous conditions (174). This unique *in situ* gelation method was the product of hydrophobic interactions between poly(ethylene glycol) methacrylate (PEGMA) and vitamin E methacrylate leading to the formation of physical crosslinks. This hydrogel's chemistry and crosslinking ability has potential in generating hydrogels capable of delivery of hydrophobic drugs.

Drug delivery coordinated with tissue replacement, such as intraocular lens implantation and vitreous substitution, is a relatively recent area of research. This work shows great promise by potentially offering a reduction in frequent administration or procedures and mitigation of post-operative complications. Tram et al. (175) proposed a solution for combatting cataract formation following vitrectomy by loading PEG-based hydrogel vitreous substitutes with the antioxidant ascorbic acid. Building off of that research, they found that glutathione may be a useful addition to ascorbic acid in ocular drug delivery (13). Polymer coatings for IOLs, made of polydopamine or synthetic polymers, are being evaluated to reduce complications after cataract surgery from infection and PCO (129, 176).

While significantly less invasive than injections and tissue replacement strategies, topical hydrogel drug delivery solutions present their own challenges, requiring prolonged contact with tissues of interest and firm shape retention. One example of a topical *in situ* forming hydrogel was reported by Anumolu et al. (177) to deliver doxycycline to the cornea using PEG octamer hydrogels (177). The hydrogels were pH-responsive, undergoing shape-retaining gelation within seconds of application. Another example of a viable *in situ* forming hydrogel used for sustained drug delivery was recently published by El-Feky et al. (178), who installed the gel into the inferior conjunctival fornix to deliver nifedipine for glaucoma treatment (178). Hydrogels were created using poloxamer 407 (P407) and HPMC, utilizing properties of P407 to incorporate thermo-responsiveness into the hydrogels. Fedorchak et al. (179) made use of a thermo-responsive PNIPAAm hydrogel eyedrop containing drug-loaded PLGA microspheres to achieve long-term delivery of brimonidine for glaucoma treatment, showing efficacy in rabbit models out to 28 days after administration.

In situ gelation provides a drug delivery solution that is tailored to the patient's ocular geometry and has great potential in reducing both treatment frequency and procedure invasiveness.

Opportunities for innovative hydrogel solutions for ocular drug delivery are ever-growing, opening doors for many more future research projects and likely commercial translation in the near future.

Fibers, Films, Rods, Extrusions

Processing polymers into fibers, films, rods, or extruded forms allows various alternative configurations for drug delivery systems. These delivery methods and geometries may even be interconnected. For example, fibers may be formed *via* electrospinning to create a rod-shaped implant, or the fibers may be spun into a sheet and hydrated to form a film.

Kelley et al. (180) detailed and compared production methods for hot-melt extrusion manufacturing of dexamethasone-loaded injectable intravitreal implants. The extruded rods were composed of PLGA with varying weight percentages of acid- and ester-terminated PLGA to control the implant degradation and drug release rate. OZURDEX® (Allergan) is an FDA-approved intravitreal implant that employs extruded PLGA (NOVADUR® technology) for sustained dexamethasone release through biodegradation (181).

One method for producing fibers is electrospinning. A recent study experimented with various configurations for conjunctival fornix inserts for sustained delivery of besifloxacin to the cornea for treatment of bacterial keratitis (182). The inserts, synthesized *via* electrospinning, were prepared as fibers of PCL and PEG and then coated with biopolymers—either sodium alginate or thiolated sodium alginate—to confer mucoadhesion. Another ocular insert composed of electrospun PCL and intended for insertion into the conjunctival fornix was developed to deliver fluocinolone acetonide to the retina and was evaluated in pre-clinical studies (183). PCL and chitosan capsules have also been prepared *via* electrospinning to fabricate a hollow bilayered design for intravitreal injection (61). Delivery systems designed with electrospun nanofibers present two specific advantages: tunable device porosity for controlled drug diffusion and a high ratio of surface area to volume for increased chemoadsorption (61).

Electrospun conjunctival fornix inserts were also investigated for the delivery of triamcinolone acetonide to the anterior and superficial segments of the eye (184). Investigators analyzed properties and release profiles of nanofiber formulations with varying concentrations of PVA, poly(vinylpyrrolidone) (PVP), zein/eudragit, and chitosan, identifying an optimal formulation of only PVP and chitosan.

Electrospinning has also been applied to develop both *in situ*-forming and pre-hydrated hydrogel systems. Göttel et al. (139) presented an *in situ* gelation system that begins as a curved lens of electrospun pullulan and gellan gum fibers. Upon application to the ocular surface, the fibrous lens hydrates to form a film/hydrogel. A different study utilized electrospun PVP and HA nanofibers to develop hydrogels for drug delivery (185). This study focused on developing an ocular insert to deliver ferulic acid and Epsiliseen®-H for treating ocular surface conditions. PVP was employed to enable electrospinning of HA while HA was the polymer responsible for the drug delivery mechanism.

Films are comparable to hydrogels for drug delivery as they hydrate to form an aqueous system. They also show potential in drug delivery, particularly for topical applications. A porous resorbable film was recently investigated as a bandage contact lens following corneal injury (186). The films were composed of bovine serum albumin (BSA) structural nanofibrils and the antioxidant kaempferol.

One recent advancement in fiber and film technology is the PRINT® technique. This technology allows researchers to precisely control a film's shape, size, surface properties/functionality, chemical composition, porosity, and moduli (187, 188). Researchers have employed PRINT® to customize drug delivery systems on the nanoscale-level to control for release profiling/kinetics and environment of application (189). The technology can use an array of biopolymers and therapeutics including peptides, nucleic acids, and antibodies (146, 187). PRINT® has been used to develop subconjunctival implants, intracameral implants, intravitreal implants, nano-and micro-suspensions, etc (190). One recent development with PRINT® technology is the AR13503 (Aerie Pharmaceuticals) implant, which utilizes PLGA, PDLA, and PEA to control delivery to the retina for more than 2 months and is in phase 1 clinical trials (190–193). Another delivery system developed with PRINT® is an Envisia Therapeutics implant (ENV515) currently in phase 2 clinical trials (194). Results thus far suggest that ENV515 is effective in lowering IOP for 28 days (195, 196). Results from a 12-month study found 25% IOP reduction compared to topical ophthalmic solution (195). PRINT® shows great promise for its ability to customize polymer-based ocular drug delivery systems at the nanoscale level.

Polymer processing techniques are well developed in other applications and are beginning to emerge in ocular drug delivery systems. These processing techniques will be required for manufacturing of several ocular drug delivery devices and give potential to explore innovative new delivery systems using already approved polymers.

ADMINISTRATION METHODS
Eyedrop Delivery

Eyedrops have seen widespread usage for delivering a variety of medications for ocular disorders, thanks to their ease of use, low cost, and relatively good patient compliance (142, 197). However, in recent years, their limitations as a drug delivery system have led to significant research effort invested in improving their capacity or developing more efficient alternatives (198). While eyedrops offer excellent delivery efficiency for topical diseases of the eye, their efficiency significantly declines when used to deliver pharmacologic agents to certain tissues in the eye. By some estimates, as little as 1–5% of an eyedrop's drug content can reach the anterior segment of the eye due to the barriers it faces in passing through the cornea to the aqueous humor (142, 158, 199). First among these is the rapid turnover of the tear film on the cornea, which leads to a significant fraction the eyedrop's volume following the tear film into nasolacrimal drainage and systemic circulation (200–202). By some estimates, as much as 80% of the tear film's volume can be turned over in a minute when eyedrops are applied to the eye, leading to significant loss of dose volume (200). This lost drug dosage then enters systemic circulation, where it may be metabolized before reaching ocular tissue and risks triggering systemic side effects that compromise patient health (202). Any drug not cleared *via* tear film drainage must still penetrate corneal tissue in order to reach the anterior chamber and have a therapeutic effect on ocular tissue. The structure of corneal tissue makes it difficult for both hydrophilic and lipophilic molecules to pass through. The corneal epithelium admits only lipophilic drugs smaller than 10 Å through cell-mediated transport mechanisms, and forces hydrophilic drugs to diffuse through paracellular pathways blocked by tight junctions (19, 158). The corneal stroma, meanwhile, is highly hydrophilic, slowing the movement of the lipophilic drugs that pass the epithelium while allowing freer movement of the few hydrophilic molecules that enter (158).

Despite these challenges to drug retention and penetration, eyedrops are still favored for the treatment of diseases in the anterior segment of the eye. Their ease of delivery has also made them attractive for delivery to the posterior of the eye, with researchers investigating a variety of eyedrop formulations with improved drug retention and penetration characteristics, with some working toward eye drop formulations for posterior ocular delivery to overcome the limits of injections (201, 203–207).

The combination of rapid clearance and the extreme difficulty of corneal penetration has led to significant research efforts aimed at increasing the delivery efficiency of eyedrops. One of the earliest options explored was to simply increase the concentration of drug delivered in the eyedrop solution, overcoming delivery barriers through essentially brute force. However, this option presents its own challenges, as such high drug doses and accompanying polymer and preservative exposure could cause local irritation or toxicity in patients (207–210). In addition, the higher drug dose per eyedrop leads to higher doses draining to the bloodstream, potentially exacerbating systemic side effects (208). As an alternative to increasing dose per eyedrop, some medications instead recommend increasing the frequency of eyedrop administration. However, this presents its own challenges, as higher frequency administration has been linked to significant reductions in patient compliance with treatment regimens (207, 211). Patients with physical or visual impairments, as well as children who are unable to administer eyedrops to themselves, may be especially non-compliant, as eyedrops rely on self-application to have an effect (210). In addition, frequent repeated application of eyedrops may still lead to local and systemic side effects associated with high dosing (207).

Because of these continued challenges in increasing delivery efficiency of eyedrops, modern research has investigated a variety of polymer-based solutions for enhancing drug penetration and residence time in the anterior eye. One solution is the development of polymer nanocarriers with mucoadhesive capabilities. These nanoparticles can entrap themselves in the mucus layer that covers the cornea, with some even capable of penetrating corneal tissue to enter the aqueous humor thanks to their small size (158, 200, 202, 205). Mucoadhesion lengthens the residence time of drug delivery systems significantly, allowing them to more effectively release their drug payload for uptake by ocular tissue. Corneal penetration is an even more desirable outcome, as the ability to effectively penetrate the cornea using a drug carrier provides immense opportunities for delivery to intraocular spaces. Recent research efforts have developed chitosan and PLGA nanoparticles capable of reaching the retinal surface, a demonstration of how nanoparticles can help solve the challenge of developing eyedrops capable of posterior ocular delivery (211, 212). Another option is the addition of polymer viscosity enhancers and gelling agents such as xanthan gum, which increase the residence time of an eyedrop atop the cornea, thereby giving more time for the drug payload to begin penetrating corneal tissue (19, 213). Both of these solutions make use of a variety of polymers. While they still face significant challenges in successful implementation and translation from laboratory to clinical use, several preclinical studies are making use of gelling systems to improve drug delivery efficiency through eyedrops. One interesting recent development has been investigation into thermosensitive polymers that form gels at physiologic temperatures (207, 214). These polymers could allow future eyedrops to be administered in solution at room temperature, then form a hydrogel reservoir on contact with the warmer tissue of the eye, providing an easily administered long-lasting form of ocular drug delivery.

Subconjunctival Injections and Implants

Injection of pharmacologic agents presents an attractive alternative route for the delivery of drugs to ocular tissue. Injection into the subconjunctival space specifically allows drugs to be released next to the sclera and avoid corneal barriers to entry (202). Drugs are able to easily penetrate the more permeable scleral layer, potentially enabling significantly more efficient delivery to the interior of the eye, particularly the posterior segment (197, 201, 209, 213). While subconjunctival drug injections and implants necessitate a relatively more invasive procedure than eyedrops, they offer the potential of prolonged drug delivery compared to eyedrops, potentially lasting months between injections or implant replacements (19, 199). This would represent a significant advantage in patient compliance, as a minimally invasive injection or implantation procedure every few months is significantly easier to maintain compared to daily eyedrop administration regimens (19, 158). This method is not without challenges, however, as the subconjunctival space, while not as severely drained as the anterior surface of the eye, is still rich in drainage routes. Conjunctival and scleral blood vessels, as well as lymphatic drainage, will interfere with delivery and cause some of the administered dose to enter systemic circulation rather than penetrate the sclera and enter the eye (201, 202). In addition, the choroidal tissue in the eye poses an additional barrier to lipophilic drug delivery, as this tissue can bind lipophilic drugs (213).

The significant potential of subconjunctival delivery to bypass the challenges of eyedrop administration in a minimally invasive manner has led to research efforts focused on overcoming the challenges of clearance and penetration while extending the duration of drug release after implantation or injection. Polymer solutions for these problems include polymer micro- and nano-particles which, similar to their role in eyedrop formulations, help improve drug residence time near ocular tissue and assist in penetrating the scleral barriers to ocular entry, thereby increasing the drug dose delivered (158, 201, 202). Alternatively, subconjunctival injections of drug-loaded hydrogels composed of polymers such as PEG, PLGA, and HA can create a reservoir capable of extended release over a course of weeks or months, offering a more easily prepared alternative to micro- and nanoparticle systems (197, 208). Finally, polymeric subconjunctival implants offer a more stable platform for drug delivery through the subconjunctival space, with research publications describing devices made of PDMS, PLGA, and polyurethane among others (19, 197, 209). Animal studies into the use polymer-based subconjunctival drug delivery systems have found promising initial data, with favorable biocompatibility and safety results for polyimide and PLGA implants and evidence of extended-release efficacy for PLGA microspheres in the subconjunctival space (215, 216). Further research into delivery through the subconjunctival space is likely to offer significant potential for improvement of drug delivery compliance and outcomes. Many of these research efforts may benefit from prior developments in subconjunctival drainage devices designed to relieve IOP and assist in glaucoma treatment, as numerous polymer drains have already received approval for market use (217).

Suprachoroidal Injections

Another alternative route for drug delivery is injection to the suprachoroidal space, a thin layer of tissue between the sclera and choroid of the eye (218). In theory, injections into this space could quickly spread across the inner surface of the eye, allowing rapid access to the posterior tissues of the eye with limited loss to the vitreous humor (201, 218). This would provide a highly specific pathway for delivery to these tissues with minimized adverse effects from off-target delivery and significantly lower invasiveness compared to intravitreal injection (213). However, the suprachoroidal space is extremely delicate, with only 30 μm of tissue thickness in the region and a recommended maximum injection volume of only 200 μl (218). Higher volumes than this risk causing choroidal edema and detachment (218). In addition, as this space has been relatively underexplored, there is a significant chance that yet-undiscovered safety challenges may emerge with the use of a broader range of polymers and injection systems. Perhaps because of these significant challenges to safe and accurate delivery, there has been relatively minimal exploration and characterization of the suprachoroidal space, with early studies beginning only in the mid-2000s and testing of suprachoroidal delivery in animal models of ocular disease by the early 2010s (219, 220).

Einmahl et al. investigated the suprachoroidal space's tolerance of POE in rabbit models, finding no evidence of complications or intolerance over the 3 weeks the polymer remained in the space (221). In recent years, microneedle-based injections to deliver drug-laden solutions into the suprachoroidal space have been frequently explored, as they are a minimally invasive method with less risk of complications and rapid sealing of the injection site (201). Polymers investigated in these suprachoroidal microneedle injections serve a variety of roles, from simple injection excipients to the focal point for investigation. Chiang et al. (222) used injections of CMC to form hydrogels capable of swelling after injection to evaluate their effect on the thickness of the suprachoroidal space. They also explored the use of polymers as injectable drug delivery excipients by evaluating the distribution of FITC-labeled CMC and HA in the suprachoroidal space following microneedle injection (223). One possible innovation in this area is the use of PRINT® technology, which has been previously used to produce microneedle arrays for transdermal drug delivery (224). This application of PRINT® has been licensed for use by Aerie Pharmaceuticals and may be employed for suprachoroidal microneedle systems in the future (189). Jung et al. (225) investigated the utility of HA hydrogels as a means of directing suprachoroidal drug delivery, using the hydrogel's swelling behavior to push drug-laden polymer microparticles toward the posterior ocular tissue. These investigations demonstrate novel potential applications of polymers in ocular drug delivery and may provide a foundation for future innovation in suprachoroidal delivery.

Intravitreal Injections and Implants

While subconjunctival and suprachoroidal injections and implants offer a more efficient alternative to eyedrops for drug delivery to the eye and are more effective at both anterior and posterior delivery, they are still subject to limitations due to the tissue and drainage barriers they face when releasing drugs (201). Delivery directly to the vitreous humor bypasses corneal and scleral tissue barriers and ensures high drug delivery efficiency, drug bioavailability, and precise control of therapeutic concentrations, especially to tissues in the posterior eye (20, 142, 200, 213). For this reason, in spite of its invasive nature, intravitreal injections are currently a popular choice for drug delivery to the posterior segment. However, injections of drug solution without controlled release systems still face rapid clearance in the vitreous, necessitating frequent injections to maintain therapeutic levels of drug in the eye (213, 226). This is problematic for patients, as this procedure requires ophthalmologists to administer the injections and risks significant side effects. These range from more manageable issues, such as elevated IOP and endophthalmitis, to severe and potentially vision-altering side effects such as retinal detachment and intravitreal or subconjunctival hemorrhage (142, 197, 201, 203). In addition, drug that has been injected must still contend with diffusion through the vitreous humor to reach target tissues, a process made more difficult by rapid clearance due to vitreal circulation, the charge of vitreal fluid interfering with the diffusion of charged molecules, and the vitreous humor's extracellular matrix hampering large molecule movement (197, 227). While this method does offer some advantages over topical and subconjunctival delivery, these challenges limit its effectiveness in current drug delivery applications.

To overcome these challenges, significant effort has been invested in the development of intravitreal drug delivery systems.

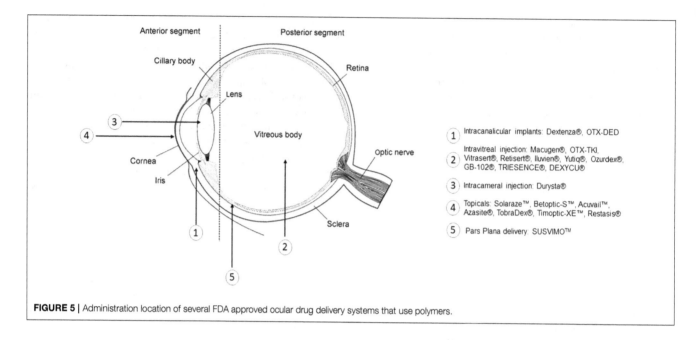

FIGURE 5 | Administration location of several FDA approved ocular drug delivery systems that use polymers.

Recent examples include a thermoresponsive polymer made of a combination of pentaerythritol, lactic acid, and ε-caprolactone functionalized with PEG and another thermoresponsive hydrogel made of PEG-poly(serinol hexamethylene urethane), which can be injected into the intraocular space to serve as a controlled-release system for extended drug delivery (226, 228). Researchers have also investigated a variety of polymer nanoparticles, using materials such as PCL and PLGA to develop drug-loaded nanoparticles for intravitreal injection (226, 227). Others have developed intravitreal implants out of materials such as PLGA, silicone, polyimide, and PVA. The goals of these systems are to increase the duration of drug release, thereby reducing injection frequency and its associated risks without exposing the eye to additional risks from the polymers themselves. This is a delicate balance, which will require significant research effort to maintain, but the potential benefits of an extended-release intravitreal drug delivery system are highly promising. Several labs are investigating additional polymer systems for intravitreal use. This includes our work developing polydopamine nanoparticles for anti-VEGF delivery, as well as efforts by other labs developing technologies such as phase-inversion mixtures of polymer and solvent, PEGylated siloxanes, and NIPAAm-based thermoresponsive polymers for intravitreal (130, 229, 230). Some of these systems are currently being translated for commercial use, such as ReVana Therapeutics' EyeLief™ and OcuLief™ injectable polymers (231). One system with particularly promising results is the Genentech Port Delivery System, SUSVIMO™ a reloadable port composed of a polysulfone body coated in silicone, which recently received FDA approval for delivery of ranibizumab for the treatment of wet AMD (232, 233). **Figure 5** contains a schematic of some of the FDA approved polymeric biomaterial products and administration location.

REGULATORY STATUS OF OCULAR DRUG DELIVERY SYSTEMS

While there is significant effort being invested in the development of polymer-based ocular drug delivery systems, a key challenge is the translation of these systems to clinical use. A number of products have successfully reached the market over the last few decades, with all four administration methods discussed previously having at least one FDA-approved drug delivery system that includes polymers to enhance their function. Notable examples are shown in **Table 3**. Eyedrops, the most mature drug delivery platform of the four, understandably have a significant number of polymer products, with numerous formulations approved for the treatment of diseases such as glaucoma, bacterial conjunctivitis, and uveitis (200, 213). Most make use of these polymers to increase the drop's residence time and release efficiency. Other applications such as polymer nanocarriers and thermosetting gels are still under investigation to evaluate their utility in extending the duration of eyedrop drug release and drug penetration (200, 202). Research into using eye drops for posterior segment delivery could have significant implications in the field of ocular drug delivery.

In the intravitreal space, progress has been much slower, with only seven intravitreal polymer systems obtaining regulatory approval for use with a small set of diseases (46, 200, 213, 244). These seven, the Iluvien®, Ozurdex®, Retisert®, Vitrasert®, Yutiq®, Dextenza, and DEXYCU® implants, use a variety of polymers in their construction. Iluvien® and Yutiq® use polyimide implants to deliver fluocinolone acetonide (46, 235). Ozurdex® uses a PLGA matrix that degrades to release dexamethasone (236). Retisert® contains a fluocinolone acetonide tablet in a silicone/PVA elastomer (46, 237). Vitrasert® releases ganciclovir from a PVA/ethylene vinyl acetate system (200). Dextenza suspends dexamethasone

TABLE 3 | Polymer-based ocular drug delivery systems with FDA approval.

Product	Polymer(s)	Pharmaceutical	Delivery route	Indication
TRIESENCE ® (234)	Carboxymethylcellulose	Triamcinolone Acetonide	Intravitreal Injection	Uveitis, temporal arteritis, sympathetic ophthalmia
Iluvien® (235)	Polyimide/Silicone/PVA	Fluocinolone Acetonide	Intravitreal Implant	Diabetic macular edema, uveitis
Ozurdex® (236)	PLGA	Dexamethasone	Intravitreal Implant	Diabetic macular edema, macular edema, uveitis
Retisert® (46, 237)	Silicone/PVA	Fluocinolone Acetonide	Intravitreal Implant	Posterior uveitis
Yutiq® (46)	Polyimide	Fluocinolone Acetonide	Intravitreal Implant	Posterior uveitis
Vitrasert (200)	PVA/Ethyl Vinyl Acetate	Ganciclovir	Intravitreal Implant	Retinitis
Dextenza (238)	PEG-Fluorescein	Dexamethasone	Intravitreal Implant	Postsurgical ocular inflammation
DEXYCU® (46)	Acetyl triethyl citrate	Dexamethasone	Intravitreal Implant	Postsurgical ocular inflammation
Durysta™ (48)	PLGA/PGA/PEG	Bimatoprost	Intravitreal Implant	Open angle glaucoma, ocular hypertension
Macugen® (21)	PEG	Pegaptanib sodium	Intravitreal Injection	Late stage AMD
SUSVIMO™ (232, 233)	Polysulfone/Silicone	Ranibizumab	Refillable Intraocular Implant	Wet AMD
ACUVUE® and others (239)	PHEMA, PMMA	None (contact lenses)	Anterior eye placement	Vision correction
Optive (85)	CMC	CMC	Eyedrop	Dry Eye Syndrome
Optive Fusion (85)	HA/CMC	HA/CMC	Eyedrop	Dry Eye Syndrome
Restasis® (77)	PAA	Cyclosporine	Eyedrop	Dry Eye Syndrome
Neopt (85)	HA	HA	Eyedrop	Dry Eye Syndrome
Vismed Multi (85)	HA	HA	Eyedrop	Dry Eye Syndrome
Tears Naturale® (240)	HPMC, Dextran 70	HPMC	Eyedrop	Dry Eye Syndrome
GenTeal® (240)	HPMC	HPMC	Eyedrop	Dry Eye Syndrome
Betoptic-S™ (200)	Polystyrene-divinylbenzene	Betaxolol	Eyedrop	Open angle Glaucoma
Acuvail™ (200)	CMC	Ketorolac Tromethamine	Eyedrop	Postsurgical ocular pain and inflammation
Azasite® (200)	Polycarbophil	Azithromycin	Eyedrop	Bacterial conjunctivitis
Lacrisert® (200)	HPMC	None (ocular insert)	Anterior eye placement	Dry Eye Syndrome
Mydriasert (200, 241)	Ammoniomethacrylate polymer	Tropicamide, phenylephrine HCl	Anterior eye placement	Induced preoperative mydriasis
TobraDex® (200, 242)	Hydroxyethylcellulose	Tobramycin, Dexamethasone	Eyedrop	Blepharitis
Timoptic-XE™ (200)	Gellan Gum	Timolol maleate	Eyedrop	Glaucoma
Xen Gel (243)	Gelatin	None (glaucoma drainage)	Subconjunctival implant	Glaucoma
Cypass (243)	Polyamide	None (glaucoma drainage)	Suprachoroidal implant	Glaucoma

in a PEG-fluorescein hydrogel (238). Finally, DEXYCU® makes use of acetyl triethyl citrate gel to deliver suspended dexamethasone (46). Four of these seven are non-degradable implants; Ozurdex®, Dextenza, and DEXYCU® are capable of resorption into the tissue of the eye. This helps to control drug release rate by providing a constant polymer membrane through which drug diffuses into the intravitreal space. However, it also presents challenge of implant removal and replacement once its therapeutic payload is expended, requires surgery and may incur additional health risks for the patient. A search of the Drugs@FDA database indicates that Iluvien, Ozurdex, Yutiq, DEXYCU, Dextenza, and Retisert remain available by prescription, while Vitrasert has been discontinued in the US. There are many more polymer implants in various phases of clinical and laboratory research making use of materials such as PLGA and PEG, indicating that there is significant progress yet to be made in clinical deployment of polymer systems in the vitreal space (20, 200, 226). In addition to recently approved systems such as the Genentech Port Delivery system, Kodiak is currently in phase 3 trials using an injectable biopolymer-antibody conjugate for the treatment of wet AMD and DME, while Aerie is testing biodegradable polymer implants for DME in a phase 2 trial (245, 246). With ongoing efforts in the development of intravitreal microparticles, nanoparticles, and injectable hydrogels, it is likely that intravitreal drug delivery options available to patients and clinicians will become significantly more diverse in the coming years (20, 142, 227, 247).

Subconjunctival drug delivery is a route that has only recently begun to be explored. Despite this, there has been progress in the development of subconjunctival polymer drug delivery systems, with the Ologen® and Xen Gel systems using collagen to construct implants and research efforts into other polymers such as PLGA showing promising results for implant performance (197, 201). However, these implants may pose challenges with discomfort and potential complications, leaving significant room for improvements in the future (197, 199).

Research into other polymer systems for subconjunctival delivery is an emerging area, with several research efforts investigating alternative implant polymer compositions, nanoparticle-based delivery systems, and injectable hydrogels for use as drug reservoirs in the subconjunctival space (197, 199, 209, 248–250). However, many of these are still in the early phases of development, and are likely to require further research showing safety and biocompatibility, as well as well-developed animal studies to show efficacy, before they can be put into clinical trials (197).

Finally, while the suprachoroidal route is the least explored for ocular drug delivery, products such as the XIPERE™ system's injectable triamcinolone acetonide solution are nearing market approval (201, 251). In addition to these promising developments in suprachoroidal injections, there are several choroidal devices that have found success in clinical uses. In particular, choroidal shunts made of polymers for the reduction of IOP in glaucoma patients have been the subject of significant investigation as an alternative to subconjunctival drainage, and choroidal port delivery systems have been successful in clinical trials evaluating their efficacy for drug delivery in retinal diseases (19, 252, 253). The ability to build on these innovations and incorporate polymers used in other ocular drug delivery systems will provide a valuable and viable path forward for the development of polymer systems for suprachoroidal injection.

Part of the reason that only a small number of synthetic polymers are being used in ocular drug delivery applications is regulatory hurdles. Even using FDA-approved therapeutics, these drug-device combinations must perform more testing than traditional medical devices through a 510(k) approval pathway with the FDA. Other challenges include the fact that the polymer delivery system likely changes the required therapeutic dose, generally leading to less therapeutic need due to reduced therapeutic waste. For example, when polymer delivery systems are employed, drug retention on the cornea improves significantly compared to non-polymer delivery systems (158). The reduction in necessary dose is not usually known until preclinical or clinical studies are conducted. Dosing at lower levels can be estimated using effective therapeutic concentrations, but long-term stability and therapeutic shelf-life are still concerns that must be addressed prior to approval.

FUTURE DIRECTIONS

While polymers have been used in ocular drug delivery for decades, with the first polymer intravitreal implants receiving approval in 1996 and topical applications making use of them since the 1970s, many applications of polymers in ocular drug delivery systems are still in the early stage of development, with significant untapped innovation that could lead to drastic improvements in the capability, quality, and ease of these treatments (213). The next decade will see a large increase in preclinical and clinical trials of polymer-based ocular drug delivery systems. Eyedrop systems have found some success in the development and clinical approval of polymers designed to extend the residence time of the drop on the corneal surface (207). However, continued challenges in corneal penetration

leave room for further exploration. Ongoing research into the translation of technologies such as nanomicelles and gelling agents to clinical applications seeks to further improve the efficacy of eyedrops as a delivery system (110, 254). Topical delivery to treat posterior segment diseases is also an area worth exploring to benefit patients. Intravitreal injections and implants have begun to embrace polymers as a method of increasing delivery duration with the development of polymer implants. Intravitreal implants, however, can be difficult to properly position and more difficult to extract once depleted. Further developments in biodegradable implants like Ozurdex®, as well as the development of alternative systems such as in-situ forming hydrogels, are likely to create less invasive intravitreal systems with similar capability to improve efficiency and reduce injection frequency. Subconjunctival and suprachoroidal injections and implants, as the youngest types of delivery systems, benefit from developments in other fields and are well-positioned to develop quickly once research locates optimal polymer formulations for both injectable solutions and implantable systems. For all of these methods, obtaining regulatory approval will be perhaps their most significant challenge. Many ocular drug delivery systems are listed in the FDA's drug databases, indicating that they were required to pass the FDA's drug approval process rather than obtaining device certification before reaching the open market. Despite this challenge in obtaining approval, dozens of polymer drug delivery systems are currently in clinical or preclinical trials for ocular applications, highlighting the immense potential many see for future growth in this field (20, 146, 255). Overall, the future is bright for the use of polymers in ocular drug delivery systems, with a solid foundation of clinical technologies, dozens of registered clinical trials evaluating next-generation delivery systems for even higher efficiency, and further investigative research developing applications of new polymer science in ocular delivery.

AUTHOR CONTRIBUTIONS

MA and KS-R were responsible for study conception. MA, RL, EH, and KS-R: literature review, analysis, interpretation of results, and writing were conducted. MA was primarily responsible for drafting the manuscript. All authors reviewed the results and approved the final version of the manuscript.

ACKNOWLEDGMENTS

We would like to acknowledge the past and present members of the Swindle-Reilly Lab for Biomimetic Polymeric Biomaterials for help and encouragement, particularly former lab members Pengfei Jiang, Nguyen Tram, and Courtney Maxwell for using polymers to advance work on ocular drug delivery.

REFERENCES

1. WHO. *World Report on Vision Executive Summary.* World Health Organization. p. 1–12 (2019).

2. Eye Health Statistics—American Academy of Ophthalmology. Available online at: https://www.aao.org/newsroom/eye-health-statistics (2019)

3. BrightFocus Foundation. *Sources for Macular Degeneration. Facts & Figures.* Available online at: https://www.brightfocus.org/sources-macular-degeneration-facts-figures (accessed Sep 13, 2021).

4. Rein DB, Wittenborn JS, Zhang X, Honeycutt AA, Lesesne SB, Saaddine J, et al. Forecasting age-related macular degeneration through the year 2050: the potential impact of new treatments. *Arch. Ophthalmol.* (2009) 127, 533–540. doi: 10.1001/archophthalmol.2009.58

5. Shahiwala A. Applications of polymers in ocular drug delivery. *Appl Polym Drug Deliv.* (2021) 355–92. doi: 10.1016/B978-0-12-819659-5.00013-6

6. Nartey A. The pathophysiology of cataract and major interventions to retarding its progression: a mini review. *MedCrave.* (2017) 6:1–3. doi: 10.15406/aovs.2017.06.00178

7. Weinreb RN, Aung T. The pathophysiology and treatment of glaucoma: a review. *JAMA.* (2014) 311:1901–11. doi: 10.1001/jama.2014.3192

8. Janson BJ, Alward WL, Kwon YH, Bettis DI, Fingert JH, Provencher LM. Glaucoma-associated corneal endothelial cell damage: a review. *Surv Ophthalmol.* (2018) 63:500–6. doi: 10.1016/j.survophthal.2017.11.002

9. Porta M. Diabetic retinopathy A clinical update. *Diabetologia.* (2002) 45:1617–34. doi: 10.1007/s00125-002-0990-7

10. Jager RD, Mieler WF. Age-related macular degeneration. *N Engl J Med.* (2008) 358:2606–17. doi: 10.1056/NEJMra0801537

11. Wang W. Diabetic retinopathy : pathophysiology and treatments. *Int J Mol Sci.* (2018) 19:1–14. doi: 10.3390/ijms19061816

12. Fogli S, Mogavero S, Egan CG, Del Re M. Pathophysiology and pharmacological targets of VEGF in diabetic macular edema. *Pharmacol Res.* (2016) 103:149–57. doi: 10.1016/j.phrs.2015.11.003

13. Tram NK, McLean RM, Swindle-Reilly KE. Glutathione improves the antioxidant activity of vitamin c in human lens and retinal epithelial cells: implications for vitreous substitutes. *Curr Eye Res.* (2021) 46:470–81. doi: 10.1080/02713683.2020.1809002

14. Kassa E, Ciulla TA, Hussain RM. Complement inhibition as a therapeutic strategy in retinal disorders. *Expert Opin Biol Ther.* (2019) 19:335–42. doi: 10.1080/14712598.2019.1575358

15. Yu B, Li X-R, Zhang X-M. Mesenchymal stem cell-derived extracellular vesicles as a new therapeutic strategy for ocular diseases. *World J. Stem Cells.* 12:178–87. doi: 10.4252/wjsc.v12.i3.178

16. Karanfil FÇ, Turgut B. Update on presbyopia-correcting *Drops Eur Ophthalmic Rev.* 11:99. (2017). doi: 10.17925/EOR.2017.11.02.99

17. Vandenberghe LH. Novel adeno-associated viral vectors for retinal gene therapy. *Gene Ther.* (2012) 19:162–8. doi: 10.1038/gt.2011.151

18. Spinozzi E, Baldassarri C, Acquaticci L, Del Bello F, Grifantini M, Cappellacci L. Adenosine receptors as promising targets for the management of ocular diseases. *Med Chem Res.* (2021) 30:353–70. doi: 10.1007/s00044-021-02704-x

19. Gote V, Sikder S, Sicotte J. Ocular drug delivery: present innovations and future challenges. *J Pharmacol Exp Ther.* (2019) 370:602–24. doi: 10.1124/jpet.119.256933

20. Kang-Mieler JJ, Rudeen KM, Liu W. Advances in ocular drug delivery systems. *Eye.* (2020) 34:1371–9. doi: 10.1038/s41433-020-0809-0

21. Basile AS, Hutmacher MM, Kowalski KG, Gandelman KY. Population pharmacokinetics of pegaptanib sodium (Macugen®) in patients with diabetic macular edema. *Clin Ophthalmol.* (2015) 9:323–35. doi: 10.2147/OPTH.S74050

22. Turecek PL, Bossard MJ, Schoetens F. PEGylation of biopharmaceuticals: a review of chemistry and nonclinical safety information of approved drugs. *J Pharm Sci.* (2016) 105:460–75. doi: 10.1016/j.xphs.2015.11.015

23. Abdelkader H, Fathalla Z, Seyfoddin A, Farahani M, Thrimawithana T, Allahham A, et al. Polymeric long-acting drug delivery systems (LADDS) for treatment of chronic diseases: Inserts, patches, wafers, and implants. *Adv Drug Deliv Rev.* (2021) 177:113957. doi: 10.1016/j.addr.2021.113957

24. Blizzard CD, Desai A, Driscoll A, Cheung M. Ocular pharmacokinetics of OTX-DED, a sustained-release intracanalicular insert delivering dexamethasone, in a canine model. *IOVS.* (2021) 62:1.

25. Hussain RM, Shaukat BA, Ciulla LM, Berrocal AM. Vascular endothelial growth factor antagonists: promising players in the treatment of neovascular age-related macular degeneration. *Drug Des Devel Ther.* (2021) 15:2653–65. doi: 10.2147/DDDT.S295223

26. Mah FSE. On gel formation time of adding topical ophthalmic medications to resure sealant, an in situ hydrogel. *J Ocul Pharmacol Ther.* (2016) 32:396–9. doi: 10.1089/jop.2015.0112

27. Foroutan SM. The *in vitro* evaluation of polyethylene glycol esters of hydrocortisone 21-succinate as ocular prodrugs. *Int J Pharm.* (1999) 182:79–92. doi: 10.1016/S0378-5173(99)00059-9

28. Eid HM, Elkomy MH, El Menshawe SF. Development, optimization, and *in vitro/in vivo* characterization of enhanced lipid nanoparticles for ocular delivery of ofloxacin: the influence of pegylation and chitosan coating. *AAPS PharmSciTech.* (2019) 20:1–14. doi: 10.1208/s12249-019-1371-6

29. Shatz W, Hass PE, Peer N, Paluch MT, Blanchette C, Han G. Identification and characterization of an octameric PEG-protein conjugate system for intravitreal long-acting delivery to the back of the eye. *PLoS ONE.* (2019) 14:1–20. doi: 10.1371/journal.pone.0218613

30. Lakhani P, Patil A, Wu K-W, Sweeney C, Tripathi S, Avula B. Optimization, stabilization, and characterization of amphotericin B loaded nanostructured lipid carriers for ocular drug delivery. *Int J Pharm.* (2019) 572:1–14. doi: 10.1016/j.ijpharm.2019.118771

31. Teodorescu M, Bercea M. Biomaterials of PVA and PVP in medical and pharmaceutical applications: Perspectives and challenges. *Biotechnol Adv.* (2019) 37:109–31. doi: 10.1016/j.biotechadv.2018.11.008

32. Kuno N. Biodegradable intraocular therapies for retinal disorders. *Drugs Aging.* (2010) 27:117–34. doi: 10.2165/11530970-000000000-00000

33. Arcinue CA, Ceró OM. A comparison between the fluocinolone acetonide (retisert) and dexamethasone (ozurdex) intravitreal implants in uveitis. *J Ocul Pharmacol Ther.* (2012) 29:501–7. doi: 10.1089/jop.2012.0180

34. Habib MS. ILUVIEN®technology in the treatment of center-involving diabetic macular edema: a review of the literature. *Ther Deliv.* (2018) 9:547–56. doi: 10.4155/tde-2018-0006

35. Schmit-Eilenberger VK. A novel intravitreal fluocinolone acetonide implant (Iluvien®) in the treatment of patients with chronic diabetic macular edema that is insufficiently responsive to other medical treatment options: a case series. *Clin Ophthalmol.* (2015) 9:801–11. doi: 10.2147/OPTH.S79785

36. Paolini MS, Fenton OS, Bhattacharya C, Andresen JL. Polymers for extended-release administration. *Biomed Microdevices 2019 212 21.* (2019) 1–24. doi: 10.1007/s10544-019-0386-9

37. Haghjou N, Soheilian M. Sustained release intraocular drug delivery devices for treatment of uveitis. *J Ophthalmic Vis Res.* (2011) 6:317–29.

38. García-Estrada P, García-Bon MA, López-Naranjo EJ, Basaldúa-Pérez DN, Santos A. Polymeric implants for the treatment of intraocular eye diseases: trends in biodegradable and non-biodegradable materials. *Pharmaceutics.* (2021) 13:1–20. doi: 10.3390/pharmaceutics13050701

39. Shin CS, Marcano DC, Park K. Application of hydrogel template strategy in ocular drug delivery. *Methods Mol Biol.* (2017) 1570:279–85. doi: 10.1007/978-1-4939-6840-4_19

40. Makadia HK. Poly lactic-co-glycolic acid (PLGA) as biodegradable controlled drug delivery carrier. *Polymers.* (2011) 3:1377–97. doi: 10.3390/polym3031377

41. Marin E, Briceño MI. Critical evaluation of biodegradable polymers used in nanodrugs. *Int J Nanomed.* (2013) 8:3071–91. doi: 10.2147/IJN.S47186

42. Farah S, Anderson DG. Physical and mechanical properties of PLA, and their functions in widespread applications—a comprehensive review. *Adv Drug Deliv Rev.* (2016) 107:367–92. doi: 10.1016/j.addr.2016.06.012

43. Kuppermann BD, Patel SS, Boyer DS, Augstin AJ, Freeman WR, Kerr KJ. Phase 2 study of the safety and efficacy of brimonidine drug delivery system (brimo dds) generation 1 in patients with geographic atrophy secondary to age-related macular degeneratiON. *Retina.* (2021) 41:144–55. doi: 10.1097/IAE.000000000000 2789

44. Baino F. Regulation of the ocular cell/tissue response by implantable biomaterials and drug delivery systems. *Bioengineering.* (2020) 7:1–31. doi: 10.3390/bioengineering7030065

45. Gentile P, Chiono V, Carmagnola I. An overview of poly(lactic-co-glycolic) acid (PLGA)-based biomaterials for bone tissue

engineering. *Int J Mol Sci.* (2014) 15:3640–59. doi: 10.3390/ijms15 033640

46. Cao Y, Samy KE, Bernards DA. Recent advances in intraocular sustained-release drug delivery devices. *Drug Discovery Today.* (2019) 24:1694–700. doi: 10.1016/j.drudis.2019. 05.031

47. Chan A, Leung L-S. Critical appraisal of the clinical utility of the dexamethasone intravitreal implant (Ozurdex®) for the treatment of macular edema related to branch retinal vein occlusion or central retinal vein occlusion. *Clin Ophthalmol.* (2011) 5:1043–9. doi: 10.2147/OPTH.S1 3775

48. Shirley M. Bimatoprost implant: first approval. *Drugs Aging.* (2020) 37:457–62. doi: 10.1007/s40266-020-00769-8

49. Liu W, Lee B-S, Mieler WF. Biodegradable microsphere-hydrogel ocular drug delivery system for controlled and extended release of bioactive aflibercept *in vitro*. *Curr Eye Res.* (2019) 44:264–74. doi: 10.1080/02713683.2018.153 3983

50. Liu W, Borrell MA, Venerus DC, Mieler WF. Characterization of biodegradable microsphere-hydrogel ocular drug delivery system for controlled and extended release of ranibizumab. *Transl Vis Sci Technol.* (2019) 8:1–13. doi: 10.1167/tvst.8.1.12

51. Osswald CR, Guthrie MJ, Avila A, Valio JA, Mieler WF, Kang-Mieler. In vivo efficacy of an injectable microsphere-hydrogel ocular drug delivery system. *Curr Eye Res.* (2017) 42:1293–301. doi: 10.1080/02713683.2017.1302590

52. Liu W, Tawakol AP, Rudeen KM, Mieler WF. Treatment efficacy and biocompatibility of a biodegradable aflibercept-loaded microsphere-hydrogel drug delivery system. *Transl Vis Sci Technol.* (2020) 9:1–14. doi: 10.1167/tvst.9.11.13

53. Mondal D, Griffith M. Polycaprolactone-based biomaterials for tissue engineering and drug delivery: current scenario and challenges. *Int J Polym Mater Polym Biomater.* (2016) 65:255–65. doi: 10.1080/00914037.2015.1103241

54. Malikmammadov E, Endogan Tanir T, Kiziltay A, Hasirci V. PCL and PCL-based materials in biomedical applications. *J Biomater Sci Polym Ed.* (2018) 29:863–93. doi: 10.1080/09205063.2017.1394711

55. Bernards DA, Bhisitkul RB, Wynn P, Steedman MR, Lee O-T, Wong F. Ocular biocompatibility and structural integrity of micro- and nanostructured poly(caprolactone) films. *J. Ocul. Pharmacol. Ther.* (2013). 29:249–57. doi: 10.1089/jop.2012.0152

56. Samy KE, Cao Y, Kim J, Konichi S. Co-delivery of timolol and brimonidine with a polymer thin-film intraocular device. *J Ocul Pharmacol Ther.* (2019) 35:124–31. doi: 10.1089/jop.2018.0096

57. Hashemi Nasr F, Khoee S, Mehdi Dehghan M, Sadeghian Chaleshtori S. Preparation and evaluation of contact lenses embedded with polycaprolactone-based nanoparticles for ocular drug delivery. *Biomolecules.* (2015) 17:485–95. doi: 10.1021/acs.biomac.5b01387

58. Zhang Z, He Z, Liang R, Ma Y, Huang W, Jiang R. Fabrication of a micellar supramolecular hydrogel for ocular drug delivery. *Biomacromolecules.* (2016) 17:798–807. doi: 10.1021/acs.biomac.5b01526

59. Shahab MS, Rizwanullah M, Alshehri S. Optimization to development of chitosan decorated polycaprolactone nanoparticles for improved ocular delivery of dorzolamide: *in vitro*, ex vivo and toxicity assessments. *Int J Biol Macromol.* (2020) 163:2392–404. doi: 10.1016/j.ijbiomac.2020.09.185

60. Jiang P, Jacobs KM, Ohr MP. Chitosan–polycaprolactone core–shell microparticles for sustained delivery of bevacizumab. *Mol Pharm.* (2020) 17:2570–84. doi: 10.1021/acs.molpharmaceut.0c00260

61. Jiang P, Chaparro FJ, Cuddington CT, Palmer AF, Ohr MP, Lannutti JJ. Injectable biodegradable bi-layered capsule for sustained delivery of bevacizumab in treating wet age-related macular degeneration. *J Control Release.* (2020) 320:442–56. doi: 10.1016/j.jconrel.2020.01.036

62. Kim J, Judisch M, Mudumba S, Asada H, Aya-Shibuya E, Bhisitkul RB. Biocompatibility and pharmacokinetic analysis of an intracameral polycaprolactone drug delivery implant for glaucoma. *Invest Ophthalmol Vis Sci.* (2016) 57:4341–6. doi: 10.1167/iovs.16-19585

63. Souto EB, Dias-ferreira J, Ana L, Ettcheto M, Elena S. Advanced formulation approaches for ocular drug delivery : state-of-the-art and recent patents. *Pharmaceutics.* (2019) 11:1–29. doi: 10.3390/pharmaceutics11090460

64. Sovadinova I, Palmermo EF, Urban M, Mpiga P, Caputo GA. Activity and mechanism of antimicrobial peptide-mimetic amphiphilic polymethacrylate derivatives. *Polymers.* (2011) 3:1512–32. doi: 10.3390/polym3031512

65. Ali U, Juhanni Bt Abd Karim K, Aziah Buang NA. Review of the properties and applications of poly (methyl methacrylate) (PMMA). *Polym Rev.* (2015) 55:678–705. doi: 10.1080/15583724.2015.1031377

66. Fan X, Torres-Luna C, Azadi M, Domszy R, Hu N, Yang A, et al. Evaluation of commercial soft contact lenses for ocular drug delivery: a review. *Acta Biomater.* (2020) 115:60–74. doi: 10.1016/j.actbio.2020.08.025

67. Kiddee W, Trope GE, Sheng L, Beltran-Agullo L, Smith M, Strungaru MH, et al. (2013). Intraocular pressure monitoring post intravitreal steroids: a systematic review. *Surv. Ophthalmol.* 58, 291–310. doi: 10.1016/j.survophthal.2012.08.003

68. Ubani-Ukoma U, Gibson D, Schultz G, Silva BO. Evaluating the potential of drug eluting contact lenses for treatment of bacterial keratitis using an ex vivo corneal model. *Int J Pharm.* (2019) 565:499–508. doi: 10.1016/j.ijpharm.2019.05.031

69. Pereira-da-Mota AF, Vivero-Lopez M, Topete A, Serro AP, Concheiro A, Alvarez-Lorenzo C. Atorvastatin-eluting contact lenses : effects of molecular imprinting and sterilization on drug loading and release. *Pharmaceutics.* (2021) 13:1–22. doi: 10.3390/pharmaceutics13050606

70. González-Chomón C, Silva M, Concheiro A. Biomimetic contact lenses eluting olopatadine for allergic conjunctivitis. *Acta Biomater.* (2016) 41:302–11. doi: 10.1016/j.actbio.2016.05.032

71. Jung HJ. Temperature sensitive contact lenses for triggered ophthalmic drug delivery. *Biomaterials.* (2012) 33:2289–300. doi: 10.1016/j.biomaterials.2011.10.076

72. Brannigan RP. Synthesis and evaluation of mucoadhesive acryloyl-quaternized PDMAEMA nanogels for ocular drug delivery. *Colloids Surfaces B Biointerfaces.* (2017) 155:538–43. doi: 10.1016/j.colsurfb.2017.04.050

73. Soni V, Pandey V, Tiwari R, Asati S, Tekade RK. Design and evaluation of ophthalmic delivery formulations. In: *Basic Fundamentals of Drug Delivery.* New york, NY: Academic Press (2019), p. 473–538.

74. Dung Nguyen D, Lai J-Y. Advancing the stimuli response of polymer-based drug delivery systems for ocular disease treatment. *Polym Chem.* (2020) 11:6988–7008. doi: 10.1039/D0PY00919A

75. Prasannan A, Tsai H-C, Chen Y-S. A thermally triggered in situ hydrogel from poly(acrylic acid-co-N-isopropylacrylamide) for controlled release of anti-glaucoma drugs. *J Mater Chem B.* (2014) 2:1988–97. doi: 10.1039/c3tb21360a

76. Prasannan A, Tsai HC. Formulation and evaluation of epinephrine-loaded poly(acrylic acid-co-N-isopropylacrylamide) gel for sustained ophthalmic drug delivery. *React Funct Polym.* (2018) 124:40–7. doi: 10.1016/j.reactfunctpolym.2018.01.001

77. Mah F, Milner M, Yiu S, Donnenfeld E, Conway TM. PERSIST: Physician's Evaluation of Restasis® Satisfaction in Second Trial of topical cyclosporine ophthalmic emulsion 0.05% for dry eye: a retrospective review. *Clin. Ophthalmol.* (2012). 6:1971–6. doi: 10.2147/OPTH.S30261

78. Lancina MG III, Yang, H. Dendrimers for ocular drug delivery. *Can J Chem.* (2017) 95:897–902. doi: 10.1139/cjc-2017-0193

79. Yavuz B, Bozdag Pehlivan S. Dendrimeric systems and their applications in ocular drug delivery. *Sci World J.* (2013) 2013:1–13. doi: 10.1155/2013/732340

80. Madaan K, Kumar S, Poonia N, Lather V, Pandita D. Dendrimers in drug delivery and targeting: drug-dendrimer interactions and toxicity issues. *J Pharm Bioallied Sci.* 6:139–50. doi: 10.4103/0975-7406.130965

81. Yavuz B, Pehlivan SB, Bolu BS, Sanyal RN, Vural I. Dexamethasone—PAMAM dendrimer conjugates for retinal delivery: preparation, characterization and *in vivo* evaluation. *J Pharm Pharmacol.* (2016) 68:1010–20. doi: 10.1111/jphp.12587

82. Iezzi R, Guru BR, Glybina IV, Mishra MJ, Kennedy A. Dendrimer-based targeted intravitreal therapy for sustained attenuation of neuroinflammation in retinal degeneration. *Biomaterials.* (2011) 33:979–88. doi: 10.1016/j.biomaterials.2011.10.010

83. Wang J, Williamson GS, Lancina MG III, Yang H. Mildly cross-linked dendrimer hydrogel prepared *via* aza-michael addition reaction for topical brimonidine delivery. *J Biomed Nanotechnol.* (2017) 13:1089–96. doi: 10.1166/jbn.2017.2436

84. Aravamudhan A, Ramos DM, Nada AA. Natural polymers: polysaccharides and their derivatives for biomedical applications. *Nat Synth Biomed Polym.* (2014) 2014:67–89. doi: 10.1016/B978-0-12-396983-5.00004-1

85. Dutescu RM, Panfil C. Comparison of the effects of various lubricant eye drops on the *in vitro* rabbit corneal healing and toxicity. *Exp Toxicol Pathol.* (2017) 69:123–9. doi: 10.1016/j.etp.2016.12.002

86. Deng S, Li X, Yang W, He K, Ye X. Injectable in situ cross-linking hyaluronic acid/carboxymethyl cellulose based hydrogels for drug release. *J Biomater Sci Polym.* Ed. 29:1643–55. doi: 10.1080/09205063.2018.1481005

87. Yuan X, Marcano DC, Shin CS, Hua X, Isenhart LC, Pflugfelder SC. Ocular drug delivery nanowafer with enhanced therapeutic efficacy. *ACS Nano.* (2015) 9:1749–58. doi: 10.1021/nn506599f

88. Coursey TG, Henriksson JT, Marcano DC, Shin CS, Isenhart LC, Ahmed F. Dexamethasone nanowafer as an effective therapy for dry eye disease. *J Control Release.* (2015) 213:168–74. doi: 10.1016/j.jconrel.2015.07.007

89. Tundisi LL, Mostaço GB, Carricondo PC. Hydroxypropyl methylcellulose: Physicochemical properties and ocular drug delivery formulations. *Eur J Pharm Sci.* (2021) 159:1–12. doi: 10.1016/j.ejps.2021.105736

90. Hu L, Sun Y. Advances in chitosan-based drug delivery vehicles. *Nanoscale.* (2013) 5:3103–11. doi: 10.1039/c3nr00338h

91. Cheng Y-H, Tsai T-H, Jhan Y-Y, Chiu AW-H, Tsai K-L, Chien C-S. Thermosensitive chitosan-based hydrogel as a topical ocular drug delivery system of latanoprost for glaucoma treatment. *Carbohydr Polym.* 144:390–9. doi: 10.1016/j.carbpol.2016.02.080

92. Rong X, Yang J, Ji Y, Zhu X, Lu Y, Mo Z. Biocompatibility and safety of insulin-loaded chitosan nanoparticles/PLGA-PEG-PLGA hydrogel (ICNPH) delivered by subconjunctival injection in rats. *J Drug Deliv Sci Technol.* (2019) 49:556–62. doi: 10.1016/j.jddst.2018.12.032

93. Başaran E. Ocular application of chitosan. *Expert Opin Drug Deliv.* (2012) 9:701–12. doi: 10.1517/17425247.2012.681775

94. Arafa MG, Girgis GNS. Chitosan-coated PLGA nanoparticles for enhanced ocular anti-inflammatory efficacy of atorvastatin calcium. *Int J Nanomed.* (2020) 15:1335–47. doi: 10.2147/IJN.S237314

95. Chaharband F, Daftarian N, Kanavi MR, Varshochian R, Hajiramezanali M, Norouzi P. Trimethyl chitosan-hyaluronic acid nano-polyplexes for intravitreal VEGFR-2 siRNA delivery: formulation and *in vivo* efficacy evaluation. *Nanomed Nanotechnol Biol Med.* (2020) 26:1–12. doi: 10.1016/j.nano.2020.102181

96. Shi H, Wang Y, Bao Z, Lin D, Liu H, Yu A. Thermosensitive glycol chitosan-based hydrogel as a topical ocular drug delivery system for enhanced ocular bioavailability. *Int J Pharm.* (2019) 570:1–7. doi: 10.1016/j.ijpharm.2019.118688

97. Zhang X, Wei D, Xu Y, Zhu Q. Hyaluronic acid in ocular drug delivery. *Carbohydr Polym.* (2021) 264:1–24. doi: 10.1016/j.carbpol.2021.118006

98. Saranraj P. Hyaluronic acid production and its applications-a review. *Int J Pharm Biol Arch.* (2013) 4:853–9.

99. Hemshekhar M, Thushara RM, Chandranayaka S, Shermen LS, Kemparaju K. Emerging roles of hyaluronic acid bioscaffolds in tissue engineering and regenerative medicine. *Int J Biol Macromol.* (2016) 86:917–28. doi: 10.1016/j.ijbiomac.2016.02.032

100. Liu Y, Wang R, Zarembinski T, Doty N, Jiang C, Regatieri C. The application of hyaluronic acid hydrogels to retinal progenitor cell transplantation. *Tissue Eng Part A.* (2013) 19:135–42. doi: 10.1089/ten.tea.2012.0209

101. Eom Y, Kim S, Huh J, Koh MY, Hwang JY, Kang B. Self-sealing hyaluronic acid-coated 30-gauge intravitreal injection needles for preventing vitreous and drug reflux through needle passage. *Sci Rep.* (2021) 11:1–10. doi: 10.1038/s41598-021-96561-8

102. Vasvani S, Kulkarni P. Hyaluronic acid: a review on its biology, aspects of drug delivery, route of administrations and a special emphasis on its approved marketed products and recent clinical studies. *Int J Biol Macromol.* (2020) 151:1012–29. doi: 10.1016/j.ijbiomac.2019.11.066

103. Jarvis B. Topical 3% diclofenac in 2.5% hyaluronic acid gel: a review of its use in patients with actinic keratoses. *Am J Clin Dermatol.* (2003) 4:203–13. doi: 10.2165/00128071-200304030-00007

104. Diaz-Montes E. Sources, structures, and properties. *Polysaccharides.* (2021) 2:554–65. doi: 10.3390/polysaccharides2030033

105. Kathuria A, Shamloo K, Jhanji V. Categorization of marketed artificial tear formulations based on their ingredients: a rational approach for their use. *J Clin Med.* (2021) 10:1–11. doi: 10.3390/jcm10061289

106. Chaiyasan W, Srinivas SP. Crosslinked chitosan-dextran sulfate nanoparticle for improved topical ocular drug delivery. *Mol Vis.* (2015) 21:1224–34.

107. Delgado D, del Pozo-Rodríguez A, Solinís MÁ, Avilés-Triqueros M, Weber BH, Fernández E, et al. (2011). Dextran and protamine-based solid lipid nanoparticles as potential vectors for the treatment of X-linked juvenile retinoschisis. *Hum Gene Ther.* 23:345–55. doi: 10.1089/hum.2011.115

108. Mudgil D, Barak S. Guar gum: processing, properties and food applications—a review. *Human Gene Therapy.* (2014) 23: 345-55.

109. Thombare N, Jha U, Mishra S. Guar gum as a promising starting material for diverse applications: a review. *Int J Biol Macromol.* (2016) 88:361–72. doi: 10.1016/j.ijbiomac.2016.04.001

110. Labetoulle M, Schmickler S, Galarreta D, Böhringer D, Ogundele A, Guillon M, Baudouin C, et al. (2018). Efficacy and safety of dual-polymer hydroxypropyl guar- and hyaluronic acid-containing lubricant eyedrops for the management of dry-eye disease: a randomized double-masked clinical study. *Clin Ophthalmol.* 12:2499–508. doi: 10.2147/OPTH.S177176

111. Shi Q, Daisy ERAC, Yang G, Zhang J, Mickymaray S, Alfaiz FA. Multifeatured guar gum armed drug delivery system for the delivery of ofloxacin drug to treat ophthalmic dieases. *Arab J Chem.* (2021) 14:1–12. doi: 10.1016/j.arabjc.2021.103118

112. Cheng K-C, Demirci A. Pullulan: biosynthesis, production, and applications. *Appl Microbiol Biotechnol.* (2011) 92:29–44. doi: 10.1007/s00253-011-3477-y

113. Prajapati VD, Jani GK. Pullulan: an exopolysaccharide and its various applications. *Carbohydr Polym.* (2013) 95:540–9. doi: 10.1016/j.carbpol.2013.02.082

114. Singh RS, Kaur N, Rana V. Recent insights on applications of pullulan in tissue engineering. *Carbohydr Polym.* (2016) 153:455–62. doi: 10.1016/j.carbpol.2016.07.118

115. Göttel B, Lucas H, Syrowatka F, Knolle W, Kuntsche J, Heinzelmann J. In situ gelling amphotericin B nanofibers: a new option for the treatment of keratomycosis. *Front Bioeng Biotechnol.* (2020) 8:384. doi: 10.3389/fbioe.2020.600384

116. Pai G. Formulation and evaluation of extended release ocular inserts prepared from synthetic and natural biodegradable-biocompatible polymers. *Res J Pharm Tech.* (2014) 7:48–51.

117. Browne S, Zeugolis DI. Collagen: finding a solution for the source. *Tissue Eng - Part A.* (2013) 19:1491–4. doi: 10.1089/ten.tea.2012.0721

118. Khan R. Use of collagen as a biomaterial: an update. *J Indian Soc Periodontol.* (2013) 17:539–42. doi: 10.4103/0972-124X.118333

119. Wong FSY, Tsang KK, Chu AMW, Chan BP, Yao KM. Injectable cell-encapsulating composite alginate-collagen platform with inducible termination switch for safer ocular drug delivery. *Biomaterials.* (2019) 201:53–67. doi: 10.1016/j.biomaterials.2019.01.032

120. Zadeh MA, Khoder M, Al-Kinani AA, Younes HM. Retinal cell regeneration using tissue engineered polymeric scaffolds. *Drug Discov Today.* (2019) 24:1669–78. doi: 10.1016/j.drudis.2019.04.009

121. Belin MW, Lim L, Rajpal RK, Hafezi F, Gomes JAP. Corneal cross-linking: Current USA status report from the cornea society. *Cornea.* (2018) 37:1218–25. doi: 10.1097/ICO.0000000000001707

122. Gómez-Guillén MC, Giménez B, López-Caballero ME. Functional and bioactive properties of collagen and gelatin from alternative sources: a review. *Food Hydrocoll.* (2011) 25:1813–27. doi: 10.1016/j.foodhyd.2011.02.007

123. Rose JB, Pacelli S, El Haj AJ, Dua HS, Hopkinson A, White LJ. Gelatin-based materials in ocular tissue engineering. *Materials.* (2014) 7:3106. doi: 10.3390/ma7043106

124. Echave MC, Burgo LS, Pedraz JL. Gelatin as biomaterial for tissue engineering. *Curr Pharm Design.* 23:3567–84 (2017). doi: 10.2174/0929867324666170511123101

125. Song V, Nagai N, Saijo S, Kaji H, Nishizawa M. In situ formation of injectable chitosan-gelatin hydrogels through double crosslinking for sustained intraocular drug delivery. *Mater Sci Eng C Mater Biol Appl.* (2018) 88:1–12. doi: 10.1016/j.msec.2018.02.022

126. Tsai CH, Wang PY, Lin IC, Huang H, Liu GS. Ocular drug delivery: role of degradable polymeric nanocarriers for ophthalmic application. *Int J Mol Sci.* (2018) 19:2830. doi: 10.3390/ijms19092830

127. Chun YY, Yap ZL, Seet LF, Chan HH, Toh LZ, Chu SWL. Positive-charge tuned gelatin hydrogel-siSPARC injectable for siRNA anti-scarring therapy in post glaucoma filtration surgery. *Sci Rep.* (2021) 11:1–14. doi: 10.1038/s41598-020-80542-4

128. Batul R, Tamanna T, Khaliq A. Recent progress in the biomedical applications of polydopamine nanostructures. *Biomater Sci.* (2017) 5:1204–29. doi: 10.1039/C7BM00187H

129. Liu S, Zhao X, Tang J, Han Y. Drug-eluting hydrophilic coating modification of intraocular lens *via* facile dopamine self-polymerization for posterior capsular opacification prevention. *ACS Biomater Sci Eng.* (2021) 7:1065–73. doi: 10.1021/acsbiomaterials.0c01705

130. Jiang P, Choi A. Controlled release of anti-VEGF by redox-responsive polydopamine nanoparticles. *Nanoscale.* (2020) 12:1–33. doi: 10.1039/D0NR03710A

131. Poinard B, Kamaluddin S, Tan AQQ, Neoh KG. Polydopamine coating enhances mucopenetration and cell uptake of nanoparticles. *ACS Appl Mater Interfaces.* (2019) 11:4777–89. doi: 10.1021/acsami.8b18107

132. Ciolacu DE, Nicu R. Cellulose-based hydrogels as sustained drug-delivery systems. *Materials.* (2020) 13:1–37. doi: 10.3390/ma13225270

133. Dubashynskaya N, Poshina D, Raik S, Urtti A. Polysaccharides in ocular drug delivery. *Pharmaceutics.* (2020) 12:1–30. doi: 10.3390/pharmaceutics12010022

134. Desfrançois C, Auzély R. Lipid nanoparticles and their hydrogel composites for drug delivery: A review. *Pharmaceuticals.* (2018) 11:1–24. doi: 10.3390/ph11040118

135. Sung YK. Recent advances in polymeric drug delivery systems. *Biomater Res.* (2020) 24:1–12. doi: 10.1186/s40824-020-00190-7

136. Tiwari S. Modified hyaluronic acid based materials for biomedical applications. *Int J Biol Macromol.* (2019) 121:556–71. doi: 10.1016/j.ijbiomac.2018.10.049

137. Tripodo G, Trapani A, Torre ML, Giammona G, Trapani G. Hyaluronic acid and its derivatives in drug delivery and imaging: recent advances and challenges. *Eur J Pharm Biopharm.* (2015) 97:400–16. doi: 10.1016/j.ejpb.2015.03.032

138. Verma D. Recent advances in guar gum based drug delivery systems and their administrative routes. *Int J Biol Macromol.* (2021) 181:653–71. doi: 10.1016/j.ijbiomac.2021.03.087

139. Göttel B, Souza de Silva C, de Oliveira CS, Syrowatka F, Fiorentzis M, Viestenz A, et al. Electrospun nanofibers—a promising solid in-situ gelling alternative for ocular drug delivery. *Eur J Pharm Biopharm.* (2019) 146:125–32. doi: 10.1016/j.ejpb.2019.11.012

140. Balasso A, Subrizi A, Salmaso S, Mastrotto F, Garofalo M, Tang M. Screening of chemical linkers for development of pullulan bioconjugates for intravitreal ocular applications. *Eur J Pharm Sci.* (2021) 161:105785. doi: 10.1016/j.ejps.2021.105785

141. Dionísio M, Braz L, Corvo M, Lourenço JP, Grenha A, Costa AM. Charged pullulan derivatives for the development of nanocarriers by polyelectrolyte complexation. *Int J Biol Macromol.* (2016) 86:129–38. doi: 10.1016/j.ijbiomac.2016.01.054

142. Liu S, Jones L. Nanomaterials for ocular drug delivery. *Macromol Biosci.* (2012) 12:608–20. doi: 10.1002/mabi.201100419

143. Maulvi FA, Soni TG. A review on therapeutic contact lenses for ocular drug delivery. *Drug Deliv.* (2016) 23:3017–26. doi: 10.3109/10717544.2016.1138342

144. Halasz K, Kelly SJ, Iqbal MT, Pathak Y, Sutariya V. Micro/nanoparticle delivery systems for ocular diseases. *Assay Drug Dev Technol.* (2019) 17:152–66. doi: 10.1089/adt.2018.911

145. Esteban-Pérez S, Bravo-Osuna I, Andrés-Guerrero V, Molina-Martínez IT. Trojan microparticles potential for ophthalmic drug delivery. *Curr Med Chem.* (2020) 27:570–82. doi: 10.2174/0929867326666190905150331

146. Gorantla S, Rapalli VK, Waghule T, Singh PP, Dubey SK, Saha RN. Nanocarriers for ocular drug delivery: current status and translational opportunity. *RSC Adv.* (2020) 10:27835–55. doi: 10.1039/D0RA04971A

147. Bravo-Osuna I, Andrés-Guerrero V, Abal PP, Molina-Martínez IT. Pharmaceutical microscale and nanoscale approaches for efficient treatment of ocular diseases. *Drug Deliv Transl Res.* (2016) 6:686–707. doi: 10.1007/s13346-016-0336-5

148. Qamar Z, Qizilbash FF, Iqubal MK, Ali A, Narang JK, Ali J. Nano-based drug delivery system: recent strategies for the treatment of ocular disease and future perspective. *Recent Pat Drug Deliv Formul.* (2019) 13:246–54. doi: 10.2174/1872211313666191224115211

149. Momin MM. Nanoformulations and highlights of clinical studies for ocular drug delivery systems: an overview. *Crit Rev Ther Drug Carrier Syst.* (2021) 38:79–107. doi: 10.1615/CritRevTherDrugCarrierSyst.2021035767

150. Li H, Palamoor M. Poly(ortho ester) nanoparticles targeted for chronic intraocular diseases: ocular safety and localization after intravitreal injection. *Nanotoxicology.* (2016) 10:1152–9. doi: 10.1080/17435390.2016.1181808

151. Fu S, Yang G, Wang J, Wang X, Cheng X, Zha Q. pH-sensitive poly(ortho ester urethanes) copolymers with controlled degradation kinetic: synthesis, characterization, and *in vitro* evaluation as drug carriers. *Eur Polym J.* (2017) 95:275–88. doi: 10.1016/j.eurpolymj.2017.08.023

152. Ug'urlu N, Aşik MD, Çakmak HB, Tuncer S, Turk M, Çag'il N, et al. Transscleral delivery of bevacizumab-loaded chitosan nanoparticles. *J Biomed Nanotechnol.* (2019) 15, 830–838. doi: 10.1166/jbn.2019.2716

153. Lu Y, Zhou N, Huang X, Cheng J, Li F, Wei R. Effect of intravitreal injection of bevacizumab-chitosan nanoparticles on retina of diabetic rats. *Int J Ophthalmol.* (2014) 7:1–7.

154. Dionísio M, Cordeiro C, Remuñán-López C, Seijo B, Rosa C. Pullulan-based nanoparticles as carriers for transmucosal protein delivery. *Eur J Pharm Sci.* (2013) 50:102–13. doi: 10.1016/j.ejps.2013.04.018

155. Garhwal R, Shady SF, Ellis EJ, Ellis JY, Leahy CD. McCarthy, SP, et al. Sustained ocular delivery of ciprofloxacin using nanospheres and conventional contact lens materials. *Investig Ophthalmol Vis Sci.* (2012) 53:1341–52. doi: 10.1167/iovs.11-8215

156. Mahor A, Prajapati SK, Verma A, Gupta R, Iyer AK. Moxifloxacin loaded gelatin nanoparticles for ocular delivery: formulation and *in-vitro*, *in-vivo* evaluation. *J Colloid Interface Sci.* (2016) 483:132–8. doi: 10.1016/j.jcis.2016.08.018

157. Grimaudo MA, Pescina S, Padula C, Santi P, Concheiro A, Alvarez-Lorenzo C. Topical application of polymeric nanomicelles in ophthalmology: a review on research efforts for the noninvasive delivery of ocular therapeutics. *Expert Opinion on Drug Deliv.* (2019) 16:397–413. doi: 10.1080/17425247.2019.1597848

158. Mandal A, Bisht R, Rupenthal ID. Polymeric micelles for ocular drug delivery: From structural frameworks to recent preclinical studies. *J Control Release.* (2017) 248:96–116. doi: 10.1016/j.jconrel.2017.01.012

159. Sun F, Zheng Z, Lan J, Li X, Li M, Song K. New micelle myricetin formulation for ocular delivery: improved stability, solubility, and ocular anti-inflammatory treatment. *Drug Deliv.* (2019) 26:575–85. doi: 10.1080/10717544.2019.1622608

160. Devi S, Saini V, Kumar M, Bhatt S, Gupta S. A novel approach of drug localization through development of polymeric micellar system containing azelastine HCl for ocular delivery. *Pharm Nanotechnol.* (2019) 7:314–27. doi: 10.2174/2211738507666190726162000

161. Grimaudo MA, Amato G, Carbone C, Diaz-Rodriguez P, Musumeci T, Concheiro A. Micelle-nanogel platform for ferulic acid ocular delivery. *Int J Pharm.* (2020) 576:118986. doi: 10.1016/j.ijpharm.2019.118986

162. Maulvi FA, Parmar RJ, Desai AR, Desai DM, Shukla MR, Ranch KM. Tailored gatifloxacin Pluronic® F-68-loaded contact lens: addressing the issue of transmittance and swelling. *Int J Pharm.* (2020) 581:119279. doi: 10.1016/j.ijpharm.2020.119279

163. Durgun ME, Kahraman E, Güngör S. Optimization and characterization of aqueous micellar formulations for ocular delivery of an antifungal drug, posaconazole. *Curr Pharm Des.* (2020) 26:1543–55. doi: 10.2174/1381612826666200313172207

164. Safwat MA, Mansour HF, Hussein AK, Abdelwahab S. Polymeric micelles for the ocular delivery of triamcinolone acetonide: preparation and *in vivo* evaluation in a rabbit ocular inflammatory model. *Drug Deliv.* (2020) 27:1115–24. doi: 10.1080/10717544.2020.1797241

165. Liu D, Wu Q, Chen W, Lin H, Zhu Y, Liu Y. A novel FK506 loaded nanomicelles consisting of amino-terminated poly(ethylene glycol)-block-poly(D,L)-lactic acid and hydroxypropyl methylcellulose for ocular drug delivery. *Int J Pharm.* (2019) 562:1–10. doi: 10.1016/j.ijpharm.2019.03.022

166. Zamboulis A, Nanaki S, Michailidou G, Koumentakou I, Lazaridou M, Ainali NM. Chitosan and its derivatives for ocular delivery formulations: recent advances and developments. *Polymers.* (2020) 12:1–67. doi: 10.3390/polym12071519

167. Xu X, Sun L, Zhou L, Cheng Y. Functional chitosan oligosaccharide nanomicelles for topical ocular drug delivery of dexamethasone. *Carbhohydr Polym.* (2020). 227:115356. doi: 10.1016/j.carbpol.2019.115356

168. Alami-Milani M, Zakeri-Milani P, Valizadeh H, Salehi R, Salatin S, Naderinia A. Novel pentablock copolymers as thermosensitive self-assembling micelles for ocular drug delivery. *Adv Pharm Bull.* (2017) 7:11–20. doi: 10.15171/apb.2017.003

169. Nasir NAA, Alyautdin RN, Agarwal R, Nukolova N, Cheknonin V. Ocular tissue distribution of topically applied PEGylated and non-PEGylated liposomes. *Adv Mater Res.* (2014) 832:1–8. doi: 10.4028/www.scientific.net/AMR.832.1

170. Danion A, Arsenault I. Antibacterial activity of contact lenses bearing surface-immobilized layers of intact liposomes loaded with levofloxacin. *J Pharm Sci.* (2007) 96:2350–63. doi: 10.1002/jps.20871

171. Swindle-Reilly KE, Maxwell CJ, Soltisz AM, Choi A, Rich W. Injectable alginate hydrogels for traumatic optic neuropathy. *Investig Ophthalmol Vis Sci.* (2021) 62:2682.

172. Reilly MA, Swindle-Reilly KE. Hydrogels for intraocular lenses and other ophthalmic prostheses. *Biomed Hydrogels.* 2011:118–48. doi: 10.1533/9780857091383.2.118

173. Xie L, Yue W, Ibrahim K. A long-acting curcumin nanoparticle/in situ hydrogel composite for the treatment of uveal melanoma. *Pharmaceutics.* (2021) 13:1335. doi: 10.3390/pharmaceutics13091335

174. Zhang J, Muirhead B, Dodd M, Liu L, Xu F, Mangiacotte N. An injectable hydrogel prepared using a PEG/Vitamin E copolymer facilitating aqueous-driven gelation. *Biomacromolecules.* (2016) 17:3648–58. doi: 10.1021/acs.biomac.6b01148

175. Tram NK, Jiang P, Torres-Flores TC, Jacobs KM, Chandler HL. A hydrogel vitreous substitute that releases antioxidant. *Macromol Biosci.* (2020) 20:1900305. doi: 10.1002/mabi.201900305

176. Tan DWN, Lim SG, Wong TT. Sustained antibiotic-eluting intra-ocular lenses: a new approach. *PLoS ONE.* (2016) 11:1–14. doi: 10.1371/journal.pone.0163857

177. Anumolu SNS, DeSantis AS, Menjoge AR, Hahn RA, Beloni JA, Gordon MK, et al. Doxycycline loaded poly(ethylene glycol) hydrogels for healing vesicant-induced ocular wounds. *Biomaterials.* (2010) 31:964–74. doi: 10.1016/j.biomaterials.2009.10.010

178. El-Feky YA, Fares AR, Zayed G, El-Telbany RFA, Ahmed KA. Repurposing of nifedipine loaded in situ ophthalmic gel as a novel approach for glaucoma treatment. *Biomed Pharmacother.* (2021) 142:112008. doi: 10.1016/j.biopha.2021.112008

179. Fedorchak MV, Conner IP, Schuman JS, Cugini A. Long term glaucoma drug delivery using a topically retained gel/microsphere eye drop. *Sci Rep.* (2017) 7:1–11. doi: 10.1038/s41598-017-09379-8

180. Kelley RA, Ghaffari A, Wang Y, Choi S, Taylor JR, Hartman RR. Manufacturing of dexamethasone–poly(d,l-Lactide-co-Glycolide) implants using hot-melt extrusion: within- and between-batch product performance comparisons. *J Ocul Pharmacol Therap.* (2020) 36:290–7. doi: 10.1089/jop.2019.0074

181. Kiss S. Sustained-release corticosteroid delivery systems. *Retin Today.* (2010) 2010:44–46.

182. Polat HK, Pehlivan SB, Özkul C, Çalamak S, Öztürk N, Aytekin E. Development of besifloxacin HCl loaded nanofibrous ocular inserts for the treatment of bacterial keratitis: *In vitro*, ex vivo and *in vivo* evaluation. *Int J Pharm.* (2020) 585:119552. doi: 10.1016/j.ijpharm.2020.119552

183. Singla J, Bajaj T, Goyal AK. Development of nanofibrous ocular insert for retinal delivery of fluocinolone acetonide. *Curr Eye Res.* (2019) 44:541–50. doi: 10.1080/02713683.2018.1563196

184. Mirzaeei S, Berenjian K. Preparation of the potential ocular inserts by electrospinning method to achieve the prolong release profile of triamcinolone acetonide. *Adv Pharm Bull.* (2018) 8:21. doi: 10.15171/apb.2018.003

185. Grimaudo MA, Concheiro A. Crosslinked hyaluronan electrospun nanofibers for ferulic acid ocular delivery. *Pharmaceutics.* (2020) 12:274. doi: 10.3390/pharmaceutics12030274

186. Yin C, Liu Y, Qi X, Guo C. Kaempferol incorporated bovine serum albumin fibrous films for ocular drug delivery. *Macromol Biosci.* (2021) 21:2100269. doi: 10.1002/mabi.202100269

187. Perry JL, Herlihy KP, Napier ME, DeSimone JM. PRINT: a novel platform toward shape and size specific nanoparticle theranostics. *Acc Chem Res.* (2011) 44:990–8. doi: 10.1021/ar2000315

188. DeSimone JM. Co-opting Moore's law: therapeutics, vaccines and interfacially active particles manufactured *via* PRINT®. *J Control Release.* (2016) 240:541–3. doi: 10.1016/j.jconrel.2016.07.019

189. Aerie Pharmaceuticals, Inc. *Drug Delivery.* Available online at: https://aeriepharma.com/rd/pipeline/drug-delivery/ (accessed Sep 29, 2021).

190. Meng T, Kulkarni V, Simmers R, Brar V. Therapeutic implications of nanomedicine for ocular drug delivery. *Drug Discov Today.* (2019) 24:1524–38. doi: 10.1016/j.drudis.2019.05.006

191. Narayana S, Ahmed MG, Gowda BHJ, Shetty PK, Nasrine A, Thriveni M. Recent advances in ocular drug delivery systems and targeting VEGF receptors for management of ocular angiogenesis: a comprehensive review. *Futur J Pharm Sci.* (2021) 7:1–21. doi: 10.1186/s43094-021-00331-2

192. Glendenning A, Crews K, Sturdivant J, deLong MA, Kopczynski C, Lin C. Sustained release, biodegradable PEA implants for intravitreal delivery of the ROCK/PKC inhibitor AR-13503. *Invest Ophthalmol Vis Sci.* (2018) 59:5672.

193. Study Assessing. *AR-13503 Implant in Subjects With nAMD or DME - Full Text View* - ClinicalTrials.gov. Available online at: https://clinicaltrials.gov/ct2/show/NCT03835884 (accessed Sep 30, 2021).

194. ClinicalTrials.gov. *Safety and Efficacy of ENV515 Travoprost Extended Release (XR) in Patients With Bilateral Ocular Hypertension or Primary Open Angle Glaucoma—Full Text View.* Available online at: https://clinicaltrials.gov/ct2/show/study/NCT02371746 (accessed Sep 30, 2021).

195. Kesav NP, Young CEC, Ertel MK, Seibold LK. Sustained-release drug delivery systems for the treatment of glaucoma. *Int J Ophthalmol.* (2021) 14:148–59. doi: 10.18240/ijo.2021.01.21

196. Mansberger SL, Conley J, Verhoeven RS, Blackwell K, Depenbusch M, Knox T. Interim analysis of low dose ENV515 travoprost XR with 11 month duration followed by dose escalation and 28 day efficacy evaluation of high dose ENV515. *Invest Ophthalmol Vis Sci.* (2017) 58:2110.

197. Rafiei F, Tabesh H. Sustained subconjunctival drug delivery systems: current trends and future perspectives. *Int Ophthalmol.* (2020) 40:2385–401. doi: 10.1007/s10792-020-01391-8

198. Jumelle C, Gholizadeh S, Annabi N. Advances and limitations of drug delivery systems formulated as eye drops. *J Control Release.* (2020) 321:1–22. doi: 10.1016/j.jconrel.2020.01.057

199. Gooch N, Molokhia SA, Condie R, Burr RM, Archer B, Ambati BK. Ocular drug delivery for glaucoma management. *Pharmaceutics.* (2012) 4:197–211.

200. Awwad S, Ahmed AHAM, Sharma G, Heng JS, Khaw PT, Brocchini S. Principles of pharmacology in the eye. *Br J Pharmacol.* (2017) 174:4205–23. doi: 10.1111/bph.14024

201. Gaballa SA, Kompella UB, Elgarhy O, Alqahtani AM, Pierscionek B, Alany RG. Corticosteroids in ophthalmology: drug delivery innovations, pharmacology, clinical applications, and future perspectives. *Drug Deliv Transl Res.* (2021) 11:866–93. doi: 10.1007/s13346-020-00843-z

202. Janagam DR, Wu L. Nanoparticles for drug delivery to the anterior segment of the eye. *Adv Drug Deliv Rev.* (2017) 122:31–64. doi: 10.1016/j.addr.2017.04.001

203. Cabrera FJ, Wang DC, Reddy K, Acharya G. Challenges and opportunities for drug delivery to the posterior of the eye. *Drug Discov Today.* (2019) 24:1679–84. doi: 10.1016/j.drudis.2019.05.035

204. Johannsdottir S, Jansook P, Stefansson E, Kristinsdottir IM, Fulop Z, Asgrimsdottir GM. Topical drug delivery to the posterior segment of the eye: Dexamethasone concentrations in various eye tissues after topical administration for up to 15 days to rabbits. *J Drug Deliv Sci Technol.* (2018) 45:449–54. doi: 10.1016/j.jddst.2018.04.007

205. Mangiacotte N, Prosperi-Porta G, Liu L, Dodd M. Mucoadhesive nanoparticles for drug delivery to the anterior eye. *Nanomaterials.* (2020) 10:1–16. doi: 10.3390/nano10071400

206. Dave RS, Goostrey TC, Ziolkowska M, Czerny-Holownia S, Hoare T. Ocular drug delivery to the anterior segment using nanocarriers: A mucoadhesive/mucopenetrative perspective. *J Control Release.* (2021) 336:71–88. doi: 10.1016/j.jconrel.2021.06.011

207. Kim YC, Shin MD, Hackett SF, Hsueh HT, Silva RLE, Date A. Gelling hypotonic polymer solution for extended topical drug delivery to the eye. *Nat Biomed Eng.* (2020) 4:1053–62. doi: 10.1038/s41551-020-00606-8

208. Voss K, Falke K, Bernsdorf A, Grabow N, Kastner C, Sternberg K. Development of a novel injectable drug delivery system for subconjunctival glaucoma treatment. *J Control Release.* (2015) 214:1–11. doi: 10.1016/j.jconrel.2015.06.035

209. Zhou C, Singh A, Qian G, Wolkow N, Dohlman CH, Vavvas DG. Microporous drug delivery system for sustained anti-vegf delivery to the eye. *Transl Vis Sci Technol.* (2020) 9:5. doi: 10.1167/tvst.9.8.5

210. Cheng Y-H, Hung KH, Tsai T-H, Lee C-J, Ku R-Y, Chiu AW-H. Sustained delivery of latanoprost by thermosensitive chitosan-gelatin-based hydrogel for controlling ocular hypertension. Acta Biomater. (2014) 10:4360–6. doi: 10.1016/j.actbio.2014.05.031

211. Li J, Tian S, Tao Q, Zhao Y, Gui R, Yang F. Montmorillonite/chitosan nanoparticles as a novel controlled-release topical ophthalmic delivery system for the treatment of glaucoma. *Int J Nanomedicine.* (2018) 13:3975–87. doi: 10.2147/IJN.S162306

212. Tahara K, Karasawa K, Onodera R. Feasibility of drug delivery to the eye's posterior segment by topical instillation of PLGA nanoparticles. *Asian J Pharm Sci.* (2017) 12:394–9. doi: 10.1016/j.ajps.2017.03.002

213. Kompella UB, Kadam RS. Recent advances in ophthalmic drug delivery. *Ther Deliv.* (2010) 1:435–56. doi: 10.4155/tde.10.40

214. Kim YC, Hsueh HT, Shin MD, Berlinicke CA, Han H, Anders NM, et al. hypotonic gel-forming eye drop provides enhanced intraocular delivery of a kinase inhibitor with melanin-binding properties for sustained protection of retinal ganglion cells. *Drug Deliv Transl Res.* (2021). doi: 10.1007/s13346-021-00987-6

215. Fedorchak MV, Conner IP, Medina CA, Wingard JB, Schuman JS. 28-day intraocular pressure reduction with a single dose of brimonidine tartrate-loaded microspheres. *Exp Eye Res.* (2014) 125:210–6. doi: 10.1016/j.exer.2014.06.013

216. Jessen BA, Shiue MHI, Kaur H, Miller P, Leedle R, Guo H. Safety assessment of subconjunctivally implanted devices containing latanoprost in dutch-belted rabbits. *J Ocul Pharmacol Ther.* (2013) 29:574–85. doi: 10.1089/jop.2012.0190

217. Lee RMH, Bouremel Y, Eames I, Brocchini S. The implications of an Ab Interno versus Ab externo surgical approach on outflow resistance of a subconjunctival drainage device for intraocular pressure control. *Transl Vis Sci Technol.* (2019) 8:58. doi: 10.1167/tvst.8.3.58

218. Rai UDJP, Young SA, Thrimawithana TR, Abdelkader H, Alani AWG, Pierscionek B. The suprachoroidal pathway: a new drug delivery route to the back of the eye. *Drug Discov Today.* (2015) 20:491–5. doi: 10.1016/j.drudis.2014.10.010

219. Olsen TW, Feng Z, Wabner K, Conston SR, Sierra DH, Folden DV. Cannulation of the suprachoroidal space: a novel drug delivery methodology to the posterior segment. *Am J Ophthalmol.* (2006) 142:777–87. doi: 10.1016/j.ajo.2006.05.045

220. Gilger BC, Abarca EM, Salmon JH. Treatment of acute posterior uveitis in a porcine model by injection of triamcinolone acetonide into the suprachoroidal space using microneedles. *Investig Ophthalmol Vis Sci.* (2013) 54:2483–92. doi: 10.1167/iovs.13-11747

221. Einmahl S, Savoldelli M, D'Hermies F, Tabatabay C, Gurny R. Evaluation of a novel biomaterial in the suprachoroidal space of the rabbit eye. *Investig Ophthalmol Vis Sci.* (2002) 43:1533–9.

222. Chiang B, Venugopal N, Grossniklaus HE, Jung JH, Edelhauser HF. Thickness and closure kinetics of the suprachoroidal space following microneedle injection of liquid formulations. *Investig Ophthalmol Vis Sci.* (2017) 58:555–64. doi: 10.1167/iovs.16-20377

223. Chiang B, Venugopal N, Edelhauser HF. Distribution of particles, small molecules and polymeric formulation excipients in the suprachoroidal space after microneedle injection. *Exp Eye Res.* (2016) 153:101–9. doi: 10.1016/j.exer.2016.10.011

224. Moga KA, Bickford LR, Geil RD, Dunn SS, Pandya AA, Wang Y. Rapidly-dissolvable microneedle patches *via* a highly scalable and reproducible soft lithography approach. *Adv Mater.* (2013) 25:5060–6. doi: 10.1002/adma.201300526

225. Jung JH, Desit P. Targeted drug delivery in the suprachoroidal space by swollen hydrogel pushing. *Investig Ophthalmol Vis Sci.* (2018) 59:2069–79. doi: 10.1167/iovs.17-23758

226. Rauck BM, Friberg TR, Medina Mendez CA, Park D, Shah V, Bilonick RA. Biocompatible reverse thermal gel sustains the release of intravitreal bevacizumab *in vivo. Investig Ophthalmol Vis Sci.* (2014) 55:469–76. doi: 10.1167/iovs.13-13120

227. Huang X. Intravitreal nanoparticles for retinal delivery. *Drug Discov Today.* (2019) 24:1510–23. doi: 10.1016/j.drudis.2019.05.005

228. Balachandra A, Chan EC, Paul JP, Ng S, Chrysostomou, Ngo S, et al. A biocompatible reverse thermoresponsive polymer for ocular drug delivery. *Drug Deliv.* (2019) 26:343–53. doi: 10.1080/10717544.2019.1587042

229. Prosperi-Porta G, Muirhead B. Tunable release of ophthalmic therapeutics from injectable, resorbable, thermoresponsive copolymer scaffolds. *J Biomed Mater Res - Part B Appl Biomater.* (2017) 105:53–62. doi: 10.1002/jbm.b.33501

230. Sheshala R, Hong GC, Yee WP, Meka VS. In situ forming phase-inversion implants for sustained ocular delivery of triamcinolone acetonide. *Drug Deliv Transl Res.* (2019) 9:534–42. doi: 10.1007/s13346-018-0491-y

231. Home-Re-Vana. *Vision In The Future.* (2021). Available online at: https://www.revanatx.com/ (accessed Sep 08, 2021).

232. Khanani AM, Callanan D, Dreyer R, Chen S, Howard JG, Hopkins JJ. End-of-study results for the ladder phase 2 trial of the port delivery system with ranibizumab for neovascular age-related macular degeneration. *Ophthalmol Retina.* (2021) 5:775–87. doi: 10.1016/j.oret.2020.11.004

233. Genentech, Inc. *Multicenter Phase II Randomized, Active Treatment-Controlled Study of the Efficacy and Safety of the Ranibizumab Port Delivery System for Sustained Delivery of Ranibizumab in Patients With Subfoveal Neovascular Age-Related Macular Degeneration.* Genentech, Inc. (2018).

234. DailyMed. *TRIESCENCE—Triamcinolone Acetonide Injection, Suspension.* (2020). Available online at: https://dailymed.nlm.nih.gov/dailymed/drugInfo.cfm?setid=3f045347-3e5e-4bbd-90f8-6c3100985ca5 (accessed Sep 31, 2021).

235. *ILUVIEN 190 Micrograms Intravitreal Implant in Applicator.* (2019). Available online at: https://iluvien.com/wp-content/uploads/2015/03/Prescribing-Information.pdf(accessed Sep 14, 2021).

236. Ozurdex. (2021). Available online at: https://www.ozurdex.com/ (accessed Sep 17, 2021).

237. Tso SC. The Chemistry Review for A/NDA 21-737 (2005). doi: 10.2476/asjaa.54.21

238. NDA 208742/S001 (2019). Available online at: https://www.accessdata.fda.gov/drugsatfda_docs/label/2019/208742s001lbl.pdf (accessed Sep 28, 2021).

239. Chaudhari P, Ghate VM. Next-generation contact lenses: towards bioresponsive drug delivery and smart technologies in ocular therapeutics. *Eur J Pharm Biopharm.* (2021) 161:80–99. doi: 10.1016/j.ejpb.2021.02.007

240. Safarzadeh M, Azizzadeh P. Comparación de la eficacia clínica de los colirios con conservantes y los colirios con contenido de hidroxipropil metilcelulosa-dextran sin conservantes. *J Optom.* (2017) 10:258–64. doi: 10.1016/j.optom.2016.11.002

241. *Mydriasert 0. 28. mg/5.4 mg Ophthalmic Insert—Summary of Product Characteristics (SmPC)—(emc).* Available online at: https://www.medicines.org.uk/emc/product/4672/smpc#gref (accessed Sep 28, 2021).

242. *Tobradex Eye Drops—Summary of Product Characteristics (SmPC)—(emc).* Available online at: https://www.medicines.org.uk/emc/product/1324/smpc#gref (accessed Sep 28, 2021).

243. Chaudhary A, Salinas L, Guidotti J, Mermoud A. XEN Gel Implant: a new surgical approach in glaucoma. *Expert Rev Med Devices.* (2018) 15:47–59. doi: 10.1080/17434440.2018.1419060

244. O'Rourke MJO. *History, Status, and Trends for the Future. Cataract & Refractive Surgery Today.* (2019). Available online at: https://crstodayeurope.com/articles/2019-june/ophthalmic-drug-delivery-history-status-and-trends-for-the-future/ (accessed Sep 09, 2021).

245. *Our Pipeline—Kodiak Sciences.* (2021). Available online at: https://kodiak.com/our-pipeline/ (accessed Sep 29, 2021).

246. Aerie Pharmaceuticals, Inc. *AR-1105 Implant.* (2020). Available online at: https://aeriepharma.com/rd/retinal-disease/ar-1105/ (accessed Sep 29, 2021).

247. Wagh V, Inamdar B. Polymers used in ocular dosage form and drug delivery systems. *Asian J Pharm.* (2008) 2:12–7. doi: 10.4103/0973-8398.41558

248. Peng Y, Ang M, Foo S, Lee WS, Ma Z, Venkatraman SS. Biocompatibility and biodegradation studies of subconjunctival implants in rabbit eyes. *PLoS ONE.* (2011) 6:22507. doi: 10.1371/journal.pone.0022507

249. Mora-Pereira M, Abarca EM, Duran S, Ravis W, McMullen RJ Jr, Fischer, BM, et al. Sustained-release voriconazole-thermogel for subconjunctival injection in horses: ocular toxicity and *in-vivo* studies. *BMC Vet Res.* (2020) 16:1–14. doi: 10.1186/s12917-020-02331-5

250. Paula JS, Ribeiro VR, Chahud F, Cannellini R, Monteiro TC,Gomes EC, et al. Bevacizumab-loaded polyurethane subconjunctival implants: effects on experimental glaucoma filtration surgery. *J Ocul Pharmacol Ther.* (2013) 29:566–573. doi: 10.1089/jop.2012.0136

251. Bausch Health And Clearside Biomedical Announce US, FDA. *Filing Acceptance For XIPERETM (Triamcinolone Acetonide Suprachoroidal Injectable Suspension)* (2021).

252. Kammer JA. Suprachoroidal devices in glaucoma surgery. *Middle East Afr J Ophthalmol.* (2015) 22:45–52. doi: 10.4103/0974-9233.148348

253. Campochiaro PA, Marcus DM, Awh CC, Regillo C, Adamis AP, Bantseev V. The port delivery system with ranibizumab for neovascular age-related macular degeneration: results from the randomized phase 2 ladder clinical trial. *Ophthalmology.* (2019) 126:1141–54. doi: 10.1016/j.ophtha.2019.03.036

254. *20 OptimEyes—Micelle Technology.* Available online at: https://www.2020optimeyes.ca/micelle-technology (accessed Sep 28, 2021).

255. Kim HM. Ocular drug delivery to the retina: current innovations and future perspectives. *Pharmaceutics.* (2021) 13:1–32. doi: 10.3390/pharmaceutics13010108

18

Periodontitis and Subsequent Risk of Cataract: Results From Real-World Practice

Li-Jen Yeh [1,2†], Te-Chun Shen [3,4†], Kuo-Ting Sun [5], Cheng-Li Lin [6] and Ning-Yi Hsia [7*]

[1] Department of Craniofacial Orthodontics, Chang Gung Memorial Hospital, Taoyuan, Taiwan, [2] Graduate Institute of Craniofacial and Dental Science, Chang Gung University, Taoyuan, Taiwan, [3] Department of Internal Medicine, China Medical University Hospital, Taichung, Taiwan, [4] School of Medicine, China Medical University, Taichung, Taiwan, [5] Department of Pediatric Dentistry, China Medical University Hospital, Taichung, Taiwan, [6] Management Office for Health Data, China Medical University Hospital, Taichung, Taiwan, [7] Department of Ophthalmology, China Medical University Hospital, Taichung, Taiwan

*Correspondence:
Ning-Yi Hsia
deepwhite1111@hotmail.com

† These authors have contributed
equally to this work

Background: Periodontitis can lead to systemic inflammation and oxidative stress, contributing to the development of various diseases. Periodontitis could also be associated with several ocular diseases.

Methods: We conducted a retrospective population-based cohort study using the National Health Insurance Research Database of Taiwan to evaluate the risk of cataract in people with and without periodontitis. We established a periodontitis cohort and a non-periodontitis cohort, which included 359,254 individuals between 2000 and 2012. Age, gender, and enrolled year were matched. All participants were monitored until the end of 2013. Cox proportional hazard models were applied to estimate hazard ratios (HRs) and confidence intervals (CIs).

Results: Patients with periodontitis had a significantly higher risk to develop cataract than those without periodontitis [10.7 vs. 7.91 per 1,000 person-years, crude HR = 1.35 (95% CI = 1.32–1.39), and adjusted HR = 1.33 (95% CI = 1.30–1.36)]. The significant levels remained the same after stratifying by age, gender, presence of comorbidity, and use of corticosteroid. In addition, we found that diabetes mellitus and hyperlipidemia had a synergistic effect in the interaction of periodontitis and cataract development.

Conclusion: Patients with periodontitis have a higher risk of cataract development than those without periodontitis. Such patients may request frequent ocular health check-up. Further studies should be performed to confirm the association and to understand the mechanisms.

Keywords: periodontitis, cataract, retrospective cohort study, epidemiology, risk factor

INTRODUCTION

Periodontitis is a common disorder that could damage the bone and tissue supporting the tooth (1). It could also induce chronic infection, systemic inflammation, and oxidative stress (2). Poor periodontal status significantly reduces life quality and general health (3). A link between periodontitis and various diseases, including cardiovascular disease (4), diabetes mellitus (5), metabolic syndrome (6), osteoporosis (7), gastrointestinal disease (8), respiratory disease (9), and autoimmune disease, is suggested (10). In addition, periodontitis can affect the development of several ocular diseases (11–13).

Cataract is caused by a build-up of protein that clouds the lens, which can lead to blurred vision and blindness (14). Around 95 million people worldwide are affected by cataract, which remains the leading cause of blindness in middle- and low-income countries (15). Many causative factors could promote the development of cataract, which include old age, female gender, smoking, sunlight exposure, family history, diabetes mellitus, cardiovascular disease, chronic airway disease, corticosteroid use, and ocular infection or inflammation (16, 17).

The association between periodontitis and cataract remains largely unknown. As we know, periodontitis may increase the systemic inflammatory reaction, and cataract could be initiated and exacerbated by the result of chronic inflammation (18–20). Furthermore, periodontitis-induced oxidative stress may also play a crucial role in the development of cataract (21–23). In a cross-sectional study, Gervasio et al. (24) examined many institutionalized geriatric residents and reported that the prevalence of periodontitis and cataract were both predominant. However, the exact relationship between these two common diseases is not well-established to date. Therefore, we aimed to conduct a retrospective population-based cohort study based on the National Health Insurance Research Database (NHIRD) in Taiwan to evaluate the association of periodontitis and subsequent development of cataract.

MATERIALS AND METHODS

Data Source

The National Health Insurance (NHI) program operated since 1995, with more than 99.9% of Taiwan citizens enrolled. The NHIRD is managed and updated by the National Health Research Institutes between 1995 and 2013. We applied the Longitudinal Health Insurance Database 2000 (LHID2000), a subset of NHIRD, to complete the study. The database included detailed medical information of 1,000,000 people randomly selected in 2000, such as demographic status, diagnostic code, medication, and procedure claims was available. The study was approved by the Research Ethics Committee of the China Medical University and Hospital (CMUH-104-REC2-115). Informed consent was unnecessary for the de-identified data and waived by the Research Ethics Committee.

Study Population

We selected newly diagnosed adult patients with periodontitis [International Classification of Diseases, 9th Revision, Clinical Modification (ICD-9-CM) codes 523.3 and 523.4] between 2000 and 2012 as the periodontitis group ($n = 179,627$). The date of diagnosis was defined as the index date. We excluded those with incomplete demographic data and those with cataract before the index date. Thus, we selected the same number of adult individuals without periodontitis as the comparison group. Age, gender, and index year were matched between the periodontitis and the non-periodontitis groups. The exclusion criteria were the same as the periodontitis group. All participants were monitored until (1) the development of cataract, (2)

TABLE 1 | Baseline characteristics for individuals with and without periodontitis.

	Periodontitis				
	No N = 179,627		Yes N = 179,627		
	n	%	n	%	p#
Age					>0.99
20–49	134,973	75.1	134,973	75.1	
50–64	36,555	20.4	36,555	20.4	
≥ 65	8,099	4.51	8,099	4.51	
Mean ±SD	40.0	±13.9	40.3	±13.5	0.001
Gender					>0.99
Women	91,658	51.0	91,658	51.0	
Men	87,969	49.0	87,969	49.0	
Comorbidity					
Hypertension	24,924	13.9	27,476	15.3	<0.001
Diabetes mellitus	4,278	2.38	4,611	2.57	<0.001
Hyperlipidemia	18,266	10.2	24,949	13.9	<0.001
Asthma/COPD	15,238	8.48	18,135	10.1	<0.001
CLD	25,978	14.5	34,272	19.1	<0.001
CKD	1,048	0.58	1,102	0.61	0.39
Rheumatic diseases	2,627	1.46	3,715	2.07	<0.001
Medication					
Corticosteroid use	4,941	2.75	5,668	3.16	<0.001

CKD, chronic kidney disease; CLD, chronic liver disease and cirrhosis; COPD, chronic obstructive pulmonary disease; SD, standard deviation.
#Chi-squired test and t-test.

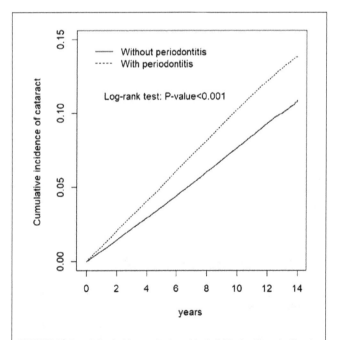

FIGURE 1 | Cumulative incidence of cataract for individuals with and without periodontitis.

withdrawal from the NHI program, (3) death, or (4) the end of 2013.

TABLE 2 | Associated factor analysis for cataract.

	Event	PY	Rate#	Crude HR (95% CI)	Adjusted HR† (95% CI)
Periodontitis					
No	10,937	1383000	7.91	1.00	1.00
Yes	15.078	1407568	10.7	1.35 (1.32–1.39)***	1.33 (1.30–1.36)***
Age					
20–49	5,394	2220424	2.43	1.00	1.00
50–64	15,098	485717	31.1	13.3 (12.9–13.7)***	10.5 (10.1–10.8)***
≥ 65	5,523	84427	65.4	28.7 (27.7–29.8)***	19.8 (19.1–20.7)***
Gender					
Women	14,487	1431226	10.1	1.19 (1.16–1.22)***	1.33 (1.30–1.36)***
Men	11,528	1359343	8.48	1.00	1.00
Comorbidity					
Hypertension					
No	14,757	2452127	6.02	1.00	1.00
Yes	11,258	338441	33.3	5.62 (5.49–5.76)***	1.39 (1.35–1.43)***
Diabetes mellitus					
No	23,094	2741295	8.42	1.00	1.00
Yes	2,921	49273	59.3	7.17 (6.90–7.46)***	1.90 (1.82–1.98)***
Hyperlipidemia					
No	17,709	2508842	7.06	1.00	1.00
Yes	8,306	281726	29.5	4.24 (4.13–4.35)***	1.28 (1.25–1.32)***
Asthma/COPD					
No	21,094	2577384	8.18	1.00	1.00
Yes	4,921	213185	23.1	2.86 (2.77–2.95)***	1.19 (1.15–1.23)***
CLD					
No	18,412	2353531	7.82	1.00	1.00
Yes	7,603	437037	17.4	2.23 (2.17–2.29)***	1.24 (1.20–1.27)***
CKD					
No	25,546	2779068	9.19	1.00	1.00
Yes	469	11500	40.8	4.50 (4.11–4.93)***	1.25 (1.14–1.37)***
Rheumatic diseases					
No	25,067	2750306	9.11	1.00	1.00
Yes	948	40263	23.6	2.61 (2.45–2.78)***	1.21 (1.13–1.29)***
Medication					
Corticosteroid use					
No	24,368	2731200	8.92	1.00	1.00
Yes	1,647	59368	27.7	3.16 (3.01–3.33)***	1.21 (1.15–1.27)***

CI, confidence interval; CKD, chronic kidney disease; CLD, chronic liver disease and cirrhosis; COPD, chronic obstructive pulmonary disease; HR, hazard ratio; PY, person-years.
#Incidence rate per 1,000 person-years.
† Multivariable analysis including age, gender, comorbidities, and corticosteroid use.
***p < 0.001.

Study Outcome and Confounders

The primary outcome of the study was the diagnosis of cataract (ICD-9-CM code 366). We further identified several comorbidities that may be potential risk factors for cataract and the most related medication, corticosteroid, as confounders. Detailed comorbidities included hypertension (ICD-9-CM codes 401–405), diabetes mellitus (ICD-9-CM code 250), hyperlipidemia (ICD-9-CM code 272), asthma/chronic obstructive pulmonary disease (COPD) (ICD-9-CM codes 493 and 496), chronic liver disease and cirrhosis (CLD; ICD-9-CM code 571), chronic kidney disease (CKD; ICD-9-CM

code 585), and rheumatic diseases (ICD-9-CM codes 446.5, 710.0–710.4, 714.0–714.2, 714.8, and 725).

Statistical Analysis

We applied chi-squared test and t-test to compare the distribution of baseline characteristics for categorical and continuous variables. We have drawn the Kaplan-Meier curves followed by testing inter-group differences with a log-rank test to evaluate the cumulative incidence of cataract in both groups. Cox proportional hazard models were used to estimate the hazard ratios (HRs) and 95% confidence intervals (CIs).

TABLE 3 | Incidences and hazard ratios of cataract for individuals with and without periodontitis by age, gender, comorbidity, and corticosteroid use.

| | Periodontitis | | | | | | | |
| | No | | | Yes | | | | |
	Event	PY	Rate#	Event	PY	Rate#	Crude HR (95% CI)	Adjusted HR† (95% CI)
Age								
20–49	2,253	1096510	2.05	3,141	1123914	2.79	1.35 (1.28–1.43)***	1.27 (1.20–1.34)***
50–64	6,512	243514	26.7	8,586	242203	35.5	1.33 (1.29–1.37)***	1.28 (1.24–1.32)***
≥ 65	2,172	42976	50.5	3,351	41451	80.8	1.59 (1.51–1.68)***	1.54 (1.45–1.62)***
Gender								
Women	6,280	711630	8.82	8,207	719596	11.4	1.29 (1.25–1.34)***	1.28 (1.24–1.33)***
Men	4,657	671370	6.94	6,871	687972	9.99	1.44 (1.39–1.49)***	1.39 (1.34–1.44)***
Comorbidity‡								
No	3,845	998982	3.85	4,496	928178	4.84	1.25 (1.20–1.31)***	1.44 (1.38–1.51)***
Yes	7,092	384018	18.5	10,582	479390	22.1	1.20 (1.16–1.23)***	1.30 (1.26–1.34)***
Corticosteroid								
No	10,289	1355838	7.59	14,079	1375362	10.2	1.35 (1.31–1.38)***	1.33 (1.29–1.36)***
Yes	648	27162	23.9	999	32206	31.0	1.30 (1.18–1.44)***	1.34 (1.22–1.48)***

CI, confidence interval; HR, hazard ratio; PY, person-years.
#Incidence rate per 1,000 person-years.
† Multivariable analysis including age, gender, comorbidities, and corticosteroid use.
‡Individuals with any comorbidity of hypertension, diabetes mellitus, hyperlipidemia, asthma/COPD, CLD, CKD, and rheumatic disease were classified into the comorbidity group.
***p < 0.001.

Multivariate Cox models were used to estimate the adjusted HRs (aHRs) and 95% CIs after controlling age, sex, comorbidities, and corticosteroid use, which were significant in the univariate model. All the analyses were performed using STATA statistical software (StataCorp. 2015, R 14, StataCorp LP). The level of significance was set at 0.05 using a two-tailed test.

RESULTS

This study included 179,627 periodontitis patients and 179,627 non-periodontitis individuals that displayed similar distributions of age and gender (**Table 1**). The mean age of the periodontitis group was 40.3 (standard deviation = 13.5) years, 51.0% of whom were women. The prevalence rates of hypertension, diabetes mellitus, hyperlipidemia, asthma/COPD, CLD, rheumatic diseases, and corticosteroid use were all greater in patients with periodontitis than those without periodontitis (p < 0.001). **Figure 1** shows that the cumulative incidence of cataract was higher in the periodontitis group than in the non-periodontitis group (p < 0.001) after a 14-year follow-up.

The incidence density of cataract was greater in the periodontitis group than in the non-periodontitis group (10.7 vs. 7.91 per 1,000 person-years) (**Table 2**). The multivariable Cox model estimated aHR of cataract was 1.33 (95% CI = 1.30–1.36) for the periodontitis group compared with the non-periodontitis group after controlling for age, gender, comorbidities, and corticosteroid use. Compared with those <50 years of age, the aHRs were 10.5 in the 50–64 years age group (95% CI = 10.1–10.8) and 19.8 in the ≥65 years age group (95% CI = 19.1–20.7). Compared with men, women had an aHR of

1.33 (95% CI = 1.30–1.36) for cataract development. Compared with non-corticosteroid users, corticosteroid users had an aHR of 1.21 (95% CI = 1.15–1.27) for cataract development. Compared with non-diabetes mellitus individuals, diabetes mellitus patients had an aHR of 1.90 (95% CI = 1.82–1.98) for cataract development. Furthermore, aHRs were 1.39 (95% CI = 1.35–1.43) for individuals with hypertension, 1.28 (95% CI = 1.25–1.32) for individuals with hyperlipidemia, 1.25 (95% CI = 1.14–1.37) for individuals with CKD, 1.24 (95% CI = 1.20–1.27) for individuals with CLD, 1.21 (95% CI = 1.13–1.29) for individuals with rheumatic diseases, and 1.19 (95% CI = 1.15–1.23) for individuals with asthma/COPD.

Table 3 shows incidences and HRs of cataract for both study groups, stratified by age, gender, the presence of comorbidity, and corticosteroid use. The incidences of cataract were higher in elders, women, those with comorbidity, and corticosteroid users between both groups. The periodontitis to non-periodontitis group aHRs were significant for the young age group (1.27, 95% CI = 1.20–1.34), middle age group (1.28, 95% CI = 1.24–1.32), and old age group (1.54, 95% CI = 1.45–1.62). The periodontitis to non-periodontitis group aHRs were significant for women (1.28, 95% CI = 1.24–1.33) and men (1.39, 95% CI = 1.34–1.44). The periodontitis to non-periodontitis group aHRs were significant for those without comorbidity (1.44, 95% CI = 1.38–1.51) and those with comorbidity (1.30, 95% CI = 1.26–1.34). The periodontitis to non-periodontitis group aHRs were significant for non-corticosteroid users (1.33, 95% CI = 1.29–1.36) and corticosteroid users (1.34, 95% CI = 1.22–1.48).

Table 4 presents the risk of cataract associated with interactions between periodontitis and the comorbidity of hypertension, diabetes mellitus, and hyperlipidemia. Those

TABLE 4 | Cox proportional hazards regression analysis for the risk of cataract-associated periodontitis and hypertension, diabetes mellitus, and hyperlipidemia.

Variables		Total N	Cataract N	Adjusted HR† (95% CI)	p$^{\#}$
Periodontitis	Hypertension				0.16
No	No	154,703	6,316	1 (Reference)	
No	Yes	24,924	4,621	1.40 (1.35–1.46)***	
Yes	No	152,151	8,441	1.38 (1.33–1.42)***	
Yes	Yes	27,476	6,637	1.84 (1.77–1.91)***	
Periodontitis	Diabetes mellitus				0.007
No	No	175,349	9,715	1 (Reference)	
No	Yes	4,278	1,222	2.08 (1.96–2.21)***	
Yes	No	175,016	13,379	1.37 (1.33–1.40)***	
Yes	Yes	4,611	1,699	2.66 (2.52–2.81)***	
Periodontitis	Hyperlipidemia				0.002
No	No	161,361	7,818	1 (Reference)	
No	Yes	18,266	3,119	1.63 (1.56–1.70)***	
Yes	No	154,678	9,891	1.37 (1.33–1.41)***	
Yes	Yes	24,949	5,187	2.00 (1.93–2.08)***	
Periodontitis	Triple H				0.08
No	0	145,595	5,090	1 (Reference)	
No	1	22,513	3,301	1.55 (1.48–1.62)***	
No	2	9,602	1,977	1.93 (1.82–2.03)***	
No	3	1,917	569	2.65 (2.43–2.90)***	
Yes	0	139,156	6,432	1.38 (1.33–1.43)***	
Yes	1	26,020	4,627	2.03 (1.95–2.12)***	
Yes	2	12,337	3,161	2.36 (2.25–2.47)***	
Yes	3	2,114	858	3.58 (3.32–3.86)***	

CI, confidence interval; HR, hazard ratio.
† Model was adjusted for age, sex, comorbidities, and corticosteroid use.
$^{\#}$ p-value for interaction.
*** p < 0.001.

with both periodontitis and diabetes mellitus (aHR = 2.66, 95% CI = 2.52–2.81, interaction p = 0.007) and those with both periodontitis and hyperlipidemia (aHR = 2.00, 95% CI = 1.93–2.08, interaction p = 0.002) presented a significantly higher risk. Moreover, patients with more comorbidities of hypertension, diabetes mellitus, and hyperlipidemia had a trend to have a higher risk of cataract (interaction p = 0.08).

DISCUSSION

This retrospective population-based cohort study analyzed the incidence of cataract in individuals with and without periodontitis. Results showed that periodontitis patients were associated with a higher risk of cataract development than non-periodontitis individuals. As expected, the incidences of cataract were higher in older people than in younger people, in women than in men, in those with comorbidity than in those without comorbidity, and in corticosteroid users than in non-corticosteroid users. Furthermore, cataract risk was significantly higher in the periodontitis group than in the comparison group even after stratifying by age, gender, the presence of comorbidity, or corticosteroid use. Moreover, we found that diabetes mellitus

and hyperlipidemia had a synergistic effect in the interaction of periodontitis and cataract development.

In the present study, we have evaluated several potential risk factors and their impacts on cataract development. Overall, diabetes mellitus played the most important role in the development of cataract, followed by hypertension, hyperlipidemia, CKD, CLD, corticosteroid use, rheumatic diseases, and asthma/COPD. Triple H (hypertension, hyperglycemia, and hyperlipidemia), metabolic syndrome, atherosclerosis, and cardiovascular diseases would have the most impact to cataract development; these findings correlated with previous studies (14, 15). However, the association between chronic liver disease and cataract or rheumatic diseases and cataract needs further investigations.

The potential mechanisms of the association between periodontitis and cataract remained unclear, but several hypotheses have been suggested. First, odontogenic ocular infections may directly influence the development of cataract. Both mouth and teeth are known reservoirs for many pathogens; therefore, periodontitis may contribute to repeated or chronic ocular infections (25). In a large-scale cohort study, Chau et al. (11). have reported that patients with periodontal disease

($n = 467,170$) are at a higher risk of infectious scleritis (aHR = 1.270, 95% CI = 1.114–1.449), uveitis (aHR = 1.144, 95% CI = 1.074–1.218), and infectious keratitis (aHR = 1.094, 95% CI = 1.030–1.161) than those without periodontal disease ($n = 467,170$). These infectious conditions have shown to be risk factors of cataract (15). Second, oral microbiome from periodontitis can cause immune responses to exacerbate cataractogenesis. Some observations implied periodontitis-induced systemic inflammation and oxidative stress in the pathogenesis of eye diseases (15, 26, 27). That is, periodontal microbiota may trigger immune dysfunction in the oro-optic-network and promote the development of cataract. Third, the impact of periodontitis in the induction and progression of ocular diseases such as diabetic retinopathy, glaucoma, and age-related macular degeneration has been identified (12, 13, 27, 28). The pathophysiology between periodontitis and these ocular complications may be similar to that of cataract. Finally, smoking, lower socioeconomic status, and shared comorbidities, such as diabetes mellitus, hypertension, hyperlipidemia, cardiovascular disease, and chronic airway disease, may also contribute to the development of cataract in periodontitis patients.

The primary strength of the study is the use of population-based data that are highly representative of the general population. No difference was found in the demographic distribution between LHID2000 and the original NHIRD. In addition, the universal coverage in the insurance system ensures that all citizens can have no access barriers to health care (29). Moreover, the NHIRD reflected a real-world scenario and the results of clinical practices.

Certain limitations should be considered in the study. First, the diagnosis is only based on ICD code, but the NHIRD has been validated and the results showed the data was reliable (30). Second, the NHIRD does not contain detailed information on smoking habits, occupational or environmental exposure, body mass index, and family history, which may be confounding factors. Third, the database did not contain clinical variables such as dental and ocular findings, disease severity and subtype, laboratory data, culture reports, and imaging findings. Fourth, the treatment effects of periodontitis could not be well-evaluated in the database. Fifth, the follow-up period may be short for cataract development. Finally, the study could be biased because of possible unmeasured or unknown confounding variables.

CONCLUSION

Patients with periodontitis are at a higher risk of cataract development than those without periodontitis. Such patients may request frequent ocular health check-up. Further studies should be performed to confirm the association and to understand the mechanisms.

AUTHOR CONTRIBUTIONS

L-JY, T-CS, K-TS, and N-YH: study concept and design. L-JY, T-CS, K-TS, C-LL, and N-YH: acquisition of data. L-JY, T-CS, C-LL, and N-YH: data analysis. L-JY, T-CS, C-LL, and N-YH: writing. All authors contributed to the article and approved the submitted version.

REFERENCES

1. Kinane DF, Stathopoulou PG, Papapanou PN. Periodontal diseases. *Nat Rev Dis Primers.* (2017) 3:17038. doi: 10.1038/nrdp.2017.38
2. Sczepanik FSC, Grossi ML, Casati M, Goldberg M, Glogauer M, Fine N, et al. Periodontitis is an inflammatory disease of oxidative stress: we should treat it that way. *Periodontol 2000.* (2020) 84:45–68. doi: 10.1111/prd.12342
3. Needleman I, McGrath C, Floyd P, Biddle A. Impact of oral health on the life quality of periodontal patients. *J Clin Periodontol.* (2004) 31:454–7. doi: 10.1111/j.1600-051X.2004.00498.x
4. Sanz M, Marco Del Castillo A, Jepsen S, Gonzalez-Juanatey JR, D'Aiuto F, Bouchard P, et al. Periodontitis and cardiovascular diseases: consensus report. *J Clin Periodontol.* (2020) 47:268–88. doi: 10.1111/jcpe.13189
5. Preshaw PM, Bissett SM. Periodontitis and diabetes. *Br Dent J.* (2019) 227:577–84. doi: 10.1038/s41415-019-0794-5
6. Srivastava MC, Srivastava R, Verma PK, Gautam A. Metabolic syndrome and periodontal disease: An overview for physicians. *J Family Med Prim Care.* (2019) 8:3492–5. doi: 10.4103/jfmpc.jfmpc_866_19
7. Penoni DC, Vettore MV, Torres SR, Farias MLF, Leão ATT. An investigation of the bidirectional link between osteoporosis and periodontitis. *Arch Osteoporos.* (2019) 14:94. doi: 10.1007/s11657-019-0643-9
8. Muhvić-Urek M, Tomac-Stojmenović M, Mijandrušić-Sinčić B. Oral pathology in inflammatory bowel disease. *World J Gastroenterol.* (2016) 22:5655–67. doi: 10.3748/wjg.v22.i25.5655
9. Moghadam SA, Shirzaiy M, Risbaf S. The associations between periodontitis and respiratory disease. *J Nepal Health Res Counc.* (2017) 15:1–6. doi: 10.3126/jnhrc.v15i1.18023
10. De Luca F, Shoenfeld Y. The microbiome in autoimmune diseases. *Clin Exp Immunol.* (2019) 195:74–85. doi: 10.1111/cei.13158
11. Chau SF, Lee CY, Huang JY, Chou MC, Chen HC, Yang SF. The existence of periodontal disease and subsequent ocular diseases: a population-based cohort study. *Medicina.* (2020) 56:621. doi: 10.3390/medicina56110621
12. Sun KT, Shen TC, Chen SC, Chang CL, Li CH, Li X, et al. Periodontitis and the subsequent risk of glaucoma: results from the real-world practice. *Sci Rep.* (2020) 10:17568. doi: 10.1038/s41598-020-74589-6
13. Sun KT, Hsia NY, Chen SC, Lin CL, Chen IA, Wu IT, et al. Risk of age-related macular degeneration in patients with periodontitis: a nationwide population-based cohort study. *Retina.* (2020) 40:2312–8. doi: 10.1097/IAE.0000000000002750
14. Lee CM, Afshari NA. The global state of cataract blindness. *Curr Opin Ophthalmol.* (2017) 28:98–103. doi: 10.1097/ICU.0000000000000340

15. Liu YC, Wilkins M, Kim T, Malyugin B, Mehta JS. Cataracts. *Lancet.* (2017) 390:600–12. doi: 10.1016/S0140-6736(17)30544-5

16. Prokofyeva E, Wegener A, Zrenner E. Cataract prevalence and prevention in Europe: a literature review. *Acta Ophthalmol.* (2013) 91:395–405. doi: 10.1111/j.1755-3768.2012.02444.x

17. Thompson J, Lakhani N. Cataracts. *Prim Care.* (2015) 42:409–23. doi: 10.1016/j.pop.2015.05.012

18. Loos BG, Van Dyke TE. The role of inflammation and genetics in periodontal disease. *Periodontol 2000.* (2020) 83:26–39. doi: 10.1111/prd.12297

19. Schaumberg DA, Ridker PM, Glynn RJ, Christen WG, Dana MR, Hennekens CH. High levels of plasma C-reactive protein and future risk of age-related cataract. *Ann Epidemiol.* (1999) 9:166–71. doi: 10.1016/S1047-2797(98)00049-0

20. Klein BE, Klein R, Lee KE, Knudtson MD, Tsai MY. Markers of inflammation, vascular endothelial dysfunction, and age-related cataract. *Am J Ophthalmol.* (2006) 141:116–22. doi: 10.1016/j.ajo.2005.08.021

21. Chen M, Cai W, Zhao S, Shi L, Chen Y, Li X, et al. Oxidative stress-related biomarkers in saliva and gingival crevicular fluid associated with chronic periodontitis: a systematic review and meta-analysis. *J Clin Periodontol.* (2019) 46:608–22. doi: 10.1111/jcpe.13112

22. Braakhuis AJ, Donaldson CI, Lim JC, Donaldson PJ. Nutritional strategies to prevent lens cataract: current status and future strategies. *Nutrients.* (2019) 11:1186. doi: 10.3390/nu11051186

23. Ahmad A, Ahsan H. Biomarkers of inflammation and oxidative stress in ophthalmic disorders. *J Immunoassay Immunochem.* (2020) 41:257–71. doi: 10.1080/15321819.2020.1726774

24. Gervasio NC, Escoto ET, Chan WY. Oral health status of institutionalized geriatric residents in Metro Manila. *J Philipp Dent Assoc.* (1998) 50:4–23.

25. Procacci P, Zangani A, Rossetto A, Rizzini A, Zanette G, Albanese M. Odontogenic orbital abscess: a case report and review of literature. *Oral Maxillofac Surg.* (2017) 21:271–9. doi: 10.1007/s10006-017-0618-1

26. Costan VV, Bogdănici CM, Gheorghe L, Obadă O, Budacu C, Grigora? C, et al. Odontogenic orbital inflammation. *Rom J Ophthalmol.* (2020) 64:116–21. doi: 10.22336/rjo.2020.22

27. Arjunan P. Eye on the enigmatic link: Dysbiotic oral pathogens in ocular diseases; the flip side. *Int Rev Immunol.* (2021) 40:409–32. doi: 10.1080/08830185.2020.1845330

28. Natesh S, Patil SR. Association between diabetic retinopathy and chronic periodontitis-A cross-sectional study. *Med Sci.* (2018) 6:104. doi: 10.3390/medsci6040104

29. Hsing AW, Ioannidis JP. Nationwide population science: lessons from the Taiwan national health insurance research database. *JAMA Intern Med.* (2015) 175:1527–9. doi: 10.1001/jamainternmed.2015.3540

30. Hsieh CY, Su CC, Shao SC, Sung SF, Lin SJ, Kao Yang YH, et al. Taiwan's National Health Insurance research database: past and future. *Clin Epidemiol.* (2019) 11:349–58. doi: 10.2147/CLEP.S196293

19

Anterior Segment Optical Coherence Tomography Angiography Following Trabecular Bypass Minimally Invasive Glaucoma Surgery

Jinyuan Gan[1], Chelvin C. A. Sng[2,3], Mengyuan Ke[2], Chew Shi Chieh[3], Bingyao Tan[2,4,5], Leopold Schmetterer[1,2,3,4,5,6,7,8] and Marcus Ang[1,2*]

[1] Duke-NUS Graduate Medical School, Singapore, Singapore, [2] Singapore National Eye Centre, Singhealth, Singapore Eye Research Institute, Singapore, Singapore, [3] Department of Ophthalmology, National University Hospital, Singapore, Singapore, [4] SERI-NTU Advanced Ocular Engineering (STANCE), Singapore, Singapore, [5] School of Chemical and Biomedical Engineering, Nanyang Technological University, Singapore, Singapore, [6] Department of Clinical Pharmacology, Medical University of Vienna, Vienna, Austria, [7] Center for Medical Physics and Biomedical Engineering, Medical University of Vienna, Vienna, Austria, [8] Institute of Molecular and Clinical Ophthalmology, Basel, Switzerland

*Correspondence:
Marcus Ang
marcus.ang@snec.com.sg

Objective: To assess anterior segment optical coherence tomography angiography (AS-OCTA) imaging of the episcleral vessels before and after trabecular bypass minimally invasive glaucoma surgery (MIGS).

Design: A prospective, clinical, single-centre, single-arm pilot feasibility study conducted at National University Hospital, Singapore.

Subjects: Patients with primary glaucomatous optic neuropathy undergoing Hydrus Microstent (Ivantis Inc., Irvine, CA, USA) implantation, who require at least one intra-ocular pressure-lowering medication. One or two eyes per patient may be enrolled.

Methods: We performed AS-OCTA (Nidek RS-3000 Advance 2, Gamagori, Japan) pre- and up to 6 months post-MIGS implantation using a standard protocol in all cornealimbal quadrants, to derive episcleral vessel densities (VD) using a previously described technique.

Main Outcome Measures: Episcleral VD pre- and post-surgery, in sectors with and without the implant.

Results: We obtained serial AS-OCTA images in 25 eyes undergoing MIGS implantation (23 subjects, mean age 70.3 $\pm$ 1.5, 61% female) with mean preoperative intraocular pressure (IOP) of 15.5 mmHg $\pm$ 4.0. We observed reductions in postoperative episcleral VD compared to preoperative VD at month 1 (mean difference −3.2, $p = 0.001$), month 3 (mean difference −2.94, $p = 0.004$) and month 6 (mean difference −2.19, $p = 0.039$) in sectors with implants (overall 6 month follow-up, $p = 0.011$). No significant changes were detected in episcleral VD in the sectors without implants ($p = 0.910$).

Conclusion: In our pilot study, AS-OCTA was able to detect changes in the episcleral VD following trabecular bypass MIGS, which may be a useful modality to evaluate surgical outcomes if validated in future studies.

Keywords: glaucoma, imaging, intraocular pressure, sclera, cornea, episclera

INTRODUCTION

Glaucoma is one of the leading causes of blindness worldwide (1). Increased intraocular pressure (IOP) is the main risk factor for glaucoma, and the mainstay of glaucoma treatment involves lowering of IOP (2, 3). The most common treatment involves the use of topical medications – however, these may be associated with adverse effects and poor compliance (4). Meanwhile conventional glaucoma surgeries such as trabeculectomy may effectively lower IOP, but can be associated with sight-threatening complications (5). To address these limitations, minimally invasive glaucoma surgery (MIGS) has gained popularity in recent years.

Currently, MIGS include a heterogeneous group of IOP-lowering devices and procedures that are generally less invasive and have a faster recovery time compared to traditional filtration surgery (6, 7). While MIGS is usually associated with a good safety profile, clinical results suggest variable efficacy in IOP reduction (8, 9). Both iStent (Glaukos, San Clemente, CA, USA) and Hydrus Microstent (Ivantis Inc., Irvine, CA, USA) are ab interno trabecular bypass products that increase aqueous outflow, with the latter scaffolding and dilating the Schlemm's canal as well. In a head-to-head study comparing Hydrus to iStent inject, the COMPARE study found Hydrus to have a greater rate of surgical success compared to iStent, with fewer subjects needing repeat glaucoma surgeries or medications (10).

When evaluating trabecular bypass MIGS devices, imaging the aqueous outflow tracts may be useful in understanding its efficacy. Aqueous angiography is a functional imaging technique utilising an ab interno approach with fluorescein or indocyanine green (ICG) as tracers, demonstrated in enucleated animal eyes (11, 12) and *in vivo* animal studies (13). However, aqueous angiography has limited clinical application as it is an invasive procedure that requires intraocular injection of dye, and is associated with potential complications such as infection and anaphylaxis (14). Recently, optical coherence tomography angiography (OCTA) has emerged as a non-invasive, rapid imaging technique that may be used to delineate vasculature in the anterior segment (15). While the role of anterior segment OCTA (AS-OCTA) has been described for episcleral, scleral and limbal vasculature (16–21), it has not been described specifically for the episcleral venous plexus in relation to MIGS to date (22). Thus, we conducted this pilot feasibility study to evaluate the role of AS-OCTA imaging following Hydrus Microstent implantation, to examine the potential effect of this trabecular bypass MIGS implant on episcleral vessel density.

Abbreviations: AHO, aqueous humour outflow; AS-OCTA, anterior segment optical coherence tomography angiography; BCVA, best-corrected visual acuity; FFT, Fast Fourier Transform; HVF, Humphrey Visual Field; ICG, indocyanine green; IOP, intraocular pressure; MD, mean deviation; MIGS, minimally invasive glaucoma surgery; OCTA, optical coherence tomography angiography; PACG, primary angle-closure glaucoma; POAG, primary open-angle glaucoma; VD, vessel density.

MATERIALS AND METHODS

This was a prospective single-centre case series of consecutive patients who underwent combined phacoemulsification with Hydrus Microstent implantation at the National University Hospital between May 2019 to Mar 2020. Approval was obtained from the National Healthcare Group Domain Specific Review Board (2016/00125) and the study was conducted in accordance with the tenets of the Declaration of Helsinki. Written informed consent was obtained from all patients prior to surgery.

Study Subjects

We included phakic subjects with primary glaucomatous optic neuropathy, as defined by Foster et al. (23), who required at least one intraocular-pressure lowering medication in this study. Exclusion criteria included advanced primary angle-closure glaucoma (PACG) (24) (as defined by cup-disc ratio ≥ 0.9 and/or a visual field defect within the central $10°$ of fixation), $>180°$ of peripheral anterior synechiae, peripheral anterior synechiae in the target quadrant of Hydrus Microstent implantation, prior incisional glaucoma surgery, secondary glaucoma (including uveitic, neovascular, traumatic glaucoma, or glaucoma secondary to raised episcleral venous pressure) and any orbital, corneal, retinal or choroidal disease which may interfere with cataract extraction or Hydrus Microstent implantation.

Study Measures

Complete ophthalmic examination by a fellowship-trained glaucoma specialist (C. A. Sng) was performed pre-operatively and on day 1, week 1, and months 1, 3, and 6. This included the best corrected Snellen visual acuity (BCVA), IOP measurement with Goldmann applanation tonometry, and a detailed slit lamp examination of the anterior and posterior segments. Humphrey perimetry (Swedish Interative Threshold Algorithm Standard 24-2 algorithm, Humphrey Visual Field, HVF Analyzer II, Carl Zeiss Meditec, Inc., Dublin, California, USA) was performed pre-operatively and 6 months post-operatively, and the mean deviation (MD) was recorded.

Surgical Technique

All surgeries were performed under topical anaesthesia or peribulbar block. Phacoemulsification and intraocular lens implantation were performed via a clear corneal incision. To implant the Hydrus Microstent, the surgical microscope was tilted $30°$ towards the patient and the patient's head was tilted $45°$ nasally or inferiorly to allow direct visualisation of the angle structures with an intra-operative gonioscopy lens (Ocular Hill Open Access Surgical Goniatomy [Left-Hand], Ocular Instruments, Bellevue, WA). An ophthalmic viscosurgical device was used to maintain the anterior chamber and widen the anterior chamber angle after phacoemulsification. The Hydrus Microstent was passed into the anterior chamber through a separate clear corneal incision (about 90 to 120° from the target site of Hydrus Microstent implantation) into the anterior chamber. The trabecular meshwork was incised with the tip of the device injector cannula and the Hydrus Microstent was inserted into the Schlemm's canal in the nasal or inferior quadrant over a span of approximately 90°. The targeted quadrants were reported to contain greater aqueous humour outflow (AHO), and selection of quadrants was based on surgical accessibility through a clear corneal temporary incision, and surgical technique of Hydrus Microstent implantation (14, 25). After visual confirmation of correct device positioning with the Schlemm's canal, the device injector was withdrawn and the ophthalmic viscosurgical device was removed. The corneal incisions were hydrated with a balanced salt solution. Vision blue (D.O.R.C. Dutch Ophthalmic Research Center [International] B.V., Zuidland, The Netherlands) was injected into the anterior chamber and the presence of the blue dye in the conjunctival vessels was noted and videoed for manual segmentation and comparison with OCTA vessels.

Anterior Segment Imaging

Anterior segment imaging was performed pre-operatively and post-operatively at week 1, month 1, month 3, and month 6 using a digital slit-lamp camera (Topcon ATE-600, Nikon Corp) with a standard diffuse illumination (×10 magnification, flash power 4) for colour photography. Next, AS-OCTA of the episcleral vessels in all cornealimbal quadrants was conducted using a previously described scan protocol (26), using a spectral domain optical coherence tomography system (Nidek RS-3000 Advance 2, Gamagori, Japan) with a central wavelength of 880 nm, axial resolution of 7 um and transverse resolution of 15 um (anterior segment module). The eye tracker function was deactivated for imaging acquisition. The lens was moved close to the area of interest at the corneal surface before optimisation of the focal length and Z position to focus on the area of interest. The scan areas were divided into six sectors: Superior, superior nasal (right eye), nasal, inferior nasal, inferior, inferior temporal (left eye) and temporal directions i.e., six scans were acquired for each eye (**Figure 1**).

AS-OCTA Image Processing

Scans were segmented manually to produce AS-OCTA enface images of (a) episcleral and (b) conjunctival to scleral i.e., full segmentation scans for each eye, before image processing as previously described (27). Essentially, motion artefacts were first removed using Fiji-J (NIH, Bethesda, MD) with a Fast Fourier Transform (FFT) bandpass filter (tolerance of direction 90%). Next, the images were processed with MATLAB (The Mathworks, Inc., Natick, Massachusetts, USA) to segment vessels by removing the speckle noise using a median filter and Gaussian smoothing, then applying Frangi filter to enhance vessel features (**Figure 2**). Finally, local adaptive thresholding was used to binarize the images. The binary images were used to calculate the vessel densities (equation label) of corneal vessels within each sector. Vessel density is defined as the segmented vessels (in white pixel) divided by the sector area (total pixels) i.e., Vessel density = $100 * P/A$; where $P = 1$ for white pixels representing blood vessels, $P = 0$ for black pixels representing the background, and A being the sector area. As a higher signal strength improves the reliability of measurement and allows for better reproducibility (28), we compared the sector with the highest OCTA vessel density with the control sectors.

For consistent comparison, inferior and temporal sectors were used as controls for superior-nasal implants. Likewise superior and temporal sectors were used as controls for inferior-nasal implants, and superior and nasal sectors for inferior-temporal implants. These same sectors were kept consistent between visits. Thus, for each Hydrus Microstent sector we have 2 opposing sectors as controls. We confirmed that vessels derived from AS-OCTA images corresponded to episcleral outflow veins, we injected trypan blue (VisionBlue®) intra-operatively into the anterior chamber after Hydrus Microstent implantation to highlight episcleral venous vessels. Corresponding AS-OCTA images at 1 month were selected from sectors with and without the implant, and compared to the intra-operative images with highlighted vessels that were manually segmented and overlaid with ImageJ (**Figure 3**).

Statistical Analysis

Vessel densities obtained from control sectors without implants were compared to vessel densities from sectors with the Hydrus Microstent in the same eye, with serial comparison analysis performed over the follow-up period (**Figure 4**). Statistical analysis was performed using Statistical Program for Social Sciences version 27.0.1.0 for MacOS© (2020 SPSS© Inc. IBM Corp, USA). Percentage differences in vessel densities were evaluated using Friedman Test (serial measurements over follow-up) and Wilcoxon Signed Rank Test (paired, compared to baseline). All data were expressed as mean ± standard deviation (SD) when applicable, and $P < 0.05$ were considered statistically significant.

RESULTS

In this pilot study, we included 25 eyes from 23 subjects undergoing Hydrus Microstent implant surgeries. Patients' mean age was 70.3 ± 1.5 years, with 74% Chinese from our predominantly Asian population, while 61% were female. The mean pre-operative intraocular pressure (IOP) was 15.5 ± 4.0 mmHg, with eyes being on an average of 1.2 glaucoma medications pre-operation, and mean HVF MD was −4.9 ± 3.2 dB. We observed a reduction in mean post-operative IOP at 1 week (11.6 ± 3.1 mmHg, $P = 0.001$), 1 month (12.8 ± 3.1 mmHg, $P = 0.002$), 3 months (12.3 ± 3.2 mmHg, $P = 0.001$), and 6 months (12.5 ± 3.1 mmHg, $P = 0.002$)—none required IOP lowering medications post-operatively during follow-up. There were no significant post-operative complications such as hyphaemia, infection or progression of glaucoma; while no eyes required a repeat surgical procedure during the follow-up period.

All eyes had intra-operative identification of episcleral vessels after Hydrus Microstent implantation to confirm drainage of aqueous humour and intra-operative images were compared with corresponding AS-OCTA images at post-operative day 1 (**Figure 3**). At baseline, implant sectors have higher vessel densities compared to control sectors for both episcleral images ($p = 0.03$, mean difference of 2.12, 95% CI [0.13, 4.11]) and full-thickness scans ($p = 0.03$, mean difference of 2.21, 95% CI [0.19, 4.23]). We analysed the month 1 AS-OCTA images that clearly corresponded with trypan blue labelled vessels (6 sectors)

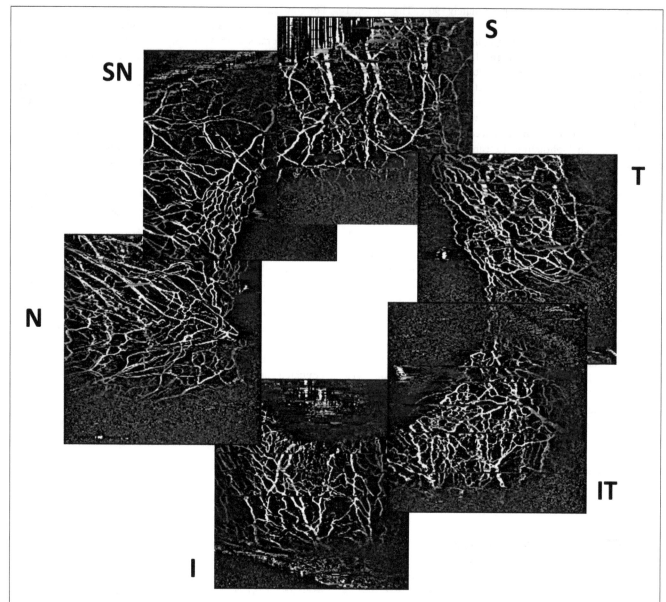

FIGURE 1 | Example of optical coherence tomography angiography scans of episcleral vessels acquired in sectors with the trabecular bypass minimally invasive glaucoma surgical device (S, superior; SN, superior nasal; N, nasal) and control sectors without the implant (I, inferior; IT, inferior temporal; T, temporal).

and observed a reduction in VD of trypan blue labelled vessels comparing sectors with the implant vs. control sectors with no implant (mean difference 1.35 ± 0.5 vs. 0.64 ± 0.2 respectively, $p = 0.008$). We also found that sectors with the Hydrus Microstent implanted showed significant reductions in episcleral vessel density over 6 months ($p = 0.011$), with specific reductions in VD observed at month 1 ($p = 0.001$, mean difference of -3.2, 95% CI $[-1.14, -5.10]$), month 3 ($p = 0.004$, mean difference of -2.94, 95% CI $[-1.12, -4.76]$) and month 6 ($p = 0.039$, mean difference of -2.19, 95% CI $[-0.29, -4.08]$) compared to pre-operative baseline. Meanwhile, control sectors remained unchanged at all time points compared to pre-operative vessel densities (**Table 1**).

Similar analysis for full segmentation of AS-OCTA scans i.e., conjunctival, episcleral and scleral layers showed a similar trend i.e., Hydrus Microstent sectors showed significant reduction in VD month 1 ($p = 0.001$, mean difference of -3.27, 95% CI -1.12, -5.42), month 3 ($p = 0.005$, mean difference of -3.24, 95% CI $[-1.33, -5.15]$) and month 6 ($p = 0.046$, mean difference of -2.18, 95% CI $[-0.12, -4.25]$) compared to baseline, while control sectors remained unchanged at all time points (**Table 2**). Of note, these differences were not significant at week 1 in both episcleral ($p = 0.326$, 95% CI -1.09, 3.07) and full segmentation scans ($p = 0.510$, 95% CI -1.45, 2.99).

Anterior Segment Optical Coherence Tomography Angiography Following Trabecular Bypass Minimally Invasive...

195

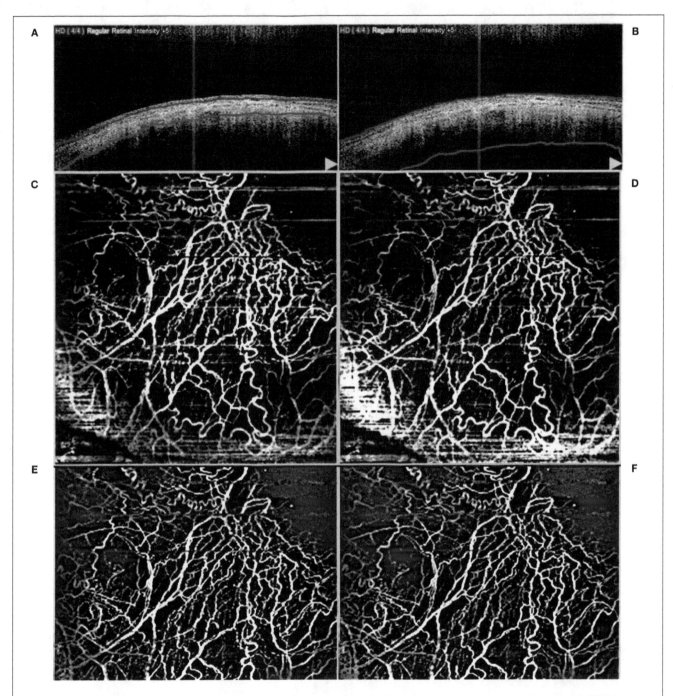

FIGURE 2 | Example of **(A)** episcleral and **(B)** full layer (conjunctival, episcleral, scleral) segmented optical coherence tomography angiography (AS-OCTA) images. Unprocessed en face AS-OCTA images of the **(C)** episcleral and **(D)** full layer vasculature, respectively, and after removal of artefacts [**(E,F)**, respectively].

DISCUSSION

In this pilot study, AS-OCTA detected a post-operative reduction in episcleral vessel density in sectors with the Hydrus Microstent implant compared to control sectors without implants. We correlated these vessels with intraoperative imaging that highlighted the aqueous outflow tracts using trypan blue. Our observations may seem counterintuitive since trabecular bypass

MIGS devices such as the Hydrus Microstent are meant to enhance flow to collector channels (29). We postulate that the apparent reduction in AS-OCTA derived vessel density measurements may be attributed to increased aqueous humour flow in the episcleral veins, thereby reducing the signal intensity or phase differences detected by the AS-OCTA (30). Changes in vessel density in the control sectors could have been a result of cataract surgery itself, which may also increase aqueous flow

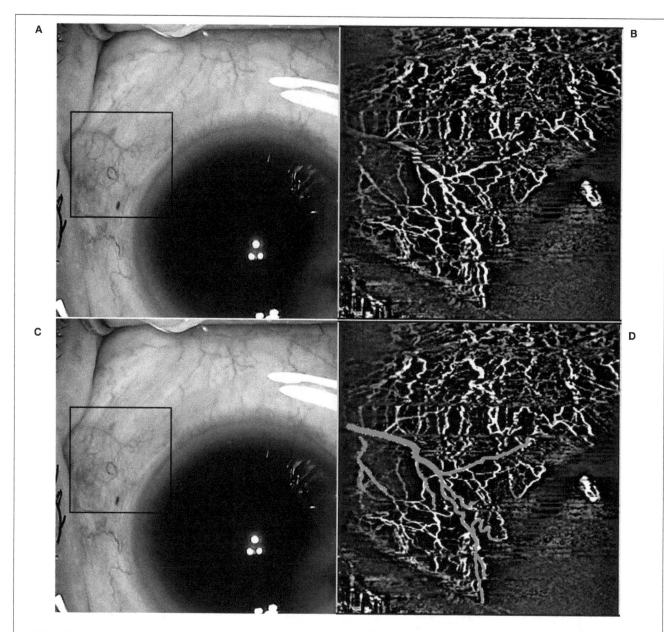

FIGURE 3 | Example of intraoperative identification of episcleral vessels using trypan blue immediately postimplant **(A)** with the corresponding optical coherence tomography angiography (OCTA) scan in the sector **(B)**. Trypan blue vessels in the region of interest were highlighted **(C)** with an overlay on the intraoperative images **(D)** before vessel density calculations.

to a lesser extent (31, 32). It is also possible that the Hydrus Microstent leads to changes in aqueous outflow in a differential manner, i.e., some vessels with greater aqueous flow, while others with decreased flow—leading to an overall AS-OCTA detection of decreased vessel density (33).

The reduction in vessel densities could also be due to the cessation of IOP-lowering medications, many of which are associated with hyperaemia (34). To control for potential confounders, we compared Hydrus Microstent sectors with control quadrants without the implant within the same eye, such that all quadrants were subjected to potential effects of

medications and cataract surgery. However, we do recognise this study's limitations and cannot exclude any local quadrant effects of prostaglandin use if applicable (35). Lastly, vessel densities were found to be higher in sectors with Hydrus Microstent compared to control sectors at baseline. One explanation could be that Hydrus Microstent sectors included more inferior-nasal sectors, which were associated with the highest vessel volume of aqueous outflow channels out of all ocular sectors, and hence greater vessel densities (36, 37). Nonetheless, we recognise that AS-OCTA cannot directly detect aqueous outflow, but instead measures episcleral vessel density as a potential surrogate (38).

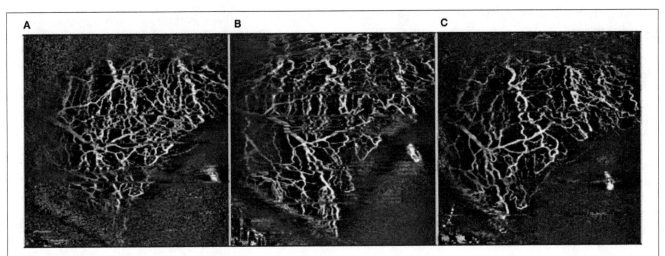

FIGURE 4 | Comparison of OCTA images of inferior temporal episcleral vessels taken **(A)** pre-operatively, **(B)** 1 month post-operatively, and **(C)** 3 months post-operatively, with artefacts removed.

TABLE 1 | Optical coherence tomography angiography vessel density measurements of episcleral vasculature in sectors with Hydrus Microstent implants and controls comparing pre-operative and post-operative week 1 and month 1, 3, and 6.

Assessment time-points	Vessel density Mean (±SD)	*P-value
Control		
Pre-operative (n = 25)	23.2 (4.3)	0.910**
Week 1 (n = 25)	23.0 (3.4)	0.946
Month 1 (n = 23)	23.3 (3.5)	0.976
Month 3 (n = 16)	22.8 (1.4)	0.538
Month 6 (n = 13)	24.0 (3.3)	0.917
Control		
Pre-operative (n = 24)	24.0 (4.4)	0.723**
Week 1 (n = 25)	23.0 (3.4)	0.241
Month 1 (n = 23)	23.3 (3.5)	0.114
Month 3 (n = 16)	23.2 (4.7)	0.836
Month 6 (n = 13)	23.0 (5.1)	0.552
Hydrus Microstent sector		
Pre-operative (n = 25)	25.6 (3.4)	0.011**
Week 1 (n = 25)	24.7 (3.9)	0.326
Month 1 (n = 23)	22.5 (3.4)	0.001
Month 3 (n = 16)	22.7 (2.8)	0.004
Month 6 (n = 13)	23.5 (3.1)	0.039

*Wilcoxon signed rank test (paired) comparing baseline VD to follow-up VD measurements.
**Friedman test for serial VD measurements over follow-up period (n = 25 eyes at baseline, 1 week and 1 month; n = 16 eyes beyond month 3).

TABLE 2 | Optical coherence tomography angiography vessel density measurements of overall vasculature (conjunctival, episcleral, scleral) in sectors with Hydrus Microstent implants and controls comparing pre-operative and post-operative week 1 and month 1, 3, and 6.

Assessment time-points	Vessel density Mean (±SD)	*P-value (compared to pre-operative)
Control		
Pre-operative (n = 25)	22.9 (4.4)	0.699**
Week 1 (n = 25)	22.8 (3.2)	0.757
Month 1 (n = 23)	23.1 (4.0)	0.761
Month 3 (n = 16)	23.1 (2.1)	0.717
Month 6 (n = 13)	24.4 (3.0)	0.701
Control		
Pre-operative (n = 24)	24.2 (4.3)	0.536**
Week 1 (n = 25)	23.2 (4.2)	0.153
Month 1 (n = 23)	23.2 (3.0)	0.153
Month 3 (n = 16)	23.3 (4.7)	0.301
Month 6 (n = 13)	24.0 (4.5)	0.601
Hydrus Microstent sector		
Pre-operative (n = 25)	25.7 (3.6)	0.021**
Week 1 (n = 25)	25.0 (4.2)	0.510
Month 1 (n = 23)	22.5 (3.8)	0.001
Month 3 (n = 16)	22.5 (2.9)	0.005
Month 6 (n = 13)	23.6 (3.5)	0.046

*Wilcoxon signed rank test (paired) comparing baseline VD to follow-up VD measurements.
**Friedman test for serial VD measurements over follow-up period (n = 25 eyes at baseline, 1 week and 1 month; n = 16 eyes beyond month 3).

As such, current AS-OCTA technology might not yet be an ideal imaging modality for the detection of conventional aqueous outflow. However, our study was a unique opportunity to confirm the location of the outflow tracts using trypan blue, and allowed us to compare pre- and post-procedure changes in vessel density in the sectors with the implant, vs. control sectors without any implant. Further validation studies using larger sampling sizes and alternative methods for aqueous outflow and episcleral vessel delineation, such as aqueous angiography, are needed to confirm our observations.

Currently, imaging the aqueous outflow tracts are not performed in the clinical setting due to the need to inject a contrast agent into the anterior chamber. Thus, AS-OCTA could provide a non-invasive alternative to imaging the episcleral venous plexus as an adjunctive or surrogate for evaluating the aqueous outflow (39). The AS-OCTA has been previously shown to detect increased episcleral vessel density due to increased episcleral venous flow leading to raised intraocular pressure (40), or reduction in episcleral vessel density following anterior segment ischemia (41). Although a previous report suggested that AS-OCT (non-angiographic) imaging did not detect changes in aqueous outflow after successful trabecular-targeted MIGS (120-degree trabectome or 360-degree suture trabeculotomy) during 3 month follow-up (42), our study specifically examined AS-OCT angiography to delineate the episcleral venous plexus following trabecular bypass MIGS. As AS-OCTA imaging is rapid and non-contact, repeated serial post-operative scans can be taken for comparison (43), and may be useful for pre-operative assessment to guide trabecular bypass device placement.

Though MIGS has been viewed as a safe surgical option for lowering IOP in carefully selected eyes, variable efficacy has been attributed to non-optimal surgical placement (44). Traditionally MIGS devices are placed in the nasal angle (45), but pre-operative imaging assessment using modalities such as AS-OCTA may be able to optimise surgical planning and the location of device implantation. Past studies have demonstrated the non-uniform nature of AHO around the limbus, which may vary over time and differ between eyes (46). Hence it is unclear how these variations might affect the surgical outcomes and decision on the most optimal location for trabecular bypass MIGS. Nonetheless, this highlights the unmet need for an imaging modality to allow for preoperative assessment to individualise MIGS implantation for patients.

Despite the promising observations from our pilot study, we would like to highlight several challenges with using the AS-OCTA to image the episcleral venous plexus. Firstly, scan techniques will have to be adjusted for the anterior segment as these systems were originally designed for the posterior segment, hence anterior segment images are motion-sensitive and regions of interest are more difficult to match in serial scans (21). In our study, we recognise the limitations of manually segmenting the episcleral layers from AS-OCTA imaging to minimise effects from conjunctival vessels on our analysis, and thus correlated our images with intraoperative dye labelled vessels and observed

reduction in overall vessel density from fully segmented scans as well. Secondly, AS-OCTA derived vessel density measurements may be underestimated due to limited detection of smaller vessels (47), or overestimated due to projection and motion artefacts (48). Thus, repeated serial measurements were performed to reduce random errors and confirm our observations. Thirdly, the AS-OCTA does not directly image the aqueous outflow tracts such as the Schlemm's canal and collector channels (49).

Ideally we should perform aqueous angiography to assess the actual flow through the collector channels—thus the Hydrus implant may not increase the flow in the collector channels. However, we used the AS-OCTA imaging of the episcleral venous plexuses as a surrogate *in vivo*, as flow may be detected because the vessels are partially filled with both clear aqueous humour and blood; and we had further confirmed increased aqueous outflow using intraoperative imaging with trypan blue. Lastly, although we have excluded patients with advanced PACG, we have included patients with both mild to moderate PACG and primary open-angle glaucoma (POAG). Ideally we would have studies with larger sample sizes that exclude PACG eyes, but as this is a pilot study primarily focused on investigating the feasibility of using AS-OCTA for imaging of episcleral vessels pre- and post-MIGS, we have decided to include PACG eyes to aid in estimation purposes. Despite these limitations, our study suggests that AS-OCTA is a promising non-invasive imaging tool that is readily available in the clinics, that may be useful in assessing changes in episcleral vessel density secondary to trabecular bypass MIGS.

In summary, our pilot study suggests that AS-OCTA detects changes in episcleral vessel density before and after trabecular bypass MIGS implantation in sectors with the implant compared to control sectors. The reduction in episcleral vessel density is observed to occur over 3 to 6 months after surgery, which requires further validation in future studies to examine the potential clinical application of AS-OCTA imaging for this indication.

AUTHOR CONTRIBUTIONS

All authors substantial contributions to conception and design, acquisition of data, or analysis and interpretation of data, drafting the article or revising it critically for important intellectual content, and final approval of the version to be published.

REFERENCES

1. Bourne RR, Taylor HR, Flaxman SR, Keeffe J, Leasher J, Naidoo K, et al. Number of people blind or visually impaired by glaucoma worldwide and in world regions 1990 - 2010: a meta-analysis. *PLoS ONE.* (2016) 11:e0162229. doi: 10.1371/journal.pone.0162229

2. Blanco A, Bagnasci L, Bagnis A, Barton K, Baudouin C, Bengtsson B. European Glaucoma Society Terminology and Guidelines for Glaucoma,

4th Edition - Chapter 3: Treatment principles and options Supported by the EGS Foundation: Part 1: Foreword; Introduction; Glossary; Chapter 3 Treatment principles and options. *Br J Ophthalmol.* (2017) 101:130–95. doi: 10.1136/bjophthalmol-2016-EGSguideline.003

3. Lavia C, Dallorto L, Maule M, Ceccarelli M, Fea AM. Minimally-invasive glaucoma surgeries (MIGS) for open angle glaucoma: a systematic review and meta-analysis. *PLoS ONE.* (2017) 12:e0183142. doi: 10.1371/journal.pone.0183142

4. Le K, Saheb H. iStent trabecular micro-bypass stent for open-angle glaucoma. *Clin Ophthalmol.* (2014) 8:1937–45. doi: 10.2147/OPTH.S45920

5. Gedde SJ, Herndon LW, Brandt JD, Budenz DL, Feuer WJ, Schiffman JC, et al. Postoperative complications in the Tube Versus Trabeculectomy (TVT) study during five years of follow-up. *Am J Ophthalmol.* (2012) 153:804–14 e1. doi: 10.1016/j.ajo.2011.10.024

6. Meier KL, Greenfield DS, Hilmantel G, Kahook MY, Lin C, Rorer EM, et al. Special commentary: Food and Drug Administration and American Glaucoma Society co-sponsored workshop: the validity, reliability, and usability of glaucoma imaging devices. *Ophthalmology.* (2014) 121:2116–23. doi: 10.1016/j.ophtha.2014.05.024

7. Wang J, Barton K. Overview of MIGS. In: Sng CCA, Barton K, editors. *Minimally Invasive Glaucoma Surgery.* Singapore: Springer Singapore (2021). p. 1–10.

8. Minckler D, Mosaed S, Dustin L, Ms BF, Trabectome Study G. Trabectome (trabeculectomy-internal approach): additional experience and extended follow-up. *Trans Am Ophthalmol Soc.* (2008) 106:149–59; discussion 59–60.

9. Huang AS, Camp A, Xu BY, Penteado RC, Weinreb RN. Aqueous angiography: aqueous humor outflow imaging in live human subjects. *Ophthalmology.* (2017) 124:1249–51. doi: 10.1016/j.ophtha.2017.03.058

10. Ahmed IIK, Fea A, Au L, Ang RE, Harasymowycz P, Jampel HD, et al. A prospective randomized trial comparing hydrus and istent microinvasive glaucoma surgery implants for standalone treatment of open-angle glaucoma: the COMPARE study. *Ophthalmology.* (2020) 127:52–61. doi: 10.1016/j.ophtha.2019.04.034

11. Saraswathy S, Tan JC, Yu F, Francis BA, Hinton DR, Weinreb RN, et al. Aqueous angiography: real-time and physiologic aqueous humor outflow imaging. *PLoS ONE.* (2016) 11:e0147176. doi: 10.1371/journal.pone.0147176

12. Burn JB, Huang AS, Weber AJ, Komaromy AM, Pirie CG. Aqueous angiography in normal canine eyes. *Transl Vis Sci Technol.* (2020) 9:44. doi: 10.1167/tvst.9.9.44

13. Huang AS, Li M, Yang D, Wang H, Wang N, Weinreb RN. Aqueous angiography in living nonhuman primates shows segmental, pulsatile, and dynamic angiographic aqueous humor outflow. *Ophthalmology.* (2017) 124:793–803. doi: 10.1016/j.ophtha.2017.01.030

14. Huang AS, Francis BA, Weinreb RN. Structural and functional imaging of aqueous humour outflow: a review. *Clin Exp Ophthalmol.* (2018) 46:158–68. doi: 10.1111/ceo.13064

15. Ang M, Sim DA, Keane PA, Sng CC, Egan CA, Tufail A, et al. Optical coherence tomography angiography for anterior segment vasculature imaging. *Ophthalmology.* (2015) 122:1740–7. doi: 10.1016/j.ophtha.2015.05.017

16. Ang M, Cai Y, Tan AC. Swept source optical coherence tomography angiography for contact lens-related corneal vascularization. *J Ophthalmol.* (2016) 2016:9685297. doi: 10.1155/2016/9685297

17. Ang M, Devarajan K, Das S, Stanzel T, Tan A, Girard M, et al. Comparison of anterior segment optical coherence tomography angiography systems for corneal vascularisation. *Br J Ophthalmol.* (2018) 102:873–7. doi: 10.1136/bjophthalmol-2017-311072

18. Ang M, Devarajan K, Tan AC, Ke M, Tan B, Teo K, et al. Anterior segment optical coherence tomography angiography for iris vasculature in pigmented eyes. *Br J Ophthalmol.* (2020) 105:929–34. doi: 10.1136/bjophthalmol-2020-316930

19. Hau SC, Devarajan K, Ang M. Anterior segment optical coherence tomography angiography and optical coherence tomography in the evaluation of episcleritis and scleritis. *Ocul Immunol Inflamm.* (2019) 29:362–9. doi: 10.1080/09273948.2019.1682617

20. Liu YC, Devarajan K, Tan TE, Ang M, Mehta JS. Optical coherence tomography angiography for evaluation of reperfusion after pterygium surgery. *Am J Ophthalmol.* (2019) 207:151–8. doi: 10.1016/j.ajo.2019.04.003

21. Ang M, Baskaran M, Werkmeister RM, Chua J, Schmidl D, Aranha Dos Santos V, et al. Anterior segment optical coherence tomography. *Prog Retin Eye Res.* (2018) 66:132–56. doi: 10.1016/j.preteyeres.2018.04.002

22. Lee WD, Devarajan K, Chua J, Schmetterer L, Mehta JS, Ang M. Optical coherence tomography angiography for the anterior segment. *Eye and Vision.* (2019) 6:4. doi: 10.1186/s40662-019-0129-2

23. Foster PJ, Buhrmann R, Quigley HA, Johnson GJ. The definition and classification of glaucoma in prevalence surveys. *Br J Ophthalmol.* (2002) 86:238–42. doi: 10.1136/bjo.86.2.238

24. Canadian Ophthalmological Society Glaucoma Clinical Practice Guideline Expert C, Canadian Ophthalmological S. Canadian Ophthalmological Society evidence-based clinical practice guidelines for the management of glaucoma in the adult eye. *Can J Ophthalmol.* (2009) 44(Suppl. 1):S7–93. doi: 10.3129/i09.080

25. Pillunat LE, Erb C, Junemann AG, Kimmich F. Micro-invasive glaucoma surgery (MIGS): a review of surgical procedures using stents. *Clin Ophthalmol.* (2017) 11:1583–600. doi: 10.2147/OPTH.S135316

26. Tey KY, Gan J, Foo V, Tan B, Ke MY, Schmetterer L, et al. Role of anterior segment optical coherence tomography angiography in the assessment of acute chemical ocular injury: a pilot animal model study. *Sci Rep.* (2021) 11:16625. doi: 10.1038/s41598-021-96086-0

27. Ang M, Foo V, Ke M, Tan B, Tong L, Schmetterer L, et al. Role of anterior segment optical coherence tomography angiography in assessing limbal vasculature in acute chemical injury of the eye. *Br J Ophthalmol.* (2021). doi: 10.1136/bjophthalmol-2021-318847. [Epub ahead of print].

28. Lim HB, Kim YW, Nam KY, Ryu CK, Jo YJ, Kim JY. Signal strength as an important factor in the analysis of peripapillary microvascular density using optical coherence tomography angiography. *Sci Rep.* (2019) 9:16299. doi: 10.1038/s41598-019-52818-x

29. Gulati V, Fan S, Hays CL, Samuelson TW, Ahmed, II, et al. A novel 8-mm Schlemm's canal scaffold reduces outflow resistance in a human anterior segment perfusion model. *Invest Ophthalmol Vis Sci.* (2013) 54:1698–704. doi: 10.1167/iovs.12-11373

30. Hays CL, Gulati V, Fan S, Samuelson TW, Ahmed, II, et al. Improvement in outflow facility by two novel microinvasive glaucoma surgery implants. *Invest Ophthalmol Vis Sci.* (2014) 55:1893–900. doi: 10.1167/iovs.13-13353

31. Mansberger SL, Gordon MO, Jampel H, Bhorade A, Brandt JD, Wilson B, et al. Reduction in intraocular pressure after cataract extraction: the Ocular Hypertension Treatment Study. *Ophthalmology.* (2012) 119:1826–31. doi: 10.1016/j.ophtha.2012.02.050

32. Berdahl JP. Cataract surgery to lower intraocular pressure. *Middle East Afr J Ophthalmol.* (2009) 16:119–22. doi: 10.4103/0974-9233.56222

33. Larkin KA, Macneil RG, Dirain M, Sandesara B, Manini TM, Buford TW. Blood flow restriction enhances post-resistance exercise angiogenic gene expression. *Med Sci Sports Exerc.* (2012) 44:2077–83. doi: 10.1249/MSS.0b013e3182625928

34. Li F, Huang W, Zhang X. Efficacy and safety of different regimens for primary open-angle glaucoma or ocular hypertension: a systematic review and network meta-analysis. *Acta Ophthalmol.* (2018) 96:e277–84. doi: 10.1111/aos.13568

35. Akagi T, Uji A, Okamoto Y, Suda K, Kameda T, Nakanishi H, et al. Anterior segment optical coherence tomography angiography imaging of conjunctiva and intrasclera in treated primary open-angle glaucoma. *Am J Ophthalmol.* (2019) 208:313–22. doi: 10.1016/j.ajo.2019.05.008

36. Carreon T, van der Merwe E, Fellman RL, Johnstone M, Bhattacharya SK. Aqueous outflow - a continuum from trabecular meshwork to episcleral veins. *Prog Retin Eye Res.* (2017) 57:108–33. doi: 10.1016/j.preteyeres.2016.12.004

37. Akagi T, Uji A, Huang AS, Weinreb RN, Yamada T, Miyata M, et al. Conjunctival and intrascleral vasculatures assessed using anterior segment optical coherence tomography angiography in normal eyes. *Am J Ophthalmol.* (2018) 196:1–9. doi: 10.1016/j.ajo.2018.08.009

38. Ang M, Cai Y, Shahipasand S, Sim DA, Keane PA, Sng CC, et al. En face optical coherence tomography angiography for corneal neovascularisation. *Br J Ophthalmol.* (2016) 100:616–21. doi: 10.1136/bjophthalmol-2015-307338

39. Stanzel TP, Devarajan K, Lwin NC, Yam GH, Schmetterer L, Mehta JS, et al. Comparison of optical coherence tomography angiography to indocyanine Green angiography and slit lamp photography for corneal vascularization in an animal model. *Sci Rep.* (2018) 8:11493. doi: 10.1038/s41598-018-29752-5

40. Ang M, Sng C, Milea D. Optical coherence tomography angiography in dural carotid-cavernous sinus fistula. *BMC Ophthalmol.* (2016) 16:93. doi: 10.1186/s12886-016-0278-1

41. Pineles SL, Chang MY, Oltra EL, Pihlblad MS, Davila-Gonzalez JP, Sauer TC, et al. Anterior segment ischemia: etiology, assessment, and management. *Eye.* (2018) 32:173–8. doi: 10.1038/eye.2017.248

42. Yoshikawa M, Akagi T, Uji A, Nakanishi H, Kameda T, Suda K, et al. Pilot study assessing the structural changes in posttrabecular aqueous humor outflow pathway after trabecular meshwork surgery using swept-source optical coherence tomography. *PLoS ONE.* (2018) 13:e0199739. doi: 10.1371/journal.pone.0199739

43. Ang M, Tan ACS, Cheung CMG, Keane PA, Dolz-Marco R, Sng CCA, et al. Optical coherence tomography angiography: a review of current and future clinical applications. *Graefes Arch Clin Exp Ophthalmol.* (2018) 256:237–45. doi: 10.1007/s00417-017-3896-2

44. Richter GM, Coleman AL. Minimally invasive glaucoma surgery: current status and future prospects. *Clin Ophthalmol.* (2016) 10:189–206. doi: 10.2147/OPTH.S80490

45. Huang AS, Penteado RC, Papoyan V, Voskanyan L, Weinreb RN. Aqueous angiographic outflow improvement after trabecular microbypass in glaucoma patients. *Ophthalmol Glaucoma.* (2019) 2:11–21. doi: 10.1016/j.ogla.2018.11.010

46. Huang AS, Saraswathy S, Dastiridou A, Begian A, Mohindroo C, Tan JC, et al. Aqueous angiography-mediated guidance of trabecular bypass improves angiographic outflow in human enucleated eyes. *Invest Ophthalmol Vis Sci.* (2016) 57:4558–65. doi: 10.1167/iovs.16-19644

47. Spaide RF, Fujimoto JG, Waheed NK. Image artifacts in optical coherence tomography angiography. *Retina.* (2015) 35:2163–80. doi: 10.1097/IAE.0000000000000765

48. Spaide RF, Fujimoto JG, Waheed NK, Sadda SR, Staurenghi G. Optical coherence tomography angiography. *Prog Retin Eye Res.* (2018) 64:1–55. doi: 10.1016/j.preteyeres.2017.11.003

49. Yao X, Tan B, Ho Y, Liu X, Wong D, chua j, et al. Full circumferential morphological analysis of schlemm's canal in human eyes using megahertz swept source OCT. *Biomedical Optics Express.* (2021) 12:3865–77. doi: 10.1364/BOE.426218

20

Associations Between the Macular Microvasculatures and Subclinical Atherosclerosis in Patients With Type 2 Diabetes: An Optical Coherence Tomography Angiography Study

Jooyoung Yoon [1], Hyo Joo Kang [2], Joo Yong Lee [1,2], June-Gone Kim [1,2], Young Hee Yoon [1,2], Chang Hee Jung [2,3*†] and Yoon Jeon Kim [1,2*†]

[1] Department of Ophthalmology, Asan Medical Center, College of Medicine, University of Ulsan, Seoul, South Korea, [2] Asan Diabetes Center, Asan Medical Center, Seoul, South Korea, [3] Department of Internal Medicine, Asan Medical Center, College of Medicine, University of Ulsan, Seoul, South Korea

*Correspondence:
Yoon Jeon Kim
anne215@gmail.com
Chang Hee Jung
chjung0204@gmail.com

†These authors have contributed equally to this work

Objective: To investigate the associations between the macular microvasculature assessed by optical coherence tomography angiography (OCTA) and subclinical atherosclerosis in patients with type 2 diabetes.

Methods: We included patients with type 2 diabetes who received comprehensive medical and ophthalmic evaluations, such as carotid ultrasonography and OCTA at a hospital-based diabetic clinic in a consecutive manner. Among them, 254 eyes with neither diabetic macular edema (DME) nor history of ophthalmic treatment from 254 patients were included. The presence of increased carotid intima-media thickness (IMT) (>1.0 mm) or carotid plaque was defined as subclinical atherosclerosis. OCTA characteristics focused on foveal avascular zone (FAZ) related parameters and parafoveal vessel density (VD) were compared in terms of subclinical atherosclerosis, and risk factors for subclinical atherosclerosis were identified using a multivariate logistic regression analysis.

Results: Subclinical atherosclerosis was observed in 148 patients (58.3%). The subclinical atherosclerosis group were older ($p < 0.001$), had a greater portion of patients who were men ($p = 0.001$) and who had hypertension ($p = 0.042$), had longer diabetes duration ($p = 0.014$), and lower VD around FAZ ($p = 0.010$), and parafoveal VD (all $p < 0.05$). In the multivariate logistic regression analysis, older age ($p \leq 0.001$), male sex ($p \leq 0.001$), lower VD around FAZ ($p = 0.043$), lower parafoveal VD of both superficial capillary plexus (SCP) ($p = 0.011$), and deep capillary plexus (DCP) ($p = 0.046$) were significant factors for subclinical atherosclerosis.

Conclusion: The decrease in VD around FAZ, and the VD loss in parafoveal area of both SCP and DCP were significantly associated with subclinical atherosclerosis in patients with type 2 diabetes, suggesting that common pathogenic mechanisms might predispose to diabetic micro- and macrovascular complications.

Keywords: carotid ultrasonography, optical coherence tomography angiography (OCTA), retinal microvasculatures, subclinical atherosclerosis, type 2 diabetes

INTRODUCTION

Carotid artery stenosis, an important, potentially life-threatening consequence of systemic atherosclerotic disease in the aging population, is responsible for 10–20% of the ischemic strokes, which are the second most common cause of death worldwide. Diabetes mellitus (DM), one of the major risk factors of carotid artery stenosis, results in systemic vascular complications: macro- and microvascular complications (1). Therefore, screening for the vascular abnormalities and prevention of irrecoverable damage in the high-risk patients are crucial to reduce the social and financial burden of DM (2). Traditionally, the macro- and microvascular complications of diabetes have been considered as the distinct and independent disorders. Recently, however, pathophysiological evidence and epidemiologic evidence suggest that these vascular complications may share common pathophysiological mechanisms (3).

Optical coherence tomography angiography (OCTA) is a new, non-invasive technology that enables the reproducible, quantitative assessment of the microcirculation of different retinal capillary layers (4–8). Unlike the fluorescein angiography, OCTA does not require intravenous dye to assess the retinal vasculature, and therefore causes less discomfort and pain, and is free from the potential systemic adverse effects (9). Characteristic retinal vascular alterations in OCTA have been well-described in patients with diabetic retinopathy (DR) from their early stage of diseases, and several reports showed that these changes were detectable even before the development of DR (10, 11). Recently, the clinical implications of the OCTA parameters for assessing associations with the carotid stenosis were investigated (12). However, not only carotid intima media thickness (IMT), but carotid plaque burden is also reported as a surrogate of atherosclerosis and predictor of future atherosclerotic cardiovascular diseases (13). Thus, we aimed

TABLE 1 | Baseline demographics and clinical characteristics of patients in this study.

	Total (n = 254)	Subclinical atherosclerosis (−) (n = 106)	Subclinical atherosclerosis (+) (n = 148)	P-value
Age (year)	57.6 ± 10.4	54.1 ± 11.2	60.1 ± 9.1	<0.001
Sex (male: female)	162: 92	55: 51	107: 41	0.001
Hypertension [n (%)]	115 (45.3)	40 (37.7)	75 (50.7)	0.041
DM duration (yr)	18.3 ± 8.1	16.8 ± 7.6	19.4 ± 8.3	0.013
DM treatment [n (%)]				0.630
OHA only	166 (65.4)	66 (62.3)	100 (67.6)	
Insulin	88 (34.5)	40 (37.7)	48 (32.4)	
Hyperlipidemia [n (%)]	141 (55.5)	52 (49.1)	89 (59.7)	0.256
Smoking status [n (%)]				0.325
Non-smoker	134 (52.8)	61 (57.5)	73 (49.3)	
Ex-smoker	69 (27.2)	27 (25.5)	42 (28.4)	
Current smoker	51 (20.1)	18 (17.0)	33 (22.3)	
HbA1C (%)	7.7 ± 1.3	7.6 ± 1.2	7.7 ± 1.4	0.517
Glucose (mg/dL)	145.2 ± 46.2	143.1 ± 46.9	146.7 ± 45.8	0.547
SBP (mmHg)	132.2 ± 18.0	131.8 ± 17.7	132.4 ± 18.3	0.768
DBP (mmHg)	74.4 ± 11.9	75.9 ± 10.7	73.4 ± 12.3	0.088
Total cholesterol (mg/dL)	145.5 ± 35.4	151.2 ± 34.2	141.3 ± 35.8	0.028
Triglyceride (mg/dL)	132.7 ± 72.9	135.2 ± 79.1	130.9 ± 68.3	0.641
HDL-cholesterol (mg/dL)	45.5 ± 10.9	46.8 ± 10.5	44.6 ± 11.2	0.122
LDL-cholesterol (mg/dL)	91.3 ± 28.5	95.0 ± 27.7	88.6 ± 28.9	0.074
UACR [n (%)]				0.149
Normal (<30 mcg/mg)	168 (66.1)	76 (71.7)	92 (62.2)	
Microalbuminuria (30~300 mcg/mg)	63 (24.8)	20 (18.9)	43 (29.1)	
Albuminuria (>300 mcg/mg)	21 (8.3)	9 (8.5)	12 (8.1)	
Creatinine (mg/dL)	1.0 ± 0.6	1.0 ± 0.7	1.0 ± 0.6	0.800
eGFR (%)	82.5 ± 20.6	84.3 ± 21.4	81.2 ± 19.9	0.237
Carotid IMT (mm)	0.73 ± 0.02	0.69 ± 0.02	0.75 ± 0.01	0.014
Presence of carotid plaque [n (%)]	155 (61.0)	15 (14.1)	140 (94.6)	<0.001

DM, diabetes mellitus; OHA, oral hypoglycemic agent; SBP, systolic blood pressure; DBP, diastolic blood pressure; HDL, high density lipid; LDL, low density lipid; UACR, urine albumin to creatinine ratio; eGFR, estimated glomerular filtration rate; IMT, intima media thickness.

to compare the retinal microvascular changes measured with OCTA in patients with type 2 diabetes in terms of the presence of carotid artery disease detected by carotid ultrasonography (US), the early indicator of systemic subclinical atherosclerosis (14). In addition, systemic and ophthalmologic factors related to subclinical atherosclerosis were evaluated.

METHODS

The research adhered to the tenets of Declaration of Helsinki. The study was approved by the international research board of Asan Medical Center (IRB No. 2020-0014). Informed consent was waived due to the retrospective nature of the study.

Study Subjects

Patients with type 2 DM who received comprehensive medical and ophthalmic evaluations during the period from January 2017 to December 2019 at a hospital-based diabetic clinic (Asan Medical Center, Seoul, Korea) were selected by medical record review in a consecutive manner. Patients underwent vascular evaluation, such as carotid US, and ophthalmic evaluation, including OCTA at regular intervals based on their medical status, and those who had both carotid US and OCTA within 6 months interval were included in this retrospective observational study. We excluded patients if they had history of ophthalmic treatment, diabetic macular edema (DME), with concomitant ocular disease other than DR, or history of ocular trauma. For image qualities, those with poor OCTA quality, with a scan quality of 6 or less out of 10, were excluded. In addition, to minimize the possible errors in image analysis, proper segmentation without errors, and removal of projection artifact are carefully considered. When both eyes met the inclusion criteria, we included the right eye, and when only one eye of the two eyes satisfied the inclusion criteria, the corresponding eye was included in the study to include one eye for each patient.

At the initial visit of endocrinology, every patient underwent detailed medical and surgical history, such as medication information and duration for diabetes and hypertension, smoking habits, and alcoholic intake. In addition, at baseline and every visit, arterial blood pressure (BP), body weight, and height were measured, and body weight and height were used to calculate the body mass index (BMI), which was used for analysis. After overnight fasting, early morning blood samples were obtained and underwent a central, certified laboratory analysis. Measurements included were hemoglobin A1C (HbA1c), serum glucose level, several lipid parameters, and creatinine. HbA1c was measured using high-performance liquid chromatography (HPLC) of a Variant II Turbo (Bio-Rad Laboratories, Hercules, CA, USA). Fasting total cholesterol, high-density lipoprotein-cholesterol (HDL-C), low-density lipoprotein-cholesterol (LDL-C), and triglyceride (TG) were measured by using an enzymatic colorimetric method (Toshiba Medical Systems). Creatinine was measured by using the Jaffe method, and estimated glomerular filtration rate (eGFR) was calculated with the modified Modification of Diet in Renal Disease (MDRD) equation. In addition, urine tests were performed and urinary albumin-to-creatinine ratio (UACR) was calculated to determine the severity of albuminuria, using a photometric method of the

Integra 800 system (Roche Diagnostics, Indianapolis, IN, USA) in a random spot urine collection.

At their initial visit and at each visit to a retina clinic, all patients underwent a comprehensive ophthalmologic examination that included a review of their ophthalmologic history, measurement of visual acuity, slit lamp biomicroscopy, and funduscopic examinations through dilated pupils by retinal specialists. The severity of DR was classified into 5 grades by the following criteria of the Early Treatment Diabetic Retinopathy Study (ETDRS): (1) no diabetic retinopathy—"no DR"; (2) mild non-proliferative diabetic retinopathy—"mild NPDR"; (3) moderate non-proliferative diabetic retinopathy—"moderate NPDR"; (4) severe non-proliferative diabetic retinopathy—"severe NPDR"; and (5) proliferative diabetic retinopathy—"PDR."

Optical Coherence Tomography Angiography

The RTVue XR Avanti (Optovue, Fremont, CA, USA) spectral-domain OCT device with phase 7 AngioVue software was used for the OCT and OCT angiography examination. A 3 mm × 3-mm macular scans centered on the fovea were acquired. Each OCTA en face image contains 304 × 304 pixels created from the intersection of the 304 vertical and the 304 horizontal B-scans. AngioVue software automatically segments the B-scan images into four layers: superficial capillary plexus (SCP), deep capillary plexus (DCP), outer retina, and choriocapillaris layer. The SCP layer was segmented with an inner boundary set at 3 μm beneath the internal limiting membrane and an outer boundary at 15 μm beneath the inner plexiform layer. The DCP layer was segmented with an inner boundary set at 15 μm beneath the inner plexiform layer and an outer boundary at 70 μm beneath the inner plexiform layer. Using SCP and DCP images, following parameters were measured with the integrated automated software. For FAZ related parameters, area (mm^2) and perimeter (mm) were measured and acircularity was calculated using those two parameters. In addition, vessel density (VD) around 300 μm boundary around FAZ and VD of each selected region (foveal and parafoveal area of four quadrants) were calculated as the percentage of area occupied by flowing blood vessels and was analyzed in both SCP and DCP, respectively.

Carotid Ultrasonography

Carotid artery examination was performed by a single specialized technician with patients in the supine position with the head elevated to 45 degrees and tilted to either side by 30 degrees and the operator seated at the head bed. High resolution ultrasound (HD 11 XE, Philips Healthcare, Andover MA) equipped with a high-frequency (5–12.5 MHz) linear transducer was used to acquire images of the left and right common carotid arteries. Carotid IMT scanning and reading was evaluated with the criteria of Mannheim Carotid Intima-Media Thickness Consensus (15). IMT was measured from the media-adventitia interface to the intima-lumen interface at the level of ∼0.5 cm below the carotid-artery bulb, over a 1-cm segment of the artery, and the degree of stenosis was assessed. The value obtained through a QLAB IMT-quantification software measurement plug-in (Philips Healthcare) was used in analysis (16). The upper

TABLE 2 | Baseline ophthalmologic characteristics and optical coherence tomography angiography (OCTA) parameters of patients.

	Total (n = 254)	Subclinical atherosclerosis (−) (n = 106)	Subclinical atherosclerosis (+) (n = 148)	P-value
BCVA (LogMAR)	0.07 ± 0.09	0.06 ± 0.08	0.08 ± 0.09	0.144
DR stage [n (%)]				0.159
No DR	33 (13.0)	18 (17.0)	15 (10.1)	
Mild NPDR	111 (43.7)	50 (47.2)	61 (41.2)	
Moderate NPDR	56 (22.1)	20 (18.9)	36 (24.3)	
Severe NPDR	42 (16.5)	13 (12.3)	29 (19.6)	
PDR	12 (4.7)	5 (4.7)	7 (4.7)	
FAZ parameters				
Area (mm^2)	0.38 ± 0.59	0.35 ± 0.11	0.40 ± 0.77	0.486
Perimeter (mm)	2.38 ± 0.43	2.43 ± 0.45	2.35 ± 0.41	0.161
VD around FAZ (%)	47.6 ± 3.7	48.3 ± 3.8	47.1 ± 3.6	0.009
Acircularity	1.16 ± 0.06	1.17 ± 0.07	1.16 ± 0.04	0.087
SCP parameters				
Fovea VD (%)	14.8 ± 5.1	14.5 ± 4.8	14.6 ± 5.4	0.817
Parafovea VD (%)	46.3 ± 3.7	47.2 ± 3.7	45.7 ± 3.6	0.002
DCP parameters				
Fovea VD (%)	27.5 ± 6.5	27.4 ± 6.2	27.7 ± 6.8	0.722
Parafovea VD (%)	49.9 ± 3.7	50.5 ± 3.5	49.5 ± 3.8	0.044
Scan quality	8.3 ± 2.2	8.2 ± 2.2	8.0 ± 2.0	0.075

BCVA, best corrected visual acuity; DR, diabetic retinopathy; NPDR, non-proliferative diabetic retinopathy; PDR, proliferative diabetic retinopathy; FAZ, foveal avascular zone; VD, vessel density; SCP, superficial capillary plexus; DCP, deep capillary plexus.

TABLE 3 | Factors associated with the presence of subclinical atherosclerosis in patients with type 2 diabetes in univariate logistic analysis.

	Odds ratio (95% CI)	P-value
Demographics		
Age	1.06 (1.03–1.09)	<0.001
Sex		
Male	2.42 (1.43–4.09)	0.001
Female	1 (Ref)	
Hypertension	1.70 (1.02–2.82)	0.042
DM duration	1.04 (1.01–1.08)	0.014
DM treatment		
OHA only	1 (Ref)	
Insulin	0.78 (0.30–2.05)	0.613
Hyperlipidemia	1.23 (0.95–1.58)	0.165
Laboratory data		
HbA1C	1.07 (0.88–1.30)	0.515
Glucose	1.00 (1.00–1.01)	0.546
SBP	1.02 (0.99–1.03)	0.622
DBP	0.98 (0.95–1.04)	0.703
Total cholesterol	0.99 (0.99–1.00)	0.030
Triglyceride	1.00 (1.00–1.00)	0.640
HDL-cholesterol	0.98 (0.96–1.01)	0.123
LDL-cholesterol	0.99 (0.98–1.00)	0.076
UACR		
Normal	1 (Ref)	
Microalbuminuria	1.78 (0.96–3.27)	0.066
Albuminuria	1.10 (0.44–2.75)	0.836
Creatinine	1.06 (0.70–1.59)	0.800
eGFR	0.99 (0.98–1.01)	0.237
Ophthalmologic data		
BCVA (LogMAR)	9.03 (0.46–175.68)	0.146
DR stage		
No DR-mild NPDR	1 (Ref)	
Worse than moderate NPDR	2.16 (0.85–5.79)	0.075
OCT angiography parameters		
FAZ parameters		
Area (mm^2)	1.25 (0.61–2.56)	0.547
Perimeter (mm)	0.66 (0.36–1.19)	0.163
VD around FAZ (%)	0.91 (0.85–0.98)	0.010
Acircularity	0.02 (0.00–1.88)	0.092
SCP parameters		
Fovea VD (%)	1.01 (0.96–1.06)	0.816
Parafovea VD (%)	0.89 (0.83–0.96)	0.002
DCP parameters		
Fovea VD (%)	1.01 (0.97–1.05)	0.721
Parafovea VD (%)	0.93 (0.87–1.00)	0.045
Scan quality	0.92 (0.85–1.05)	0.116

DM, diabetes mellitus; OHA, oral hypoglycemic agent; SBP, systolic blood pressure; DBP, diastolic blood pressure; HDL, high density lipid; LDL, low density lipid; UACR, urine albumin to creatinine ratio; eGFR, estimated glomerular filtration rate; BCVA, best corrected visual acuity; DR, diabetic retinopathy; NPDR, non-proliferative diabetic retinopathy; PDR, proliferative diabetic retinopathy; OCT, optical coherence tomography; FAZ, foveal avascular zone; VD, vessel density; SCP, superficial capillary plexus; DCP, deep capillary plexus.

normal limit of IMT was 1.0 mm, and focal lesions with increased carotid IMT (>1.0 mm) or the presence of carotid plaque was defined as subclinical atherosclerosis (17).

Statistical Analysis

The following variables were analyzed in each patient: (i) demographic variables (i.e., age, sex, comorbidities with hypertension or hyperlipidemia, DM duration, and DM treatment), (ii) laboratory variables (i.e., carotid IMT, presence of carotid plaque, HbA1C, glucose, systolic BP (SBP) and diastolic BP (DBP), total cholesterol, TG, HDL and LDL-cholesterol, UACR, creatinine, and eGFR), (iii) ocular characteristics (i.e., BCVA and DR severity), and (iv) OCTA parameters (FAZ related parameters; area, perimeter, acircularity, and VD around FAZ, foveal and parafoveal VD in SCP and DCP).

Descriptive statistics were demonstrated in numbers and percentages for categorical variables and mean ± SD of continuous variables to present the baseline characteristics of study subjects. For comparison in terms of the presence of subclinical atherosclerosis (the subclinical atherosclerosis group and the non-subclinical atherosclerosis group), independent *t*-test or Mann–Whitney *U*-test was used depending on the normality of their distribution. Chi-squared test was used to compare the categorical data. To explore the factors significantly associated with subclinical atherosclerosis, logistic regression analyses were conducted. Univariate analyses were separately performed for each variable and those with $p < 0.1$ were included in the multivariate analysis with the forward elimination process. Odds ratios (*ORs*) with 95% *CIs* were calculated. All statistical analyses were performed using SPSS version 21.0 software (SPSS Inc., Chicago, IL, USA).

RESULTS

Of a total of 254 patients included in this analysis, 148 patients (58.3%) had subclinical atherosclerosis. Patients with subclinical atherosclerosis were older than those without (60.1 ± 9.1 vs. 54.1 ± 11.2 years, $p < 0.001$). Baseline characteristics in this study are summarized in **Table 1**. Patients with subclinical atherosclerosis had greater portion of male sex (72.3 vs. 52.9%, $p = 0.001$), hypertension (50.7 vs. 37.7%, $p = 0.041$), and longer duration of type 2 DM (19.4 ± 8.3 vs. 16.9 ± 7.6 years, $p = 0.013$). All the study participants were receiving either oral hypoglycemic agents or insulin injection or both, and the proportion of patients on insulin treatment and smoking status were not significantly different between the two groups. HbA1C, serum glucose, SBP, DBP, UACR, creatinine, and eGFR were not different between the two groups.

Regarding the ophthalmologic data, BCVA, DR stage, and OCTA signal strength were not significantly different in terms of subclinical atherosclerosis (**Table 2**). Whereas, the area, perimeter, and acircularity of FAZ were not different between the two groups, VD around FAZ was significantly more impaired in the subclinical atherosclerosis group (47.1 ± 3.6 vs. 48.3 ± 3.8, $p = 0.009$). While foveal VD in the SCP and DCP was not different between two groups, parafoveal VD in the SCP (45.7 ± 3.6 vs. 47.2 ± 3.7, P = 0.002) and DCP (49.5 ± 3.6 vs. 50.5 ± 3.5, P = 0.044) was significantly reduced in the subclinical atherosclerosis group. There was no significant difference in scan quality in terms of subclinical atherosclerosis to identify the factors associated with presence of the subclinical atherosclerosis, univariate and multivariate logistic regression analyses were conducted including the baseline variables and OCTA parameters. In the univariate analysis (**Table 3**), old age [*OR* = 1.06 (95% *CI* 1.03-1.09), $p < 0.001$], male sex [*OR* = 2.42 (95% *CI* 1.43-4.09), $p = 0.001$], longer duration of DM

[*OR* = 1.04 (95% *CI* 1.01-1.08), $p = 0.014$], and the presence of hypertension [*OR* = 1.70 (95% *CI* 1.02-2.82), $p = 0.042$] were associated with the presence of subclinical atherosclerosis. When all patients were divided into two groups according to DR severity, marginal association was confirmed in the univariate analysis [*OR* = 2.16 (95% *CI* 0.85-5.79), $p = 0.075$]. Among the OCTA parameters, decrease in foveal VD around FAZ [*OR* = 0.91 (95% *CI* 0.85-0.98), $p = 0.010$] and parafoveal VD in SCP [*OR* = 0.89 (95% *CI* 0.83-0.96), $p = 0.002$] and DCP [*OR* = 0.93 (95% *CI* 0.87-1.00), $p = 0.045$] was associated with subclinical atherosclerosis.

We performed three models of multivariate analyses (**Table 4**) to obviate the confounding effects of the multicollinearity of the OCTA parameters (correlation coefficients >0.8). Old age and male sex were consistently remained as the significant factors for subclinical atherosclerosis (all $p < 0.05$) in all three models. Low foveal VD around FAZ [*OR* = 0.92 (95% *CI* 0.86-1.00), $p = 0.043$], parafoveal VD in both SCP [*OR* = 0.91 (95% *CI* 0.85-0.98), $p = 0.011$], and DCP [*OR* = 0.93 (95% *CI* 0.86-1.00), $p = 0.046$] were significant factors for subclinical atherosclerosis in each of three models. **Figure 1** shows the different averages and distributions in the significant OCTA parameters according to the presence of subclinical atherosclerosis. And **Figure 2** demonstrated the difference in the foveal and parafoveal capillary vessel density of an age-sex matched control and a patient with subclinical atherosclerosis.

DISCUSSION

This study demonstrates that the decreases in VD of macular microvasculatures were associated and the presence of subclinical atherosclerosis in type 2 DM, suggesting associations between macro- and microvascular diabetes complications. Based on our findings, the alterations of macular microvasculatures in OCTA which are implicative of higher risk of subclinical atherosclerosis, could be used as one of the non-invasive imaging biomarkers for the higher risk of macrovascular diseases which requires careful monitoring.

Our results showing the associations between the carotid disease and retinal vasculatures in diabetes were in line with the

TABLE 4 | Factors significantly associated with the presence of subclinical atherosclerosis in patients with type 2 diabetes in multivariate logistic analysis.

	Model 1 including foveal VD around FAZ		Model 2 including SCP Parafovea VD		Model 3 including DCP Parafovea VD	
	Odds ratio (95% CI)	*P*-value	Odds ratio (95% CI)	*P*-value	Odds ratio (95% CI)	*P*-value
Age (year)	1.06 (1.03–1.10)	<0.001	1.06 (1.03–1.09)	0.001	1.06 (1.03–1.10)	<0.001
Male sex	2.67 (1.51–4.75)	0.001	2.77 (1.56–4.93)	0.001	2.77 (1.56–4.90)	<0.001
DM duration (yr)	1.02 (0.98–1.06)	0.456	1.02 (0.98–1.06)	0.425	1.02 (0.98–1.06)	0.409
Hypertension	1.24 (0.71–2.18)	0.448	1.27 (0.72–2.23)	0.412	1.34 (0.76–2.35)	0.311
Foveal VD around FAZ	0.92 (0.86–1.00)	0.043				
SCP Parafovea VD			0.91 (0.84–0.98)	0.011		
DCP Parafovea VD					0.93 (0.86–1.00)	0.046

Model 1, 2, and 3 contains each of OCTA parameters which showed associations with subclinical atherosclerosis in univariate analyses.
DM, diabetes mellitus; VD, vessel density; FAZ, foveal avascular zone; SCP, superficial capillary plexus; DCP, deep capillary plexus.

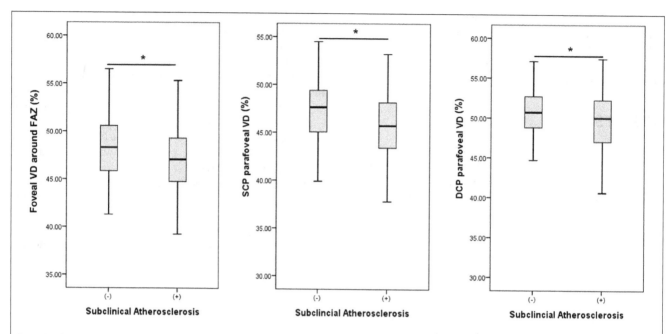

FIGURE 1 | Bar graphs showing the different averages and 95% distributions of the significantly associated optical coherence tomography angiography (OCTA) parameters (foveal vessel density (VD) around foveal avascular zone (FAZ) and parafoveal VD in superficial and deep capillary plexuses (DCP) according to the presence of subclinical atherosclerosis. An asterisk means a statistical significance ($p < 0.05$) between two groups in an independent t-test. VD, vessel density; FAZ, foveal avascular zone; SCP, superficial capillary plexus; DCP, deep capillary plexus.

previous studies that proved the increased cardiovascular risks in patients with DR. DR is an independent risk factor for carotid plaques, and the severity of carotid atherosclerosis correlates with the severity of microangiopathy. In this study, we could provide stronger evidence for those findings through access to a more sensitive retinal imaging modality than the conventionally used color fundus photography. Morphologic changes assessed by OCTA in DR, i.e., retinal microvasculature abnormalities, such as capillary dropout, reduced capillary VD, tortuous capillary branches, dilated average vascular caliber, FAZ enlargement, and irregular FAZ contour, were present before the beginning of the clinically diagnosed DR and become more obvious as DR progress. As a result, we revealed general reduction in VD in terms of subclinical atherosclerosis.

Interestingly, however, we could not find significant differences in area and contour of FAZ and foveal VD in terms of subclinical atherosclerosis. These differences imply that the overall hemodynamic changes of retinal vasculatures may reflect systemic risk factors related to subclinical atherosclerosis more sensitively, compared with the localized deformation of retinal vessels in FAZ. Moreover, foveal VD which means VD within a fovea centered circle of 1 mm diameter is mostly influenced by the FAZ area. In other words, when the FAZ area is large, the foveal VD is small, and when the FAZ area is small, the foveal VD is large. Therefore, parafoveal VD or VD around FAZ reflects vascular impairment more accurately than foveal VD, which is related to the FAZ area with large individual variability.

Our results showing the close associations between retinal microvasculature obtained by OCTA and diabetic macrovascular complications were in line with those by Drinkwater et al. (12). On the other hand, it is differentiated by the fact that not only carotid stenosis represented by carotid IMT thickening but also carotid plaque, which is a predictor of atherosclerotic cardiovascular diseases. Most of our patients classified as the subclinical atherosclerosis group had carotid plaques without IMT thickening. Moreover, when we evaluated the VD changes of each layer, we noted that parafoveal VDs in both SCP and DCP were all correlated with subclinical atherosclerosis. These results were different from their study which concluded that the decrease VD in only DCP correlates to the increased IMT and the grade of stenosis and VD in SCP did not show significant association with the carotid parameters (17). This difference primarily may be due to the different patient characteristics, particularly in the distribution of DR stages between two studies. While our study included the patients with variable stages of DR (13.1% patients with no DR), the study by Drinkwater et al. (12) mainly included the patients with no DR (83.8% patients with no DR). Since it is widely reported that the vascular changes in DCP occur in the early stage of DR (even before the development of DR) and those in SCP occur in the later stage, patients with no DR or early stage of DR might not have the significant changes in SCP (18). Rather, our data showed that the degree of association between subclinical atherosclerosis and reduction in VD was slightly higher in SCP compared with that of DCP. While metabolic diseases, i.e., diabetes mainly affect DCP with slower blood flow, where toxic materials take longer to contact the blood vessels, arterial diseases, i.e., hypertension, act more on precapillary arterioles where shear stress and oxidative stress work well (19).

The pathogenic mechanism of how carotid diseases associates with retinal microvascular disease is not well-established, although there are several hypotheses. Similar risk factors

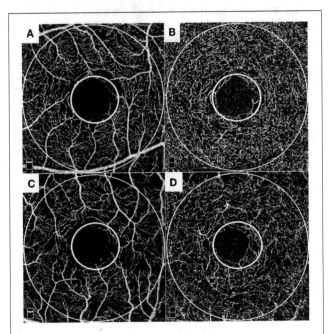

FIGURE 2 | Representative cases of an age-sex matched control **(A,B)** and a patient with subclinical atherosclerosis **(C,D)**. Each of small and large circles denote foveal and parafoveal area. Control: A 56-year- old male patient with 18-years history of diabetes showed 0.63 mm of carotid intima media thickness (IMT) with plaque-free in carotid ultrasonography (US). He had well-preserved foveal VD around foveal avascular zone FAZ (49.7%), parafoveal VD in superficial capillary plexus (49.3%), and parafoveal VD in deep capillary plexus (50.3%) in OCTA. A patient with subclinical atherosclerosis: a 57-year- old male patient with 5-years history of diabetes showed 1.11 mm of carotid IMT with plaque in carotid US. He had impaired foveal VD around FAZ (45.9%), parafoveal VD in superficial capillary plexus (40.8%), and parafoveal VD in deep capillary plexus (46.5%) in OCTA.

may contribute to both diseases. In addition, microcirculation damage caused by diabetes serves as the "common soil" for macro- and microangiopathy of diabetes, since diabetic macroangiopathy evolves from the microvascular damage within the major arterial wall (the vasa vasorum) (20). Recent evidence has shown that the vasa vasorum of the major vessels in patients with diabetes undergoes the similar process as the microvascular changes of the DR. Endothelial dysfunction and increase of vascular permeability occur at first, followed by hypoxia, which leads to the angiogenesis and neovascularization. Therefore, this shared vascular pathophysiology proves that microangiopathy and macroangiopathy of the diabetes are not entirely separated entities.

In our analysis, we could not confirm the differences in BP, blood lipid, glucose control level, and treatment thereof, known factors which affect retinal vasculatures, according to the presence of subclinical atherosclerosis. This can be explained by several reasons. First, this study was conducted on patients who had undergone medical treatment for BP, blood lipid, and glucose. The second reason is that the systemic clinical data included in this study were measured on the day of the visit to the internal medicine clinic, not on the exact date of OCTA acquisition. Considering the variability of medical indicators, the possibility that the time difference affected in the lack of associations cannot be excluded.

The present study has some limitations, including its retrospective nature of study design. The other limitation is that our measurements based on a small field of view (3 mm × 3 mm) of OCT angiography, which may not represent the whole retinal circulation. Despite these limitations, this approach could provide the important clinical implications of predicting the systemic status with widely available ocular images captured in a short time. The other strength of this study is that we focused only on patients with no DR or treatment naïve patients with DR to obviate the possible effects of ocular treatments on retinal vasculatures. Since previous studies reported changes in macular vasculatures after laser photocoagulation or intravitreal injections (21, 22), we believe that this point has an importance for the accurate analysis. In addition, to minimize the possible errors in image analysis, we included only patients with good OCTA image quality of scan quality ≥ 7, proper segmentation without errors, and the removal of projection artifact, which are all major factors that must be carefully considered in an OCTA imaging study. Last, the number of patients was sufficient for the analysis of risk factors for subclinical atherosclerosis.

In conclusion, we found that decreased VD around FAZ and parafoveal VD in OCTA were significantly associated with subclinical atherosclerosis with other risk factors, such as male sex and old age. Non-invasive *in vivo* retinal vascular imaging captured by OCTA could be used to assess DR but also as the early indicator of macrovascular complications, which suggests that diabetic microangiopathy and macroangiopathy may share the common pathophysiology. Therefore, ophthalmologists should keep in mind such close relationship between ocular changes and systemic diseases and consider evaluations for other comorbidities, such as carotid US, when they examine the patients with impaired macular vasculatures.

AUTHOR CONTRIBUTIONS

All authors listed have made a substantial, direct, and intellectual contribution to the work and approved it for publication.

FUNDING

This study was supported by a grant from the Technology Innovation Program (or Industrial Strategic Technology Development Program) (1415175064, Development of portable fundus imaging and diagnosis device equipped with artificial intelligence and edge computing) funded by the Ministry of Trade, Industry & Energy (MOTIE, South Korea), and the Asan Institute for Life Sciences (2020IP0103-1), Asan Medical Center, Seoul, South Korea.

REFERENCES

1. Nathan DM. Long-term complications of diabetes mellitus. *N Engl J Med.* (1993) 328:1676–85. doi: 10.1056/NEJM199306103282306

2. Zhang P, Gregg E. Global economic burden of diabetes and its implications. *Lancet Diab Endocrinol.* (2017) 5:404–5. doi: 10.1016/S2213-8587(17)30100-6

3. Krentz AJ, Clough G, Byrne CD. Interactions between microvascular and macrovascular disease in diabetes: pathophysiology and therapeutic implications. *Diab Obes Metab.* (2007) 9:781–91. doi: 10.1111/j.1463-1326.2007.00670.x

4. Agrawal R, Xin W, Keane PA, Chhablani J, Agarwal A. Optical coherence tomography angiography: a non-invasive tool to image end-arterial system. *Expert Rev Med Devices.* (2016) 3:519–21. doi: 10.1080/17434440.2016.1186540

5. Jia Y, Bailey ST, Wilson DJ, Tan O, Klein ML, Flaxel CJ, et al. Quantitative optical coherence tomography angiography of choroidal neovascularization in age-related macular degeneration. *Ophthalmology.* (2014) 121:1435–44. doi: 10.1016/j.ophtha.2014.01.034

6. Matsunaga D, Yi J, Puliafito CA, Kashani AH. OCT angiography in healthy human subjects. *Ophthal Surg Lasers Imaging Retina.* (2014) 45:510–5. doi: 10.3928/23258160-20141118-04

7. Spaide RF, Klancnik JM, Cooney MJ. Retinal vascular layers imaged by fluorescein angiography and optical coherence tomography angiography. *JAMA Ophthalmol.* (2015) 133:45–50. doi: 10.1001/jamaophthalmol.2014.3616

8. Spaide RF, Klancnik JM, Cooney MJ. Retinal vascular layers in macular telangiectasia type 2 imaged by optical coherence tomographic angiography. *JAMA Ophthalmol.* (2015) 133:66–73. doi: 10.1001/jamaophthalmol.2014.3950

9. Kwiterovich KA, Maguire MG, Murphy RP, Schachat AP, Bressler NM, Bressler SB, et al. Frequency of adverse systemic reactions after fluorescein angiography: results of a prospective study. *Ophthalmology.* (1991) 98:1139–42. doi: 10.1016/S0161-6420(91)32165-1

10. E.T.D.R.S.R. Group. Fluorescein angiographic risk factors for progression of diabetic retinopathy: ETDRS report number 13. *Ophthalmology.* (1991) 98:834–40. doi: 10.1016/S0161-6420(13)38015-4

11. E.T.D.R.S.R. Group. Classification of diabetic retinopathy from fluorescein angiograms: ETDRS report number 11. *Ophthalmology.* (1991) 98:807–22. doi: 10.1016/S0161-6420(13)38013-0

12. Drinkwater JJ, Chen FK, Brooks AM, Davis BT, Turner AW, Davis TM, et al. Carotid disease and retinal optical coherence tomography angiography parameters in type 2 diabetes: the fremantle diabetes study phase II. *Diabetes Care.* (2020) 43:3034–41. doi: 10.2337/dc20-0370

13. Sillesen H, Sartori S, Sandholt B, Baber U, Mehran R, Fuster V. Carotid plaque thickness and carotid plaque burden predict future cardiovascular events in asymptomatic adult Americans. *Eur Heart J Cardiovasc Imaging.* (2018) 19:1042–50. doi: 10.1093/ehjci/jex239

14. O'Leary DH, Polak JF, Kronmal RA, Manolio TA, Burke GL, Wolfson SK Jr. Carotid-artery intima and media thickness as a risk factor for myocardial infarction and stroke in older adults. *N Engl J Med.* (1999) 340:14–22. doi: 10.1056/NEJM199901073400103

15. Touboul PJ, Hennerici MG, Meairs S, Adams H, Amarenco P, Bornstein N, et al. Mannheim carotid intima-media thickness and plaque consensus (2004-2006-2011). An update on behalf of the advisory board of the 3rd, 4th and 5th watching the risk symposia, at the 13th, 15th and 20th European Stroke Conferences, Mannheim, Germany, 2004, Brussels, Belgium, 2006, and Hamburg, Germany, 2011. *Cerebrovasc Dis.* (2012) 34:290–6. doi: 10.1159/000343145

16. Jung CH, Lee WJ, Lee MJ, Kang YM, Jang JE, Leem J, et al. Association of serum angiopoietin-like protein 2 with carotid intima-media thickness in subjects with type 2 diabetes. *Cardiovasc Diabetol.* (2015) 14:35. doi: 10.1186/s12933-015-0198-z

17. Cobble M, Bale B. Carotid intima-media thickness: knowledge and application to everyday practice. *Postgraduate Med.* (2010) 122:10–8. doi: 10.3810/pgm.2010.01.2091

18. J Ting DSW, Tan GSW, Agrawal R, Yanagi Y, Sie NM, Wong CW, et al. Optical coherence tomographic angiography in type 2 diabetes and diabetic retinopathy. *JAMA Ophthalmol.* (2017) 135:306–12. doi: 10.1001/jamaophthalmol.2016.5877

19. Yang M, Park CS, Kim SH, Noh TW, Kim JH, Park S, et al. Dll4 Suppresses transcytosis for arterial blood-retinal barrier homeostasis. *Circ Res.* (2020) 126:767–83. doi: 10.1161/CIRCRESAHA.119.316476

20. Rubinat E, Ortega E, Traveset A, Arcidiacono MV, Alonso N, Betriu A, et al. Microangiopathy of common carotid vasa vasorum in type 1 diabetes mellitus. *Atherosclerosis.* (2015) 241:334–8. doi: 10.1016/j.atherosclerosis.2015.05.024

21. Kim YJ, Yeo JH, Son G, Kang H, Sung YS, Lee JY, et al. Efficacy of intravitreal AFlibercept injection For Improvement of retinal Nonperfusion In diabeTic retinopathY (AFFINITY study). *BMJ Open Diabetes Res Care.* (2020) 8:e001616. doi: 10.1136/bmjdrc-2020-001616

22. Fawzi AA, Fayed AE, Linsenmeier RA, Gao J, Yu F. Improved macular capillary flow on optical coherence tomography angiography after panretinal photocoagulation for proliferative diabetic retinopathy. *Am J Ophthalmol.* (2019) 206:217–27. doi: 10.1016/j.ajo.2019.04.032

21

Lipidomics Analysis of the Tears in the Patients Receiving LASIK, FS-LASIK, or SBK Surgery

Yan Gao [1†], Yuanyuan Qi [2†], Yue Huang [2], Xiaorong Li [2], Lei Zhou [1,3,4*] and Shaozhen Zhao [2*]

[1] Ocular Proteomics Platform, Singapore Eye Research Institute, Singapore, Singapore, [2] Tianjin Key Laboratory of Retinal Functions and Diseases, Tianjin Branch of National Clinical Research Center for Ocular Disease, Eye Institute and School of Optometry, Tianjin Medical University Eye Hospital, Tianjin, China, [3] Department of Ophthalmology, Yong Loo Lin School of Medicine, National University of Singapore, Singapore, Singapore, [4] Ophthalmology and Visual Sciences Academia Clinical Program, Duke-National University of Singapore Medical School, Singapore, Singapore

Purpose: Tear film lipid layer (TFLL) plays a vital role in maintaining the tear film stability and, thus, the lipid composition of the tears could greatly affect the physiological function and biophysical integrity of the tear film. The objective of this study is to assess the tear lipid composition of the patients receiving laser-assisted *in situ* keratomileusis (LASIK), femtosecond LASIK (FS-LASIK), or sub-Bowman's keratomileusis (SBK) surgery preoperatively and postoperatively.

Methods: Tear samples were collected from the left eye of the patient who receiving LASIK ($n = 10$), FS-LASIK ($n = 10$), or SBK ($n = 10$) surgery in week 0, week 1, week 4, and week 52. A rapid direct injection shotgun lipidomics workflow, MS/MS^{ALL} (<2 min/sample), was applied to examine the tear lipidome.

Correspondence:
Lei Zhou
zhou.lei@seri.com.sg
Shaozhen Zhao
zhaosz1997@sina.com

† These authors have contributed equally to this work and share first authorship

Results: In week 52, the SBK group demonstrated a similar lipidome profile compared to week 0, while the FS-LASIK and LASIK groups shifted away from week 0. Two lipids, ganglioside (GD3) 27:4 and triacylglycerol (TAG) 59:3, were found to be associated with the lipidome changes preoperatively and postoperatively. No statistical significance was found in the overall lipid classes from the FS-LASIK group. The LASIK group showed significant alteration in the phospholipid and sphingolipid over time, while the SBK group demonstrated a significant difference in the (O-acyl)-ω-hydroxy fatty acid (OAHFA) and phospholipid.

Conclusion: LASIK showed the greatest impact on the tear lipidome changes over time, while SBK demonstrated minimal impact among the three types of refractive surgeries after 1 year.

Keywords: lipidomics, refractive surgery, LASIK, FS-LASIK, SBK, PLS-DA

INTRODUCTION

The thin layer of the tear film covers the anterior surface of the cornea and serves the critical functions in maintaining the proper ocular function and health. Its main roles include moistening the mucous membrane, nourishing the avascular corneal, flushing out the contaminants and irritants, and providing a smooth surface for the visual acuity (1, 2).

It has been proposed that the tear film is composed of three layers: an inner mucin layer, a middle aqueous layer, and an outer tear film lipid layer (TFLL). Lam et al. further divided the lipid layer into two sublayers: the superficial sublayer mainly consisting of the non-polar lipids and an inner amphiphilic sublayer facilitating the interaction between the polar and non-polar components of the tears (3). TFLL is vital for a stable tear film by preventing the tear film from evaporation (4). Therefore, the physiological function and biophysical integrity of the tear film would be greatly affected by the lipid composition. It was a challenging task to fully evaluate the lipid profile of the tear samples considering the small amount of the materials obtained from the humans, the diversity of the lipid species, and the complexities of the qualitative and quantitative lipidomics analysis (5). Nevertheless, the lipid composition of the tear film has been extensively studied (6–8). The high sensitivity of the mass spectrometry (MS) in analyzing the low sample volumes makes it a preferred approach in the biomedical research to decipher the fine changes of the lipid metabolism in the ocular and nonocular disorders, for example, Meibomian gland dysfunction, dry eye syndrome (9), and multiple sclerosis (10).

There are two techniques used for the excimer laser refractive correction procedures: surface or stromal ablation. The shallow cornea disruption in the surface ablation procedures such as photorefractive keratectomy (PRK), laser epithelial keratomileusis (LASEK), and epithelial laser-assisted *in situ* keratomileusis (Epi-LASIK) results in a lower incidence of the surgery-induced dry eye and provides more stability for the thinner cornea, implicating the better biomechanical outcomes. However, greater discomfort caused by the wound response and delayed vision recovery would still be the major problems for the surface ablation technique (11, 12). In contrast, the stromal ablation surgeries such as LASIK, femtosecond LASIK (FS-LASIK), and sub-Bowman's keratomileusis (SBK) have the advantages of essentially immediate vision correction, quick recovery, and very little to no discomfort (13). These three types of the refractive surgery use the corneal flap creation procedure to maintain the integrity of the corneal structures such as the Bowman's layer and the epithelium (14). However, the risk of post-LASIK keratectasia was elevated for the patients with moderate to high myopia due to the thicker flap (110–160 μm) (15, 16). SBK was developed from LASIK by using a mechanical microkeratome to create a thinner corneal flap (90–110 μm) and more planar in shape compared with the conventional LASIK approach (17). This approach is an evolutive procedure that increased the biomechanical stability of LASIK and reduced the pain experience of PRK (18, 19). The variation of the flap thicknesses and flap diameters by using a mechanical microkeratome in LASIK and SBK approaches was still a problem, despite their safeness and effectiveness. Corneal flap creation has become a more predictable and safe procedure with the introduction of FS-LASIK (20, 21).

Dry eye is a common symptom after LASIK surgery. It is believed that postsurgical development of the dry eye is closely related to the surgical cut of the corneal nerve fibers during the flap creation (22) and associated with the degree of preoperative myopia and the depth of laser treatment (23). The loss of the corneal innervation could affect the lacrimal function unit (LFU) (24), corneal blinking, and blinking of the Meibomian gland reflexes, resulting in the decreased aqueous and lipid tear secretion and mucin expression (25). Patel et al. showed that the tear lipid layer became thinner after LASIK (26). In general, patients receiving FS-LASIK surgery demonstrated the stable tear film compared with the mechanical microkeratome group (27, 28).

Although the tear lipids have been widely studied, a comprehensive lipidomics study examining the tear lipid profiles before and after the refractive surgery is still lacking. In this study, a technique specifically designed for the global lipidomics, MS/MS^{ALL}, was used to assess the tear lipidome prior to and after the refractive surgery (29–31). This technique collects all the precursor ions in the Q1 quadrupole and the collision-induced dissociation is carried out in Q2 quadrupole while collecting all the high-resolution MS/MS spectra at a high speed (29, 30). MS/MS^{ALL} is highly reproducible, bias free, and requires no method development (32). Given the important role of TFLL in maintaining the proper ocular function and easy accessibility of the tear samples, the tear lipid compositions of the patients taken FS-LASIK, LASIK, or SBK surgery preoperatively (week 0) and postoperatively (week 1, week 4, and week 52) were investigated by using MS/MS^{ALL} in this study.

METHODS AND MATERIALS

Sample Collection

The study was approved by the Tianjin Medical University Institutional Review Board and was conducted according to the Declaration of Helsinki. The signed consent forms were obtained from the participating volunteers. The criteria for this study include: (1) the age of the participants should be over 18 years old; (2) a stable refractive error in the last 1 year; (3) soft contact lenses had not been worn for more than 1 week; (4) rigid contact lenses had not been worn for more than 2 weeks; (5) no history of eye disease or eye surgery; (6) no systemic connective tissue disease or autoimmune disease; (7) no other systemic diseases (such as diabetes, seborrheic dermatitis, or hyperlipidemia); (8) postoperative corneal stromal bed thickness was >250 μm; and (9) no breastfeeding or pregnancy. All the patients were explained about the advantages, disadvantages, and the risk of the three types of surgeries. The type of surgery to be carried out in each patient was based on the preference of the patient. Clinical examinations for the patients receiving FS-LASIK ($n = 10$), LASIK ($n = 10$), or SBK ($n = 10$) surgery included Schirmer test (without anesthesia), tear breakup time (TBUT), and corneal fluorescein staining. Corneal staining was graded from 0 to 5 according to the Oxford schema (33). Tear samples were collected by using the Schirmer strips from both the eyes of the patients and the strips were stored at −80°C until further analysis. Postregime for all the patients is the same. Topical medications after surgery consisted of fluorometholone eye drops four times daily for 1 week and tapered over 4 weeks, levofloxacin eye drops three times per day for 3 days, and artificial tears four times daily for 1–3 months depending on the severity of the postsurgical dry eye symptoms.

A metal spatula was used to collect the expressed meibum, which was generated by gentle squeezing the eyelids of the volunteers. Meibum lipids were eluted by washing the spatula thoroughly with chloroform and the lipid extracts were subjected to dry by using a miVac sample concentrator (Genevac, Ipswich, UK). The dried samples were stored at −80°C until further analysis.

Lipid Extraction

The protocol for the lipid extraction was adopted from the previous work with some modifications (34). The first 15 mm of Schirmer strips were cut into the fine pieces (∼2 mm) in the glass tubes. About 200 µL of methanol containing 50 µg/ml butylated hydroxytoluene (BHT) and 25 ng/ml myristic-d27 acid were added to the glass tube followed by 600 µL methyl tert-butyl ester (MTBE). The mixture was then incubated at 20°C for 30 min with a mixing speed of 900 rpm. About 180 µL of water was added for the phase separation. After thoroughly mixing the sample, the suspension is centrifuged for 10 min at 10°C with a speed of 2,000 g. The upper phase containing lipid was then transferred into a collection vial and dried down.

Direct Injection MS/MS^{ALL} Data Acquisition

Lipid extract was reconstituted in 100 µL methanol/chloroform (2:1, v/v) with 5 mM ammonium acetate and the sample was automatically loaded and directly delivered to the electrospray ionization (ESI) source by using the ACQUITY UPLC I-Class System (Waters Corporation, Milford, Massachusetts, USA). The running buffer was methanol/isopropanol (3:1, v/v) with 5 mM ammonium acetate and the flow rate was 30 µL/min. The MS/MS^{ALL} acquisition experiment was carried out on the SCIEX TripleTOF 5600 System (SCIEX, Framingham, Massachusetts, USA) in both the positive and negative polarities for the complete lipidome coverage. The parameter settings for ESI source included nebulizing gases (GS1) at 25, heating gases (GS2) at 10, curtain gas (CUR) at 20, temperature at 250°C, and ion spray voltage floating at 5,500 V for positive ionization and −4,500 V for negative ionization, respectively. The atmospheric pressure chemical ionization (APCI) probe and inlet were connected to an external calibrant delivery system (CDS) delivering the mass calibration solution for MS and MS/MS. The Analyst® TF 1.7 software (SCIEX, Framingham, Massachusetts, USA) was used to acquire the data from MS/MS^{ALL}. The mass range for time-of-flight MS (TOFMS) was from 200 to 1,200 m/z and the accumulation time was 300 ms, followed by 1,000 MS/MS spectra from 200.050 to 1,200.049 m/z in 1 Da steps. The accumulation time for the product ion scan was 100 ms and the collision energy was set to 50 ± 30 eV for positive polarity and −45 ± 30 eV for negative polarity, respectively. The total run time for one MS/MS^{ALL} acquisition was <2 min.

Raw Data Processing

The lipid identification and quantitation were performed by using the LipidView™ software 1.2 (SCIEX, Framingham, Massachusetts, USA) with a built-in library containing glycerolipids, phospholipids, sphingolipids, sterol lipids, and fatty acyls. A targeted search list for the wax esters was also

TABLE 1 | Characteristics of the patients receiving FS-LASIK, LASIK, or SBK surgery.

	FS-LASIK	LASIK	SBK	p-value
Patients, n	10	10	10	-
Age, years, mean ± SD	21 ± 3	25 ± 5	23 ± 5	0.311
Sex, male, n (%)	5 (50%)	5 (50%)	5 (50%)	1.00
Refractive status				
Spherical (mean ± SD)	−4.58 ± 1.65	−4.43 ± 1.39	−3.53 ± 1.80	0.311
Cylindrical (mean ± SD)	−0.80 ± 0.40	−1.25 ± 0.53	−1.03 ± 1.39	0.142
Clinical examinations				
TBUT (s)[a]	11.30 ± 5.44	10.70 ± 4.11	7.90 ± 2.96	0.186
Schirmer I (mm)	20.60 ± 11.06	15.50 ± 9.82	19.40 ± 10.65	0.534
Corneal staining	0.0 (0.0)	0.0 (0.25)	0.0 (0.25)	0.328

[a]FS-LASIK, femtosecond laser-assisted in situ keratomileusis; SBK, sub-Bowman's keratomileusis; TBUT, tear breakup time.

included. A background subtraction by using the Schirmer strip and solvent was applied to the sample.

Statistical Analysis

The results are expressed as mean ± SD. Clinical characteristics were compared among LASIK, FS-LASIK, and SBK participants by the chi-squared test, a one-way ANOVA, or the Kruskal–Wallis one-way ANOVA as appropriate. The analysis of the lipids over the course of time was conducted by using the ANOVA by R programming (35). The principal component analysis (PCA) and partial least squares-discriminant analysis (PLS-DA) were carried out by the MetaboAnalyst 4.0 (Xia Lab@McGill, Quebec, Canada) (36) and the SIMCA 13.0.3 (Umetrics, Sweden, UK).

RESULTS

Clinical Characteristics of the Patients

Table 1 shows the characteristics of the recruited patients in this study. There is no significant difference in age, gender, spherical, cylindrical, TBUT, Schirmer test, or corneal staining results among LASIK, FS-LASIK and SBK group prior to the refractive surgery. The assessment of TBUT, Schirmer test, and corneal staining for the patients receiving FS-LASIK, LASIK, or SBK surgery in week 0, week 1, week 4, and week 52 was shown in **Figure 1**. A significant difference in the corneal staining was noted in the FS-LASIK group over time. There was also a significant difference in the Schirmer test for the SBK group.

Lipid Detection by Using MS/MS^{ALL}

To demonstrate the reasonable coverage of the lipid species detected by this ultra-fast MS/MS^{ALL} method, several normal human tears and the meibum samples were evaluated. In this study, a list of the lipid species detected in the tears or meibum by using MS/MS^{ALL} technique was compared with the previous publications (3, 5, 37–41) and the result was shown in **Table 2** indicating that this technique is capable of detecting the major lipid classes. We also found 76 new lipid species by using MS/MS^{ALL} method including (O-acyl)-ω-hydroxy fatty acids (OAHFAs), wax ester (WE), triacylglycerol (TAG),

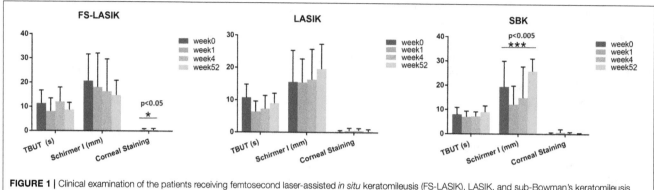

FIGURE 1 | Clinical examination of the patients receiving femtosecond laser-assisted *in situ* keratomileusis (FS-LASIK), LASIK, and sub-Bowman's keratomileusis (SBK) surgery in week 0, week 1, week 4, and week 52, respectively. *$p < 0.05$, **$p < 0.01$, ***$p < 0.005$.

TABLE 2 | Summary of the lipids detected in the tears or meibum by using MS/MS^{ALL}.

Lipid group	Lipid class[a]	Ionization polarity	Number of species		
			Reported in tears/ meibum[b]	Tears	Meibum
Fatty acyls	OAHFA	Negative	74	10	33
	WE	Positive	65	44	67
Glycerolipids	TAG	Positive	44	17	0
Glycerophospholipids	PE	Negative	45	0	1
	PI	Negative	18	0	1
	PC	Positive	51	5	0
	LPC	Positive	13	10	0
Sphingolipids	SM	Positive	23	9	0
Sterol lipids	CE	Positive	56	30	40

[a]*OAHFA, (O-acyl)-ω-hydroxy fatty acid; WE, wax ester; TAG, triacylglycerol; PE, phosphatidylethanolamine; PI, phosphatidylinositol; PC, phosphatidylcholine; LPC, lysophosphatidylcholine; SM, sphingomyelin; CE, cholesteryl ester; MS, mass spectrometry.*
[b]*Based on work by Butovich (5), Butovich et al. (37), Hancock et al. (39), Chen et al. (38, 40), Rantamäki et al. (41), and Lam et al. (3) groups.*

TABLE 3 | New lipid species detected by using MS/MS^{ALL} workflow.

Lipid group	Lipid class[a]	Ionization polarity	Number of species newly detected in tears/meibum (# = 76)
Fatty acyls	OAHFA	Negative	13
	WE	Positive	14
Glycerolipids	TAG	Positive	9
	DAG	Positive	1
Glycerophospholipids	PE	Negative	0
	PI	Negative	0
	PC	Positive/Negative	3
	PA	Negative	11
	PS	Negative	5
	PG	Negative	4
	LPC	Positive	7
Sphingolipids	SM	Positive	1
	GM3	Positive	5
Sterol lipids	CE	Positive	3

[a]*OAHFA, (O-acyl)-ω-hydroxy fatty acid; WE, wax ester; TAG, triacylglycerol; DAG, diacylglycerol; PE, phosphatidylethanolamine; PI, phosphatidylinositol; PC, phosphatidylcholine; PA, phosphatidic acid; PS, phosphatidylserine; PG, phosphatidylglycerol; LPC, lysophosphatidylcholine; SM, sphingomyelin; GM3, monosialodihexosylganglioside; CE, cholesteryl ester.*

diacylglycerol (DAG), phosphatidylcholine (PC), phosphatidic acid (PA), phosphatidylserine (PS), phosphatidylglycerol (PG), lysophosphatidylcholine (LPC), sphingomyelin (SM), monosialodihexosylganglioside (GM3), and cholesteryl ester (CE) (**Table 3**). In total, around 300 lipid species that are present in ≥75% of the samples were detected in this study.

Multivariate Analysis of the Lipidomic Profile

Multivariate analysis including PCA and PLS-DA was applied in this study to examine the pattern of the lipidomic profiles over time (week 0, week 1, week 4, and week 52). The tight cluster of the quality control (QC) samples in PCA score plot indicated the robustness of our direct injection MS/MS^{ALL} data acquisition platform (**Supplementary Figure 1**). An overview of the lipidomic profiles preoperatively and postoperatively from

the FS-LASIK, LASIK, and SBK groups was shown in **Figure 2** by using the PLS-DA score plots. There was ample overlap among week 0, week 1, and week 4 in the FS-LASIK group, implicating there was no clear difference among these three time points. In contrast, the lipidomic profiles of the LASIK and SBK groups in week 1 and 4 were distinctly separated compared to week 0. Interestingly, an overlap between week 0 and 52 was observed in the SBK group. On the other hand, the LASIK group showed a larger difference compared to the FS-LASIK group between week 0 and 52. In addition, the first two components of the PLS-DA model for the three types of surgeries can only explain ∼20% of covariance among the different time points. Individual variations and small sample size might be one reason for this covariance.

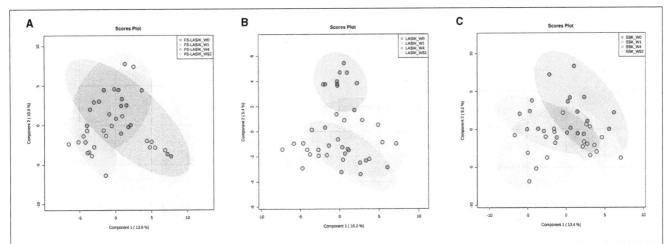

FIGURE 2 | The partial least squares-discriminant analysis (PLS-DA) score plots showing the lipid profiles in week 0, week 1, week 4, and week 52 from the FS-LASIK, LASIK, and SBK groups, respectively. **(A)** FS-LASIK; **(B)** LASIK; **(C)** SBK. Red circle: week 0; Green circle: week 1; Purple circle: week 4; and Blue circle: week 52.

The above findings revealed that in week 52, the SBK group demonstrated a similar lipidome profile compared to week 0, while the FS-LASIK and LASIK groups shifted away from week 0.

The loading plot of the PLS-DA model is complementary to the score plot and summarizes how the lipids relate to each subgroup. By examining the corresponding loading plot of the PLS-DA model (**Supplementary Figure 2**), TAG 59:3 is closely associated with the FS-LASIK and LASIK groups in week 52. In addition, GD3 27:4, a disialoganglioside with the three glycosyl groups, is closely associated with the FS-LASIK and SBK groups in week 1. Interestingly, this lipid is associated with the lipidomics profile of the LASIK group in week 4. The levels of these two lipids in the FS-LASIK, LASIK, and SBK groups preoperatively and postoperatively were shown in **Figure 3**.

Comparison of the Lipid Classes and Lipid Species Among the Refractive Surgeries

The levels of the major lipid classes found in the FS-LASIK, LASIK, and SBK groups in week 0, week 1, week 4, and week 52 were shown in **Figure 4**. In this study, the major lipid classes include OAHFAs, non-polar lipid, phospholipid, sphingolipid, and lysophospholipid. No statistical significance was found in the overall lipid classes from the FS-LASIK group. The LASIK group showed significant alteration in the phospholipid and sphingolipid over time, while the SBK group demonstrated a significant difference in the OAHFA and phospholipid.

Individual lipid species belonging to non-polar lipid, phospholipid, and lysophospholipid in week 0, week 1, week 4, and week 52 were also examined in this study and the quantitative comparison from the FS-LASIK, LASIK, and SBK groups was shown in **Figure 5**. The levels of DAG in the FS-LASIK and WE in the SBK groups were significantly changed over time (**Figures 5A,C**). Most of the difference in the phospholipids was observed in PC from the LASIK and SBK groups with statistical significance. No significant change was detected in lysophospholipid.

DISCUSSION

Tear samples have gained popularity in the investigation of disease pathogenesis (1), progression (7), and treatment response (42) due to its quick and non-invasive collection. The content of tear is a dynamic reflection of the ocular surface and, therefore, the lipidomic profiling analysis of the tear could provide information of the physiological, nutritional, and health status of an individual. A high-resolution MS/MS^{ALL} shotgun lipidomics analysis was applied here to investigate the tear samples from the patients receiving LASIK, FS-LASIK, or SBK surgery preoperatively and postoperatively.

In this study, direct injection-based MS shotgun lipidomics combined with liquid pump and autosampler from liquid chromatography (LC) with MS to perform the rapid lipidomic profiling. Comprehensive profiling and quantitation of lipid species could be achieved by this approach without the front-end chromatography separation (43). It captured every precursor ion by high-resolution MS/MS without missing any information. Therefore, MS/MS^{ALL} could obtain quantification information with no method development required for all the species in a single analysis. The use of a fully automated sampler and short run time (around 2 min for each sample) makes high-throughput sample analysis applicable for future clinical applications. Lastly, this approach allows for the detection of most lipid species reported in the literature and some new lipid species, implicating the feasibility of the direct injection based-MS shotgun lipidomics.

Dry eye after the stromal ablation surgeries is closely related to the corneal denervation. The stromal and sub-basal nerves are both severed during the flap creation, except those located at the flap hinge. As a consequence of the severed nerves, a reduction in the tear film stability and dry eye symptoms may occur (44). In this study, we only detected the significant changes in the corneal staining that results in the FS-LASIK group and the Schirmer test in the SBK group. Dry eye after the laser corneal refractive surgery is considered the most common complication with clinical signs

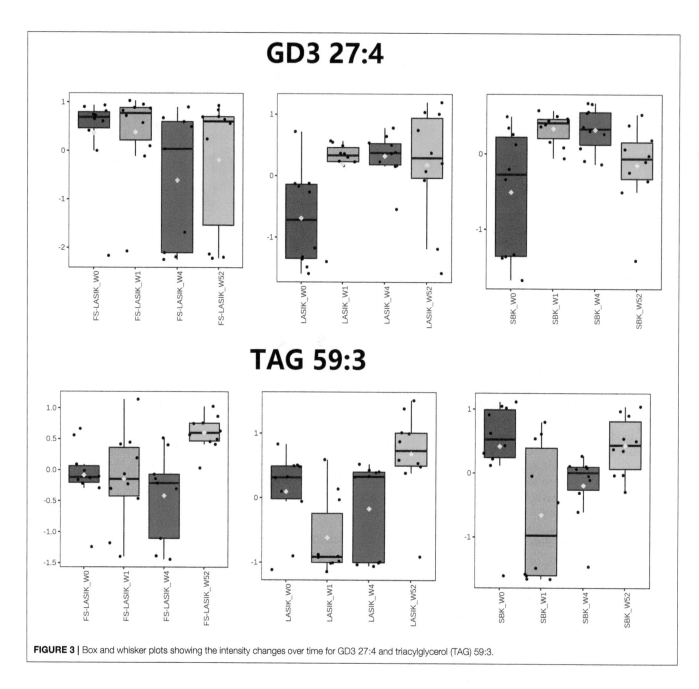

FIGURE 3 | Box and whisker plots showing the intensity changes over time for GD3 27:4 and triacylglycerol (TAG) 59:3.

such as positive vital staining of the ocular surface, decreased TBUT and Schirmer test value, reduced corneal sensitivity, and decreased functional visual acuity (45). However, previous literature is inconsistent with respect to the tear film stability after the refractive surgery. Some have reported that TBUT and Schirmer test value were diminished in both the microkeratome and femtosecond laser-created flaps (46–49), while others found no significant changes in TBUT and Schirmer test or noted a slight but insignificant increase in TBUT (50–53). There is also a discrepancy in the corneal staining that results after the refractive surgery. Some research groups observed the elevated corneal staining after 1 week of the refractive surgery and it recovered to the baseline levels after 1 month (54, 55). In contrast, Bower

et al. reported significantly higher cornea staining for up to 12 months (56). In this study, corneal staining was elevated in week 1 and almost returned to the preoperative levels in week 52 among all the three types of refractive surgery. The sub-basal nerves left in the flap will undergo a degenerative process other than a sudden vanishing after surgery (57, 58). Furthermore, Wilson suggested that the punctate epithelial erosions after surgery may be attributed to the neurotrophic epitheliopathy (50). The creation of the flap by using the microkeratome was irregular and thick compared with the femtosecond laser (59) and, thus, more sub-basal nerves were disrupted and undergoing regeneration after the microkeratome application. The total number of the sub-basal nerve was reported to be negatively

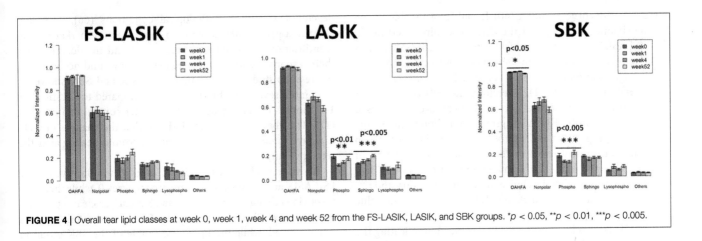

FIGURE 4 | Overall tear lipid classes at week 0, week 1, week 4, and week 52 from the FS-LASIK, LASIK, and SBK groups. $*p < 0.05$, $**p < 0.01$, $***p < 0.005$.

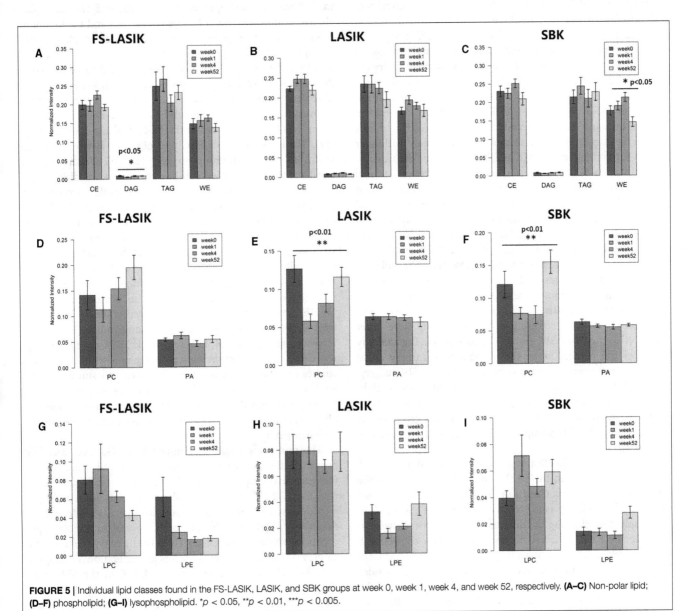

FIGURE 5 | Individual lipid classes found in the FS-LASIK, LASIK, and SBK groups at week 0, week 1, week 4, and week 52, respectively. **(A–C)** Non-polar lipid; **(D–F)** phospholipid; **(G–I)** lysophospholipid. $*p < 0.05$, $**p < 0.01$, $***p < 0.005$.

correlated with corneal staining (60). It could be a possible reason for the significant changes of the corneal staining overtime in the FS-LASIK group. Another factor to be considered for this observation is the difference in suction time. A femtosecond laser had a longer suction time (~56 s) compared to laser (~40 s) and microkeratome (~20 s) (61). Therefore, the cells of the ocular surface including conjunctival goblet cells may have an increased risk of damage in the FS-LASIK group. In addition, the energy attenuation property of the femtosecond laser during the flap creation process may result in the incomplete dissociation of the corneal flap margin. Lastly, small sample size and individual variation may also affect the clinical observations in this study.

The SBK group showed higher TBUT and Schirmer test value in week 52 compared with preoperation, while the FS-LASIK and LASIK groups had lower TBUT in week 52, implicating the recovery of the SBK group in week 52. This finding is consistent with the PLS-DA score plot results, which demonstrated a similar lipidome profile in week 52 and 0 for the SBK group. The accordance between the clinical examination and lipidomics results indicated that the occurrence and development of dry eye after the refractive surgery are closely related to the lipidome alteration. The creation of the corneal flap is the most critical element in LASIK surgery. FS-LASIK performed the corneal flap creation by using the femtosecond laser, while LASIK and SBK used a mechanical microkeratome. SBK can create a thinner corneal flap compared to LASIK and, hence, increase the available residual stromal bed, preserve corneal tissue, and reduce stromal nerve damage (62, 63). It has been reported that the femtosecond laser could directly trigger the apoptosis of the keratocytes and the corneal flap must be separated bluntly after the application of the femtosecond laser (64). This additional mechanical flap dissection might induce an extra injury for the corneal nerve or tissue cell and, thus, affect the recovery rate. The different patterns of lipidome among the three types of surgeries might also be due to the various tissue reactions caused by the laser or microkeratome application. Zhang et al. found that the corneal sub-basal nerve fibers repairing in the SBK group were faster compared to the FS-LASIK group (17). In addition, the anatomy results of the corneal nerve showed that SBK surgery could conserve more nerve branches compared to FS-LASIK surgery. This study indicates that the thinner corneal flap creation might accelerate the recovery of the lipidomic profile to preoperation after 1 year compared to the lipidome of the SBK group to the FS-LASIK and LASIK groups in week 0 and 52, respectively (**Figure 2**).

In this study, GD3 27:4 was highly expressed in week 1 compared to week 0 in the LASIK and SBK groups, while the difference between week 0 and 1 in the FS-LASIK group was not obvious. This finding was in accordance with the PLS-DA score plot results that showing the different patterns between week 0 and 1 in the FS-LASIK, LASIK, and SBK groups, respectively. Gangliosides are a family of acidic glycosphingolipids and GD3 is a minor ganglioside in most normal tissue. Gangliosides might play a role in the biological processes related to the retinal physiology and vision disorders involving the loss of photoreceptors or pathological retinal neovascularization (65). The expression of GD3 ganglioside increases during the

development and in pathological conditions (66). The 3G5 antigen, a ganglioside, is reported to be a useful marker for the identification of the corneal keratocytes and for documenting their response to stress associated with the wound healing (67). A previous study reported that FS-LASIK and SBK showed a little more severe keratocyte reaction compared to LASIK after 1–3 months of surgery due to the thinner corneal flap creation (17). The above observations indicate that the changes of GD3 27:4 levels might be associated with the wound healing after the refractive surgery.

An increased level of TAG 59:3 in week 52 was observed in the FS-LASIK and LASIK group compared to week 0, while there was no obvious change in the SBK group. Similarly, a clear separation between week 0 and 52 in the FS-LASIK and LASIK groups was observed, while the lipidomic profile of the SBK group in week 0 and 52 overlapped as shown in the PLS-DA score plot. No association was found between TAG 59:3 and the lipidomic profile of the SBK group in week 52. Chen et al. reported the upregulated TAGs in the meibum of the patients with dry eyes (68). Higher TAG has been demonstrated to be related to the corneal nerve damage in the patients with idiopathic small fiber neuropathy (69). In addition, it has been reported that the recovery rate of the corneal sub-basal nerve fibers in the SBK group was faster compared to the FS-LASIK and LASIK groups (17). The higher levels of TAG 59:3 observed at week 52 in the FS-LASIK and LASIK groups suggest that TAG 59:3 might play a negative role in the corneal sub-basal nerve fiber repairing.

(O-acyl)-ω-hydroxy fatty acid, an amphiphilic component in tears, plays a role in orienting the molecules at the lipid/water interface and facilitating the interaction between the polar and non-polar components of the tears to maintain the tear film stability (70). Lam et al. reported that the level of OAHFA was positively correlated with TBUT, reductions in ocular evaporation rate, and degree of ocular discomfort in the patients with dry eyes (3, 42). In this study, an obvious decrease of OAHFA intensity in week 52 was observed, while the intensity at week 0, week 1, and week 4 did not change much (**Figure 4C**). However, an increase of TBUT in week 52 in the SBK groups was detected (**Table 2**) showing a discrepancy with the previous studies (3, 42). The inconsistency between this study and Lam study might be due to the different cohorts of the patients. Their findings were based on a cohort of the patients with Meibomian gland dysfunction, while this study recruited only the patients with myopia.

The non-polar lipids, including CE, DAG, TAG, and WE, reside on the surface of an aqueous film and, thus, prevent the excessive evaporation of the aqueous component in the tear film. The deficiencies of the non-polar lipids may play a critical role in the evaporative dry eye (71). We did not detect any significant changes of the overall non-polar lipids preoperatively and postoperatively in the three types of refractive surgery (**Figure 4**). Only a significant alteration of DAG in the FS-LASIK group (**Figure 5A**) and WE in the SBK group (**Figure 5C**) was observed when examining the lipid species of an individual within the non-polar lipids. WEs are a major component of TFLL and recent studies have shown that WE film can effectively retard the evaporation of water (72, 73). Lam et al. reported a positive correlation between high molecular mass of the WEs with unsaturated FA chains and corneal staining, implying that the alteration of WEs level in the patients with dry eye syndrome was dependent on their molecular masses and fatty acyl chain saturation (9). However, different patterns were observed between the expression levels of WE and TBUT and Schirmer test in the SBK group. The assessment of overall levels of WE despite the fatty acyl saturations and molecular mass in this study might be a possible reason for this observation. Therefore, further evidence is required to determine the role of WE prior to and after the refractive surgery.

Phospholipids, accounting for 5–20 mol% of all the lipids in tears (74), play an essential role in the surface-active behavior of the meibum-like lipid compositions (75) and, thus, maintain the function of TFLL. This class of lipid could act as an interface between the Meibomian oil and the aqueous layer, since it lies anterior to the aqueous components. The presence of this polar phospholipid interface is critical to the spreading of the non-polar lipid film over the aqueous layer (76). Lysophospholipids were released by the hydrolysis of the phospholipid and this process was catalyzed by phospholipase A2. We have detected the significant changes in the phospholipids in the LASIK and SBK groups. Peters et al. found that TBUT was improved by the presence of the phospholipids by using a model eye (77). The trends of TBUT in the LASIK and SBK groups over time are similar compared to the PCs, which is a major component of the phospholipid. Those facts implicated that PC is responsible for the alterations of the overall phospholipids in the LASIK and SBK groups.

Our study findings must be considered in light of their limitations. First, a relatively small sample size was assessed in this study. Most clinical examination characteristics preoperatively and postoperatively did not achieve the statistical significance, most likely due to the small sample size. Furthermore, the inclusion of several time points between week 4 and 52 would provide more information for the lipidomic profile changes over time.

In this study, a rapid direct injection shotgun lipidomics workflow (<2 min/sample) was developed to examine the human tear lipidome from the patients receiving LASIK, FS-LASIK, or SBK surgery preoperatively and postoperatively (week 0, week 1, week 4, and week 52). The PLS-DA score plots revealed that the lipidome of the SBK group in week 52 was similar compared to week 0, while the FS-LASIK and LASIK groups showed distinct separation between week 0 and 52. Two lipids, TAG 59:3 and GD3 27:4, were found to be associated with the pattern changes among the FS-LASIK, LASIK, and SBK groups. LASIK showed the greatest impact on the lipidome changes over time. SBK demonstrated minimal impact among the three types of the refractive surgery after 1 year of surgery. Those findings in this longitudinal study could potentially aid in the understanding of the impact of the refractive surgery on the stability of the tear film by examining the human tear lipidome.

AUTHOR CONTRIBUTIONS

SZ and LZ designed the study and verify the underlying data. Preoperative patients were screened and surgeries were performed by SZ. YQ followed up the patients, collected tears from patients, and led the data collection. YG led the tear lipid layer analysis. YH and XL oversaw the research. YQ and YG wrote the first draft of the manuscript. All authors contributed to the article and approved the submitted version.

ACKNOWLEDGMENTS

This study is grateful for the experimental technical support provided by the Tianjin Medical University Eye Hospital and the Singapore Eye Research Institute.

REFERENCES

1. Zhou L, Beuerman RW. Tear analysis in ocular surface diseases. *Prog Retin Eye Res.* (2012) 31:527–50. doi: 10.1016/j.preteyeres.2012.06.002
2. Yazdani M, Elgstøen KBP, Rootwelt H, Shahdadfar A, Utheim ØA, Utheim TP. Tear metabolomics in dry eye disease: a review. *Int J Mol Sci.* (2019) 20:3755. doi: 10.3390/ijms20153755
3. Lam SM, Tong L, Duan X, Petznick A, Wenk MR, Shui G. Extensive characterization of human tear fluid collected using different techniques unravels the presence of novel lipid amphiphiles. *J Lipid Res.* (2014) 55:289–98. doi: 10.1194/jlr.M044826
4. Pflugfelder SC, Stern ME. Biological functions of tear film. *Exp Eye Res.* (2020) 197:108115. doi: 10.1016/j.exer.2020.108115
5. Butovich IA. On the lipid composition of human meibum and tears: comparative analysis of nonpolar lipids. *Invest Ophthalmol Vis Sci.* (2008) 49:3779–89. doi: 10.1167/iovs.08-1889
6. Cwiklik L. Tear film lipid layer: a molecular level view. *Biochim Biophys Acta.* (2016) 1858:2421–30. doi: 10.1016/j.bbamem.2016.02.020
7. Walter SD, Gronert K, McClellan AL, Levitt RC, Sarantopoulos KD, Galor A. ω-3 tear film lipids correlate with clinical measures of dry eye. *Invest Ophthalmol Vis Sci.* (2016) 57:2472–8. doi: 10.1167/iovs.16-19131
8. Sassa T, Tadaki M, Kiyonari H, Kihara A. Very long-chain tear film lipids produced by fatty acid elongase ELOVL1 prevent dry eye disease in mice. *FASEB J.* (2018) 32:2966–78. doi: 10.1096/fj.201700947R
9. Lam SM, Tong L, Reux B, Duan X, Petznick A, Yong SS, et al. Lipidomic analysis of human tear fluid reveals structure-specific lipid alterations in dry eye syndrome. *J Lipid Res.* (2014) 55:299–306. doi: 10.1194/jlr.P041780
10. Cicalini I, Rossi C, Pieragostino D, Agnifili L, Mastropasqua L, Di Ioia M, et al. Integrated lipidomics and metabolomics analysis of tears in multiple sclerosis: an insight into diagnostic potential of lacrimal fluid. *Int J Mol Sci.* (2019) 20:1265. doi: 10.3390/ijms20061265
11. Wen D, McAlinden C, Flitcroft I, Tu R, Wang Q, Alió J, et al. Postoperative efficacy, predictability, safety, and visual quality of laser corneal refractive surgery: a network meta-analysis. *Am J Ophthalmol.* (2017) 178:65–78. doi: 10.1016/j.ajo.2017.03.013
12. Althomali TA. Comparison of microkeratome assisted sub-Bowman keratomileusis with photorefractive keratectomy. *Saudi J Ophthalmol.* (2017) 31:19–24. doi: 10.1016/j.sjopt.2017.01.004

13. Shortt AJ, Bunce C, Allan BDS. Evidence for superior efficacy and safety of LASIK over photorefractive keratectomy for correction of myopia. *Ophthalmology*. (2006) 113:1897–908. doi: 10.1016/j.ophtha.2006.08.013

14. Xu Z, Shen M, Hu L, Zhuang X, Peng M, Hu D, et al. The impact of flap creation methods for Sub-Bowman's Keratomileusis (SBK) on the central thickness of bowman's layer. *PLoS ONE*. (2015) 10:e0124996. doi: 10.1371/journal.pone.0124996

15. Tatar MG, Kantarci FA, Yildirim A, UsluH, Colak HN, Goker H, et al. Risk factors in post-LASIK corneal ectasia. *J Ophthalmol*. (2014) 2014:204191. doi: 10.1155/2014/204191

16. Harissi-Dagher M, Frimmel SAF, Melki S. High myopia as a risk factor for post-LASIK ectasia: a case report. *Digit J Ophthalmol*. (2009) 15:9–13. doi: 10.5693/djo.01.2009.003

17. Zhang F, Deng S, Guo N, Wang M, Sun X. Confocal comparison of corneal nerve regeneration and keratocyte reaction between FS-LASIK, OUP-SBK, and conventional LASIK. *Invest Ophthalmol Vis Sci*. (2012) 53:5536–44. doi: 10.1167/iovs.11-8786

18. Durrie DS, Slade SG, Marshall J. Wavefront-guided excimer laser ablation using photorefractive keratectomy and sub-Bowman's keratomileusis: a contralateral eye study. *J Refract Surg*. (2008) 24:S77–84. doi: 10.3928/1081597X-20080101-14

19. Slade SG. Thin-flap laser-assisted *in situ* keratomileusis. *Curr Opin Ophthalmol*. (2008) 19:325–9. doi: 10.1097/ICU.0b013e328302cc77

20. Vaddavalli PK, Yoo SH. Femtosecond laser *in-situ* keratomileusis flap configurations. *Curr Opin Ophthalmol*. (2011) 22:245–50. doi: 10.1097/ICU.0b013e3283479ebd

21. Yuen LH, Chan WK, Koh J, Mehta JS, Tan DT. A 10-year prospective audit of LASIK outcomes for myopia in 37,932 eyes at a single institution in Asia. *Ophthalmology*. (2010) 117:1236–44. doi: 10.1016/j.ophtha.2009.10.042

22. Shtein RM. Post-LASIK dry eye. *Expert Rev Ophthalmol*. (2011) 6:575–82. doi: 10.1586/eop.11.56

23. De Paiva CS, Chen Z, Koch DD, Hamill MB, Manuel FK, Hassan SS, et al. The incidence and risk factors for developing dry eye after myopic LASIK. *Am J Ophthalmol*. (2006) 141:438–45. doi: 10.1016/j.ajo.2005.10.006

24. Bron AJ, de Paiva CS, Chauhan SK, Bonini S, Gabison EE, Jain S, et al. TFOS DEWS II pathophysiology report. *Ocul Surf*. (2017) 15:438–510. doi: 10.1016/j.jtos.2017.05.011

25. Yu C, Li Y, Wang Z, Jiang Y, Jin Y. Comparison of corneal nerve regeneration and dry eye condition after conventional LASIK and femtosecond-assisted LASIK. *Zhonghua Yan Ke Za Zhi*. (2015) 51:188–92. doi: 10.3760/cma.j.issn.0412-4081.2015.03.008

26. Patel S, Perez-Santonja JJ, Alio JL, Murphy PJ. Corneal sensitivity and some properties of the tear film after laser *in situ* keratomileusis. *J Refract Surg*. (2001) 17:17–24. doi: 10.3928/1081-597X-2001 0101-02

27. Xia L-K, Yu J, Chai G-R, Wang D, Li Y. Comparison of the femtosecond laser and mechanical microkeratome for flap cutting in LASIK. *Int J Ophthalmol*. (2015) 8:784–90. doi: 10.3980/j.issn.2222-3959.2015.04.25

28. Sun C-C, Chang C-K, Ma DH-K, Lin Y-F, Chen K-J, Sun M-H, et al. Dry eye after LASIK with a femtosecond laser or a mechanical microkeratome. *Optom Vis Sci*. (2013) 90:1048–56. doi: 10.1097/OPX.0b013e31829d9905

29. Simons B, Kauhanen D, Sylvänne T, Tarasov K, Duchoslav E, Ekroos K. Shotgun lipidomics by sequential precursor ion fragmentation on a hybrid quadrupole time-of-flight mass spectrometer. *Metabolites*. (2012) 2:195–213. doi: 10.3390/metabo2010195

30. Rockwell HE, Gao F, Chen EY, McDaniel J, Sarangarajan R, Narain NR, et al. Dynamic assessment of functional lipidomic analysis in human urine. *Lipids*. (2016) 51:875–86. doi: 10.1007/s11745-016-4142-0

31. Gao F, McDaniel J, Chen EY, Rockwell H, Lynes MD, Tseng YH, et al. Monoacylglycerol analysis using MS/MSALL quadruple time of flight mass spectrometry. *Metabolites*. (2016) 6:25. doi: 10.3390/metabo 6030025

32. Gao F, McDaniel J, Chen EY, Rockwell HE, Nguyen C, Lynes MD, et al. Adapted MS/MSALL shotgun lipidomics approach for analysis of cardiolipin molecular species. *Lipids*. (2018) 53:133–42. doi: 10.1002/lipd. 12004

33. Bron AJ, Evans VE, Smith JA. Grading of corneal and conjunctival staining in the context of other dry eye tests. *Cornea*. (2003) 22:640–50. doi: 10.1097/00003226-200310000-00008

34. Matyash V, Liebisch G, Kurzchalia TV, Shevchenko A, Schwudke D. Lipid extraction by methyl- tert -butyl ether for high-throughput lipidomics. *J Lipid Res*. (2008) 49:1137–46. doi: 10.1194/jlr.D700041-JLR200

35. R Core Team. *A Language and Environment for Statistical Computing*. Vienna: R Foundation for Statistical Computing (2018). Available online at: https:// www.r-project.org (accessed September 26, 2021).

36. Chong J, Soufan O, Caraus I, Xia J, Li C, Wishart DS, et al. MetaboAnalyst 40: towards more transparent and integrative metabolomics analysis. *Nucleic Acids Res*. (2018) 46:W486–94. doi: 10.1093/nar/gky310

37. Butovich IA, Uchiyama E, Di Pascuale MA, McCulley JP. Liquid chromatography-mass spectrometric analysis of lipids present in human meibomian gland secretions. *Lipids*. (2007) 42:765–76. doi: 10.1007/s11745-007-3080-2

38. Chen J, Green-Church KB, Nichols KK. Shotgun lipidomic analysis of human meibomian gland secretions with electrospray ionization tandem mass spectrometry. *Invest Ophthalmol Vis Sci*. (2010) 51:6220–31. doi: 10.1167/iovs.10-5687

39. Hancock SE, Ailuri R, Marshall DL, Brown SHJ, Saville JT, Narreddula VR, et al. Mass spectrometry-directed structure elucidation and total synthesis of ultra-long chain (O-acyl)-ω-hydroxy fatty acids. *J Lipid Res*. (2018) 59:1510–8. doi: 10.1194/jlr.M086702

40. Chen J, Green KB, Nichols KK. Quantitative profiling of major neutral lipid classes in human meibum by direct infusion electrospray ionization mass spectrometry. *Investi Ophthalmol Vis Sci*. (2013) 54:5730–53. doi: 10.1167/iovs.12-10317

41. Rantamäki AH, Seppänen-Laakso T, Oresic M, Jauhiainen M, Holopainen JM. Human tear fluid lipidome: from composition to function. *PLoS ONE*. (2011) 6:1–7. doi: 10.1371/journal.pone.0019553

42. Lam SM, Tong L, Duan X, Acharya UR, Tan JH, Petznick A, et al. Longitudinal changes in tear fluid lipidome brought about by eyelid-warming treatment in a cohort of meibomian gland dysfunction. *J Lipid Res*. (2014) 55:1959–69. doi: 10.1194/jlr.P051185

43. Gao F, McDaniel J, Chen EY, Rockwell HE, Drolet J, Vishnudas VK, et al. Dynamic and temporal assessment of human dried blood spot MS/MSALL shotgun lipidomics analysis. *Nutr Metab*. (2017) 14:1–12. doi: 10.1186/s12986-017-0182-6

44. Ang RT, Dartt DA, Tsubota K. Dry eye after refractive surgery. *Curr Opin Ophthalmol*. (2001) 12:318–22. doi: 10.1097/00055735-200108000-00013

45. Toda I. Dry eye after LASIK. *Invest Ophthalmol Vis Sci*. (2018) 59:DES109–115. doi: 10.1167/iovs.17-23538

46. Kalyvianaki MI, Katsanevaki VJ, Kavroulaki DS, Kounis GA, Detorakis ET, Pallikaris IG. Comparison of corneal sensitivity and tear function following Epi-LASIK or laser *in situ* keratomileusis for myopia. *Am J Ophthalmol*. (2006) 142:669–71. doi: 10.1016/j.ajo.2006.04.054

47. Barequet IS, Hirsh A, Levinger S. Effect of thin femtosecond LASIK flaps on corneal sensitivity and tear function. *J Refract Surg*. (2008) 24:897–902. doi: 10.3928/1081597X-20081101-08

48. Tanaka M, Takano Y, Dogru M, Toda I, Asano-Kato N, Komai-Hori Y, et al. Effect of preoperative tear function on early functional visual acuity after laser *in situ* keratomileusis. *J Cataract Refract Surg*. (2004) 30:2311–5. doi: 10.1016/j.jcrs.2004.02.086

49. Goto T, Zheng X, Klyce SD, Kataoka H, Uno T, Yamaguchi M, et al. Evaluation of the tear film stability after laser *in situ* keratomileusis using the tear film stability analysis system. *Am J Ophthalmol*. (2004) 137:116–20. doi: 10.1016/S0002-9394(03)00901-2

50. Wilson SE. Laser *in situ* keratomileusis–induced (presumed) neurotrophic epitheliopathy. *Ophthalmology*. (2001) 108:1082–7. doi: 10.1016/S0161-6420(01)00587-5

51. Donnenfeld ED, Solomon K, Perry HD, Doshi SJ, Ehrenhaus M, Solomon R, et al. The effect of hinge position on corneal sensation and dry eye after LASIK. *Ophthalmology*. (2003) 110:1023–30. doi: 10.1016/S0161-6420(03) 00100-3

52. Foo SK, Kaur S, Abd Manan F, Low AJ. The changes of tear status after conventional and wavefront-guided intraLASIK. *Malaysian J Med Sci*. (2011) 18:32–9. Available online at: https://www.ncbi.nlm.nih.gov/pmc/ articles/PMC3216215/

53. Petznick A, Chew A, Hall RC, Chan CML, Rosman M, Tan D, et al. Comparison of corneal sensitivity, tear function and corneal staining

following laser *in situ* keratomileusis with two femtosecond laser platforms. *Clin Ophthalmol.* (2013) 7:591–8. doi: 10.2147/OPTH.S42266

54. Zhang C, Ding H, He M, Liu L, Liu L, Li G, et al. Comparison of early changes in ocular surface and inflammatory mediators between femtosecond lenticule extraction and small-incision lenticule extraction. *PLoS ONE.* (2016) 11:e0149503. doi: 10.1371/journal.pone.0149503

55. Mian SI, Shtein RM, Nelson A, Musch DC. Effect of hinge position on corneal sensation and dry eye after laser *in situ* keratomileusis using a femtosecond laser. *J Cataract Refract Surg.* (2007) 33:1190–4. doi: 10.1016/j.jcrs.2007.03.031

56. Bower KS, Sia RK, Ryan DS, Mines MJ, Dartt DA. Chronic dry eye in photorefractive keratectomy and laser *in situ* keratomileusis: manifestations, incidence, and predictive factors. *J Cataract Refract Surg.* (2015) 41:2624–34. doi: 10.1016/j.jcrs.2015.06.037

57. Linna TU, Vesaluoma MH, Pérez-Santonja JJ, Petroll WM, Alió JL, Tervo TMT. Effect of myopic LASIK on corneal sensitivity and morphology of subbasal nerves. *Invest Ophthalmol Vis Sci.* (2000) 41:393–7. Available online at: https://iovs.arvojournals.org/article.aspx?articleid=2199874

58. Nettune GR, Pflugfelder SC. Post-LASIK tear dysfunction and dysesthesia. *Ocul Surf.* (2010) 8:135–45. doi: 10.1016/S1542-0124(12)70224-0

59. Zhou Y, Zhang J, Tian L, Zhai C. Comparison of the Ziemer FEMTO LDV femtosecond laser and Moria M2 mechanical microkeratome. *J Refract Surg.* (2012) 28:189–94. doi: 10.3928/1081597X-20120208-01

60. Latifi G, Afshan AB, Beheshtnejad AH, Zarei-Ghanavati M, Mohammadi N, Ghaffari R, et al. Changes in corneal subbasal nerves after punctal occlusion in dry eye disease. *Curr Eye Res.* (2020) 46:777–83. doi: 10.1080/02713683.2020.1833349

61. Salomão MQ, Ambrósio Jr R, Wilson SE. Dry eye associated with laser *in situ* keratomileusis: mechanical microkeratome vs. femtosecond laser. *J Cataract Refract Surg.* (2009) 35:1756–60. doi: 10.1016/j.jcrs.2009.05.032

62. Sun Y, Deng Y-P, Wang L, Huang Y-Z, Qiu L-M. Comparisons of morphologic characteristics between thin-flap LASIK and SBK. *Int J Ophthalmol.* (2012) 5:338–42. doi: 10.3980/j.issn.2222-3959.2012.03.17

63. Dawson DG, Grossniklaus HE, Edelhauser HF, McCarey BE. Biomechanical and wound healing characteristics of corneas after excimer laser keratorefractive surgery. *J Refract Surg.* (2008) 24:S90–6. doi: 10.3928/1081597X-20080101-16

64. Lee BH, McLaren JW, Erie JC, Hodge DO, Bourne WM. Reinnervation in the cornea after LASIK. *Invest Ophthalmol Vis Sci.* (2002) 43:3660–4. Available online at: https://iovs.arvojournals.org/article.aspx?articleid=2162391

65. Lydic TA, Busik J V, Reid GE. A monophasic extraction strategy for the simultaneous lipidome analysis of polar and non-polar retina lipids. *J Lipid Res.* (2014) 55:1797–809. doi: 10.1194/jlr.D050302

66. Malisan F, Testi R. GD3 ganglioside and apoptosis. *Biochim Biophys Acta.* (2002) 1585:179–87. doi: 10.1016/S1388-1981(02)00339-6

67. Stramer BM, Kwok MGK, Farthing-Nayak PJ, Jung J-C, Fini ME, Nayak RC. Monoclonal antibody (3G5)–defined ganglioside: cell surface marker of corneal keratocytes. *Invest Ophthalmol Vis Sci.* (2004) 45:807–12. doi: 10.1167/iovs.03-0256

68. Chen J, Keirsey J, Basso K, Nichols KK. Differentially expressed non-polar lipids in human meibum of dry eye disease. *Invest Ophthalmol Vis Sci.* (2015) 56:342. Available online at: https://iovs.arvojournals.org/article.aspx?articleid=2333286

69. Tavakoli M, Marshall A, Pitceathly R, Fadavi H, Gow D, Roberts ME, et al. Corneal confocal microscopy: a novel means to detect nerve fibre damage in idiopathic small fibre neuropathy. *Exp Neurol.* (2010) 223:245–50. doi: 10.1016/j.expneurol.2009.08.033

70. Butovich IA. Tear film lipids. *Exp Eye Res.* (2013) 117:4–27. doi: 10.1016/j.exer.2013.05.010

71. Bruna M, Breward CJW. The influence of non-polar lipids on tear film dynamics. *J Fluid Mech.* (2014) 746:565–605. doi: 10.1017/jfm.2014.106

72. Rantamäki AH, Javanainen M, Vattulainen I, Holopainen JM. Do lipids retard the evaporation of the tear fluid? *Invest Ophthalmol Vis Sci.* (2012) 53:6442–7. doi: 10.1167/iovs.12-10487

73. Rantamäki AH, Wiedmer SK, Holopainen JM. Melting points—the key to the anti-evaporative effect of the tear film wax esters. *Invest Ophthalmol Vis Sci.* (2013) 54:5211–7. doi: 10.1167/iovs.13-12408

74. Millar TJ, Schuett BS. The real reason for having a meibomian lipid layer covering the outer surface of the tear film - a review. *Exp Eye Res.* (2015) 137:125–38. doi: 10.1016/j.exer.2015.05.002

75. Rantamäki AH, Holopainen JM. The effect of phospholipids on tear film lipid layer surface activity. *Invest Ophthalmol Vis Sci.* (2017) 58:149–54. doi: 10.1167/iovs.16-20468

76. Ham BM, Cole RB, Jacob JT. Identification and comparison of the polar phospholipids in normal and dry eye rabbit tears by MALDI-TOF mass spectrometry. *Invest Ophthalmol Vis Sci.* (2006) 47:3330–8. doi: 10.1167/iovs.05-0756

77. Peters K, Millar TJ. The role of different phospholipids on tear break-up time using a model eye. *Curr Eye Res.* (2002) 25:55–60. doi: 10.1076/ceyr.25.1.55.9965

22

Magnesium and its Role in Primary Open Angle Glaucoma: A Novel Therapeutic

Mirna Elghobashy[1†], Hannah C. Lamont[1,2†], Alexander Morelli-Batters[1], Imran Masood[1] and Lisa J. Hill[1]*

[1] School of Biomedical Sciences, Institute of Clinical Sciences, University of Birmingham, Birmingham, United Kingdom,
[2] School of Chemical Engineering, Healthcare Technologies Institute, University of Birmingham, Birmingham, United Kingdom

Correspondence:
Lisa J. Hill
l.j.hill@bham.ac.uk

[†]*These authors have contributed equally to this work and share first authorship*

Glaucoma is the leading cause of irreversible blindness globally, with Primary open angle glaucoma (POAG) being the commonest subtype. POAG is characterized by an increase in intraocular pressure (IOP), leading to optic nerve damage and subsequent visual field defects. Despite the clinical burden this disease poses, current therapies aim to reduce IOP rather than targeting the underling pathogenesis. Although the pathogenesis of POAG is complex, the culprit for this increase in IOP resides in the aqueous humour (AH) outflow pathway; the trabecular meshwork (TM) and Schlemm's canal. Dysfunction in these tissues is due to inherent mitochondrial dysfunction, calcium influx sensitivity, increase in reactive oxygen species (ROS) production, TGFβ-2 induction, leading to a sustained inflammatory response. Magnesium is the second most common intracellular cation, and is a major co-factor in over 300 reactions, being highly conserved within energy-dependent organelles such as the mitochondria. Magnesium deficiency has been observed in POAG and is linked to inflammatory and fibrotic responses, as well as increased oxidative stress (OS). Magnesium supplementation been shown to reduce cellular ROS, alleviate mitochondrial dysregulation and has further antifibrotic and anti-inflammatory properties within ocular tissues, and other soft tissues prone to fibrosis, suggesting that magnesium can improve visual fields in patients with POAG. The link between magnesium deficiency and glaucoma pathogenesis as well as the potential role of magnesium supplementation in the management of patients with POAG will be explored within this review.

Keywords: glaucoma, magnesium, oxidative stress, trabecular meshwork, retinal ganglion cells

INTRODUCTION

Glaucoma is the most common cause of irreversible blindness globally, affecting over 70 million people worldwide (1). This disease encompasses many conditions which contributes to progressive optic neuropathy, resulting from progressive retinal ganglion cell (RGC) degeneration and optic disc cupping (2). The commonest subtypes of glaucoma are; primary open angle glaucoma (POAG) and acute angle closure glaucoma (AACG), with POAG accounting for 70% of worldwide total glaucoma cases (3). Currently, the only modifiable risk factor, elevated intraocular pressure (IOP), contributes to this optic neuropathy and subsequent visual loss (4). The culprit for this increase in IOP lies within the anterior chamber of the eye, where aqueous humor (AH) outflow is regulated by the trabecular meshwork tissue (TM) (5). In POAG, the induction of a fibrotic response occurs within the TM, creating heightened resistance to fluid outflow, subsequently elevating IOP beyond normal levels (6). Furthermore, due to POAG having a multifactorial nature, vascular dysregulation and endothelial dysfunction within the Schlemm's canal (SC), further contribute to the induction of a fibrotic response by increasing extracellular matrix (ECM) deposition, oxidative stress (OS), and apoptosis within the within the TM (7). With current therapies focusing on alleviating symptoms, such as lowering IOP, rather than targeting the underlying causes that contribute towards the pathogenesis of POAG (8), this has led to POAG bearing a high prevalence and posing a significant clinical burden (9). Therefore, it is important to consider alternative therapeutics that could be utilized to treat glaucoma.

Previous research has indicated that magnesium has the potential to be a promising therapeutic for fibrotic diseases due to its antioxidant and anti-fibrotic effects in the body within different organs (10, 11). In ocular tissues, magnesium is present mainly in the cornea, lens, retina and in the anterior chamber (12), with deficiency being linked to ionic and antioxidant imbalances (13). Furthermore, significant magnesium deficiency has been identified in patients with glaucoma (14, 15), with magnesium supplementation having been shown to improve the visual field of glaucoma patients (16).

This review will explore the link between POAG pathogenesis, and the role that magnesium could potentially play in the management of POAG focusing on its mechanism of action in mediating cellular homeostasis. As it is widely regarded that POAG originates in the anterior chamber of the eye, emphasis is placed on TM and vascular dysfunction occurring during AH outflow.

GLAUCOMA PATHOPHYSIOLOGY

Several mechanisms have been proposed for the pathogenesis of POAG, with TM fibrosis leading to impaired drainage of AH being widely regarded as a large contributor to this multi-faceted disease (17). Studies have identified a link between elevated TGF-β2 levels in the AH and extracellular matrix (ECM) of patients with POAG (18–21). It has been established that TGF-β isoforms regulate TM cellular fate due to their mesenchymal nature (22–24), with a heightened presence of TGF-β2 stimulating a myofibroblast phenotype, increasing contractile features, pro-fibrotic protein expression (α-SMA, fibronectin) and ECM deposition (25, 26). Overall, these factors contribute to a loss of cell-cell contact, increased stiffness, and fibrosis of the TM, leading to AH outflow resistance and increased IOP (26).

Being highly metabolizing cells, TM cells are also sensitive to overproduction of reactive oxidative species (ROS) (27). Increased production of ROS can be generated from cells within the anterior chamber of the eye from several organelles,

such as; the mitochondria, endoplasmic reticulum, and cytosol, in response to exogenous stress such as UV damage, further leading to protein and cellular damage (28, 29). Similar events occur within the TM, with an imbalance in ROS production causing mitochondrial dysfunction, ECM accumulation, cytoskeletal changes and induction of apoptosis (28). This has been reflected in POAG patients, with a significant reduction in TM cellularity compared to age matched controls (30). Prolonged ROS production in POAG is also associated with inflammation and inflammatory stress to the TM (31). There is a release of proinflammatory cytokines such as IL-1β *via* the activation of the nuclear factor kappa b (NF-κB) pathway (32). NF-κB is a transcription factor which promotes genes related to inflammation to produce an inflammatory response (33). Chronic inflammation is pathognomonic of ocular hypertension, and the development of POAG (32, 34). Overall, these processes contribute to increased outflow resistance and thus increased IOP (35, 36).

MAGNESIUM AND ITS ROLE WITHIN THE EYE

Magnesium (Mg^{2+}) is the fourth most abundant cation in the body, acting as a co-factor in over 300 enzymatic reactions (37), particularly those required in ATP-generating reactions and regulating mitochondrial functions (13, 38). Intracellular magnesium concentrations remain virtually unaltered due to tight intracellular regulation, despite significant gradients across cell membranes and being the second most abundant intracellular cation. This gives appreciation into how tightly regulated magnesium intracellular stores are, with the mitochondria, endoplasmic reticulum and nucleus holding the largest stores of magnesium, with around 15-18mM magnesium present in each organelle (39–41). While it has been noted in studies that there are several conserved magnesium co-transport mechanisms across cell membranes, there are also compensatory mechanisms that allow the cell to effectively buffer any loss or overaccumulation of this cation (41, 42). With magnesium having a high impact on energy metabolism, inevitably effecting cellular responses (13), it is also considered a potent antagonist against the stimulatory effects of calcium, an important cation associated with the implications of POAG (13, 43). Thus, what should be considered in future studies is how magnesium can directly and indirectly effect POAG patients and what mechanism(s) of action will be affected for maintaining homeostasis and normal cellular functions.

Within the eye, magnesium is present in high concentrations within the cornea, lens, retina and the anterior chamber (12). In the cornea, magnesium is shown to be essential in preventing dry eye disease and infection (44) and acts as a neuroprotective and anti-apoptotic agent by reducing nitric oxide synthase and the induction of calcium channels in RGCs (15, 45, 46). Furthermore, as TM cells are highly metabolic and can possess a smooth muscle phenotype, the cells express several known transporters that are known to mediate the tissues contractility by enhancing intracellular calcium stores, hence mediating fluid outflow (47, 48). Thus, with magnesium being essential in cellular metabolism, and regulation of intracellular anionic balance, it is likely to be vital for the maintenance of ocular structural and cellular integrity (15). This is further evident in the case of magnesium concentrations in the AH of healthy patients being estimated at 6.7mg/L, compared to patients with POAG, at around 3mg/L (14). While current studies into magnesium levels in POAG patients is limited, it is worth highlighting that a potential relationship could be correlated from the existing literature. The current evidence emphasizes the importance of physiological magnesium levels for normal ocular tissue function, further suggesting that research into how magnesium can directly and indirectly manage POAG through various mechanisms of action could be explored for therapeutic potential.

This review will discuss several roles in which magnesium deficiency is linked to POAG pathogenesis (**Figure 1**), with major outcomes of this deficiency consisting of mitochondrial dysfunction, inflammatory stress and endothelial dysfunction.

ROLE OF MAGNESIUM IN OXIDATIVE STRESS AND OCULAR PATHOLOGIES

Oxidative stress (OS) is defined as an imbalance of oxidants to antioxidants, leading to lipid peroxidation and protein damage, further perpetuating an ongoing cycle of OS, causing aberrant ECM deposition, cytoskeletal changes within TM cell, and eventual apoptosis (49). The majority of intracellular ROS are generated in the mitochondria, as a by-product of cellular respiration (50), with the accumulation of intracellular ROS

production being influenced by mitochondrial functionality. Likewise, magnesium deficiency can also affect mitochondrial function due to being a major co-factor necessary in energy production (13). This holds true within the eye, as OS is associated with the pathogenesis of several ocular pathologies; cataracts, retinopathies, age-related macular degeneration and glaucoma (27). Specifically, within POAG, it is widely regarded that mitochondrial dysfunction and genetic abnormalities are associated with complex I of the electron transport chain and are common attributes found within patients (51, 52). It is hypothesized that it is this defect in the electron transport chain that contributes to the progressive loss of TM cells in POAG, abnormal ATP production, increased ROS production and heightened vulnerability to calcium ion stress (52, 53). It has previously proposed that the introduction of antioxidants may help subside these effects and decrease IOP (54, 55).

Specifically, magnesium deficiency disrupts the electron transport chain within the mitochondria by facilitating the uncoupling of oxidative phosphorylation leading to electron loss (56, 57). As previously mentioned, magnesium is vital with regards to ATP and its production. *In vitro* studies have identified that many magnesium-dependent enzymes and dehydrogenases are necessary in the mitochondria to maintain cellular homeostasis, with computer simulation models of the Krebs cycle showing that mitochondrial magnesium levels are essential for the regulation of these enzymes and the Krebs cycle itself (13, 58, 59), indicating that magnesium is a vital regulator of mitochondrial homeostasis and, by extension, metabolic status. The known magnesium deficiency in patients with POAG could be contributing to mitochondrial dysfunction within various ocular cell types, giving rise to ROS, calcium

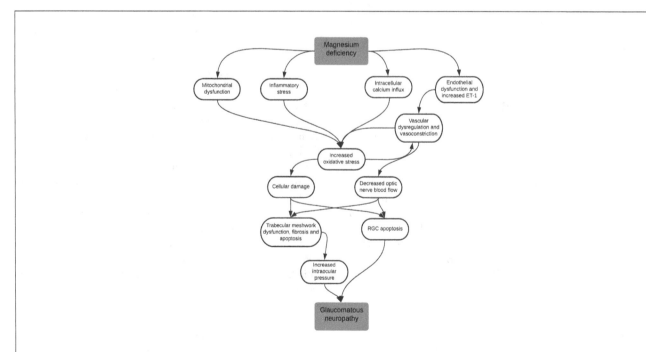

FIGURE 1 | Flowchart depicting the role of magnesium deficiency in the pathogenesis of glaucomatous neuropathy. It is important to note that all pathways lead to increased oxidative stress, a major driver of glaucomatous neuropathy. Oxidative stress also leads to a cycle of increased vascular dysregulation and vasoconstriction which, in turn, causes further oxidative stress to cells.

ion sensitivity and subsequent tissue impairment (14, 58). Current evidence illustrates the importance of conserving magnesium in the mitochondria, with deficiency indirectly influencing OS through the induction of stress responses by effecting the calcium (Ca^{2+}) intracellular homeostasis (60). It has been observed that magnesium deficiency leads to increased intracellular calcium influx and thus a decreased ratio of magnesium to calcium (11). Increased intracellular calcium causes a myriad of cellular imbalances, inducing intracellular swelling and apoptosis, with this dysfunction observed in POAG TM cells (43, 61). This is also important when considering the RGC loss observed in glaucoma, leading to visual defects (61, 62).

While magnesium deficiency has been associated with POAG, a direct link between magnesium deficiency and increased OS in the eyes has not yet been fully elucidated (14). The impact of magnesium related modulation of OS has been explored through the use of rodent models; magnesium deficient rats are more susceptible to oxidative damage than control rats and have higher levels of circulating oxidized lipoproteins (63). Furthermore, in a rodent glaucoma model, magnesium acetyltaurate has been shown to reduce OS and reduce RGC apoptosis (64). While these studies have created a foundation in forming a link between the presence of magnesium of OS levels, further understanding its therapeutic potential in minimizing ROS production and overall cellular health in the TM samples of patients still remains to be elucidated.

MAGNESIUM AND VASCULAR REGULATION

Several studies have suggested a link between magnesium deficiency and vascular dysfunction (65–67), with general dysfunction of the microvascular endothelium being identified as a contributing factor of glaucomatous optic neuropathy (66). Studies have shown that blood flow is reduced in several ocular tissues in patients with glaucoma including the retina, optic nerve and choroid due to systematic hypertension (68, 69). This can further cause ocular endothelial damage and ocular hypertension leading to dysfunctional TM and hence increase IOP in POAG (70–72).

POAG has been associated with primary vascular dysregulation, wherein ocular and retinal vascular tissue responds abnormally to stimuli, due to low blood pressure and disturbed vascular homeostasis, causing abnormal AH outflow (73). Moreover, decreased available blood flow leads to an hypoxia-induced increase in OS within these tissues (74). These scenarios have shown to cause a marked increase in endothelin-1 (ET-1), a potent vasoconstrictor dependent on voltage-gated calcium channels to exert its actions. This can be potentially modulated by magnesium, which has been observed to attenuate such events that may arise from aberrant calcium homeostasis (75–77). It has also been theorized that ET-1 acts on the distal vascular post-TM and SC to increase resistance (78, 79), as activation of ET-1 receptors in the TM induces tissue contraction, increasing fluid outflow resistance, and raises IOP. Magnesium has been identified in ex vivo studies as a substance which reduces the vasoconstrictive effect of ET-1 and

inhibiting ET-1 vasoconstriction in porcine ciliary arteries (80, 81). Although the evidence for the use of magnesium as a preventative vasorelaxant is largely theoretical when discussing ocular vasculature, there is a significant correlation between magnesium's role as a physiological calcium channel blocker and its action in ET-1 inhibition and has been shown to be beneficial for chronic hypertension (15, 77, 80).

Magnesium deficiency is also associated with endothelial dysfunction (82). Normally, the endothelium of ocular blood vessels produces signaling molecules which control the balance between thrombin and fibrinolysis as well as the synthesis of proinflammatory cytokines and reduction of nitric oxide (11, 83, 84). It has been suggested that paracrine signaling between the TM and SC regulates vascular tone and is similar to that found in vascular smooth muscle endothelium, in the presence of ET-1 and nitric oxide (85). Moreover, in magnesium deficiency, it has been shown there is increased intracellular nitric oxide and peroxynitrite production, giving rise to an increased levels of ROS (86, 87). A study assessing the use of magnesium on glaucoma patients as a 'physiological calcium channel blocker', found that supplementation led to significant improvements in peripheral circulation and visual fields (16). Although further studies have not been conducted assessing the validity of this finding, it adds weight to the argument that supplementation with magnesium could induce vasodilation and reduce the vasoconstrictor effects of ROS in glaucoma patients (88).

ROLE OF MAGNESIUM IN INFLAMMATION AND FIBROSIS

Magnesium deficiency has been linked with inflammation in the context of chronic disease and it has been theorized that the development of POAG, as TM dysfunction and ocular hypertension is mediated by chronic low-level inflammation (32, 34, 89). It has been suggested that there is a release of proinflammatory cytokines such as IL-1β via the activation of the NF-κB pathway in patients with POAG (32, 90). NF-κB being a primary transcription factor which promotes genes related to inflammation, has an intimate cross-talk with the TGFβ-2 signaling pathway (33, 91, 92). Studies have identified elevated TGF-β2 levels in the AH of POAG patients, with a heightened presence associated with the induction of ROS, and overproduction of profibrotic proteins in TM cells (18, 91, 93, 94). Furthermore, TGF-β2 has been shown to contribute to the myofibroblastic properties and increased ECM deposition seen in glaucomatous TM (95). Although there is no evidence linking the specific role of magnesium in TM fibrosis, it may have the potential to reduce fibrosis indirectly in the TM through alternative pathways previously discussed. As magnesium is a primary mediator in metabolic processes and mitochondrial functionality, the effects this cation has on ROS production, could be beneficial in reducing TGFβ-2 production, as it has been previously shown that the presence of mitochondrial targeted antioxidants has the potential to attenuate TGFβ-2 in TM cells (96). This may in turn, have an indirect, and advantageous effect on the inflammatory response that is induced through the NF-κB pathway.

As magnesium deficiency is common in POAG patients, it can also be observed in other fibrotic diseases, with supplementation currently being trialed in soft tissues, such as liver and lungs (10, 97). In a rat model, magnesium deficiency led to development of systemic inflammatory disease, and magnesium supplementation resulted in decreased inflammatory and immunological responses (98). Moreover, in a trial of middle-aged women, lower serum magnesium levels were associated with a significantly raised C-reactive protein (CRP), an acute phase protein which is a valuable marker for inflammatory stress (99). It was also found that short-term magnesium supplementation reduced inflammatory cytokine production in both mothers and neonates, including a reduction in NF-κB and IL-6 (100). This adds weight to the argument that magnesium supplementation can also be beneficial for POAG patients as anti-inflammatory agent although it is yet to be seen whether the effects observed would also be seen in the eye.

In terms of fibrosis, hepatic fibrosis has a similar pathogenesis to POAG including excess ECM accumulation, as hepatocytes are also highly metabolic cells (101–103). Insults to the liver stimulate hepatic stellate cells to become pro-fibrotic and adopt myofibroblastic properties *via* the NF-κB pathway, alike the TM (101, 104). Paik et al. (2011) has shown that magnesium supplementation in rats with hepatic fibrosis reduced α-SMA, TGF-β and collagen expression, all profibrotic proteins overexpressed by TM cells during POAG pathogenesis (10, 105). Additionally, ROS generation was suppressed, and transcriptional activation of NF-κB was reduced (10). Similar findings with magnesium supplementation has been shown to alleviate pulmonary fibrosis in mouse models through similar pathways related to POAG (97, 106). It was later indicated by Luo et al. (2021) that magnesium inhibited TGF-β-induced myofibroblastic changes in primary lung cells and decreased collagen deposition in human lung fibroblasts *via* regulation of the TGF-β/SMAD pathway (97). These findings suggest that magnesium has an influence in mediating an anti-fibrotic effect that is similar to the fibrotic pathogenesis seen in the TM and may show promise as a potential anti-fibrotic treatment.

CONCLUSION

As glaucoma is a multi-factorial disease, there are several pathways that have been considered that contribute towards disease pathogenesis, such as inherent mitochondrial dysfunction, subsequent OS stress, calcium influx sensitivity, pro-fibrotic protein induction and vascular dysregulation. It has been presented within this review that the functionality of these same pathways have been shown to be restored with magnesium supplementation in POAG and other fibrotic disease types such as hepatic and pulmonary fibrosis. This suggests that magnesium could be potentially promising in its applications for reducing POAG symptoms by reducing oxidative damage, vascular dysfunction, inflammation and fibrosis, alike other fibrotic diseases.

Overall, it is established that magnesium is vitally important in the regulation and homeostasis of ocular tissues by maintaining cellular functionality. The association of magnesium deficiency in POAG patients and the pathogenesis of glaucoma potentially attributed to magnesium's role as an important cofactor in enzymatic reactions, metabolic and OS regulation, all associated with TM dysregulation, POAG and AH fluid outflow. It has not yet been fully determined the exact impact of magnesium deficiency on the development and progression of glaucoma, however it should be emphasized that there is room in the field for further investigation into its beneficial effects.

AUTHOR CONTRIBUTIONS

ME and HL; preparation of original draft and review of the manuscript. AM-B, IM, and LH; edited and reviewed the manuscript. All authors contributed to the article and approved the submitted version.

ACKNOWLEDGMENTS

The authors would like to thank the British Division of the International Academy of Pathology and the Arthur Thomson Trust for their support of ME.

REFERENCES

1. Quigley H. Number of People With Glaucoma Worldwide. *Br J Ophthalmol* (1996) 80(5):389–93. doi: 10.1136/bjo.80.5.389
2. Weinreb RN, Aung T, Medeiros FA. The Pathophysiology and Treatment of Glaucoma: A Review. *JAMA* (2014) 311(18):1901–11. doi: 10.1001/jama.2014.3192
3. Beidoe G, Mousa S. Current Primary Open-Angle Glaucoma Treatments and Future Directions. *Clin Ophthalmol* (2012) 6:1699–707.
4. Morrison J, Johnson E, Cepurna W, Jia L. Understanding Mechanisms of Pressure-Induced Optic Nerve Damage. *Prog Retin Eye Res* (2005) 24 (2):217–40. doi: 10.1016/j.preteyeres.2004.08.003
5. Stamer W, Clark A. The Many Faces of the Trabecular Meshwork Cell. *Exp Eye Res* (2017) 158:112–23. doi: 10.1016/j.exer.2016.07.009
6. Lamont H, Masood I, Grover L, El Haj A, Hill L. Fundamental Biomaterial Considerations in the Development of a 3D Model Representative of Primary Open Angle Glaucoma. *Bioeng (Basel)* (2021) 8(11):147. doi: 10.3390/bioengineering8110147
7. Buffault J, Labbé A, Hamard P, Brignole-Baudouin F, Baudouin C. The Trabecular Meshwork: Structure, Function and Clinical Implications. A Review of the Literature. *J Francais D'ophtalmologie* (2020) 43(7):e217–30. doi: 10.1016/j.jfo.2020.05.002
8. Sheybani A, Scott R, Samuelson T, Kahook M, Bettis D, Ahmed I, et al. Open-Angle Glaucoma: Burden of Illness, Current Therapies, and the Management of Nocturnal IOP Variation. *Ophthalmol Ther* (2020) 9(1):1–14. doi: 10.1007/s40123-019-00222-z
9. Zhang N, Wang J, Li Y, Jiang B. Prevalence of Primary Open Angle Glaucoma in the Last 20 Years: A Meta-Analysis and Systematic Review. *Sci Rep* (2021) 11(1):13762. doi: 10.1038/s41598-021-92971-w
10. Paik Y, Yoon Y, Lee H, Jung M, Kang S, Chung S, et al. Antifibrotic Effects of Magnesium Lithospermate B on Hepatic Stellate Cells and Thioacetamide-

Induced Cirrhotic Rats. *Exp Mol Med* (2011) 43(6):341–9. doi: 10.3858/emm.2011.43.6.037

11. Zheltova A, Kharitonova M, Iezhitsa I, Spasov A. Magnesium Deficiency and Oxidative Stress: An Update. *BioMedicine* (2016) 6(4):20. doi: 10.7603/s40681-016-0020-6

12. Li X, Xie L, Pan F, Wang Y, Liu H, Tang Y, et al. A Feasibility Study of Using Biodegradable Magnesium Alloy in Glaucoma Drainage Device. *Int J Ophthalmol* (2018) 11(1):135–42. doi: 10.18240/ijo.2018.01.21

13. Pilchova I, Klacanova K, Tatarkova Z, Kaplan P, Racay P. The Involvement of Mg 2+ in Regulation of Cellular and Mitochondrial Functions. *Oxid Med Cell Longev* (2017) 2017:6797460. doi: 10.1155/2017/6797460

14. Iomdina E, Arutyunyan L, Khorosheva E. Analyzing Trace Elements in the Structures of Glaucomatous Eyes. *Int J Biomed* (2019) 9(1):23–5. doi: 10.21103/Article9(1)_OA3

15. Ajith T. Possible Therapeutic Effect of Magnesium in Ocular Diseases. *J Basic Clin Physiol Pharmacol* (2019) 31(2):20190107. doi: 10.1515/jbcpp-2019-0107

16. Gaspar A, Gasser P, Flammer J. The Influence of Magnesium on Visual Field and Peripheral Vasospasm in Glaucoma. *Ophthalmologica* (1995) 209 (1):11–3. doi: 10.1159/000310566

17. Wordinger R, Sharma T, Clark A. The Role of TGF-β2 and Bone Morphogenetic Proteins in the Trabecular Meshwork and Glaucoma. *J Ocul Pharmacol Ther* (2014) 30(2-3):154–62. doi: 10.1089/jop.2013.0220

18. Tripathi R, Li J, Chan W, Tripathi B. Aqueous Humor in Glaucomatous Eyes Contains an Increased Level of TGF-Beta 2. *Exp Eye Res* (1994) 59(6):723–7. doi: 10.1006/exer.1994.1158

19. Fuchshofer R, Tamm E. The Role of TGF-β in the Pathogenesis of Primary Open-Angle Glaucoma. *Cell Tissue Res* (2012) 347(1):279–90. doi: 10.1007/s00441-011-1274-7

20. Inatani M, Tanihara H, Katsuta H, Honjo M, Kido N, Honda Y. Transforming Growth Factor-Beta 2 Levels in Aqueous Humor of Glaucomatous Eyes. *Graefes Arch Clin Exp Ophthalmol* (2001) 239 (2):109–13. doi: 10.1007/s004170000241

21. Ozcan A, Ozdemir N, Canataroglu A. The Aqueous Levels of TGF-Beta2 in Patients With Glaucoma. *Int Ophthalmol* (2004) 25(1):19–22. doi: 10.1023/B:INTE.0000018524.48581.79

22. Tripathi R, Li J, Borisuth N, Tripathi B. Trabecular Cells of the Eye Express Messenger RNA for Transforming Growth Factor-Beta 1 and Secrete This Cytokine. *Invest Ophthalmol Vis Sc* (1993) 34(8):2562–9.

23. Chakraborty M, Sahay P, Rao A. Primary Human Trabecular Meshwork Model for Pseudoexfoliation. *Cells* (2021) 10(12):3448. doi: 10.3390/cells10123448

24. Zhang Y, Cai S, Tseng S, Zhu Y. Isolation and Expansion of Multipotent Progenitors From Human Trabecular Meshwork. *Sci Rep* (2018) 8(1):2814. doi: 10.1038/s41598-018-21098-2

25. Braunger B, Fuchshofer R, Tamm E. The Aqueous Humor Outflow Pathways in Glaucoma: A Unifying Concept of Disease Mechanisms and Causative Treatment. *Eur J Pharm Biopharm* (2015) 95(Pt B):173–81. doi: 10.1016/j.ejpb.2015.04.029

26. Takahashi E, Inoue T, Fujimoto T, Kojima S, Tanihara H. Epithelial Mesenchymal Transition-Like Phenomenon in Trabecular Meshwork Cells. *Exp Eye Res* (2014) 118:72–9. doi: 10.1016/j.exer.2013.11.014

27. Wang M, Zheng Y. Oxidative Stress and Antioxidants in the Trabecular Meshwork. *PeerJ* (2019) 7:e8121. doi: 10.7717/peerj.8121

28. Zhao J, Wang S, Zhong W, Yang B, Sun L, Zheng Y. Oxidative Stress in the Trabecular Meshwork (Review). *Int J Mol Med* (2016) 38(4):995–1002. doi: 10.3892/ijmm.2016.2714

29. Beckman K, Ames B. Mitochondrial Aging: Open Questions. *Ann N Y Acad Sci* (1998) 854:118–27. doi: 10.1111/j.1749-6632.1998.tb09897.x

30. Alvarado J, Murphy C, Juster R. Trabecular Meshwork Cellularity in Primary Open-Angle Glaucoma and Nonglaucomatous Normals. *Ophthalmology* (1984) 91(6):564–79. doi: 10.1016/S0161-6420(84)34248-8

31. Pantalon A, Obadă O, Constantinescu D, Feraru C, Chiseliță D. Inflammatory Model in Patients With Primary Open Angle Glaucoma and Diabetes. *Int J Ophthalmol* (2019) 12(5):795–801. doi: 10.18240/ijo.2019.05.15

32. Yerramothu P, Vijay A, Willcox M. Inflammasomes, the Eye and Anti-Inflammasome Therapy. *Eye (Lond)* (2018) 32(3):491–505. doi: 10.1038/eye.2017.241

33. Meier-Soelch J, Jurida L, Weber A, Newel D, Kim J, Braun T, et al. RNAi-Based Identification of Gene-Specific Nuclear Cofactor Networks Regulating Interleukin-1 Target Genes. *Front Immunol* (2018) 9:775. doi: 10.3389/fimmu.2018.00775

34. Yasuda M, Takayama K, Kanda T, Taguchi M, Someya H, Takeuchi M. Comparison of Intraocular Pressure-Lowering Effects of Ripasudil Hydrochloride Hydrate for Inflammatory and Corticosteroid-Induced Ocular Hypertension. *PLos One* (2017) 12(10):e0185305. doi: 10.1371/journal.pone.0185305

35. Toris C, Yablonski M, Wang Y, Camras C. Aqueous Humor Dynamics in the Aging Human Eye. *Am J Ophthalmol* (1999) 127(4):407–12. doi: 10.1016/S0002-9394(98)00436-X

36. Tian B, Geiger B, Epstein D, Kaufman P. Cytoskeletal Involvement in the Regulation of Aqueous Humor Outflow. *Invest Ophthalmol Vis Sci* (2000) 41 (3):619–23.

37. Al Alawi AM, Majoni SW, Falhammar H. Magnesium and Human Health: Perspectives and Research Directions. *Int J Endocrinol* (2018) 2018:9041694. doi: 10.1155/2018/9041694

38. Aikawa J. *Magnesium: Its Biologic Significance.* (1st ed.). New York: CRC Press. (2019). doi: 10.1201/9780429276101

39. Vink R, Nechifor M. *Magnesium in the Central Nervous System.* Adelaide (AU): University of Adelaide Press (2011).

40. Romani A. Intracellular Magnesium Homeostasis. In: R Vink and M Nechifor, editors. *Magnesium in the Central Nervous System.* Adelaide (AU): University of Adelaide Press (2011).

41. Wolf F, Torsello A, Fasanella S, Cittadini A. Cell Physiology of Magnesium. *Mol Aspects Med* (2003) 24(1-3):11–26. doi: 10.1016/S0098-2997(02)00088-2

42. Romani A. Regulation of Magnesium Homeostasis and Transport in Mammalian Cells. *Arch Biochem Biophys* (2007) 458(1):90–102. doi: 10.1016/j.abb.2006.07.012

43. He Y, Ge J, Tombran-Tink J. Mitochondrial Defects and Dysfunction in Calcium Regulation in Glaucomatous Trabecular Meshwork Cells. *Invest Ophthalmol Vis Sci* (2008) 49(11):4912–22. doi: 10.1167/iovs.08-2192

44. Kirkpatrick H. The Use of Magnesium Sulphate as a Local Application in Inflammation of the Conjunctiva and Cornea. *Br J Ophthalmol* (1920) 4 (6):281. doi: 10.1136/bjo.4.6.281

45. Dubé L, Granry J. The Therapeutic Use of Magnesium in Anesthesiology, Intensive Care and Emergency Medicine: A Review. *Can J Anaesth* (2003) 50 (7):732–46. doi: 10.1007/BF03018719

46. Agarwal R, Iezhitsa I, Agarwal P, Spasov A. Mechanisms of Cataractogenesis in the Presence of Magnesium Deficiency. *Magnes Res* (2013) 26(1):2–8. doi: 10.1684/mrh.2013.0336

47. Stumpff F, Wiederholt M. Regulation of Trabecular Meshwork Contractility. *Ophthalmologica* (2000) 214(1):33–53. doi: 10.1159/000027471

48. Uchida T, Shimizu S, Yamagishi R, Tokuoka S, Kita Y, Honjo M, et al. Mechanical Stretch Induces Ca 2+ Influx and Extracellular Release of PGE 2 Through Piezo1 Activation in Trabecular Meshwork Cells. *Sci Rep* (2021) 11 (1):4044. doi: 10.1038/s41598-021-83713-z

49. Sies H. Oxidative Stress: Oxidants and Antioxidants. *Exp Physiol* (1997) 82 (2):291–5. doi: 10.1113/expphysiol.1997.sp004024

50. Murphy M. How Mitochondria Produce Reactive Oxygen Species. *Biochem J* (2009) 417(1):1–13. doi: 10.1042/BJ20081386

51. Izzotti A, Saccà S, Longobardi M, Cartiglia C. Mitochondrial Damage in the Trabecular Meshwork of Patients With Glaucoma. *Arch Ophthalmol* (2010) 128(6):724–30. doi: 10.1001/archophthalmol.2010.87

52. He Y, Leung K, Zhang Y, Duan S, Zhong X, Jiang R, et al. Mitochondrial Complex I Defect Induces ROS Release and Degeneration in Trabecular Meshwork Cells of POAG Patients: Protection by Antioxidants. *Invest Ophthalmol Vis Sci* (2008) 49(4):1447–58. doi: 10.1167/iovs.07-1361

53. Wu H, Shui Y, Liu Y, Liu X, Siegfried C. Trabecular Meshwork Mitochondrial Function and Oxidative Stress: Clues to Racial Disparities of Glaucoma. *Ophthalmol Sci* (2022) 2(1):100107. doi: 10.1016/j.xops.2021.100107

54. Mutolo M, Albanese G, Rusciano D, Pescosolido N. Oral Administration of Forskolin, Homotaurine, Carnosine, and Folic Acid in Patients With Primary Open Angle Glaucoma: Changes in Intraocular Pressure, Pattern Electroretinogram Amplitude, and Foveal Sensitivity. *J Ocul Pharmacol Ther* (2016) 32(3):178–83. doi: 10.1089/jop.2015.0121

55. Jabbehdari S, Chen J, Vajaranant T. Effect of Dietary Modification and Antioxidant Supplementation on Intraocular Pressure and Open-Angle Glaucoma. *Eur J Ophthalmol* (2021) 31(4):1588–1605. doi: 10.1177/1120672120960337

56. Goubern M, Rayssiguier Y, Miroux B, Chapey M, Ricquier D, Durlach J. Effect of Acute Magnesium Deficiency on the Masking and Unmasking of the Proton Channel of the Uncoupling Protein in Rat Brown Fat. *Magnes Res* (1993) 6(2):135–43.

57. Zhao R, Jiang S, Zhang L, Yu Z. Mitochondrial Electron Transport Chain, ROS Generation and Uncoupling (Review). *Int J Mol Med* (2019) 44(1):3–15. doi: 10.3892/ijmm.2019.4188

58. Yamanaka R, Tabata S, Shindo Y, Hotta K, Suzuki K, Soga T, et al. Mitochondrial Mg(2+) Homeostasis Decides Cellular Energy Metabolism and Vulnerability to Stress. *Sci Rep* (2016) 6:30027. doi: 10.1038/srep30027

59. Piskacek M, Zotova L, Zsurka G, Schweyen R. Conditional Knockdown of Hmrs2 Results in Loss of Mitochondrial Mg(2+) Uptake and Cell Death. *J Cell Mol Med* (2009) 13(4):693–700. doi: 10.1111/j.1582-4934.2008.00328.x

60. Park S, Johnson M, Fischer J. Vitamin and Mineral Supplements: Barriers and Challenges for Older Adults. *J Nutr Elder* (2008) 27(3-4):297–317. doi: 10.1080/01639360802265855

61. Yap T, Donna P, Almonte M, Cordeiro M. Real-Time Imaging of Retinal Ganglion Cell Apoptosis. *Cells* (2018) 7(6):60. doi: 10.3390/cells7060060

62. Tchedre K, Yorio T. Sigma-1 Receptors Protect RGC-5 Cells From Apoptosis by Regulating Intracellular Calcium, Bax Levels, and Caspase-3 Activation. *Invest Ophthalmol Vis Sci* (2008) 49(6):2577–88. doi: 10.1167/iovs.07-1101

63. Gueux E, Azais-Braesco V, Bussière L, Grolier P, Mazur A, Rayssiguier Y. Effect of Magnesium Deficiency on Triacylglycerol-Rich Lipoprotein and Tissue Susceptibility to Peroxidation in Relation to Vitamin E Content. *Br J Nutr* (1995) 74(6):849–56. doi: 10.1079/BJN19950011

64. Nor Arfuzir N, Agarwal R, Iezhitsa I, Agarwal P, Sidek S, Spasov A, et al. Effect of Magnesium Acetyltaurate and Taurine on Endothelin1-Induced Retinal Nitrosative Stress in Rats. *Curr Eye Res* (2018) 43(8):1032–40. doi: 10.1080/02713683.2018.1467933

65. DiNicolantonio J, Liu J, O'Keefe J. Magnesium for the Prevention and Treatment of Cardiovascular Disease. *Open Heart* (2018) 5(2):e000775. doi: 10.1136/openhrt-2018-000775

66. Grieshaber M, Mozaffarieh M, Flammer J. What is the Link Between Vascular Dysregulation and Glaucoma? *Surv Ophthalmol* (2007) 52 Suppl 2:S144–54. doi: 10.1016/j.survophthal.2007.08.010

67. Kostov K, Halacheva L. Role of Magnesium Deficiency in Promoting Atherosclerosis, Endothelial Dysfunction, and Arterial Stiffening as Risk Factors for Hypertension. *Int J Mol Sci* (2018) 19(6):1724. doi: 10.3390/ijms19061724

68. Flammer J, Orgül S. Optic Nerve Blood-Flow Abnormalities in Glaucoma. *Prog Retin Eye Res* (1998) 17(2):267–89. doi: 10.1016/S1350-9462(97)00006-2

69. Kaiser H, Flammer J, Graf T, Stümpfig D. Systemic Blood Pressure in Glaucoma Patients. *Graefes Arch Clin Exp Ophthalmol* (1993) 231(12):677–80. doi: 10.1007/BF00919280

70. Nakabayashi M. Review of the Ischemia Hypothesis for Ocular Hypertension Other Than Congenital Glaucoma and Closed-Angle Glaucoma. *Ophthalmologica* (2004) 218(5):344–9. doi: 10.1159/000079477

71. Kaiser H, Flammer J. Systemic Hypotension: A Risk Factor for Glaucomatous Damage? *Ophthalmologica* (1991) 203(3):105–8. doi: 10.1159/000310234

72. Dang Y, Wang C, Shah P, Waxman S, Loewen R, Loewen N. RKI-1447, a Rho Kinase Inhibitor, Causes Ocular Hypotension, Actin Stress Fiber Disruption, and Increased Phagocytosis. *Graefes Arch Clin Exp Ophthalmol* (2019) 257(1):101–09. doi: 10.1007/s00417-018-4175-6

73. Flammer J, Konieczka K, Flammer A. The Primary Vascular Dysregulation Syndrome: Implications for Eye Diseases. *EPMA J* (2013) 4(1):14. doi: 10.1186/1878-5085-4-14

74. McGarry T, Biniecka M, Veale D, Fearon U. Hypoxia, Oxidative Stress and Inflammation. *Free Radic Biol Med* (2018) 125:15–24. doi: 10.1016/j.freeradbiomed.2018.03.042

75. Orgül S, Cioffi G, Wilson D, Bacon D, Van Buskirk E. An Endothelin-1 Induced Model of Optic Nerve Ischemia in the Rabbit. *Invest Ophthalmol Vis Sci* (1996) 37(9):1860–9.

76. Hartzell H, White R. Effects of Magnesium on Inactivation of the Voltage-Gated Calcium Current in Cardiac Myocytes. *J Gen Physiol* (1989) 94(4):745–67. doi: 10.1085/jgp.94.4.745

77. Mu Y, Huang Q, Zhu J, Zheng S, Yan F, Zhuang X, et al. Magnesium Attenuates Endothelin-1-Induced Vasoreactivity and Enhances Vasodilatation in Mouse Pulmonary Arteries: Modulation by Chronic Hypoxic Pulmonary Hypertension. *Exp Physiol* (2018) 103(4):604–16. doi: 10.1113/EP086655

78. McDonnell F, Dismuke W, Overby D, Stamer W. Pharmacological Regulation of Outflow Resistance Distal to Schlemm's Canal. *Am J Physiol Cell Physiol* (2018) 315(1):C44–C51. doi: 10.1152/ajpcell.00024.2018

79. Zhao Y, Zhu H, Yang Y, Ye Y, Yao Y, Huang X, et al. AQP1 Suppression by ATF4 Triggers Trabecular Meshwork Tissue Remodelling in ET-1-Induced POAG. *J Cell Mol Med* (2020) 24(6):3469–80. doi: 10.1111/jcmm.15032

80. Dettmann E, Lüscher T, Flammer J, Haefliger I. Modulation of Endothelin-1-Induced Contractions by Magnesium/Calcium in Porcine Ciliary Arteries. *Graefes Arch Clin Exp Ophthalmol* (1998) 236(1):47–51. doi: 10.1007/s004170050041

81. Laurant P, Berthelot A. Endothelin-1-Induced Contraction in Isolated Aortae From Normotensive and DOCA-Salt Hypertensive Rats: Effect of Magnesium. *Br J Pharmacol* (1996) 119(7):1367–74. doi: 10.1111/j.1476-5381.1996.tb16048.x

82. Maier J, Malpuech-Brugère C, Zimowska W, Rayssiguier Y, Mazur A. Low Magnesium Promotes Endothelial Cell Dysfunction: Implications for Atherosclerosis, Inflammation and Thrombosis. *Biochim Biophys Acta* (2004) 1689(1):13–21. doi: 10.1016/j.bbadis.2004.01.002

83. Bunte M, Patnaik M, Pritzker M, Burns L. Pulmonary Veno-Occlusive Disease Following Hematopoietic Stem Cell Transplantation: A Rare Model of Endothelial Dysfunction. *Bone Marrow Transplant* (2008) 41(8):677–86. doi: 10.1038/sj.bmt.1705990

84. Corti R, Fuster V, Badimon J. Pathogenetic Concepts of Acute Coronary Syndromes. *J Am Coll Cardiol* (2003) 41(4 Suppl S):7S–14S. doi: 10.1016/S0735-1097(02)02833-4

85. Dismuke W, Liang J, Overby D, Stamer W. Concentration-Related Effects of Nitric Oxide and Endothelin-1 on Human Trabecular Meshwork Cell Contractility. *Exp Eye Res* (2014) 120:28–35. doi: 10.1016/j.exer.2013.12.012

86. Mak I, Komarov A, Wagner T, Stafford R, Dickens B, Weglicki W. Enhanced NO Production During Mg Deficiency and its Role in Mediating Red Blood Cell Glutathione Loss. *Am J Physiol* (1996) 271(1 Pt 1):C385–90. doi: 10.1152/ajpcell.1996.271.1.C385

87. Rock E, Astier C, Lab C, Malpuech C, Nowacki W, Gueux E, et al. Magnesium Deficiency in Rats Induces a Rise in Plasma Nitric Oxide. *Magnes Res* (1995) 8(3):237–42.

88. Murata T, Dietrich H, Horiuchi T, Hongo K, Dacey R. Mechanisms of Magnesium-Induced Vasodilation in Cerebral Penetrating Arterioles. *Neurosci Res* (2016) 107:57–62. doi: 10.1016/j.neures.2015.12.005

89. Ekici F, Korkmaz Ş, Karaca E, Sül S, Tufan H, Aydın B, et al. The Role of Magnesium in the Pathogenesis and Treatment of Glaucoma. *Int Sch Res Notices* (2014) 2014:745439. doi: 10.1155/2014/745439

90. Tabak S, Schreiber-Avissar S, Beit-Yannai E. Crosstalk Between MicroRNA and Oxidative Stress in Primary Open-Angle Glaucoma. *Int J Mol Sci* (2021) 22(5):2421. doi: 10.3390/ijms22052421

91. Hernandez H, Medina-Ortiz W, Luan T, Clark A, McDowell C. Crosstalk Between Transforming Growth Factor Beta-2 and Toll-Like Receptor 4 in the Trabecular Meshwork. *Invest Ophthalmol Vis Sci* (2017) 58(3):1811–23. doi: 10.1167/iovs.16-21331

92. Hernandez H, Roberts A, McDowell C. Nuclear Factor-Kappa Beta Signaling is Required for Transforming Growth Factor Beta-2 Induced Ocular Hypertension. *Exp Eye Res* (2020) 191:107920. doi: 10.1016/j.exer.2020.107920

93. Guo T, Guo L, Fan Y, Fang L, Wei J, Tan Y, et al. Aqueous Humor Levels of Tgfβ2 and SFRP1 in Different Types of Glaucoma. *BMC Ophthalmol* (2019) 19(1):170. doi: 10.1186/s12886-019-1183-1

94. Rao V, Stubbs E. TGF-β2 Promotes Oxidative Stress in Human Trabecular Meshwork Cells by Selectively Enhancing NADPH Oxidase 4 Expression. *Invest Ophthalmol Vis Sci* (2021) 62(4):4. doi: 10.1167/iovs.62.4.4

95. Meng X, Nikolic-Paterson D, Lan H. TGF-β: The Master Regulator of Fibrosis. *Nat Rev Nephrol* (2016) 12(6):325–38. doi: 10.1038/nrneph.2016.48

96. Rao V, Lautz J, Kaja S, Foecking E, Lukács E, Stubbs E. Mitochondrial-Targeted Antioxidants Attenuate TGF-β2 Signaling in Human Trabecular Meshwork Cells. *Invest Ophthalmol Vis Sci* (2019) 60(10):3613–24. doi: 10.1167/iovs.19-27542

97. Luo X, Deng Q, Xue Y, Zhang T, Wu Z, Peng H, et al. Anti-Fibrosis Effects of Magnesium Lithospermate B in Experimental Pulmonary Fibrosis: By Inhibiting TGF-βri/Smad Signaling. *Molecules* (2021) 26(6):1715. doi: 10.3390/molecules26061715

98. Spasov A, Iezhitsa I, Kravchenko M, Kharitonova M. Study of Anti-Inflammatory Activity of Some Organic and Inorganic Magnesium Salts in Rats Fed With Magnesium-Deficient Diet. *Vopr Pitan* (2007) 76(5):67–73.

99. Moslehi N, Vafa M, Rahimi-Foroushani A, Golestan B. Effects of Oral Magnesium Supplementation on Inflammatory Markers in Middle-Aged Overweight Women. *J Res Med Sci* (2012) 17(7):607–14.

100. Sugimoto J, Romani A, Valentin-Torres A, Luciano A, Ramirez Kitchen C, Funderburg N, et al. Magnesium Decreases Inflammatory Cytokine Production: A Novel Innate Immunomodulatory Mechanism. *J Immunol* (2012) 188(12):6338–46. doi: 10.4049/jimmunol.1101765

101. Bataller R, Brenner D. Liver Fibrosis. *J Clin Invest* (2005) 115(2):209–18. doi: 10.1172/JCI24282

102. Grierson I, Lee W. The Fine Structure of the Trabecular Meshwork at Graded Levels of Intraocular Pressure. (1) Pressure Effects Within the Near-Physiological Range (8-30 mmHg). *Exp Eye Res* (1975) 20(6):523–30. doi: 10.1016/0014-4835(75)90218-3

103. Boon R, Kumar M, Tricot T, Elia I, Ordovas L, Jacobs F, et al. Amino Acid Levels Determine Metabolism and CYP450 Function of Hepatocytes and Hepatoma Cell Lines. *Nat Commun* (2020) 11(1):1393. doi: 10.1038/s41467-020-15058-6

104. Lee K, Buck M, Houglum K, Chojkier M. Activation of Hepatic Stellate Cells by TGF Alpha and Collagen Type I is Mediated by Oxidative Stress Through C-Myb Expression. *J Clin Invest* (1995) 96(5):2461–8. doi: 10.1172/JCI118304

105. Han H, Wecker T, Grehn F, Schlunck G. Elasticity-Dependent Modulation of TGF-β Responses in Human Trabecular Meshwork Cells. *Invest Ophthalmol Vis Sci* (2011) 52(6):2889–96. doi: 10.1167/iovs.10-6640

106. Yang Q, Zhang P, Liu T, Zhang X, Pan X, Cen Y, et al. Magnesium Isoglycyrrhizinate Ameliorates Radiation-Induced Pulmonary Fibrosis by Inhibiting Fibroblast Differentiation via the P38mapk/Akt/Nox4 Pathway. *BioMed Pharmacother* (2019) 115:108955. doi: 10.1016/j.biopha.2019.108955

23

Problems in CSF and Ophthalmic Disease Research

Ryan Machiele[1], Benjamin Jay Frankfort[2], Hanspeter Esriel Killer[3,4]
and David Fleischman[1*]

[1] Department of Ophthalmology, University of North Carolina at Chapel Hill, Chapel Hill, NC, United States, [2] Department of
Ophthalmology, Baylor College of Medicine, Houston, TX, United States, [3] Department of Ophthalmology, Kantonsspital
Aarau, Aarau, Switzerland, [4] Center for Biomedicine University of Basel, Basel, Switzerland

*Correspondence:
David Fleischman
david_fleischman@med.unc.edu

There has been significant interest and progress in the understanding of cerebrospinal
fluid pressure and its relationship to glaucoma and other ophthalmic diseases. However,
just as every physiologic fluid pressure fluctuates, cerebrospinal fluid pressure (CSFP) is
similarly dynamic. Coupling this with the difficulty in measuring the pressure, there are
many obstacles in furthering this field of study. This review highlights some of the
difficulties in CSFP research, including fluid compartmentalization, estimation equations,
and pressure fluctuation. Keeping these limitations in mind will hopefully improve the
quality and context of this burgeoning field.

Keywords: translaminar pressure difference, translaminar pressure gradient, cerebrospinal fluid, glaucoma,
lamina cribrosa

INTRODUCTION

Glaucoma is the second leading cause of blindness worldwide and is characterized by a specific
pattern of nerve damage with corresponding visual field loss. Elevated intraocular pressure (IOP) is
the only clinically modifiable risk factor and as such is central to diagnosis and treatment. Many
theories exist to explain the pathophysiology of pressure-driven nerve damage including vascular
dysfunction (1), metabolic and axonal dysregulation (2), and mechanical damage (3). In general,
there is agreement that damaging IOP injures the optic nerve at the nerve head, where it disrupts
axonal flow to cause retrograde retinal ganglion cell (RGC) loss.

A growing body of research supports the notion that IOP is only part of the equation in the
process of pressure-driven optic nerve damage. In this paradigm, RGC damage is the product of the
net imbalance between two pressurized compartments: the intraocular space and the optic nerve
sheath subarachnoid space. These compartments typically have different pressures, and the force
exerted by IOP at the optic nerve head is opposed by the cerebrospinal fluid pressure (CSFP), or
intracranial pressure (ICP).

The difference between these two compartments is termed the translaminar pressure difference (TLPD). An increased TLPD (IOP>CSFP) is postulated to precipitate glaucomatous nerve damage, perhaps contributing to posterior bowing of the lamina cribrosa (4–6). Elevations in IOP can certainly cause this imbalance, but low ICP in the presence of a "normal" IOP has also been linked with glaucomatous nerve damage. Several studies have found a strong correlation between lower ICP and glaucoma, while numerous animal-model studies have identified a causal relationship. Ren et al. prospectively studied patients with normal tension glaucoma (NTG) and primary open angle glaucoma (POAG), and found that visual field loss was strongly associated with an increased TLPD (7). Berdahl et al. has published several large-scale retrospective reviews of patients who had undergone lumbar puncture (LP), and found that lower ICP and higher TLPG is associated with POAG and NTG (8, 9). In 1979, Yablonski et al. sought to develop a model for causality in cats by lowering ICP and unilaterally lowering IOP, and found that eyes with a greater difference between IOP and ICP (TLPD) developed more cupping and posterior bowing of the LC (10). Twenty-six years later, Zhao et al. used the electroretinogram to measure changes in retinal function when varying IOP in rats with normal ICP compared with reduced ICP, and found a larger TLPG resulted in worse retinal function (11). Most recently, Zhu et al. conducted an *in vivo* study of monkeys using optical coherence tomography to image and quantify real-time deformations of the LC, and found that lowering ICP resulted in larger amplitude bowing of the LC in response to IOP variations (12). Further evidence of a relationship of optic nerve cupping related to changes in CSF pressure and flow dynamics is highlighted by works by Gallina and colleagues that examined the development of NTG in patients with shunt-treated normal pressure hydrocephalus (13).

The relevant biomechanics of the LC include two key stress forces with significantly different vectors: the forces acting from opposing sides of the LC (IOP and CSFP) and the hoop stress within the sclera, acting circumferentially around the LC (14). Stress is defined as the force across a small boundary per unit area of that boundary (15). Stress force when applied causes strain, or measurable deformation. At the most fundamental level, deformation of the LC is thought to directly damage nerve and vascular tissue. The opposing forces of IOP and CSFP cause stress at the level of the LC that is inversely proportional to the thickness of the LC: stress decreases with increasing LC thickness. Circumferential hoop stress at the level of the LC is directly proportional to the IOP and inversely proportional to the scleral thickness (or rigidity): as IOP increases, the hoop stress translated to the LC increases, while as scleral thickness increases, LC stress is decreased. It is worth noting that of the two primary stress forces, the trans-laminar force is influenced by CSFP whereas the hoop stress is not. Baneke and colleagues point out that since hoop stress decreases with increasing scleral rigidity, the increased scleral rigidity seen in aging can be thought to make hoop stress less of a factor, and CSFP mediated stress more significant (14).

While much research has been dedicated to the role of CSFP in the pathogenesis of glaucoma and the biomechanics of the LC, the fluid pressure is very difficult to study. The purpose of this review is to highlight some of the difficulties in the study of the contribution of CSF in glaucomatous pathogenesis.

MEASUREMENT OF CSF PRESSURE

Central to our understanding of the translaminar pressure gradient is accurate measurement of CSF pressure. This has proven a challenge for the scientific community due to limitations in techniques for invasive pressure monitoring as well as shifting definitions of CSFP.

CSFP is classically assessed *via* the lumbar puncture (LP). The LP was first introduced by Heinrich Quincke in 1891 but the technique was not immediately adopted in clinical practice (16). In 1950, Pierre Janny shed light on the clinical applications of CSFP measurement in his examination of the relationship between ophthalmologic signs and CSFP (17). The LP remains the mainstay to the present day for clinical assessment of CSFP. This technique provides an instantaneous measurement of the intrathecal CSFP, which indirectly describes intracranial CSFP under Pascal's principle which assumes that CSF circulates freely throughout the subarachnoid space. For much of the 20th century, the intracranial CSFP was, by definition, synonymous with intrathecal CSFP as alternative methods for assessing intracranial CSFP did not exist. It should not be overlooked, however, that the LP, while used ubiquitously to assess *intracranial* CSFP, is ultimately an indirect measurement. Lundberg was the first to attempt direct and continuous measurement of ventricular CSFP in 1960 (18). Continued developments in direct measurement of ventricular and brain-tissue pressure have redefined true intracranial CSFP and spawned several studies which examine the variation between intrathecal CSFP and ICP measured by brain tissue pressure-sensing transducers in patients in intensive care units with continuous electrode monitoring (19). These studies have been performed exclusively in neurocritical patients, the only clinical population where such invasive monitoring is routinely justified. Unfortunately, the results of these studies are difficult to generalize as several other studies have demonstrated that measurement of CSFP in critical care and sedation settings may be unreliable, due to factors such as hypercarbia and direct action of anesthetic agent (20). Additionally, instrumentation in critically ill populations confers additional risks including infection, hemorrhage and development of neurological deficits, which make prospective studies nonviable. Outside of the critically ill population, Lenfeldt and colleagues performed a novel study which employed a pressure control strategy in patients with communicating hydrocephalus and found a high degree of agreement between intracranial CSFP and CSFP measured by LP (21). Again, these results are difficult to generalize given the unique physiology of the population studied.

The LP faces three key limitations as a reliable tool for studies involving CSFP: it is an invasive sterile procedure which requires a high level of skill, it is indirect in its assessment of intracranial CSFP, and it is highly temporal, providing only a snapshot of intrathecal CSFP (19). To tackle the problem of the impracticability of an invasive, sterile technique in most outpatient clinical settings, a myriad of non-invasive techniques for CSFP estimation are currently being developed. These innovations typically follow one of two paths and provide either *qualitative* markers that suggest the possibility of increased cranial CSFP or *quantitative* measurements of intracranial CSFP or estimations based on previous measurements (22). Optic nerve edema is commonly employed as a qualitative indicator of elevated CSFP. By extension, many studies have sought to quantify optic nerve changes as a surrogate measurement of CSFP, typically through measurement of optic nerve sheath diameter (ONSD) *via* ultrasound, CT or MRI. Chen et al. performed ultrasound measurement of ONSD 5 minutes before and after LP and found that ONSD correlated closely with real-time changes in CSFP (23). Weidner et al. performed ultrasonographic measurement of ONSD in awake, spontaneously breathing patients with continuous invasive ICP monitoring, finding a strong correlation between ONSD and CSFP (24). Bauerle et al. compared ultrasound and MRI derived values of ONSD, and found a high degree of agreement (25). As IOP measurement is readily obtained in the outpatient setting without a sterile field and without risk of harm to the patient, further exploration of the role TLPD plays in the pathogenesis of glaucoma will be best served by CSFP measurement techniques that are similarly non-invasive. Thus far, ultrasound imaging of the ONSD certainly shows the most promise as a potential surrogate for general estimates of CSFP status.

THE RELATIONSHIP BETWEEN INTRACRANIAL AND ORBITAL CSF PRESSURE

One of the key questions facing CSF and ophthalmic disease research is whether CSFP measured within the lumbar space reliably represents the CSFP within the optic nerve sheath. In most clinical studies examining the TLPG, the pressure measured during LP was used as a surrogate for the pressure posterior to the lamina cribrosa, or the orbital CSFP. Considering the distance and differences in the anatomy between the lumbar spine and the orbital subarachnoid space, it is logical to question the utility of an LP to estimate orbital CSFP. In a study on 10 patients with idiopathic normal pressure hydrocephalus, Lenfeldt et al. compared the lumbar pressure to parenchymal pressure in the brain and found an agreement between the measurements (21). The authors conclude their study with a caveat: the results depend on a communicating CSF system. Clinically, especially in the elderly population,

there is good reason to doubt whether such a communicating CSF system exists (26). Studies applying CT myelography demonstrate that a variety of processes like vertebral degenerations, disc herniations, arachnoiditis and other anatomic variations or obstructions can markedly narrow this CSF pathway—and possibly completely obstruct CSF flow (27). But even if the CSF pathway from the lumbar site to the intracranial CSF spaces is patent, there is yet another restriction point. The optic canal, within the lesser wing of the Sphenoid, can be a critical bottleneck for free communication from the intracranial compartment to the lamina cribrosa. Computer-assisted imaging studies revealed that the optic canal can be particularly narrow in some patients with normal tension glaucoma when compared to nonglaucoma controls (28). Similarly, computer-assisted cisternography demonstrated impaired CSF dynamics between the intracranial CSF spaces and the orbital subarachnoid space in a series of patients with papilledema and normal tension glaucoma, which proved the existence of an optic nerve compartment syndrome (29, 30). Studies of animal models have utilized an array of subarachnoid pressure-sensitive probes placed at the level of the optic nerve to assess for variations between intracranial and intraorbital CSFP and found variability (31). Other studies have used various tracer dyes to assess for continuity of the subarachnoid space into the optic nerve and confirmed various bottlenecks (32). In general, these studies suggest a positive relationship between CSFP within the optic nerve and intracranial CSFP obtained *via* LP, but also demonstrate highly variable intraorbital CSF inflow, suspected to be due to fibrillar tissue and CSF compartmentalization in the subarachnoid space. To assume that the lumbar pressure is a reliable surrogate for the pressure posterior to the lamina cribrosa is therefore speculative, likely inaccurate in many subjects, and in need of further study by new measurement technologies. But even if the pressure on both sides of the lamina cribrosa was known accurately, the area of the lamina cribrosa – an important component in the definition of pressure, is not. Indeed, because of the space occupying trabeculae in the subarachnoid space, the area of the lamina cribrosa resembles a fractal ring anulus with a high variability between individuals (33). Another potential confounding variable is the thickness of the lamina cribrosa and the transmission and action of pressure across this tissue. The lamina is known to be thinner in patients with glaucoma, possibly increasing the transmissibility of pressures (34). Studying the role of CSFP and IOP counterbalance factoring lamina cribrosa thickness and biomechanics is very difficult, and an area in need of further study. Only William Morgan has studied the TLPG in earnest, taking into account the thickness of the lamina with the pipette-manometer measurement technique, and it was clear that the thickness of this structure was critical (35). These factors confound the accurate measurement of TLPG.

Lastly, we question the importance of the "translaminar pressure." The translaminar pressure gradient or difference would be between the eye and the retrolaminar optic nerve tissue. If we consider the optic nerve subarachnoid space (ONSAS) and the eye, the correct terminology would be the transscleral pressure (**Figure 1**). Of course, the fluid pressure around the nerve also affects the nerve tissue pressure itself, so it is possible that any or all of these pressure relationships are most critical (**Figure 2**).

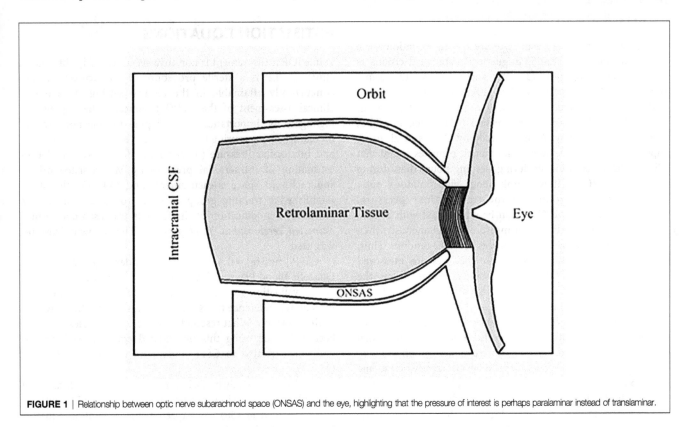

FIGURE 1 | Relationship between optic nerve subarachnoid space (ONSAS) and the eye, highlighting that the pressure of interest is perhaps paralaminar instead of translaminar.

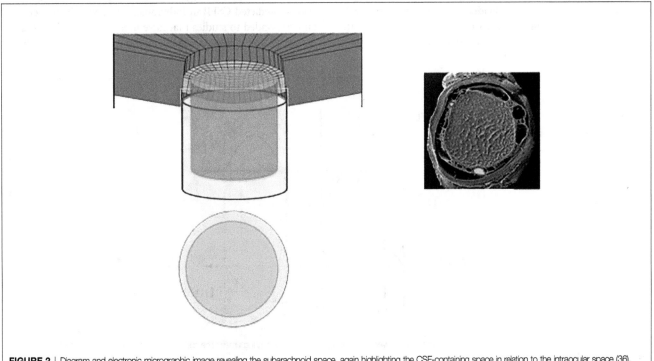

FIGURE 2 | Diagram and electronic micrographic image revealing the subarachnoid space, again highlighting the CSF-containing space in relation to the intraocular space (36).

UTILITY OF SINGULAR PRESSURE READINGS: WHAT IS KNOWN ABOUT DIURNAL, LONGITUDINAL AND POSITIONAL CHANGES IN CSFP

Glaucoma specialists are acutely aware of the limitations of a single snap-shot IOP reading in guiding treatment decisions as IOP fluctuates over time (37, 38). and is subject to normal physiologic diurnal variation (39, 40). Furthermore, several studies have identified exaggerated diurnal variation as an independent risk factor for progression (41). Much like IOP, CSFP fluctuates widely. A recent study by Downs et al. using implanted telemetry devices in nonhuman primates found that ICP was 92%–166% higher during sleeping hours than during waking hours (42). If we think about glaucomatous optic neuropathy as a product of the translaminar pressure, fluctuations in IOP and CSFP can be represented with a wave form. If IOP and CSFP are not measured simultaneously, then the alignment between these two forces becomes random. Thus, even in an ideal setting where both pressures are measured simultaneously the TLPG will constantly change unless the variations of IOP and CSFP are in perfect alignment – a dubious expectation (**Figures 3**, **4**).

Studies have validated the LP obtained in lateral decubitus for the measurement of ICP, but have also found that intracranial CSFP decreases to zero—or even subzero values—when standing (21). In general, CSFP is found to be in the low teens when supine and sub-atmospheric, and approaches equilibrium when sitting. As such, the TLPD is expected to be highest when upright. A study by Qvarlander et al. found a high degree of CSFP variation in the upright position compared with a low degree of variation in supine positioning, suggesting interindividual variation in capacity to regulate upright CSFP (43). These variations in tandem with the posture-dependence of CSFP further question the utility of a singular LP measurement without accounting for its diurnal and positional context.

ESTIMATION EQUATIONS

While IOP measurement is non-invasive and readily obtained in clinic, an LP is a sterile procedure of its own and is not concurrently attainable in the clinical setting. This makes clinical assessment of the TLPD technically challenging and highlights the importance of developing reliable non-invasive modalities for measuring CSF pressure. The Beijing Intracranial and Intraocular Pressure (iCOP) study developed a model for estimation of intracranial pressure by MRI-assisted orbital subarachnoid space measurement, and (44, 45) the study established a training group in order to validate its utility. However, a modification of the formula was used and termed *estimated cerebrospinal fluid pressure*. The following formula was used:

CSFP [mmHg] = 0.44 × Body Mass Index [kg/m(2)] + 0.16 × Diastolic Blood Pressure [mmHg]-0.18 × Age[Years]

No validation for this formula was ever given, and many inaccurately reference the Xie et al. manuscript as the derivation of this equation. What resulted was a series of studies that have been published using this unvalidated equation, contributing faulty data related to CSFP and ophthalmic disease research (46–57).

A subsequent study by Fleischman et al. identified limitations in multiple regression models to estimate CSFP without radiographic data (58). As expected, the estimation equation (and similarly-derived regression formulas from large datasets) poorly predicted CSFP in individuals. While we have identified and responded to studies that have used unvalidated estimation equations for CSFP-associated ophthalmic research, reviewers

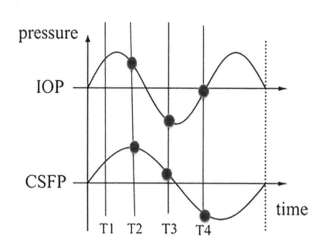

FIGURE 3 | Possible wave forms of IOP and CSFP over time. The vertical lines represent the measuring times. The distance between the two curves at different times differ. The TLPG therefore varies over time.

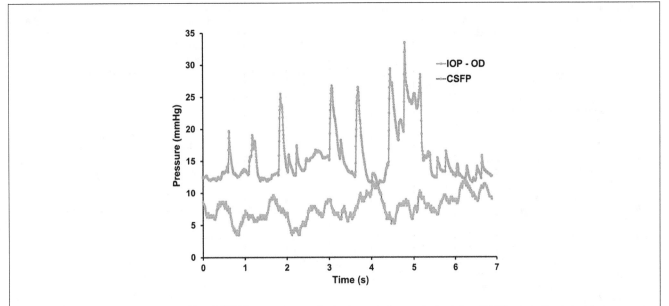

FIGURE 4 | Seven seconds of continuous IOP and CSFP from non-human primate. demonstrating constant variation of TLPG and significant physiologic pressure variability. (Courtesy of Crawford Downs, PhD).

and journal editors should take note that these are not valid methods of conducting CSF-related research.

CONCLUSION

IOP and CSFP are two highly dynamic pressures, which in clinical practice are assessed with snap-shot measurements of varying accuracy and applicability. The current methods used for the determination of the TLPD need to be improved in order to render more reliable data including modalities which allow for continuous measurement of IOP and CSFP. Similarly, appreciating the difference between orbital CSFP and lumbar

CSFP is important and methods to easily and accurately report these fluid pressures need to be established. Discretization of the fluid pressure curves need to be performed in order to process the TLPD or gradient over time. As the role of the TLPD in the pathogenesis of glaucoma and other eye diseases continues to be explored, the nuances of CSF behavior and the technical limitations in measuring intra-orbital CSFP must be appreciated.

AUTHOR CONTRIBUTIONS

All authors listed have made a substantial, direct, and intellectual contribution to the work, and approved it for publication.

REFERENCES

1. Flammer J, Orgül S, Costa VP, Orzalesi N, Krieglstein GK, Metzner Serra L, et al. The Impact of Ocular Blood Flow in Glaucoma. *Prog Retinal Eye Res* (2002) 21(4):359–93. doi: 10.1016/S1350-9462(02)00008-3
2. Fahy ET, Chrysostomou V, Crowston JG. Mini-Review: Impaired Axonal Transport and Glaucoma. *Curr Eye Res* (2016) 41(3):273–83. doi: 10.3109/02713683.2015.1037924
3. Stowell C, Burgoyne CF, Tamm ER. The Lasker/ IRRF Initiative on Astrocytes and Glaucomatous Neurodegeneration Participants. Biomechanical Aspects of Axonal Damage in Glaucoma: A Brief Review. *Exp Eye Res* (2017) 157:13–9. doi: 10.1016/j.exer.2017.02.005
4. Tong J, Ghate D, Kedar S, Gu L. Relative Contributions of Intracranial Pressure and Intraocular Pressure on Lamina Cribrosa Behavior. *J Ophthalmol* (2019) 2019:3064949. doi: 10.1155/2019/3064949
5. Feola AJ, Myers JG, Raykin J, Mulugeta L, Nelson ES, Samuels BC, et al. Finite Element Modeling of Factors Influencing Optic Nerve Head Deformation Due to Intracranial Pressure. *Invest Ophthalmol Visual Science* (2016) 57 (4):1901–11. doi: 10.1167/iovs.15-17573

6. Downs JC, Roberts MD, Burgoyne CF. Mechanical Environment of the Optic Nerve Head in Glaucoma. *Optom Vis Sci* (2008) 85(6):425–35. doi: 10.1097/OPX.0b013e31817841cb
7. Ren R, Jonas JB, Tian G, Zhen Y, Ma K, Li S, et al. Cerebrospinal Fluid Pressure in Glaucoma: A Prospective Study. *Ophthalmology* (2010) 117 (2):259–66. doi: 10.1016/j.ophtha.2009.06.058
8. Berdahl JP, Fautsch MP, Stinnett SS, Allingham RR. Intracranial Pressure in Primary Open Angle Glaucoma, Normal Tension Glaucoma, and Ocular Hypertension: A Case-Control Study. *Invest Ophthalmol Visual Science* (2008) 49(12):5412–8. doi: 10.1167/iovs.08-2228
9. Berdahl JP, Allingham RR, Johnson DH. Cerebrospinal Fluid Pressure is Decreased in Primary Open-Angle Glaucoma. *Ophthalmology* (2008) 115 (5):763–8. doi: 10.1016/j.ophtha.2008.01.013
10. Yablonski ME, Ritch R, Pokorny KS. Effect of Decreased Intracranial-Pressure on Optic Disk. In Investigative Ophthalmology & Visual Science. (1979) 227:165.
11. Zhao D, He Z, Vingrys AJ, Bui BV, Nguyen CTO. The Effect of Intraocular and Intracranial Pressure on Retinal Structure and Function in Rats. *Physiol Rep* (2015) 3(8). doi: 10.14814/phy2.12507

12. Zhu Z, Waxman S, Wang B, Wallace J, Schmitt SE, Tyler-Kabara E, et al. Interplay Between Intraocular and Intracranial Pressure Effects on the Optic Nerve Head In Vivo. Exp Eye Res (2021) 213:108809. doi: 10.1016/j.exer.2021.108809

13. Gallina P, Savastano A, Becattini E, Orlandini S, Scollato A, Rizzo S, et al. Glaucoma in Patients With Shunt-Treated Normal Pressure Hydrocephalus. J Neurosurg (2018) 129(4):1078–84. doi: 10.3171/2017.5.JNS163062

14. Baneke AJ, Aubry J, Viswanathan AC, Plant GT. The Role of Intracranial Pressure in Glaucoma and Therapeutic Implications. Eye (London England) (2020) 34(1):178–91. doi: 10.1038/s41433-019-0681-y

15. Chen W-F, Han D-J. Plasticity for Structural Engineers. (2007). Fort Lauderdale, FL: J. Ross Publishing

16. Quincke H. Berliner Klinische Wochenschrift. In: Die Lumbalpunction Des Hydrocephalus. Berlin, Germany: August Hirschwald (1891).

17. Janny P. La Pression Intracranienne Chez L'homme. In: Méthode D'enregistrement: Etude De Ses Variations Et De Ses Rapports Avec Les Signes Cliniques Et Ophtalmologiques (1950). New York City, NY: Springer Editions.

18. Lundberg N. Continuous Recording and Control of Ventricular Fluid Pressure in Neurosurgical Practice. Acta Psychiatrica Scandinavica Supplementum (1960) 36(149):1–193. doi: 10.3171/jns.1965.22.6.0581

19. Czosnyka M, Pickard JD. Monitoring and Interpretation of Intracranial Pressure. J Neurology Neurosurgery Psychiatry (2004) 75(6):813–21. doi: 10.1136/jnnp.2003.033126

20. Eidlitz-Markus T, Stiebel-Kalish H, Rubin Y, Shuper A. CSF Pressure Measurement During Anesthesia: An Unreliable Technique. Paediatric Anaesthesia (2005) 15(12):1078–82. doi: 10.1111/j.1460-9592.2005.01675.x

21. Lenfeldt N, Koskinen LO, Bergenheim AT, Malm J, Eklund A, et al. CSF Pressure Assessed by Lumbar Puncture Agrees With Intracranial Pressure. Neurology (2007) 68(2):155–8. doi: 10.1212/01.wnl.0000250270.54587.71

22. Bruce BB. Noninvasive Assessment of Cerebrospinal Fluid Pressure. J Neuro-Ophthalmology Off J North Am Neuro-Ophthalmology Society (2014) 34(3):288–94. doi: 10.1097/WNO.0000000000000153

23. Chen LM, Wang LJ, Hu Y, Jiang X-H, Wang Y-Z, Xing Y-Q. Ultrasonic Measurement of Optic Nerve Sheath Diameter: A Non-Invasive Surrogate Approach for Dynamic, Real-Time Evaluation of Intracranial Pressure. Br J Ophthalmol (2019) 103(4):437–41. doi: 10.1136/bjophthalmol-2018-312934

24. Weidner N, Kretschmann J, Bomberg H, Antes S, Leonhardt S, Tschan C, et al. Real-Time Evaluation of Optic Nerve Sheath Diameter (ONSD) in Awake, Spontaneously Breathing Patients. J Clin Med (2021) 10(16). doi: 10.3390/jcm10163549

25. Bäuerle J, Schuchardt F, Schroeder L, Egger K, Weigel M, Harloff A, et al. Reproducibility and Accuracy of Optic Nerve Sheath Diameter Assessment Using Ultrasound Compared to Magnetic Resonance Imaging. BMC Neurol (2013) 13:187. doi: 10.1186/1471-2377-13-187

26. Killer HE, Pircher A. What Do We Really Know About Translaminar Pressure? J Neuro-Ophthalmology Off J North Am Neuro-Ophthalmology Society (2016) 36(1):112–3. doi: 10.1097/WNO.0000000000000365

27. Patel DM, Weinberg BD, Hoch MJ. CT Myelography: Clinical Indications and Imaging Findings, Vol. 40. (2020). pp. 470–84. doi: 10.1148/rg.2020190135

28. Pircher A, Montali M, Berberat J, Remonda L, Killer HE. The Optic Canal: A Bottleneck for Cerebrospinal Fluid Dynamics in Normal-Tension Glaucoma? Front Neurol (2017) 8:47–7. doi: 10.3389/fneur.2017.00047

29. Killer HE, Miller NR, Flammer J, Meyer P, Weinreb RN, Remonda L, et al. Cerebrospinal Fluid Exchange in the Optic Nerve in Normal-Tension Glaucoma. Br J Ophthalmol (2012) 96(4):544–8. doi: 10.1136/bjophthalmol-2011-300663

30. Killer HE, Jaggi GP, Miller NR, Huber AR, Landolt H, Mironov A, et al. Cerebrospinal Fluid Dynamics Between the Basal Cisterns and the Subarachnoid Space of the Optic Nerve in Patients With Papilloedema. Br J Ophthalmol (2011) 95(6):822–7. doi: 10.1136/bjo.2010.189324

31. Hou R, Zhang Z, Yang D, Wang H, Chen W, Li Z, et al. Intracranial Pressure (ICP) and Optic Nerve Subarachnoid Space Pressure (ONSP) Correlation in the Optic Nerve Chamber: The Beijing Intracranial and Intraocular Pressure (iCOP) Study. Brain Res (2016) 1635:201–8. doi: 10.1016/j.brainres.2016.01.011

32. Mathieu E, Gupta N, Paczka-Giorgi LA, Zhou X, Ahari A, Lani R, et al. Reduced Cerebrospinal Fluid Inflow to the Optic Nerve in Glaucoma. Invest Ophthalmol Visual Science (2018) 59(15):5876–84. doi: 10.1167/iovs.18-24521

33. Killer HE, Laeng HR, Flammer J, Groscurth P. Architecture of Arachnoid Trabeculae, Pillars, and Septa in the Subarachnoid Space of the Human Optic Nerve: Anatomy and Clinical Considerations. Br J Ophthalmol (2003) 87(6):777–81. doi: 10.1136/bjo.87.6.777

34. Tian H, Li L, Song F. Study on the Deformations of the Lamina Cribrosa During Glaucoma. Acta Biomaterialia (2017) 55:340–8. doi: 10.1016/j.actbio.2017.03.028

35. Morgan WH, Yu DY, Cooper RL, Alder VA, Cringle SJ, Constable IJ. The Influence of Cerebrospinal Fluid Pressure on the Lamina Cribrosa Tissue Pressure Gradient. Invest Ophthalmol Visual Science (1995) 36(6):1163–72.

36. Morgan WH, Yu DY, Balaratnasingam C. The Role of Cerebrospinal Fluid Pressure in Glaucoma Pathophysiology: The Dark Side of the Optic Disc. J Glaucoma (2008) 17(5):408–13. doi: 10.1097/IJG.0b013e31815c5f7c

37. Mansouri K, Shaarawy T. Continuous Intraocular Pressure Monitoring With a Wireless Ocular Telemetry Sensor: Initial Clinical Experience in Patients With Open Angle Glaucoma. Br J Ophthalmol (2011) 95(5):627–9. doi: 10.1136/bjo.2010.192922

38. Bradley KC. Cerebrospinal Fluid Pressure. J Neurology Neurosurgery Psychiatry (1970) 33(3):387–97. doi: 10.1136/jnnp.33.3.387

39. Wilensky JT. Diurnal Variations in Intraocular Pressure. Trans Am Ophthalmological Society (1991) 89:757–90.

40. Kaufman PL. Diurnal Fluctuation of Intraocular Pressure. Invest Ophthalmol Visual Science (2016) 57(14):6427–7. doi: 10.1167/iovs.16-20997

41. Asrani S, Zeimer R, Wilensky J, Gieser D, Vitale S, Lindenmuth K. Large Diurnal Fluctuations in Intraocular Pressure are an Independent Risk Factor in Patients With Glaucoma. J Glaucoma (2000) 9(2):134–42. doi: 10.1097/00061198-200004000-00002

42. Jasien JV, Samuels BC, Johnston JM, Crawford Downs J. Diurnal Cycle of Translaminar Pressure in Nonhuman Primates Quantified With Continuous Wireless Telemetry. Invest Ophthalmol Visual Science (2020) 61(2):37–7. doi: 10.1167/iovs.61.2.37

43. Qvarlander S, Sundström N, Malm J, Eklund A. Postural Effects on Intracranial Pressure: Modeling and Clinical Evaluation. J Appl Physiol (Bethesda Md 1985) (2013) 115(10):1474–80. doi: 10.1152/japplphysiol.00711.2013

44. Wang N, Yang D, Jonas JB. Low Cerebrospinal Fluid Pressure in the Pathogenesis of Primary Open-Angle Glaucoma: Epiphenomenon or Causal Relationship? The Beijing Intracranial and Intraocular Pressure (iCOP) Study. J Glaucoma (2013) 22(Suppl 5):S11–12. doi: 10.1097/IJG.0b013e31829349a2

45. Wang YX, Jonas JB, Wang N, You QS, Yang D, Xie XB, et al. Intraocular Pressure and Estimated Cerebrospinal Fluid Pressure. The Beijing Eye Study 2011. PLoS One (2014) 9(8):e104267. doi: 10.1371/journal.pone.0104267

46. Jonas JB, Wang N, Wang S, Wang YX, You QS, Yang D, et al. Retinal Vessel Diameter and Estimated Cerebrospinal Fluid Pressure in Arterial Hypertension: The Beijing Eye Study. Am J Hypertension (2014) 27(9):1170–8. doi: 10.1093/ajh/hpu037

47. Jonas JB, Wang N, Wang YX, Wang YX, You QS, Yang D, et al. Incident Retinal Vein Occlusions and Estimated Cerebrospinal Fluid Pressure. The Beijing Eye Study. Acta Ophthalmologica (2015) 93(7):e522–526. doi: 10.1111/aos.12575

48. Li L, Li C, Zhong H, Tao Y, Yuan Y, Pan C-W. Estimated Cerebrospina Fluid Pressure and the 5-Year Incidence of Primary Open-Angle Glaucoma in a Chinese Population. PLoS One (2016) 11(9):e0162862. doi: 10.1371/journal.pone.0162862

49. Jonas JB, Wang N, Xu J, Wang YX, You QS, Yang D, et al. Diabetic Retinopathy and Estimated Cerebrospinal Fluid Pressure. The Beijing Eye Study 2011. PLoS One (2014) 9(5):e96273. doi: 10.1371/journal.pone.0096273

50. Jonas JB, Wang N, Xu Jie, Wang YX, You QS, Yang D, et al. Body Height, Estimated Cerebrospinal Fluid Pressure and Open-Angle Glaucoma. The Beijing Eye Study 2011. PLoS One (2014) 9(1):e86678. doi: 10.1371/journal.pone.0086678

51. Lee SH, Kwak SW, Kang EM, Kim GA, Lee SY, Bae HW, et al. Estimated Trans-Lamina Cribrosa Pressure Differences in Low-Teen and High-Teen Intraocular Pressure Normal Tension Glaucoma: The Korean National Health

and Nutrition Examination Survey. *PLoS One* (2016) 11(2):e0148412. doi: 10.1371/journal.pone.0148412

52. Jonas JB, Wang NL, Xu J, Wang YX, You QS, Yang D, et al. Estimated Trans-Lamina Cribrosa Pressure Difference Versus Intraocular Pressure as Biomarker for Open-Angle Glaucoma. The Beijing Eye Study 2011. *Acta Ophthalmologica* (2015) 93(1):e7–13. doi: 10.1111/aos.12480

53. Horwitz A, Petrovski BE, Torp-Pedersen C, Kolko M. Danish Nationwide Data Reveal a Link Between Diabetes Mellitus, Diabetic Retinopathy, and Glaucoma. *J Diabetes Res* (2016) 2016:2684674. doi: 10.1155/2016/2684674

54. Landi L, Casciaro F, Telani S, Traverso CE, Harris A, Verticchio AC, et al. Evaluation of Cerebrospinal Fluid Pressure by a Formula and Its Role in the Pathogenesis of Glaucoma. *J Ophthalmol* (2019) 2019:1840481. doi: 10.1155/2019/1840481

55. Jonas JB, Wang N, Xu J, Wang YX, You QS, Yang D, et al. Ocular Hypertension: General Characteristics and Estimated Cerebrospinal Fluid Pressure. The Beijing Eye Study 2011. *PLoS One* (2014) 9(7):e100533. doi: 10.1371/journal.pone.0100533

56. Yang JY, Yang X, Li Y, Xu J, Zhou Y, Wang AX, et al. Carotid Atherosclerosis, Cerebrospinal Fluid Pressure, and Retinal Vessel Diameters: The Asymptomatic Polyvascular Abnormalities in Community Study. *PLoS One* (2016) 11(12):e0166993. doi: 10.1371/journal.pone.0166993

57. Yang DY, Guo K, Wang Y, Guo YY, Yang XR, Jing XX, et al. Intraocular Pressure and Associations in Children. The Gobi Desert Children Eye Study. *PLoS One* (2014) 9(10):e109355. doi: 10.1371/journal.pone.0109355

58. Fleischman D, Bicket AK, Stinnett SS, Berdahl JP, Jonas JB, Wang NL. Analysis of Cerebrospinal Fluid Pressure Estimation Using Formulae Derived From Clinical Data. *Invest Ophthalmol Visual Science* (2016) 57(13):5625–30. doi: 10.1167/iovs.16-20119

Permissions

All chapters in this book were first published by Frontiers; hereby published with permission under the Creative Commons Attribution License or equivalent. Every chapter published in this book has been scrutinized by our experts. Their significance has been extensively debated. The topics covered herein carry significant findings which will fuel the growth of the discipline. They may even be implemented as practical applications or may be referred to as a beginning point for another development.

The contributors of this book come from diverse backgrounds, making this book a truly international effort. This book will bring forth new frontiers with its revolutionizing research information and detailed analysis of the nascent developments around the world.

We would like to thank all the contributing authors for lending their expertise to make the book truly unique. They have played a crucial role in the development of this book. Without their invaluable contributions this book wouldn't have been possible. They have made vital efforts to compile up to date information on the varied aspects of this subject to make this book a valuable addition to the collection of many professionals and students.

This book was conceptualized with the vision of imparting up-to-date information and advanced data in this field. To ensure the same, a matchless editorial board was set up. Every individual on the board went through rigorous rounds of assessment to prove their worth. After which they invested a large part of their time researching and compiling the most relevant data for our readers.

The editorial board has been involved in producing this book since its inception. They have spent rigorous hours researching and exploring the diverse topics which have resulted in the successful publishing of this book. They have passed on their knowledge of decades through this book. To expedite this challenging task, the publisher supported the team at every step. A small team of assistant editors was also appointed to further simplify the editing procedure and attain best results for the readers.

Apart from the editorial board, the designing team has also invested a significant amount of their time in understanding the subject and creating the most relevant covers. They scrutinized every image to scout for the most suitable representation of the subject and create an appropriate cover for the book.

The publishing team has been an ardent support to the editorial, designing and production team. Their endless efforts to recruit the best for this project, has resulted in the accomplishment of this book. They are a veteran in the field of academics and their pool of knowledge is as vast as their experience in printing. Their expertise and guidance has proved useful at every step. Their uncompromising quality standards have made this book an exceptional effort. Their encouragement from time to time has been an inspiration for everyone.

The publisher and the editorial board hope that this book will prove to be a valuable piece of knowledge for researchers, students, practitioners and scholars across the globe.

List of Contributors

Jianhua Wu, Han Zhang, Xiaoguang Zhang and Guisen Zhang
Inner Mongolia Chaoju Eye Hospital, Inner Mongolia Chaoju Institute of Eye Disease Control, Hohhot, China

Xiaomei Wu
Department of Clinical Epidemiology and Center of Evidence-Based Medicine, The First Hospital of China Medical University, Shenyang, China

Jie Zhang
School of Public Health, Weifang Medical University, Weifang, China
Tobacco Control, Chinese Center for Disease Control and Prevention, Beijing, China

Yanqiu Liu
Department of Ophthalmology, Anshan Central Hospital, Anshan, China

Jun Liu
Department of Ophthalmology, Changzhi People's Hospital, Changzhi, China

Lu Lu
Department of Ophthalmology, The Fourth Affiliated Hospital of China Medical University, Shenyang, China

Song Zhang
The First Hospital of China Medical University, Shenyang, China

Lei Liu
Department of Ophthalmology, Guangdong Eye Institute, Guangdong Provincial People's Hospital, Guangdong Academy of Medical Sciences, Guangzhou, China
School of Medicine, South China University of Technology, Guangzhou, China
Department of Ophthalmology, The First Affiliated Hospital of China Medical University, Shenyang, China

Riccardo Vinciguerra
Humanitas San Pio X Hospital, Milan, Italy

Robert Herber and Frederik Raiskup
Department of Ophthalmology, University Hospital Carl Gustav Carus, Dresden, Germany

Yan Wang
Tianjin Eye Hospital, Tianjin Key Laboratory of Ophthalmology and Visual Science, Nankai University Affiliated Eye Hospital, Tianjin, China
Clinical College of Ophthalmology, Tianjin Medical University, Tianjin, China

Fengju Zhang
Beijing Tongren Eye Center, Beijing Tongren Hospital, Beijing Ophthalmology and Visual Sciences Key Lab, Capital Medical University, Beijing, China

Xingtao Zhou
EYE & ENT Hospital of Fudan University, Shanghai, China

Ji Bai
BAI JI Ophthalmology, Chongqing, China

Keming Yu
Zhongshan Ophthalmic Center, Sun Yat-Sen University, Guangzhou, China

Shihao Chen
Eye Hospital, Wenzhou Medical University, Zhejiang, China

Xuejun Fang
Shenyang Aier Eye Hospital, Shenyang, China

Paolo Vinciguerra
Department of Biomedical Sciences, Humanitas University, Milan, Italy
IRCCS Humanitas Research Hospital, Rozzano, Italy

Jing Xu, Peng Chen, Chaoqun Yu, Yaning Liu, Shaohua Hu and Guohu Di
School of Basic Medicine, Qingdao University, Qingdao, China

Hon Shing Ong
Department of Corneal & External Eye Diseases, Singapore National Eye Centre, Singapore, Singapore
Singapore Eye Research Institute, Singapore, Singapore
Duke-NUS Medical School, Singapore, Singapore

Hla M. Htoon
Singapore Eye Research Institute, Singapore, Singapore
Duke-NUS Medical School, Singapore, Singapore

Maryam Eslami
Department of Ophthalmology and Visual Sciences, University of British Columbia, Vancouver, BC, Canada

Blanca Benito-Pascual and Saadiah Goolam
Sydney Eye Hospital, Sydney, NSW, Australia
Save Sight Institute, University of Sydney, Sydney, NSW, Australia

Tanya Trinh
Sydney Eye Hospital, Sydney, NSW, Australia
Save Sight Institute, University of Sydney, Sydney, NSW, Australia
Mosman Eye Centre and Narellan Eye Specialists, Sydney, NSW, Australia

Greg Moloney
Department of Ophthalmology and Visual Sciences, University of British Columbia, Vancouver, BC, Canada
Sydney Eye Hospital, Sydney, NSW, Australia
Save Sight Institute, University of Sydney, Sydney, NSW, Australia
Mosman Eye Centre and Narellan Eye Specialists, Sydney, NSW, Australia

Shuang Song, Yidan Chen, Feng Wang and Ying Su
Department of Ophthalmology, The First Affiliated Hospital of Harbin Medical University, Harbin, China

Ying Han
Department of Geriatric, The First Affiliated Hospital of Harbin Medical University, Harbin, China

Kai Yuan Tey
Singapore Eye Research Institute, Singapore, Singapore
Tasmanian Medical School, University of Tasmania, Hobart, TAS, Australia

Sarah Yingli Tan
Tasmanian Medical School, University of Tasmania, Hobart, TAS, Australia

Darren S. J. Ting
Academic Ophthalmology, Division of Clinical Neuroscience, University of Nottingham, Nottingham, United Kingdom
Department of Ophthalmology, Queen's Medical Centre, Nottingham, United Kingdom

Li Lian Foo, Chee Wai Wong, Daniel Ting and Marcus Ang
Singapore National Eye Centre, Singapore, Singapore
Singapore Eye Research Institute, Singapore, Singapore
Duke–NUS Medical School, National University of Singapore, Singapore, Singapore

Carla Lanca
Singapore Eye Research Institute, Singapore, Singapore
Escola Superior de Tecnologia da Saúde de Lisboa (ESTeSL), Instituto Politécnico de Lisboa, Lisboa, Portugal
Comprehensive Health Research Center (CHRC), Escola Nacional de Saúde Pública, Universidade Nova de Lisboa, Lisboa, Portugal

Ecosse Lamoureux
Singapore Eye Research Institute, Singapore, Singapore
Duke–NUS Medical School, National University of Singapore, Singapore, Singapore

Seang-Mei Saw
Singapore Eye Research Institute, Singapore, Singapore
Duke–NUS Medical School, National University of Singapore, Singapore, Singapore
NUS Saw Swee Hock School of Public Health, Singapore, Singapore

Mark A. Chia
Lions Outback Vision, Lions Eye Institute, Nedlands, WA, Australia
Institute of Ophthalmology, Faculty of Brain Sciences, University College London, London, United Kingdom

Angus W. Turner
Lions Outback Vision, Lions Eye Institute, Nedlands, WA, Australia
Centre for Ophthalmology and Visual Science, University of Western Australia, Nedlands, WA, Australia

Thanh-Tin P. Nguyen, Susan Ostmo and J. Peter Campbell
Casey Eye Institute, Oregon Health and Science University, Portland, OR, United States

Shuibin Ni, Guangru Liang, Shanjida Khan, Xiang Wei, Yali Jia, David Huang and Yifan Jian
Casey Eye Institute, Oregon Health and Science University, Portland, OR, United States
Department of Biomedical Engineering, Oregon Health and Science University, Portland, OR, United States

Alison Skalet
Casey Eye Institute, Oregon Health and Science University, Portland, OR, United States
Knight Cancer Institute, Oregon Health and Science University, Portland, OR, United States
Department of Radiation Medicine, Oregon Health and Science University, Portland, OR, United States
Department of Dermatology, Oregon Health and Science University, Portland, OR, United States

Michael F. Chiang
National Eye Institute, National Institutes of Health, Bethesda, MD, United States

Xiang Gu, Minyue Xie, Renbing Jia and Shengfang Ge
Department of Ophthalmology, Ninth People's Hospital, Shanghai JiaoTong University School of Medicine, Shanghai, China
Shanghai Key Laboratory of Orbital Diseases and Ocular Oncology, Shanghai JiaoTong University School of Medicine, Shanghai, China

Anahita Kate
The Cornea Institute, KVC Campus, LV Prasad Eye Institute, Vijayawada, India

Sayan Basu
The Cornea Institute, KAR Campus, LV Prasad Eye Institute, Hyderabad, India
Prof. Brien Holden Eye Research Centre (BHERC), LV Prasad Eye Institute, Hyderabad, Telangana, India

T. Y. Alvin Liu
Wilmer Eye Institute, Johns Hopkins University, Baltimore, MD, United States

Jo-Hsuan Wu
Shiley Eye Institute and Viterbi Family Department of Ophthalmology, University of California, San Diego, La Jolla, CA, United States

Giulio Petronio Petronio, Roberto Di Marco and Ciro Costagliola
Department of Medicine and Health Science "V. Tiberio", Università degli Studi del Molise, Campobasso, Italy

Darren Shu Jeng Ting
Academic Ophthalmology, School of Medicine, University of Nottingham, Nottingham, United Kingdom
Department of Ophthalmology, Queen's Medical Centre, Nottingham, United Kingdom
Anti-Infectives Research Group, Singapore Eye Research Institute, Singapore, Singapore

Imran Mohammed
Academic Ophthalmology, School of Medicine, University of Nottingham, Nottingham, United Kingdom

Rajamani Lakshminarayanan and Roger W. Beuerman
Anti-Infectives Research Group, Singapore Eye Research Institute, Singapore, Singapore

Harminder S. Dua
Academic Ophthalmology, School of Medicine, University of Nottingham, Nottingham, United Kingdom
Department of Ophthalmology, Queen's Medical Centre, Nottingham, United Kingdom

Anshu Arundhati and Jodhbir S. Mehta
Singapore National Eye Centre, Singapore, Singapore
Singapore Eye Research Institute, Singapore, Singapore
Department of Ophthalmology and Visual Sciences, Duke-NUS Medical School, Singapore, Singapore

Feng He
Singapore Eye Research Institute, Singapore, Singapore

Stephanie Lang
Singapore National Eye Centre, Singapore, Singapore

Charumathi Sabanayagam and Ching-Yu Cheng
Singapore Eye Research Institute, Singapore, Singapore
Department of Ophthalmology and Visual Sciences, Duke-NUS Medical School, Singapore, Singapore

Megan M. Allyn
William G. Lowrie Department of Chemical and Biomolecular Engineering, The Ohio State University, Columbus, OH, United States

Richard H. Luo and Elle B. Hellwarth
Department of Biomedical Engineering, The Ohio State University, Columbus, OH, United States

Katelyn E. Swindle-Reilly
William G. Lowrie Department of Chemical and Biomolecular Engineering, The Ohio State University, Columbus, OH, United States
Department of Biomedical Engineering, The Ohio State University, Columbus, OH, United States
Department of Ophthalmology and Visual Sciences, The Ohio State University, Columbus, OH, United States

Li-Jen Yeh
Department of Craniofacial Orthodontics, Chang Gung Memorial Hospital, Taoyuan, Taiwan
Graduate Institute of Craniofacial and Dental Science, Chang Gung University, Taoyuan, Taiwan

Te-Chun Shen
Department of Internal Medicine, China Medical University Hospital, Taichung, Taiwan
School of Medicine, China Medical University, Taichung, Taiwan

Kuo-Ting Sun
Department of Pediatric Dentistry, China Medical University Hospital, Taichung, Taiwan

Cheng-Li Lin
Management Office for Health Data, China Medical University Hospital, Taichung, Taiwan

Ning-Yi Hsia
Department of Ophthalmology, China Medical University Hospital, Taichung, Taiwan

Jinyuan Gan
Duke-NUS Graduate Medical School, Singapore, Singapore

Chelvin C. A. Sng
Singapore National Eye Centre, Singhealth, Singapore Eye Research Institute, Singapore, Singapore
Department of Ophthalmology, National University Hospital, Singapore, Singapore

Mengyuan Ke
Singapore National Eye Centre, Singhealth, Singapore Eye Research Institute, Singapore, Singapore

Chew Shi Chieh
Department of Ophthalmology, National University Hospital, Singapore, Singapore

Bingyao Tan
Singapore National Eye Centre, Singhealth, Singapore Eye Research Institute, Singapore, Singapore
SERI-NTU Advanced Ocular Engineering (STANCE), Singapore, Singapore
School of Chemical and Biomedical Engineering, Nanyang Technological University, Singapore, Singapore

Leopold Schmetterer
Duke-NUS Graduate Medical School, Singapore, Singapore
Singapore National Eye Centre, Singhealth, Singapore Eye Research Institute, Singapore, Singapore
Department of Ophthalmology, National University Hospital, Singapore, Singapore
SERI-NTU Advanced Ocular Engineering (STANCE), Singapore, Singapore
School of Chemical and Biomedical Engineering, Nanyang Technological University, Singapore, Singapore
Department of Clinical Pharmacology, Medical University of Vienna, Vienna, Austria
Center for Medical Physics and Biomedical Engineering, Medical University of Vienna, Vienna, Austria
Institute of Molecular and Clinical Ophthalmology, Basel, Switzerland

Jooyoung Yoon
Department of Ophthalmology, Asan Medical Center, College of Medicine, University of Ulsan, Seoul, South Korea

Hyo Joo Kang
Asan Diabetes Center, Asan Medical Center, Seoul, South Korea

Joo Yong Lee, June-Gone Kim, Young Hee Yoon and Yoon Jeon Kim
Department of Ophthalmology, Asan Medical Center, College of Medicine, University of Ulsan, Seoul, South Korea
Asan Diabetes Center, Asan Medical Center, Seoul, South Korea

Chang Hee Jung
Asan Diabetes Center, Asan Medical Center, Seoul, South Korea
Department of Internal Medicine, Asan Medical Center, College of Medicine, University of Ulsan, Seoul, South Korea

Yan Gao
Ocular Proteomics Platform, Singapore Eye Research Institute, Singapore, Singapore

Yuanyuan Qi, Yue Huang, Xiaorong Li and Shaozhen Zhao
Tianjin Key Laboratory of Retinal Functions and Diseases, Tianjin Branch of National Clinical Research Center for Ocular Disease, Eye Institute and School of Optometry, Tianjin Medical University Eye Hospital, Tianjin, China

Lei Zhou
Ocular Proteomics Platform, Singapore Eye Research Institute, Singapore, Singapore
Department of Ophthalmology, Yong Loo Lin School of Medicine, National University of Singapore, Singapore, Singapore
Ophthalmology and Visual Sciences Academia Clinical Program, Duke-National University of Singapore Medical School, Singapore, Singapore

Mirna Elghobashy, Alexander Morelli-Batters, Imran Masood and Lisa J. Hill
School of Biomedical Sciences, Institute of Clinical Sciences, University of Birmingham, Birmingham, United Kingdom

Hannah C. Lamont
School of Biomedical Sciences, Institute of Clinical Sciences, University of Birmingham, Birmingham, United Kingdom
School of Chemical Engineering, Healthcare Technologies Institute, University of Birmingham, Birmingham, United Kingdom

Ryan Machiele and David Fleischman
Department of Ophthalmology, University of North Carolina at Chapel Hill, Chapel Hill, NC, United States

Benjamin Jay Frankfort
Department of Ophthalmology, Baylor College of Medicine, Houston, TX, United States

Hanspeter Esriel Killer
Department of Ophthalmology, Kantonsspital Aarau, Aarau, Switzerland
Center for Biomedicine University of Basel, Basel, Switzerland

Index

Printed in the USA
CPSIA information can be obtained
at www.ICGtesting.com
JSHW051410091023
49903JS00006B/361

9 781646 475124